ADVANCES IN

Pathology and Laboratory Medicine®

VOLUME 8

ADVANCES IN

Pathology and Laboratory Medicine®

VOLUME 1–4 (OUT OF PRINT)

VOLUME 5

VOLUME 6

The following is a list of authors who have contributed to *Advances in Pathology* and *Advances in Pathology and Laboratory Medicine*. The number(s) in parentheses indicate the volumes in which their chapters appeared.

Osama M.A. Abdelatif, M.D. (7)
Joseph F. Aceto, Ph.D. (7)
Randa Alsabeh, M.D. (8)
Sebastian R. Alston, M.D. (4)
Robert E. Anderson, M.D. (2, 4)
Virginia M. Anderson, M.D. (6)
Barbara L. Bane, M.D. (5)
Raymond L. Barnhill, M.D. (6)
Hector Battifora, M.D. (8)
William T. Bellamy, Ph.D. (6, 8)
Rodger L. Bick, M.D. (8)
Paul W. Biddinger, M.D. (4)
Jack R. Bierig, J.D. (7)
David D. Biggs, M.D. (7)
William C. Black, M.D. (4)
Kenneth J. Bloom, M.D. (6)
G. Tim Bowden, Ph.D. (8)
Paul D. Bozzo, M.D. (6)
John J. Brooks, M.D. (5)
Barbara A. Burke, M.D. (5)
M. Desmond Burke, M.D. (3)
R. Jean Campbell, M.B., Ch.B. (6)
Terence T. Casey, M.D. (6)
George S. Cembrowski, M.D., Ph.D. (7)
Daniel W. Chan, Ph.D. (6)
Douglas B. Cines, M.D. (7)
Joanne Comerford, M.S., M.T. (5)
Donald P. Connelly, M.D., Ph.D. (5)
John S. Coon, M.D., Ph.D. (1, 4)
Ramzi S. Cotran, M.D. (3)
John E. Craighead, M.D. (1)
Anne E. Cress, Ph.D. (8)
John D. Crissman, M.D. (5, 7)
Christopher P. Crum, M.D. (5)
Umberto De Girolami, M.D. (7)
Ronald F. Dorfman, M.D. (1)
Sandra L. Drake, Ph.D. (5)
Stuart B. Dubin, M.D., Ph.D. (7)
Paul H. Duray, M.D. (7)
Paul H. Edelstein, M.D. (8)

J. Roger Edson, M.D. (1)
Jesse E. Edwards, M.D. (5)
Steven N. Emancipator, M.D. (8)
Stanley L. Erlandsen, Ph.D. (5)
David S. Ettenson, M.Sc. (6)
Anne E. Faassen, Ph.D. (5)
Ronald J. Falk, M.D. (8)
A.M. Fanizza-Orphanus, M.D. (3)
Elizabeth L. Fasola, M.D. (5)
Cecilia M. Fenoglio-Preiser, M.D. (2, 3, 8)
Judith A. Ferry, M.D. (7)
Jonathan A. Fletcher, M.D. (4)
Andrew Flint, M.D. (6)
Anne L. Frattali, M.D., Ph.D. (8)
Rafael Fridman, Ph.D. (7)
Carleton T. Garrett, M.D., Ph.D. (5)
James C. Garriott, Ph.D. (7)
David R. Genest, M.D. (7)
Robert M. Genta, M.D., D.T.M. & H., F.A.C.G. (7)
David F.C. Gibson, Ph.D. (3)
Sidney A. Goldblatt, M.D. (6)
Avrum I. Gotlieb, M.D., C.M. (6)
Allen Gown, M.D. (8)
Anna R. Graham, M.D. (7)
Scott R. Granter, M.D. (6)
M. Alba Greco, M.D. (6)
Thomas M. Grogan, M.D. (4, 6, 8)
John G. Gruhn, M.D. (3)
Karen R. Halliday, M.D. (2)
Curtis A. Hanson, M.D. (3)
Nancy L. Harris, M.D. (7)
John Hart, M.D. (6)
Jean-Jacques Hauw, M.D. (7)
Robert L. Hawley, M.D. (4)
Reid R. Heffner, Jr., M.D. (8)
Dominique Hènin, M.D. (7)
Rolla B. Hill, M.D. (2, 4)
Brian Hjelle, M.D. (4)
Peter A. Humphrey, M.D., Ph.D. (7)

Joji Iida, Ph.D. (5)
Kamal G. Ishak, M.D., Ph.D. (8)
Shriram M. Jakate, M.D. (4)
Peter I. Jatlow, M.D. (6)
Kay Ann Jenkins, H.T.(A.S.C.P.),
  H.T.L. (8)
J. Charles Jennette, M.D. (8)
V. Craig Jordan, Ph.D., D.Sc. (3)
Ellen Kahn, M.D. (6)
Raj P. Kapur, M.D., Ph.D. (8)
Harold A. Kessler, M.D. (2)
Frederick L. Kiechle, M.D., Ph.D.
  (7)
Gordon K. Klintworth, M.D., Ph.D.
  (3)
Larry F. Kluskens, M.D., Ph.D. (4)
Jennifer R. Knutson (5)
Michael N. Koss, M.D. (7)
George Koukoulis, M.D. (3)
Beverly Balfour Kraemer, M.D. (5)
Larry J. Kricka, D.Phil. (6)
Elizabeth A. Krupinski, Ph.D. (6)
Jerome R. Kuszak, Ph.D. (4)
Janice M. Lage, M.D. (5)
Michael E. Lamm, M.D. (8)
Alan L. Landay, Ph.D. (2)
Chris Lawrence, M.B.B.S. (6)
Klaus J. Lewin, M.D. (6)
Margaret B. Listrom, M.D. (2)
James Linder, M.D. (6)
James V. Little, III, M.D. (1)
Vincent Marks, D.M. (1)
Ralph Martel (8)
James B. McCarthy, Ph.D. (5)
Keith R. McCrae, M.D. (7)
Darin McDaniel (8)
Brian McGraw (8)
Bruce M. McManus, M.D., Ph.D.
  (3)
Aurelia M. Meloni, Ph.D. (5)
Toby L. Merlin, M.D. (1, 3)
Richard D. Meyer, M.D. (8)
Phillip C. Miller, B.S. (6)
Roger E. Mittleman, M.D. (4)
George F. Murphy, M.D. (1)
William M. Murphy, M.D. (7)
Irving Nachamkin, Dr. P.H. (7)
Raymond B. Nagle, M.D. (6, 8)
Amy E. Noffsinger, M.D. (8)
David W. Nunnery, B.S. (6)

Gerard J. Nuovo, M.D. (8)
Jan Marc Orenstein, M.D., Ph.D. (8)
David M. Parham, M.D. (8)
Lance R. Peterson, M.D. (5)
Barry Portugal (8)
Michael F. Press, M.D. (6)
James Radosevich, Ph.D. (3)
Bruce D. Ragsdale, M.D. (6)
Petrie M. Rainey, M.D., Ph.D. (6)
Naomi E. Rance, M.D., Ph.D. (7)
Catherine S. Rangel, H.T.L. (6, 8)
William Richards (8)
Lynne Richter (8)
Lisa Rimsza (8)
Foster Robberson, J.D. (7)
Paula Rodgers (8)
E. Rene Rodriguez, M.D. (5)
Victor B. Roggli, M.D. (2)
Steven T. Rosen, M.D. (3)
Charles W. Ross, M.D. (3)
L. Susan Rozek, R.N. (6)
James Rybski (8)
Caliope Sarago, B.S., M.T. (5)
Fazlul H. Sarkar, Ph.D. (5, 7)
Hironobu Sasano, M.D. (7)
Robert E. Schmidt, M.D., Ph.D. (6)
Deborah E. Schofield, M.D. (7)
Arnold M. Schwartz, M.D., Ph.D.
  (5)
Daniel Schwartz, M.D. (1)
Melvin M. Schwartz, M.D. (6)
Morton K. Schwartz, Ph.D. (6)
Danielle Seilhean, M.D. (7)
Darryl Shibata, M.D. (8)
Wayne Showalter (8)
Leslie E. Silberstein, M.D. (7)
Laurel O. Sillerud, Ph.D. (2)
Ernest R. Simon, M.D. (7)
Toby L. Simon, M.D. (4, 7)
Jean F. Simpson, M.D. (7)
Dale C. Snover, M.D. (5)
Thomas M. Sodeman, M.D. (5)
Gregory T. Spear, Ph.D. (2)
Carl E. Speicher, M.D. (8)
Steven L. Spitalnik, M.D. (8)
Jim Standefer, Ph.D. (2)
Paul E. Steele, M.D. (4)
Paul E. Swanson, M.D. (5)
Sally G. Swenson, M.T. (4)
Clive R. Taylor, M.D., Ph.D. (7)

Henry Dale Tazelaar, M.D. (3)
Jack L. Titus, M.D., Ph.D. (5)
John E. Tomaszewski, M.D. (8)
Thomas B. Tomasi, M.D., Ph.D. (1)
Joel Umlas, M.D. (1)
Elizabeth R. Unger, M.D., Ph.D. (6)
Elizabeth Vela (8)
Daniel W. Visscher, M.D. (5, 7)
F. Stephen Vogel, M.D. (1)
Roger A. Warnke, M.D. (1)
Ronald S. Weinstein, M.D. (1, 4, 6)
Lawrence M. Weiss, M.D. (1)

Carol L. Wells, Ph.D. (5)
Charles V. Wetli, M.D. (4)
Mark R. Wick, M.D. (5)
David S. Wilkinson, M.D., Ph.D. (6)
Ralph C. Williams, Jr., M.D. (8)
Robert B. Wilson, M.D., Ph.D. (8)
Douglas M. Wolf, B.S. (3)
Nancy A. Young, M.D. (8)
Jorge J. Yunis, M.D. (2)
Ron Zeheb (8)
Lanmin Zhang, M.D. (7)
Ross E. Zumwalt, M.D. (3)

ADVANCES IN

Pathology and Laboratory Medicine®

VOLUME 8

Editor-in-Chief
Ronald S. Weinstein, M.D.
Professor and Head, Department of Pathology, University of Arizona Health
Sciences Center, Tucson, Arizona

Associate Editor
Anna R. Graham, M.D.
Professor, Department of Pathology, University of Arizona Health Sciences
Center, Tucson, Arizona

Editorial Board
Robert E. Anderson, M.D.
Professor, Department of Laboratory Medicine and Pathology, University of
Minnesota Medical School, Minneapolis, Minnesota

Ellis S. Benson, M.D.
Professor, Department of Laboratory Medicine and Pathology, University of
Minnesota Medical School, Minneapolis, Minnesota

Ramzi S. Cotran, M.D.
F.B. Mallory Professor of Pathology, Harvard Medical School; Chairman,
Department of Pathology, Brigham and Women's Hospital; Chairman,
Department of Pathology, Children's Hospital, Boston, Massachusetts

Leonard Jarett, M.D.
Simon Flexner Professor and Chairman, Department of Pathology and
Laboratory Medicine, University of Pennsylvania Medical Center, Philadelphia,
Pennsylvania

Mark R. Wick, M.D.
Director of Surgical Pathology, Professor of Pathology, Washington University
Medical Center, St. Louis, Missouri

Ross E. Zumwalt, M.D.
Chief Medical Investigator, State of New Mexico; Professor of Pathology,
University of New Mexico School of Medicine, Albuquerque, New Mexico

Mosby

St. Louis Baltimore Berlin Boston Carlsbad Chicago London Madrid
Naples New York Philadelphia Sydney Tokyo Toronto

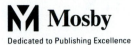

Mosby

Dedicated to Publishing Excellence

Vice President and Publisher, Continuity Publishing: Kenneth H. Killion
Director, Editorial Development: Gretchen C. Murphy
Developmental Editor: Amy L. Reynaldo
Acquisitions Editor: Jennifer Roche
Manager, Continuity—EDP: Maria Nevinger
Project Specialist: Denise M. Dungey
Assistant Project Supervisor: Sandra Rogers
Proofreading Supervisor: Barbara M. Kelly
Vice President, Professional Sales and Marketing: George M. Parker
Senior Marketing Manager: Eileen M. Lynch
Marketing Specialist: Lynn D. Stevenson

Printed in the United States of America
Composition by The Clarinda Company
Printing/binding by The Maple-Vail Book Manufacturing Group

Mosby–Year Book, Inc.
11830 Westline Industrial Drive
St. Louis, Missouri 63146

Editorial Office:
Mosby–Year Book, Inc.
200 North LaSalle Street
Chicago, IL 60601

International Standard Serial Number: 1057-1256
International Standard Book Number: 0-8151-3398-7

Contributors

Randa Alsabeh, M.D.
Division of Pathology, City of Hope National Medical Center, Duarte, California

Hector Battifora, M.D.
Chairman, Division of Pathology, City of Hope National Medical Center, Duarte, California

William T. Bellamy, Ph.D.
Department of Pathology, University of Arizona, Tucson, Arizona

Rodger L. Bick, M.D.
Clinical Professor of Medicine and Pathology, University of Texas Southwestern Medical Center, and Medical Director of Hematology and Oncology, Presbyterian Comprehensive Cancer Center, Presbyterian Hospital of Dallas, Dallas, Texas

G. Tim Bowden, Ph.D.
Professor of Radiation Oncology, University of Arizona Health Sciences Center, Tucson, Arizona

Anne E. Cress, Ph.D.
Associate Professor of Radiation Oncology, University of Arizona Health Sciences Center, Tucson, Arizona

Paul H. Edelstein, M.D.
Clinical Microbiology Laboratory, Departments of Pathology and Laboratory Medicine, Department of Medicine, Hospital of the University of Pennsylvania, University of Pennsylvania School of Medicine, Philadelphia, Pennsylvania

Steven N. Emancipator, M.D.
Institute of Pathology, Case Western Reserve University, Cleveland, Ohio

Ronald J. Falk, M.D.
Associate Professor of Medicine, School of Medicine, University of North Carolina, Chapel Hill, North Carolina

Cecilia M. Fenoglio-Preiser, M.D.
MacKenzie Professor and Director, Department of Pathology and Laboratory Medicine, University of Cincinnati College of Medicine, Cincinnati, Ohio

Anne L. Frattali, M.D., Ph.D.
Assistant Instructor, The University of Pennsylvania Medical Center, Hospital of the University of Pennsylvania, Department of Pathology and Laboratory Medicine, Philadelphia, Pennsylvania

Allen Gown, M.D.
Department of Pathology, University of Washington School of Medicine, Seattle, Washington

Thomas M. Grogan, M.D.
Department of Pathology, University of Arizona College of Medicine, Tucson, Arizona

Reid R. Heffner, Jr., M.D.
Professor and Associate Chairman, Department of Pathology, School of Medicine and Biomedical Sciences, State University of New York at Buffalo, Buffalo, New York

Kamal G. Ishak, M.D., Ph.D.
Department of Hepatic and Gastrointestinal Pathology, Armed Forces Institute of Pathology, Washington, D.C.

Kay Ann Jenkins, H.T.(A.S.C.P.), H.T.L.
Division of Pathology, City of Hope National Medical Center, Duarte, California

J. Charles Jennette, M.D.
Professor of Pathology and Medicine, School of Medicine, University of North Carolina, Chapel Hill, North Carolina

Raj P. Kapur, M.D., Ph.D.
Assistant Professor, Department of Pathology, University of Washington School of Medicine, Children's Hospital and Medical Center, Seattle, Washington

Michael E. Lamm, M.D.
Institute of Pathology, Case Western Reserve University, Cleveland, Ohio

Ralph Martel, Ph.D.
Ventana Medical Systems, Tucson, Arizona

Darin McDaniel, B.S.
Ventana Medical Systems, Tucson, Arizona

Brian McGraw, B.S.
Ventana Medical Systems, Tucson, Arizona

Richard D. Meyer, M.D.
Department of Medicine, University of California, Los Angeles, UCLA School of Medicine, Los Angeles, California

Ray B. Nagle, M.D., Ph.D.
Professor of Pathology and Anatomy, University of Arizona Health Sciences Center, Tucson, Arizona

Amy E. Noffsinger, M.D.
Assistant Professor, Department of Pathology and Laboratory Medicine, University of Cincinnati College of Medicine, Cincinnati, Ohio

Gerard J. Nuovo, M.D.
Associate Professor of Pathology and Obstetrics and Gynecology, Director, Cytopathology, State University of New York at Stony Brook, Health Sciences Center School of Medicine, Stony Brook, New York

Jan Marc Orenstein, M.D., Ph.D.
Professor of Pathology, Department of Pathology, George Washington University Medical Center, Washington, D.C.

David M. Parham, M.D.
Department of Pathology and Laboratory Medicine, St. Jude Children's Research Hospital, Memphis, Department of Pathology, University of Tennessee, Memphis, College of Medicine, Memphis, Tennessee

Barry Portugal, M.B.A.
President, Health Care Development Services, Inc., Northbrook, Illinois

Catherine Rangel, B.A., H.T.L. (A.S.C.P.)
Department of Pathology, University of Arizona, Tucson, Arizona

William Richards, B.S.E.E.
Ventana Medical Systems, Tucson, Arizona

Lynne Richter, B.A., M.T. (A.S.C.P.) S.H.
Department of Pathology, University of Arizona, Tucson, Arizona

Lisa Rimsza, M.D.
Department of Pathology, University of Arizona, Tucson, Arizona

Paula Rodgers, M.S.
Ventana Medical Systems, Tucson, Arizona

James Rybski, Ph.D.
Ventana Medical Systems, Tucson, Arizona

Darryl Shibata, M.D.
Assistant Professor of Pathology, University of Southern California School of Medicine, Los Angeles, California

Wayne Showalter, B.S.
Ventana Medical Systems, Tucson, Arizona

Carl E. Speicher, M.D.
Professor and Director, Clinical Services, Vice-Chair, Department of Pathology, Ohio State University College of Medicine, Ohio State University Medical Center, Columbus, Ohio

Steven L. Spitalnik, M.D.
Co-Vice Chair, Division of Laboratory Medicine, Associate Professor, The University of Pennsylvania Medical Center, Hospital of the University of Pennsylvania, Department of Pathology and Laboratory Medicine, Philadelphia, Pennsylvania

John E. Tomaszewski, M.D.
Associate Professor of Pathology and Laboratory Medicine, Department of Pathology and Laboratory Medicine, University of Pennsylvania Medical Center, Philadelphia, Pennsylvania

Elizabeth Vela, M.S.
Department of Pathology, University of Arizona, Tucson, Arizona

Ralph C. Williams, Jr., M.D.
Eminent Scholar, Marcia Whitney Schott Chair in Rheumatoid Arthritis Research and Professor and Chief, Division of Rheumatology, Department of Medicine, University of Florida College of Medicine, Gainesville, Florida

Robert B. Wilson, M.D., Ph.D.
Assistant Professor, Division of Molecular Diagnosis, The University of Pennsylvania Medical Center, Hospital of the University of Pennsylvania, Department of Pathology and Laboratory Medicine, Philadelphia, Pennsylvania

Nancy A. Young, M.D.
Department of Pathology, Fox Chase Cancer Center, Clinical Associate
Professor, Hahnemann University School of Medicine, Philadelphia,
Pennsylvania

Ron Zeheb, Ph.D.
Ventana Medical Systems, Tucson, Arizona

In addition to members of the Editorial Board, the following individuals reviewed papers in this volume:

Preface

Volume 8 of *Advances in Pathology and Laboratory Medicine* consists of 21 chapters by 44 authors and examines a diverse group of topics relevant to the practice of pathology. On behalf of the Editorial Board, I would like to thank the authors both for their initial willingness to take on these writing assignments and for their subsequently excellent chapters.

Selecting topics for inclusion in each annual volume of *Advances* is both a pleasure and a challenge. To accomplish this task, the Editorial Board must be up to date on what is new in pathology as well as on who is an appropriate spokesperson for a specific field. Once the "what" and "who" issues are settled, additional decisions have to be made. The tricky part is establishing a goal for the length of each article and making it stick.

Establishing chapter length goals for authors may sound mundane but it isn't. Since many consequences result from the manipulation of this single parameter, we fancy it's a bit like the Fed setting interest rates. Various considerations go into recommending a specific chapter length. From the perspective of the Editorial Board, readers' needs are the first priority. Therefore, the Board discusses depth of coverage and speculates on the time readers would devote to the topic. Admittedly, these judgments are based more on intuition than on hard data. Demographic information and questionnaires identify those who buy *Advances*, but they don't tell us which chapters are actually read. Furthermore, questionnaires don't verify the correlation of reading habits and good intentions for any of us.

The issue of chapter length often brings a different set of considerations to the minds of authors. *Advances* authors have many opportunities to present their topics in various forums. While readers' needs are of some interest to authors, they often see the body of literature in their respective fields as having a life of its own. Creating and nurturing the literature can be uppermost in an author's mind. I'm impressed that many outstanding authors, with large followings, are relatively uninfluenced by their readers. Such authors may not write an article based on what readers need or want to know, but rather on what he or she wishes to tell them. On the whole, that just may be the best approach for certain review articles, despite the fact that Editorial Boards may think otherwise.

Do authors consider the relationship of length of article to eventual size of readership? I doubt that this is often the case. I don't have hard data, but it's interesting how rarely we encounter authors who are concerned about the size of *Advances* readership. I suspect that many authors would be quite satisfied to know that copies of their articles are archived, in perpetuity, in the great medical libraries of the world. A large readership would only be a bonus.

Operationally, final decisions on length and content are left largely to the authors' discretion. The Editorial Board chooses first-rate authors, typically suggests that an article of 25 to 35 pages in length would be an appropriate objective, and then allows the authors to do as they see fit. This generally results in papers 10 to 50 pages in length. Each year, we ask one or two authors to write more extensive articles because we believe that each volume benefits from the inclusion of a few longer articles. Articles by Dr. Carl E. Speicher and Dr. Kamal G. Ishak fill that bill in Volume 8, and we are grateful to them for their special contributions. Taking the entire volume into account, I think it confirms the effectiveness of *Advances'* authors in satisfying the needs of our readers. Give fine and knowledgeable authors a free rein, and they get the job done, *par excellence*.

Ronald S. Weinstein, M.D.
Editor−in−Chief

Contents

Quality Assurance Issues and Problems Specific to Autopsies.
By Nancy A. Young

PART II. Diagnostic Pathology

Kinetic-Mode, Automated Double-Labeled Immunohistochemistry and in situ Hybridization in Diagnostic Pathology.
By Thomas M. Grogan, Catherine Rangel, Lisa Rimsza, William Bellamy, Ralph Martel, Darin McDaniel, Brian McGraw, William Richards, Lynne Richter, Paula Rodgers, James Rybski, Wayne Showalter, Elizabeth Vela, and Ron Zeheb

Antineutrophil Cytoplasmic Autoantibodies: Discovery, Specificity, Disease Associations, and Pathogenic Potential.

PCR-DNA Utilization: General Laboratory Usage for Mismatched Specimens.

Mosby Document Express

Copies of the full text of journal articles referenced in this book are available by calling Mosby Document Express, toll-free, at 1-800-55-MOSBY.

With Mosby Document Express, you have convenient 24-hour-a-day access to literally every journal reference within this book. In fact, through Mosby Document Express, virtually any medical or scientific article can be located and delivered by FAX, overnight delivery service, international airmail, electronic transmission of bit-mapped images (via Internet), or regular mail. The average cost of a complete delivered copy of an article, including copyright clearance charges and first-class mail delivery, is $12.

For inquiries and pricing information, please call the toll-free number shown above.

PART I

Laboratory Practice

Laboratory Utilization: A Discussion of the Appropriate Use of Clinical Laboratory Tests by Physicians

Carl E. Speicher, M.D.

Professor and Director, Clinical Services, Vice-Chair, Department of Pathology, Ohio State University College of Medicine, Ohio State University Medical Center, Columbus, Ohio

I n 1994 the United States spent about $1 trillion on health care—14% of the gross domestic product, a proportion far higher than that of any other nation. And the Congressional Budget Office says that under current law the share will grow to 20% in the year 2003.[1] Estimates of the cost of clinical laboratory tests range up to 10%.[2] No one knows how much of this testing is wasteful, and some boldly predict that in an optimally managed, capitated care system, approximately 50% of the tests can be eliminated.[3]

The use of clinical laboratory tests by physicians is a topic of great interest not only because of escalating health care costs but also because laboratory testing has a profound effect on the quality of patient care. The goal of appropriate testing is conceptualized in Table 1. The goal is not A, B, or even C. It is X. To achieve the ideal result, not only must physicians choose the right tests, but they must also have the tests performed in an accredited laboratory. Moreover, the test results must be properly interpreted, and the correct therapy must be implemented. Through appropriate laboratory testing—not too little, not too much—physicians practice high-quality, cost-conscious medicine, which is philosophically consistent with the concept that good medicine is cost-effective.[4]

In the author's opinion, the United States has embarked on an era that may be termed the industralization of American medicine. In this era business techniques that were developed and honed in industry are being increasingly applied to the practice of medicine.[5] Although the ostensible goals are to improve medical outcomes and control costs, there is concern that price will be the dominant factor. In fact, a recent survey revealed that for managed care organizations, this is already the case (Fig 1). It will be unfortunate if excessive restriction of laboratory tests based

Advances in Pathology and Laboratory Medicine®, vol. 8
© 1995, Mosby–Year Book, Inc.

TABLE 1.
Goal of Appropriate Testing*

Amount and Kind of Testing	Outcomes			
	Poor	Average	Good	Excellent
Too little	A			
About right			C	X (the ideal result)
Too much		B		

*From Speicher CE: *The Right Test: A Physician's Guide to Laboratory Medicine*, ed 2. Philadelphia, WB Saunders, 1993, p 2. Used by permission.

on cost interferes with the achievement of excellent outcomes because of inappropriate/insufficient testing.[6]

Under managed care and capitation, the clinical laboratory changes from a profit center to a cost center. In the pursuit of low-cost testing the production of test results will be decentralized and regionalized, which will have an impact on test utilization. Benchmarking relative financial and operational performance will be essential.[7] Practice parameters will serve as a benchmark to eliminate wasteful testing. Pathologists must be

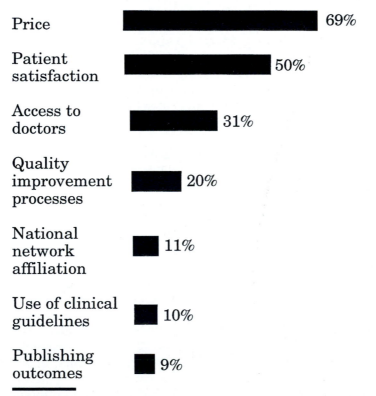

Price	69%
Patient satisfaction	50%
Access to doctors	31%
Quality improvement processes	20%
National network affiliation	11%
Use of clinical guidelines	10%
Publishing outcomes	9%

FIGURE 1.
How 102 managed care organizations ranked factors important to success in the market place; percentage of plans ranking a factor first or second. (From Winslow R: *Wall Street Journal*, p B1, Jan 18, 1994. Used by permission.)

proactive in this rapidly changing environment. They can do this by aggressively pursuing high-quality, low-cost testing as well as functioning as the "gatekeepers" of the clinical laboratory for appropriate testing. A variety of coping strategies will be required to respond to reduced funding.[8]

In the discussion that follows, a review of medical decision making by laboratory tests is followed by an approach to laboratory testing based on medical problem solving and decision making. Recommendations for the use of laboratory tests are based on practice parameters and other credible advice, which should be adapted for each health care organization by local experts. A method is described for improving these recommendations through outcome studies in the spirit of total quality improvement. Suggestions for implementing these recommendations include a medical decision-oriented test request system that will function best through the use of physician computer workstations. An integrated laboratory database that can be used by physicians and administrators is essential.

MEDICAL DECISION MAKING BY LABORATORY TESTS

Medical decision making by laboratory tests involves not only the way physicians use tests but also the way tests are produced. Test utilization and test production are interrelated. In this regard, the brain-to-brain turn-around time loop is a useful concept (Fig 2). One can see that laboratory utilization begins and ends in the physician's brain and that four processes are active[9]:

1. Choosing laboratory tests
2. Performing laboratory tests
3. Interpreting laboratory test results
4. Deliberating and acting on laboratory test results

One can also see that there are two distinct aspects of clinical laboratory testing, namely, test production and test utilization. Although the thrust of this discussion is focused on test utilization, one should also understand the variables that affect test production.

TEST UTILIZATION

Physicians order laboratory tests for many reasons, including the following: confirmation of clinical opinion, diagnosis, establishing a baseline, monitoring, completing a database, fraud and kickbacks, public relations, curiosity, insecurities, hospital policy, screening, legal requirements, medicolegal needs, documentation, peer pressure, patient pressure, recent literature pressure, a previous abnormal result, questionable accuracy of a previous test, unavailability of a prior result, prognosis, habit, buying time, CYA (covering your alternatives), "hunting" or "fishing" expeditions, personal education, research, personal reassurance, personal or institutional profit, demonstration for an attending physician, frustration at nothing else to do, and availability or ease of performance.[10] Operational factors such as "turnaround time too long" are an important

Physician's Brain

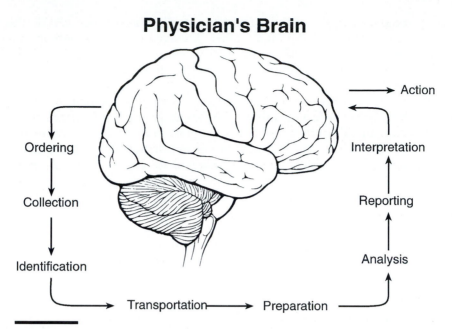

FIGURE 2.

The nine steps in the performance of any laboratory test; the brain-to-brain turn-around time loop. (From Lundberg GD: *JAMA* 245:1762–1763, 1981. Used by permission.)

cause of unnecessary testing.[11] Legitimate reasons for ordering tests are to help physicians make diagnostic, monitoring, and screening medical decisions.[4, 9]

Since the legitimate use of laboratory tests is to help make medical decisions, the decision-making model is a useful framework for characterizing the role of laboratory tests in medical problem solving (Fig 3). In addition to their use for diagnosis and monitoring, laboratory tests are used for screening, of which there are two different types: (1) wellness screening, in which the individuals are asymptomatic and basically healthy, and (2) case finding, in which individuals are screened for un-related symptoms or diseases (i.e., they are patients).[4, 9] In a survey, physicians indicated that they use laboratory tests almost equally for these three reasons: screening (32%), diagnosis (37%), and monitoring (33%).[12]

Wellness screening is the testing of asymptomatic individuals who are basically healthy. General screening of everyone for every disorder may lead to false-positive test results and fruitless follow-up testing with little gain and potential for real harm. Selective screening refers to testing of asymptomatic persons who are at risk for the target condition. Baseline information against which to compare future test results, data that make other studies unnecessary, and reassurance that the patient is free of disease are legitimate reasons for requesting screening tests. One should screen for diseases that are relatively common, that can be detected before clinical findings develop, that are easy to treat, and that have harmful consequences if left untreated.[4]

Diagnosis involves more than just the type of logic that is needed for ruling a condition in and out. Diagnostic reasoning proceeds from effect

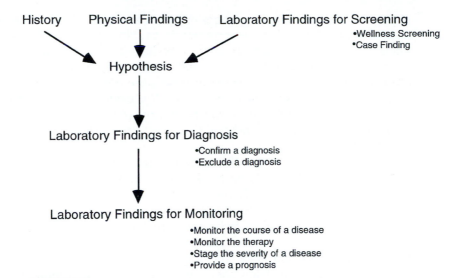

FIGURE 3.
The medical decision-making model as a framework for laboratory testing. (From Speicher CE: *The Right Test: A Physician's Guide to Laboratory Medicine*, ed 2. Philadelphia, WB Saunders, 1993, p 3. Used by permission.)

to cause, that is, from symptoms, signs, and laboratory data to etiology. On the other hand, pathogenetic reasoning (the method by which medical students are usually taught) proceeds from cause to effect, that is, from etiology to symptoms, signs, and laboratory findings. Medical students and physicians in training tend to adopt an exhaustive approach to medical diagnosis and rely heavily on the laboratory rather than on clinical testing. In contrast, experienced physicians favor a more pointed and abbreviated approach. They use a minimum number of tests, often clinical, and are parsimonious in requesting laboratory studies; that is, they use a rifle, not a shotgun approach.[13] It is possible that because experienced physicians have developed a better intuitive sense of the probability of a given diagnosis with less data, they are able to function with fewer laboratory measurements. In addition to confirming or excluding a diagnosis, diagnostic reasons for initiating testing strategies include clarifying a diagnosis and providing clues when the diagnosis is unclear.[4, 9, 14, 15]

In some settings tests are used to make monitoring decisions more often than commonly realized. Sixty percent of the laboratory tests performed at the Upstate Medical Center in Syracuse, New York, were carried out to monitor therapy.[16] In many settings 60% to 80% of the most common laboratory tests are performed to monitor therapy rather than to make an initial diagnosis.[17] Primary care health care facilities may differ from tertiary care hospitals and may have tests performed more often for diagnostic than monitoring purposes. It is in the area of monitoring that good testing strategies are particularly lacking.[18]

The medical decision-oriented view of laboratory testing is a powerful one, and the effective use of laboratory tests can be best understood in the context of the medical decisions they influence. In addition to a requirement for generic problem solving, specific medical decision-making strategies for using laboratory tests are needed. The physician's task of managing a particular patient's problem comprises a series of medical decisions. Some decisions rely heavily on laboratory tests for their solution; some decisions use test results as ancillary information to clinical, radiographic, or electrocardiographic data; and other decisions do not depend on laboratory tests at all. For example, when caring for a patient with an acute myocardial infarction (AMI), physicians are confronted with a number of medical decisions that vary in their test dependency (Table 2).[4, 19]

Although in the future this may change, certain medical decisions cannot presently be made with laboratory tests. For example, the decision to use thrombolytic therapy in a patient with probable AMI must presently be made clinically—not by laboratory tests. A test for the earlier diagnosis of AMI needs to be developed and used (perhaps an analysis for creatine kinase [CK] isoforms or troponin T).[20] Thrombolytic therapy has significant risks, and if an earlier diagnosis of AMI could be made, the medical decision about whether or not this therapy is appropriate for a particular patient could be improved. In the emergency department, the diagnosis of probable AMI used to be made clinically—now better tests are available. In the hospital coronary care unit, serial measurements of creatine kinase, isoenzyme MB (CK-MB), have high diagnostic sensitivity and specificity for diagnosing AMI, whereas in the emergency department setting, the diagnostic sensitivity and specificity of a single measurement of CK-MB for diagnosing AMI are much lower because there is usually time for only one measurement of CK-MB. This emergency department dilemma is being approached by either using bet-

TABLE 2.

Discrete Medical Decisions Concerning the Problem of Acute Myocardial Infarction*

Medical Decision	Dependence on Laboratory Tests
Deciding to admit an emergency department patient with chest pain	*No*—although a positive CK/CK-MB† test result could detect an unexpected AMI‡
Diagnosing AMI in the coronary care unit	*Yes*—serial CK/CK-MB tests are the gold standard for diagnosis
Estimating the size of an AMI	*Partially*—although the prognostic information may not be very good
Diagnosing AMI in a patient after noncardiac surgery	*Yes*—similar to diagnosing AMI in a patient in the coronary care unit
Deciding to use thrombolytic therapy in a patient with AMI	*No*—therapy should be initiated before CK/CK-MB elevations
Evaluating the effectiveness of thrombolytic therapy for AMI	*Partially*—an early rise in serum CK/CK-MB can signal reperfusion of ischemic muscle

*From Speicher CE: *Clin Lab Med* 11:255–265, 1991. Used by permission.
†CK-MB = creatine kinase, isoenzyme MB; AMI = acute myocardial infarction.
‡New tests for an earlier diagnosis of AMI have made this decision test dependent.

ter tests for the earlier diagnosis of AMI or holding the patient for serial CK-MB determinations.[4, 21]

A variety of statistical techniques are available for understanding how a laboratory test changes the pretest probability of a medical decision to the post-test probability (predictive value). These techniques are mostly based on Bayes' theorem and include likelihood ratios, odds, receiver operating curves, and dot plots. These techniques have also been used to develop a formal method of structuring a medical problem in the form of a decision tree, i.e., formal decision analysis. The decision tree delineates management choices, which allow a calculation of the probability that each clinical outcome will occur if a particular strategy is used. Moreover, the relative worth of each outcome is depicted.[14, 22-24]

TEST PRODUCTION

The production of test results involves a number of different steps in the brain-to-brain turnaround time loop, and the quality of test results can be judged by several different criteria.[9]

Steps in the Brain-to-Brain Turnaround Time Loop

The brain-to-brain turnaround time loop represents an enlarged model of clinical laboratory testing. Instead of viewing the laboratory as the physical place where testing takes place (starting when a specimen is received by the laboratory and ending when a report is sent out), one should think of the brain-to-brain turnaround time loop as embracing all that happens from the time a physician decides to order a test until the result of the test is placed in the physician's hands.[9, 25] It is now recognized that analytic quality control is only one component of the overall quality of laboratory services. Quality assurance—as opposed to quality control—demands attention to all phases of the laboratory testing sequence, beginning with the clinician's formation of testing strategy and ending with clinical action in response to the test result.[14] There are three limbs.

THE PREANALYTIC LIMB.—The preanalytic limb encompasses all steps that occur from the time the physician decides to order a test until a specimen is received in the laboratory. Problems in the preanalytic limb can seriously affect the accuracy, precision, and turnaround time of laboratory data. Adverse effects causing increased turnaround time include delays in executing the physician's order, in collecting the specimen, and in transporting the specimen to the laboratory. Most physicians are familiar with the deterioration of accuracy secondary to poor specimen collection and handling, such as decreased serum glucose levels in specimens not refrigerated or not collected in fluoride-containing tubes, increased serum potassium levels in specimens allowed to stand for hours on a desk or bench top at room temperature, and prolonged plasma prothrombin times or activated partial thromboplastin times in specimens not properly collected and preserved. Many physicians, however, are not aware of the manner in which problems in the preanalytic limb can cause deterioration of precision. For example, the variation in serum creatinine measurements can be as large for the preanalytic limb as for the analytic limb.[9]

Ideally, specimen collection and handling should be the responsibility of the laboratory and under its control. Proper identification, collection, preservation, and transportation of specimens are as important to generating timely, accurate, and precise data as are well-performed, well-controlled technical procedures. The importance of proper identification of specimens has been emphasized by good clinical laboratories. Misidentification of patients' specimens and test results is a risk factor for the occurrence of bad patient outcomes.[9]

Long physical distances between the sites of specimen collection and the laboratory can cause specimen deterioration and increased turnaround times. The larger and more spread-out the health care facility or system, the greater the problems. Expediting test requests through electronic communication is essential. There are a number of ways of overcoming the problems of long physical distances[9]:

1. Improved methods of specimen preservation, such as the addition of fluoride to blood specimens for glucose analysis or the use of ice to preserve specimens for lactate analysis. Although these methods decrease specimen deterioration, they do nothing to decrease turnaround time.

2. Improved transportation of specimens to the laboratory. Developments such as special vertical lifts (dumbwaiters) and automated mechanical and pneumatic transportation systems are helpful. Most specimens for routine laboratory studies can be safely transported by pneumatic tube if the system has the correct engineering characteristics.[26]

3. Decentralization of the laboratory and utilization of alternate-site laboratory testing such as point-of-care testing. This causes the additional problems of quality control and increased costs in decentralized locations. Nevertheless, this solution is increasingly applied in a variety of settings.[27–29]

THE ANALYTIC LIMB.—All steps that occur from the time a specimen is received in the laboratory until a report is released from the laboratory are part of the analytic limb.

THE POSTANALYTIC LIMB.—This limb includes all steps that occur from the time a report is released from the laboratory until a result is placed in the hands of the ordering physician.[9] The brain-to-brain turnaround time loop is not closed until the test result is communicated to the ordering physician. To affect patient care in a meaningful way, the test result must be communicated in a timely manner. A variety of communication methods are available, and the method of communication should fit the required turnaround time. Because the results of certain laboratory tests have lifesaving implications for patient care, policies have been devised for the immediate communication of critical information, i.e., critical values.[30, 31] Therapeutic drug monitoring exemplifies the necessity of closing the brain-to-brain turnaround time information loop. If the result of a given drug blood level measurement is not received in time to adjust the next dose, the measurement is worthless for patient care and a waste of money.[32]

Criteria for the Quality of Test Results

One can assess the quality of test results produced by the laboratory through the brain-to-brain turnaround time loop by four criteria: accuracy, precision, timeliness, and interpretability.[9]

ACCURACY.—Accuracy is how closely the data conform to the true values. Laboratory data are not always accurate, and a small number of mistakes occur. Good laboratories make fewer mistakes than poor laboratories. Estimates of the cumulative probability of mistakes may approach 1% to 2%.[33] One suspects that physicians have learned to ignore data that do not fit with their clinical impressions. The problem with this behavior is that physicians may ignore accurate data because the data do not make sense when in reality the data may provide clues to diagnoses they never considered. This tendency to ignore unexpected abnormalities in laboratory test results has been well documented.[34–40]

PRECISION.—Precision relates to how well the data can be reproduced. Precision is commonly quantified in terms of the coefficient of variation (CV). The CV is simply another way of expressing the standard deviation (SD) of a series of measurements on the same sample. It is defined as 100 times the SD divided by the mean and it is expressed as a percentage.[41] Its chief value is that it relates the SD to the level at which the measurements are made. It is important when critically using the CV to ensure that it was determined at the level at which it is being used. For example, if 1 SD for the measurement of serum aspartate aminotransferase (AST) is 5 units/mL, this represents a CV of 12.5% at a serum AST level of 40 units/mL (the approximate upper limit of the reference level), but a CV of only 2.5% at a serum AST level of 200 units/mL. The CV for the measurement of any single analyte is expressed in terms of either within-day CV or day-to-day CV. Usually the day-to-day CV is larger than the within-day CV. It is commonly accepted by statistical argument that a change of three times day-to-day CV for any given analyte indicates a real day-to-day change in the concentration of that analyte in the body fluids or tissues of a patient.[42] For example, if the day-to-day CV for a patient's serum glucose is 6% at a level of 100 mg/100 mL, a change of 18 mg/100 mL in the day-to-day concentration of serum glucose is required to indicate a real change in the day-to-day serum glucose level.[9]

TIMELINESS.—Timeliness is the appropriateness of the test turnaround time for the medical decision that confronts the physician. Requirements for different kinds of turnaround times are reflected in the following terms (the times listed are based on the author's perceptions of physicians' typical needs)[9, 43]:

- *Life-threatening:* less than 15 minutes, preferably less than 5 minutes
- *Stat:* as soon as possible, usually within 1 hour
- *Expedite:* as soon as possible after stat, usually within 3 hours
- *Today:* as soon as possible after expedite, usually within 8 hours
- *Routine:* varies from more than 8 hours to days or weeks

The intensity of medical practice, especially at tertiary care hospitals, continues to increase. Physicians need test results in ever-decreasing turnaround times (e.g., arterial blood gas and serum potassium results in critically ill patients or patients in surgery).[44, 45] In 1981 it was stated that "the cause of the lack of oxygen" (i.e., arterial blood gases) "should be assessed in less than 5 minutes by a good laboratory."[46] There is an increasing requirement for point-of-care testing to perform tests for life-threatening situations, especially in large acute care hospitals. By consensus, the most common tests needed in emergency situations include blood gases, oxygen saturation, hemoglobin, hematocrit, and determinations of serum sodium, potassium, glucose, osmolality, and colloidal osmotic pressure. Others would include basic blood clotting tests and measurements of serum amylase and urea nitrogen.[9]

Limitations on turnaround time depend on how quickly specimens can be delivered to the laboratory, how quickly tests can be performed, and how quickly test results can be delivered to the physician. Because present test performance is rapid and reporting of results can be accomplished electronically, the usual limiting step is the speed with which specimens can be delivered to the laboratory. In spite of dedicated specimen carriers and mechanical specimen delivery systems, the distance of laboratories from patients remains the major impediment to very rapid turnaround times (i.e., less than 5 minutes). For this reason, point-of-care testing has emerged as a solution for patients who require very quick results. Recent developments in testing technology makes this an increasingly attractive option.[27] For tests to be useful in an acute care monitoring situation, they must be understood in depth (including potential sources of error) and repeated frequently so that trends may be noted and defensive action taken.[47]

INTERPRETABILITY.—Interpretability involves relevance to patient care (i.e., the ease with which the data can be applied to patient diagnosis and monitoring). Even accurate and precise test results produced within acceptable turnaround times may not be interpretable. Laboratory data are typically expressed in terms of values consisting of numbers and units (e.g., a creatinine value of 1.2 mg/100 mL). The data are useless unless one knows the correct reference intervals, i.e., 0.6 to 1.2 mg/100 mL for males and 0.5 to 1.0 mg/100 mL for females for specific creatinine methods—true creatinine (total chromogen) methods are about 0.3 mg/100 mL higher.[48] Decision levels that correlate the data with other laboratory data or clinical signs and symptoms can be helpful. For instance, a creatinine value of 4.0 mg/100 mL correlates approximately with a creatinine clearance that is 25% of the healthy value and is also the level above which serum electrolyte changes (an increased anion gap) secondary to renal failure occur.[49, 50] Interpretive reports may be helpful.[51, 52]

COMMON MEDICAL PROBLEMS THAT REQUIRE LABORATORY TESTS

Physicians have more than 1,000 individual tests available each time they face a medical decision that requires laboratory tests. Moreover, the number of new tests grows weekly. The physician's task of learning about tests can be frustrating and time-consuming. Why not organize an approach to choosing laboratory tests in terms of a limited number of common and costly medical problems and component medical decisions rather than an almost endless list of individual laboratory tests?[4]

The laboratory request slip is like a restaurant menu in need of better decision-making choices.[53] Presently it consists of long "a la carte" lists of individual tests together with multitest panels (also called batteries or profiles). These panels or combinations of tests have often been predetermined by instrument manufacturers and may have no pathophysiologic basis.[15] The use of panels has been critized as inappropriate and wasteful; however, it is the content of the panel—not the concept of the panel—that has been problematic.[54]

In some settings pathologists are available for consultation, but their assistance may be infrequently used. "Chance" informal consultative assistance happens in hallways, dining rooms, locker rooms, and other such places, but these chance encounters affect only a small percentage of total laboratory testing. Pathologists have not done enough to improve this situation. They need to be the "gatekeepers" of the laboratory. Interpretive reporting is fine, but interpretive reports represent the end of the laboratory testing process. If the wrong tests were chosen, then effective interpretations are impossible.[51, 52] Moreover, if unnecessary tests were ordered along with appropriate tests, then effective interpretations may be possible, but cost-effectiveness is not.

It is possible to describe and categorize the common and costly medical problems and component medical decisions that depend on laboratory testing for their solutions. These decisions entail diagnosis, monitoring, and screening, and a list of them can be used in several ways[4, 9, 15, 19]:

1. To educate medical students and physicians in how to use laboratory tests to help make medical decisions
2. To communicate to physicians the various medical decisions for which pathologists can be of assistance
3. To develop a "dinner" menu for laboratory testing whereby the physician would not only be able to choose from the "a la carte" menu of individual tests but would also be able to choose from a menu of testing strategies for medical decisions that are both effective for patient care and cost-efficient

In applying a medical decision-making approach to the use of laboratory tests, sound, scientifically based recommendations for test ordering in common patient care situations, although urgently needed, are not always available. Testing standards, guidelines, options, and nonoptions must be developed.[4]

- *Standards* should be followed exactly; strictly speaking, there are very few real standards.
- *Guidelines* give limits that allow some freedom of choice.
- *Options* provide a wider spectrum of choice than guidelines.
- *Nonoptions* describe choices that are inappropriate or obsolete.

Because physicians see patients in either an ambulatory care (outpatient) setting or in a hospital (inpatient) setting, it makes sense to iden-

TABLE 3.
Common Medical Problems in the Hospital (Inpatient) Setting*

Rank	Description	Total	%	Cumulative %
1	Normal delivery/live born	4,392,000	14.8	14.8
2	Complications of birth, puerperium	2,265,000	7.6	22.4
3	Ischemic heart disease	1,617,000	5.4	27.8
4	Complications during pregnancy	911,000	3.1	30.9
5	Pneumonia and influenza	879,000	3.0	33.9
6	Cerebrovascular disease	808,000	2.7	36.6
7	Fractures (not hip)	784,000	2.6	39.2
8	Congestive heart failure	685,000	2.3	41.5
9	Respiratory infections (not tuberculosis)	688,000	2.3	43.8
10	Spondylosis, intervertebral disk disorders, cervical disorders, miscellaneous back pain	681,000	2.3	46.1

*Adapted from *Trends in Hospital Procedures Performed on Black Patients and White Patients: 1980–87*. Washington, DC, U.S. Department of Health and Human Services, Agency for Health Care Policy and Research Publication No 94-0003, April 1994, pp 202–204.

TABLE 4.
Common Medical Problems in the Ambulatory Care (Outpatient) Setting*

Rank	Description	Total	%	Cumulative %
1	Other medical examination for preventive and presymptomatic purposes	43,951	8.4	8.4
2	Benign or unspecified hypertension with or without heart and/or renal disease	30,235	5.7	14.1
3	Lacerations, amputations, contusions, and abrasions	21,137	4.0	18.1
4	Pharyngitis (including febrile sore throat and tonsillitis)	20,176	3.8	21.9
5	Bronchitis, acute	13,511	2.6	24.5
6	Sprains and strains	12,830	2.4	26.9
7	Diabetes mellitus	12,435	2.4	29.3
8	Coryza (nonfebrile common cold)	10,951	2.1	31.4
9	Obesity	10,679	2.0	33.4
10	Febrile cold and influenza-like illness	9,366	1.8	35.2

*Adapted from Marsland DW, Wood M, Mayo F: *J Fam Pract* 3:37–68, 1976.

tify common medical problems and component medical decisions in each setting. By concentrating on these common problems, one can reduce the issue of appropriate laboratory test utilization from an endless number of individual laboratory tests to a finite list of medical problems and component medical decisions of manageable proportions (Tables 3 and 4). Since the variety of inpatient and outpatient medical problems may differ from one location to another, the problem lists and component decisions should be individualized for each health care organization.

RECOMMENDATIONS FOR THE USE OF LABORATORY TESTS

In an attempt to provide scientifically based recommendations for test ordering in common patient care situations, medical societies, health care organizations, and other groups have developed practice parameters, consensus statements, and miscellaneous advice for appropriate laboratory testing. Of these various kinds of recommendations, practice parameters have been the most prominent.[55] The problem with these recommendations is that few have been subjected to rigorous scientific evaluation to measure outcomes and costs. Many are based on expert opinion with little experimental data.[56] Rigorous evaluations need to be conducted.[57, 58]

Among the many available consensus statements, the National Cholesterol Education Program recommendations for managing patients with elevated blood cholesterol levels is one of the best known.[59] These recommendations have recently been updated and continue to emphasize low-density lipoprotein (LDL)-cholesterol as the primary target of cholesterol-lowering therapy and to recommend dietary changes as initial therapy, with drug therapy reserved for those at high risk for coronary artery disease.[60]

Besides practice parameters and consensus statements, the medical literature is full of recommendations about laboratory testing emanating from experts, health care organizations, and miscellaneous sources.[4, 61-63]

PRACTICE PARAMETERS

Practice parameters are recommendations for patient management developed to assist physicians in medical decision making. Based on a thorough evaluation of the scientific literature and relevant clinical experience, practice parameters describe the range of acceptable approaches to diagnose, monitor, or prevent specific diseases or conditions. Practice parameters are educational tools that enable physicians to (1) obtain the advice of recognized clinical experts, (2) stay abreast of the latest clinical research, and (3) assess the clinical significance of conflicting research findings. Practice parameters provide a rational foundation for quality assurance, utilization review, facility accreditation, and other review activities.[64, 65]

Consider two examples. Practice parameters developed by the American College of Cardiology clarified and improved the appropriate use of cardiac pacemakers. These parameters received widespread acceptance by physicians, and subsequently, the utilization rates for pacemakers among Medicare patients declined from 2.44 per 1,000 Medicare beneficiaries in 1983 to 1.76 in 1988, an approximate 25% reduction in utilization rates. In another experience, use of the American Society of Anesthesiologists' practice parameters for basic intraoperative monitoring in Massachusetts was associated with a marked reduction in hypoxic injuries. This allowed the Massachusetts Medical Malpractice Joint Underwriting Association to offer a 20% premium reduction to anesthesiologists who agreed to follow the parameters.[55]

THE EMERGENCE OF PRACTICE PARAMETERS

The development of practice parameters represents the latest attempt of physicians, through their professional societies, to improve the quality of health care and respond to mounting pressure to contain health care costs. Recently, some studies have identified unexplained variations in health care services, and other studies have indicated that in certain instances medical care may be inappropriate or marginally beneficial.[66] The perception is that much of medical care is unnecessary, and the assumption is that practice parameters represent a way to improve the quality of health care and at the same time eliminate waste.[55]

The American Medical Association (AMA) is working cooperatively with national medical specialty societies, including the American Society of Clinical Pathologists (ASCP) and the College of American Pathologists (CAP), to guide the development and implementation of practice parameters. About 1,600 practice parameters developed by 70 physician groups and organizations are already available. Additional practice parameters are under development, and it is anticipated that the number of practice parameters will increase significantly.[65]

The quality of existing practice parameters is unknown. Most have never been critically reviewed. Few have been evaluated to determine their effects on patient outcomes and costs. Some call practice parameters "cookbook" medicine and argue against their development and use on the theory that such parameters may be used perversely as evidence against individual physicians in malpractice cases in which the defendant has deviated from the standards. Others say that the answer to this concern lies not in avoiding practice parameters on the grounds of an exaggerated fear of possible liability but in ensuring the following:

- The recommendations are substantively defensible in light of current respectable scientific evidence.
- The recommendations have been arrived at through an open, fair, and credible process.
- Proper explanatory commentary accompanies the dissemination of recommendations to practitioners who must implement them.[55]

In this way, physicians who comply with practice parameters may cite them as presumptive evidence of appropriate conduct should the need to defend their actions in a malpractice case arise.[55] Notwithstanding these reassurances, medical practitioners are finding that they can get hurt by practice parameters. In a 1990–1992 study of 259 malpractice claims, 17 of these claims involved using practice parameters to exonerate the defendant physician, whereas another 12 of these claims involved using practice parameters to implicate the defendant physician.[67] Another potential problem with practice parameters is the inhibition of new and promising strategies for patient care.

PRACTICE PARAMETERS FOR PATHOLOGY AND LABORATORY MEDICINE

Both ASCP and CAP have established committees for the development of practice parameters for laboratory medicine, i.e., the ASCP Practice Parameters/Outcome Measurements Committee and the CAP Practice Guidelines Committee. The two societies have agreed to cooperate in this important endeavor, and a joint steering committee has been established to coordinate the work of the two committees. The AMA is cooperating with the two committees to facilitate the development of laboratory medicine practice parameters. The task before the ASCP and CAP is as follows:

1. Become proactive with other national medical specialty societies in the codevelopment of practice parameters that pertain to laboratory medicine.

2. Develop practice parameters that are *exclusively for laboratory medicine*, e.g., practice parameters for the workup of a lymph node excision biopsy specimen.

3. Review existing practice parameters that pertain to laboratory medicine to provide constructive feedback for revisions. Although many existing practice parameters contain some reference to laboratory medicine services, it is unlikely that pathologists have had any influence on them.[55]

After practice parameters for laboratory medicine have been developed and approved, the next challenge will be to implement them and evaluate their effects on health care quality and costs. Practice parameters require regular review and revision as new technology becomes available. It appears that the Joint Commission on Accreditation of Healthcare Organizations will incorporate practice parameters into its quality assurance agenda and that many of us will encounter practice parameters in the context of our quality assurance programs.

Two points about practice parameters deserve additional comment:

1. Practice parameters often deal with the "average patient" with the "typical disease." With time and experience, more but not all variations will be covered. Therefore physicians must be free to exercise judgment when a particular patient's problem falls outside the purview of a given practice parameter.

2. Practice parameters must be timely, updated frequently, and updated promptly when necessary. This is a strong argument for the development and updating of practice parameters by medical organizations.[55]

IMPLEMENTATION OF PRACTICE PARAMETERS

A problem with the national practice parameter effort is that for the most part, groups and societies that write practice parameters are working alone. There is little cooperation aimed at producing a single practice parameter on a given topic that represents the consensus recommendations of all parties. This is illustrated by the example of practice parameters for wellness screening: the American College of Physicians, the U.S. Preventive Services Task Force, the Canadian Task Force on Periodic Health Examination, and others have developed separate and different recommendations. The recommendations of these separate groups have been tabulated and summarized in a recent publication.[68]

Because local physician preferences can differ from those of national groups,[69] practice parameters developed by national societies and groups should be evaluated by local medical experts in the context of local expertise and resources for the purpose of producing local recommendations on specific patient care problems. Pathologists should participate with local medical experts to generate guidelines for laboratory testing. This is the process used at The Ohio State University Medical Center (OSUMC), and three examples of this process will be given in the form of recommendations for wellness screening of asymptomatic adults; recommendations to prevent, detect, and monitor complications of diabetes mellitus after the initial diagnosis has been established; and recommendations for the use of serum prostate-specific antigen (PSA) to screen for prostate cancer.

Recommendations for Wellness Screening of Adults

Starting in 1989, the faculty of OSUMC, in the context of the OSUMC Faculty and Staff Health Plan, began to formulate practice guidelines that incorporated recommendations for appropriate laboratory testing. One of the first of these was guidelines for wellness screening of adults[70] (Figs 4 and 5). These guidelines decreased inappropriate chest radiograms, electrocardiograms, and laboratory tests. The average cost for a physical examination before the guidelines was $173.30 and after the guidelines, $129.14, thus providing a saving of $44.15 per examination (1989 dollars).*[71]

Recommendations to Prevent, Detect, and Manage Complications of Diabetes Mellitus

Another OSUMC guideline addressed the prevention, detection, and management of the following complications of diabetes mellitus:

1. *Retinopathy* leading to blindness.
2. *Nephropathy* leading to renal failure.
3. *Uncontrolled diabetes* resulting in ketoacidosis, a hyperosmolar non-ketotic state, and hypoglycemia leading to hospitalization, coma, and death.
4. *Cardiovascular disease* resulting in hypertension, cerebral vascular disease, coronary artery disease, and peripheral vascular disease. Smoking accelerates the seriousness of all of the cardiovascular complications.
5. *Adverse outcomes of pregnancy* leading to prematurity, fetal demise, congenital anomalies, accelerated maternal complications, and neonatal morbidity.
6. *Peripheral vascular disease and neuropathy* leading to amputations.

---

*All OSUMC tests and services are designated in terms of costs, not charges.

Age

Elements of the exam	20 21 22 23 24 25 26 27 28 29 30 31 32 33 34 35 36 37 38 39 40 41 42 43 44 45 46 47 48 49 50 51 52 53 54 55 56 57 58 59 60 61 62 63 64 65
History, physical and counselling regarding risk factors, every 5 years to age 40, then every year.	□ □ □ ...
Gyn Exam: Begin age 18, yearly thereafter, or every 2 years after 3 negative Pap smears, until age 40. After age 40 every year or every other year.	± □ ± ...
Clinical Breast Exam, Same frequency as Gyn exam. Teach monthly self exam.	± □ ± ...
Pap smear, Same frequency as Gyn exam.	± □ ± ...
Blood Pressure Check, each visit.	± ± ...
Vision, dilated eye exam, age 20-39; every 3-5 years; age 40-64 every 2-4 years. (Covered under Vision Plan.)	□ ...
Hearing, pure tone audiometry if exposed chronically to excessively loud noises, every 1-3 years, begin age 40.	

Diagnostic/Screening Tests:

Mammogram, 35-39 baseline. 40-49 every 1-2 years. Age 50 yearly.	(ONE EXAM) ± ...
Stool for occult blood. Yearly after age 40, 3 consecutive stools, using Hemoccult II cards. Follow recommended diet and sampling procedure.	
Urinalysis, multi-combination dip-stick, same frequency as Gyn exam.	± □ ± ...
Sigmoidoscopy, with 60 cm flexible scope; age 50 or older, for individuals with first degree relatives with colorectal cancer, or other high risk conditions. Repeat every 5 years after 2 negative exams.	
Blood Work: FBS, Cholesterol, CBC, BUN, Cr., Electrolytes. Every 5-10 yrs.	± ONE EKG ...
EKG, Baseline before age 40, every 5 years thereafter or at the physician's discretion.	(ONE EKG ...

□ Recommended age to be performed.

± Can be performed at the discretion of patient or physician.

FIGURE 4.

Ohio State University Medical Center health maintenance "physical examination" guidelines for asymptomatic adult females at low medical risk. *FBS* = fasting blood sugar; *CBC* = complete blood count; *BUN* = blood urea nitrogen; *Cr* = creatine; *EKG* = electrocardiogram. (From Ohio State Faculty: Wellness screening and case finding, in *The Ohio State University Health Plan Clinical Notes*, vol 2, no 1. Columbus, Ohio State University, 1992. Used by permission.)

Elements of the exam

Age: 20 21 22 23 24 25 26 27 28 29 30 31 32 33 34 35 36 37 38 39 40 41 42 43 44 45 46 47 48 49 50 51 52 53 54 55 56 57 58 59 60 61 62 63 64 65

History, physical and counselling regarding risk factors, every 5 years to age 40, then every year.

Blood Pressure Check, each visit.

Rectal/Prostate exam included with physical exam.

Vision, dilated eye exam age 20-39: every 3-5 years; age 40-64 every 2-4 years. (Covered under Vision Plan.)

Hearing, pure tone audiometry if exposed chronically to excessively loud noises, every 1-3 years, begin age 40.

Diagnostic/Screening Tests:

Stool for Occult Blood. Yearly after age 40, 3 consecutive stools, using Hemoccult II cards. Follow recommended diet and sampling procedure.

Urinalysis, multi-combination dipstick, every 5-10 years.

Sigmoidoscopy, with 60 cm flexible scope; age 50 or older, for individuals with first degree relatives with colorectal cancer, or other high risk conditions. Repeat every 5 years after 2 negative exams.

Blood Work: FBS, Cholesterol, CBC, BUN, Cr., Electrolytes. Every 5-10 years. CBC, PSA every year after age 50.

EKG, Baseline before age 40, every 5 years thereafter, or at the physicians discretion.

ONE EKG

□ Recommended age to be performed.

± Can be performed at the discretion of patient or physician.

FIGURE 5.

Ohio State University Medical Center health maintenance "physical examination" guidelines for asymptomatic adult males at low medical risk. *PSA* = prostate-specific antigen. (From Ohio State Faculty: Wellness screening and case finding, in *The Ohio State University Health Plan Clinical Notes*, vol 2, no 1. Columbus, Ohio State University, 1992. Used by permission.)

See Figures 6 and 7 for these detailed recommendations.[72]

Before these guidelines, in a survey at OSUMC among more than 50 physicians, the majority did not follow the American Diabetes Association (ADA) national guidelines for managing diabetics. However, after our clinicians "fine-tuned" the ADA guidelines to produce local guidelines by local experts, most of our physicians said that they would follow them.[73]

Recommendations for Using Serum Prostate-Specific Antigen to Screen for Prostate Cancer

An OSUMC guideline on the use of serum PSA to screen for prostate cancer illustrates the importance of local medical experts producing recommendations on a specific patient care problem.

The American Cancer Society recommends annual serum PSA measurements on men 50 years and older and the American Urological Association agrees. However, the National Cancer Institute and the American Academy of Family Physicians disagree. The OSUMC guideline takes the position that serum PSA is a useful screening strategy and includes this test in its screening recommendations for asymptomatic adult men as seen in Figure 5.[74-76]

UPDATING PRACTICE PARAMETERS

Practice parameters must be frequently reviewed and updated so that they are consistent with the latest available scientific information. See Figure 8 to review how laboratory testing for the diagnosis of AMI has changed over the years.[77, 78]

IMPROVING THE USE OF LABORATORY TESTS

Unfortunately, definitive information to determine the appropriateness of laboratory testing for all medical decisions is not presently available. Far too little effort has been spent in determining the effectiveness of what we already know on patient care. The investment in effectiveness research needs to grow from less than 0.01% of our health care budget to probably 2% to 3%. We need to know much more about what does and what does not work.[79]

The Joint Commission on the Accreditation of Healthcare Organizations encourages us to perform outcome studies to improve patient care and control costs. An outcome is the result of a process, and a good outcome is a result that achieves the goal of the process. Goals that relate directly to the patient's health include avoiding adverse effects, improving physiologic status, reducing signs and symptoms, and improving functional status and well-being. Goals that are not directly health-related include achieving patient satisfaction, minimizing cost of care, and maximizing revenues.[80] In outcome studies, practice parameters can be used as a benchmark for appropriate practice.[65]

Although outcome studies are typically conducted on the total patient care process, it is possible to perform outcome studies on individual test-dependent medical decisions. At OSUMC this is accomplished in the spirit of total quality improvement, and the following

Elements of Care	Initial	1	2	3	4	5	6 MONTHS	7	8	9	10	11	12	As Needed	Compli-cations
Comprehensive Evaluation*	☐	(may require frequent contact until stable)													☐
Routine Examination, stable patients may only require examination every 6 months	☐		☐	☐	☐		☐			☐			☐	☐	
Nutrition Evaluation and Teaching	☐												☐	☐	
Eye Examination (visual acuity, intraocular pressure, ophthalmic exam through dilated pupil in darkened room)	☐												☐	☐	
Foot Examination	☐		☐	☐	☐		☐			☐			☐	☐	☐
Dental Examination	☐						☐						☐	☐	☐
Gynecologic Exam	☐												☐	☐	☐
Pre-conception Counseling and Obstetrical Care	☐												☐	☐	☐
Home Glucose Monitoring *Continuously 2-8 times per day, Record mean glucose at each visit.*	☐		☐	☐	☐		☐			☐			☐		
Fasting Plasma Glucose	☐														
HbA1c	☐		☐	☐	☐		☐			☐			☐	☐	
Fast Lipid Profile (tot chol, HDL, trigly)	☐												☐	☐	
Lytes, H&H, WBC, BUN, Creat	☐												☐		
UA per multistick, protein, ketones, leukocytes, etc.	☐												☐		
EKG	☐														
24 hour urine albumin and creatinine clearance (5 years after diagnosis, then annually)	☐												☐		

☐ Date / Result

* According to ADA guidelines, annual visit to diabetes specialist is encouraged

FIGURE 6.

Diabetes mellitus type I (insulin dependent) and type II (insulin requiring) initial and ongoing evaluation and care; annual flow sheet and care guidelines. *Lytes* = electrolytes; *chol* = cholesterol; *HDL* = high-density lipoprotein; *H&H* = hematocrit and hemoglobin; *WBC* = white blood cell count; *UA* = urinalysis. (From Ohio State Faculty: Diabetes mellitus, in *The Ohio State University Health Plan Clinical Notes*, vol 1, no 3. Columbus, Ohio State University, 1991. Used by permission.)

FIGURE 7.

Diabetes mellitus type II (non—insulin requiring) initial and ongoing evaluation and care; annual flow sheet and care guidelines. (From Ohio State Faculty: Diabetes mellitus. in *The Ohio State University Health Plan Clinical Notes*, vol 1, no 3. Columbus, Ohio State University, 1991. Used by permission.)

Complete blood count/Erythrocyte sedimentation rate
↓
Aspartate aminotransferase (AST previously SGOT)/
Alanine aminotransferase (ALT previously SGPT)
↓
Creatine kinase (CK)/Lactate dehydrogenase (LDH)
↓
Creatine kinase-MB (CK-MB)/
Lactate dehydrogenase isoenzymes (LD1:LD2)
↓
Creatine kinase-MB subforms (CK-MB subforms)
and Troponin T

FIGURE 8.
The evolution of laboratory testing for the diagnosis of acute myocardial infarction.

discussion illustrates this approach through a number of test-dependent medical decisions that occur in the context of the hospital (inpatient) setting, the ambulatory care (outpatient) setting, and the clinical laboratory itself.

MEDICAL DECISIONS IN THE HOSPITAL (INPATIENT) SETTING

Consider three testing strategies for medical decisions in hospitalized patients with cardiac disorders that illustrate inappropriate practice. The strategies were used to diagnose AMI in the coronary care unit, monitor digoxin therapy, and monitor the reversal of heparin therapy.

Diagnosing Acute Myocardial Infarction in the Coronary Care Unit

This is an example of a diagnostic testing strategy that is inappropriate because it took too long to execute. Until 1991, it was our practice to perform CK isoenzyme assays once a day with results available by late afternoon. Clinicians told us that they make their decisions to discharge patients in the morning; if the CK results were not available in the morning, patients could wait until the next day to be discharged. In response, performance of CK assays was initiated around the clock so that results were available in the morning. Although an extra day in the coronary unit did not produce a significant adverse effect on the patient, it did cost $595.97.

Another example of the "right strategy/too long to execute" is failure to perform chest radiography within 1 hour of arrival and sputum culture evaluation within 2 hours of arrival on patients with pneumonia admitted to the hospital.[81]

Monitoring Digoxin Therapy

This is an example of a monitoring strategy that is inappropriate. In 1991, OSUMC chemistry technologists noticed that there were frequent measurements of serum digoxin levels in patients with results of 0 ng/mL. When the medical staff was questioned about ordering digoxin levels on patients with 0 serum digoxin values, it was learned that these patients were on standing orders that usually required digitalization but for a number of reasons certain patients were excepted. However, the orders for serum digoxin levels, which were also included in the standing orders, were not canceled. When notified of the situation, the medical staff gladly canceled the orders. Since then, each serum level of digoxin or another drug of 0 initiates a telephone call to the medical staff. See Figure 9 for the results of this effort. In addition, this incorrect strategy caused unnecessary phlebotomies, which may potentially have serious adverse effects.[82] Moreover, each phlebotomy cost $3.50 and each digoxin test cost $3.82. A careful analysis of standing orders can be useful in identifying inappropriate testing strategies.

Reversing Heparin Therapy

This is an example of an inappropriate therapy and testing strategy that has the potential for adverse effects for the patient as well as increased costs. Instances were discovered of attempts to reverse heparin therapy with fresh frozen plasma instead of protamine. This inappropriate therapy can have several poor outcomes. First, fresh frozen plasma is not effective. Second, fresh frozen plasma can transmit disease (e.g., hepatitis C), cause allergic reactions, and produce a possible volume overload. Moreover, whereas the cost of protamine is $0.68 a dose (the correct therapy), the cost of 2 units of fresh frozen plasma is $101.20. Finally, this ineffective therapy causes unnecessary phlebotomies with potential adverse effects and costs as well as unnecessary prothrombin time measurements at a cost of $3.13 each.[82]

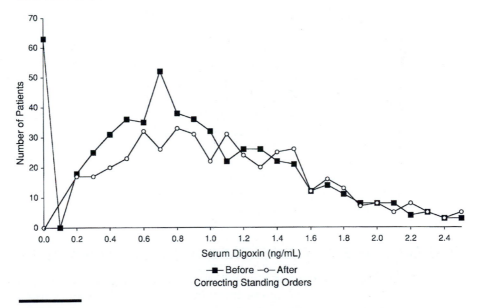

FIGURE 9.

Results of an appropriate digoxin testing quality assurance monitor. Comparison periods equal two weeks each.

MEDICAL DECISIONS IN THE AMBULATORY CARE (OUTPATIENT) SETTING

Inappropriate testing for ambulatory patients can cause poor outcomes and excessive costs. Consider an adult patient with acute pharyngitis. In this situation, the clinician attempts from the history and physical examination to determine whether the patient needs antibiotic treatment.[4, 83]

In the presence of four key clinical findings—pharyngeal exudate, cervical lymphadenopathy, lack of cough, and temperature over 100°C—the probability of the sore throat being due to streptococcal infection is more than 40%. In this case, a decision to treat can be made on clinical criteria alone. A throat culture will add little since it can have a false-negative rate of 10% to 24%.[84] Because of false negatives, performance of a throat culture can cause patients with streptococcal pharyngitis to not be treated with potential for a bad outcome. Moreover, a throat culture costs $5.96. A related error would be to use a rapid streptococcal test, which is even less sensitive than a throat culture and costs $16.52.

In the reverse situation—a patient with a sore throat who has no fever, no exudate, no swollen lymph nodes, and a cough—the likelihood of streptococcal infection is less than 3%. In this instance, a throat culture may identify false positives (carriers), who may be treated unnecessarily with the possibility of an allergic reaction. Increased costs include a throat culture and unnecessary antibiotic therapy.

It is only when some of these four key clinical findings are positive and some are negative that a throat culture is appropriate. In this instance, according to Bayes' rule, a throat culture can improve the medical decision to use antibiotic therapy and avoid allergic reactions.

MEDICAL DECISIONS IN THE CLINICAL LABORATORY SETTING

Not only physicians practicing clinical medicine but also physicians (pathologists) practicing laboratory medicine need to study their test-dependent medical decisions concerning outcomes and costs. There are many settings for medical decisions arising in the clinical laboratory that require the right testing strategies (Table 5).

Consider two examples—one in anatomic pathology (surgical pathology) and one in clinical pathology (hematology/immunology)—that require appropriate testing strategies. The first involves sampling the correct amount of tissue in radical prostatectomy specimens.[85, 86] The second involves the laboratory diagnosis of lupus erythematosus where the lupus erythematosus cell test, an obsolete test, is inappropriate—when more definitive immunologic tests are available.[87]

CHANGING THE WAY PHYSICIANS USE LABORATORY TESTS

It is difficult to change physicians' behavior. Efforts to combat laboratory overuse have included education in appropriate laboratory use, feedback concerning utilization and charge data to the clinician, administrative changes including display of guidelines and redesign of request forms, physician participation in limiting strategies, and penalties and rewards.[14] Although each method has shown some success on its own, in-

---
TABLE 5.
Clinical Laboratory Settings
in Which Medical Decisions
Arise

Anatomic Pathology
  Autopsy service
  Cytology
  Surgical pathology
Clinical Pathology
  Clinical chemistry
  Hematology
  Immunology
  Microbiology
  Transfusion service

---

terventions that rely on more than one method appear to be the most successful.[88]

DECISION-ORIENTED LABORATORY TESTING

The use of decision-oriented laboratory testing represents an effective way to encourage physicians to use the right tests and eliminate unnecessary ones. Historically, efforts to modify physicians' behavior by various techniques, including education, have not been very successful.[14] Interestingly, when house officers were reminded about the charges for tests, they ordered 14% fewer tests—apparently, without adverse effects on patient outcomes.[89]

In a recent study it was possible to decrease inappropriate serum triiodothyronine (T_3) testing by 38% and thyrotropin (thyroid-stimulating hormone [TSH]) testing by 61% through an educational program plus implementation of a medical decision-oriented test request form for hyperthyroidism and hypothyroidism in place of a menu of individual thyroid tests (Fig 10). This new form accomplished the reduction by eliminating inappropriate testing. Moreover, the physicians were ensured of obtaining the correct tests for the diagnosis they had in mind. A similar effort to improve the use of serum CK and lactate dehydrogenase isoenzyme tests for the diagnosis of AMI failed when the educational program was conducted but the medical decision-oriented test request form was omitted.[90] New test request forms were also useful in reducing unnecessary ordering of tumor marker tests.[91]

In another study, clerical and laboratory staff improved the appropriateness of physicians' requests for thyroid function tests—apparently because computer terminal operators had access to help screens and technologists had some knowledge of appropriate test strategy.[92]

The development of a medical decision-oriented testing program not only benefits discrete medical choices but also enhances serially linked, test-dependent medical decisions. Some test-dependent medical decisions are not performed independently of one another but are linked in

	T_3 uptake
	T_4 (RIA)
	T_3 (RIA)
A	TSH

❑	Thyroid function screen (T_4 [RIA], T_3 uptake, plus index)
❑	Hyperthyroid panel (T_4 [RIA], T_3 uptake, plus indexes)
❑	Hypothyroid panel (T_4 [RIA], T_3 uptake, TSH, plus index
❑	Other thyroid tests
B	Specify

FIGURE 10.

A, thyroid function tests as listed on the previous comprehensive laboratory test request form. **B,** problem-oriented format for thyroid function tests on the new request form. T_3 = triiodothyronne; T_4 = thyroxine; *RIA* = radioimmunoassay; *TSH* = thyrotropin. (From Wong ET, McCarron MM, Shaw ST Jr: *JAMA* 249:3076–3080, 1983. Used by permission.)

the context of an algorithm (for instance, maternal serum α-fetoprotein [MsAFP] testing, wherein one decision is linked to the results of a previous decision [Fig 11]). In 1985 at OSUMC, laboratory and clinical specialists collaborated to develop a decision-oriented MsAFP program. Following a communitywide educational effort conducted by the departments of obstetrics and pathology, physicians became aware of the OSU MsAFP testing program and began using it. Like the testing strategy for thyroid dysfunction discussed earlier, an educational program was conducted and a medical decision-oriented test request/report system was implemented. Physicians appreciate the program because OSUMC maintains a readily accessible database that can be used for outcome studies. Test results are communicated in the context of a medical decision-oriented test request/report system. Every report includes not only the test result but also an interpretation of the meaning of the test result, as well as a "prompt"—to direct the physician about what to do next.[19]

By analogy, other serially linked, test-dependent medical decisions can benefit by the development of similar testing programs. For example, implementation of the National Cholesterol Education Program Expert Panel's recommendations could be expedited by a cholesterol testing program that would educate the physicians, implement a medical decision-oriented request/report system, maintain the database, ensure quality, and "prompt" the physician about what to do next.[59, 60]

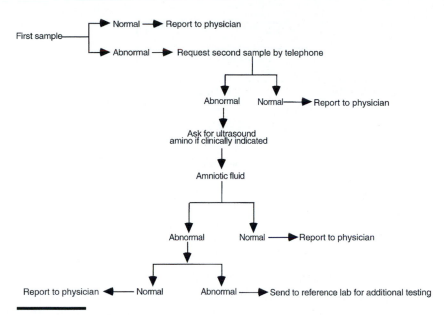

FIGURE 11.

Algorithm for maternal serum α-fetoprotein testing. (From Speicher CE: *Clin Lab Med* 11:255–265, 1991. Used by permission.)

CARE PLANS, CLINICAL PATHWAYS, AND PATIENT CARE MANAGEMENT

A new vocabulary has emerged to describe management of the patient care process. *Care plans* represent a way to map each step in the process so as to ensure that it occurs at the right time and in the right way. *Care plan managers* are individuals charged with seeing that the care plan is carried out.[93] At OSUMC, care plan managers are called *patient care resource managers*.

Patient care resource managers have two levels of expertise: level 1 managers are mainly administrators, whereas level 2 managers, in addition to functioning as administrators, are credentialed to perform a number of medical procedures. Patient care resource managers at OSUMC are paid jointly by the hospital and physicians. They report to the medical staff and are assigned to a particular service, i.e., cardiovascular surgery, nephrology, neurosurgery, and pulmonary. They have been well received by everyone, especially patients, and have effected significant improvements in outcomes, including decreased length of stay and increased patient satisfaction.

Care plans are composed of pathways that are called clinical pathways or critical pathways (Fig 12).[94] One can analyze a care plan and isolate the component test-dependent medical decisions. Practice parameters can be used to benchmark these decisions and conduct outcome studies. Pathologists should actively participate in the development and improvement of care plans and test-dependent clinical pathways as one way of ensuring appropriate laboratory utilization. This activity will enhance physicians' laboratory-ordering practices in the context of total quality improvement.[95, 96]

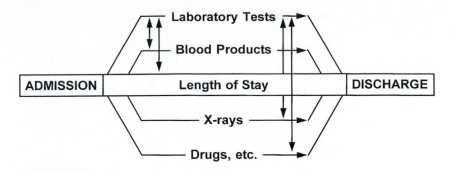

FIGURE 12.

Care plan showing clinical pathways and interrelationships for laboratory tests, blood products, patient length of stay, radiographs, drugs, etc. Effective and cost-efficient clinical pathways are important not only in themselves but also in their effects on other clinical pathways, especially the length of patient stay.

CLINICAL PROTOCOL SOFTWARE

In the future, physicians will use computer workstations to validate their diagnostic testing, affirm optimum treatments, and reduce the use of expensive and ineffective procedures.[97] One cannot possibly remember all the guidelines—computer-based prompts are essential. At OSUMC we have chosen the Kurzweil AI (Waltham, Mass) workstation to accomplish surgical pathology reports and intend to explore the use of this device for autopsy reports and clinical pathology consultations. These physician workstations will contain guidelines to help pathologists execute appropriate laboratory medicine testing strategies.

Clinical protocol software is currently under development to assist physicians in their diagnostic, monitoring, and cost-saving efforts. Several software packages are now available: Quality First, developed by Health Risk Management, Inc., of Minneapolis; Help, offered by Minnesota Mining and Manufacturing Co., Minneapolis; and protocol guidance systems by Value Health Sciences of Santa Monica, Calif, and GMIS, Inc., of Malvern, Pa.[98] Strong evidence suggests that computer-based medical decision support systems can improve physician performance. Additional well-designed studies are needed to assess their effects and cost-effectiveness, especially on patient outcomes.[99]

MANAGED CARE, CAPITATION, AND LABORATORY TESTS

Managed care and capitation significantly affect the production and utilization of laboratory tests because they change the clinical laboratory from a profit center to a cost center. This causes decentralization and regionalization of testing with migration of test production to low-cost, high-volume test providers. This migration will continue unless rapid turnaround times or other considerations force exceptions.[100–104]

EFFECTS ON PRODUCTION AND UTILIZATION OF LABORATORY TESTS

Realignment of testing sites based on costs and turnaround times will affect laboratory test utilization. In a recent OSUMC experience, an insurer decided to contract ambulatory care (outpatient) testing to another laboratory than the OSUMC laboratory. This caused a number of problems:

1. Some patients (e.g., oncology patients receiving chemotherapy) have their laboratory tests performed shortly before seeing their physician. This is not easily accomplished in a system where the laboratory is not on site in the same location as the physician's office.
2. Other patients with routine laboratory test turnaround time requirements may be required to travel to a site for phlebotomy that is different from the location of their physicians' offices.
3. Special tests performed in different laboratories may have different reference ranges and decision levels. This seriously interferes with physicians' ability to follow trends in certain test results such as serum tumor markers and hormone levels. Not all laboratory tests are created equal.[105]
4. Another difficulty is that the results of tests performed in outside laboratories may be less easily integrated into a single laboratory database.[106]

The complexity of dealing with multiple third-party payers that specify different laboratories can be significant, especially when one considers that the OSUMC currently works with more than 45 different health care plans.

PATHOLOGISTS AS "GATEKEEPERS" OF THE CLINICAL LABORATORY

Pathologists should function as "gatekeepers" of the clinical laboratory. In addition to striving for high-quality, low-cost test production in their laboratories, they are in an excellent position to take a leadership role in the development of appropriate testing. A simple formulation of recommendations for laboratory testing will not suffice. A dynamic program for practice parameters with strong pathologist involvement has potential for success. It could be as valuable in validating the pathologist's role in clinical pathology as the tissue committee was for surgical pathology.[55]

Practice parameters have important implications for reimbursement. In this regard, it is well to consider the statement made by the Physician Payment Review Commission in its 1990 report to Congress that will largely determine how increases in expenditures for physicians' services paid under Medicare are to be determined. "The medical profession must take the leading role in changing the way the physicians and patients think about using medical resources. The perceived obligation for physicians to provide and for patients to receive every service that has some marginal value regardless of cost must change." By becoming proactive in the development and use of practice parameters, pathologists can be the beneficiaries of change, not the victims.[55]

Pathologists can provide leadership for appropriate laboratory utilization in a number of ways:

1. Function as clinical consultants on the choice and interpretation of laboratory tests. Standing orders should be reviewed. Pathologists should be available for consultation by telephone and have a site in the laboratory where clinicians can see them and discuss patient care

decisions as well as review laboratory test materials, e.g., Wright-stained blood smears, Gram stains, etc.

2. Work with clinical colleagues in the process of adapting national practice parameters to local versions based on local expertise and resources.

3. Be available to analyze the test-dependent medical decision of various care plans through an analysis of outcomes.

4. Evaluate new technology before introduction for patient care, including systematic evaluation of technical validity, diagnostic value, and clinical usefulness.

5. Function as health care professionals responsible for the processing, storage, and transmission of information, as well as for its generation.

Decentralization and regionalization of testing sites create a need for an integrated laboratory database that can be used to provide a regional value-added laboratory information system. Independent laboratories and tertiary care hospitals are the most likely candidates to create these value-added systems. This information will prove valuable not only to physicians but also to administrators.[106, 107]

Through these contributions, pathologists will ensure themselves a "seat at the table" when important medical and business decisions are being made.

CONCLUSION

Driven by a mandate to contain escalating health care costs, a wave of managed care and capitation is inexorably moving across the United States. Low-cost laboratory test production and appropriate test utilization are the "order of the day." A medical decision-making approach to test utilization is a promising approach. In this milieu pathologists have an opportunity to provide leadership in the development, implementation, and evaluation of practice parameters. Through outcome studies in the context of total quality improvement, better, more cost-efficient guidelines can be constructed. Finally, pathologists should spearhead the development of an integrated laboratory database that can be used to provide patient care information to physicians and management data to health care administrators. As the clinical laboratory is completing this transition from technical to managerial leadership, the stage is set for pathologists to function as medical consultants and managers to implement the skills and tools of total quality management.[108]

ACKNOWLEDGMENT

Special thanks are extended to Donald A. Senhauser, M.D., and Mary Grose for their critical reading of the manuscript and to Chris Anderson for her meticulous attention to committing these concepts to paper.

REFERENCES

1. Pear R: Cost is obscured in health debate. *New York Times*, p 1, Aug 7, 1994.
2. Shaw ST Jr, Miller JM: Cost containment and the use of reference laboratories. *Clin Lab Med* 5:725–752, 1985.

3. *Capitation I: The New American Medicine.* Washington, DC, The Advisory Board Company, The Governance Committee, 1994.
4. Speicher CE: *The Right Test: A Physician's Guide to Laboratory Medicine,* ed 2. Philadelphia, WB Saunders, 1993.
5. Tenery RM Jr: Should doctors treat patients like we make cars? *Am Med News,* p 20, Oct 10, 1994.
6. Anders G: Required surgery: Health plans force even elite hospitals to cut costs sharply. *Wall Street Journal,* p A1, March 8, 1994.
7. Portugal B: Benchmarking hospital laboratory financial and operational performance. Technology series—Special Report. *Am Hosp Assoc* 12:1–21, 1993.
8. Winkelman JW, Hill RB: Clinical laboratory responses to reduced funding. *JAMA* 252:2435–2440, 1984.
9. Speicher CE, Smith JW: *Choosing Effective Laboratory Tests.* Philadelphia, WB Saunders, 1983.
10. Lundberg GD (ed): *Using the Clinical Laboratory in Medical Decision-Making.* Chicago, American Society of Clinical Pathologists, 1983.
11. Speicher CE: So duplicate chemistry profiles correlate with multiple physicians: Let's not blame the doctors! *Arch Pathol Lab Med* 112:235–236, 1988.
12. Wertman BG, Sostrin SV, Pavlova Z, et al: Why do physicians order laboratory tests? A study of laboratory test request and use patterns. *JAMA* 243:2080–2082, 1980.
13. Moser R: No more "battered" patients: Blue Cross urges curb on hospital tests. *Time,* p 80, Feb 19, 1979.
14. Burke DM: Clinical decision making and laboratory use, in Fenoglio-Preiser C, Weinstein RS (eds): *Advances in Pathology,* vol 3. St Louis, Mosby, 1990, pp 207–231.
15. Speicher CE, Smith JW: Helping physicians use laboratory tests. *Clin Lab Med* 5:653–663, 1985.
16. Murphy J, Henry JB: Effective utilization of clinical laboratories. *Hum Pathol* 9:625–633, 1978.
17. Brecher G: Laboratory medicine 1953–1978 and the next ten years. *Hum Pathol* 9:615–618, 1978.
18. Burke MD: Clinical decision-making: The role of the laboratory, in Benson ES, Rubin M (eds): *Logic and Economics of Clinical Laboratory Use.* New York, Elsevier, 1978, pp 59–64.
19. Speicher CE: Decision-oriented test request forms: A system for implementing practice parameters in laboratory medicine. *Clin Lab Med* 11:255–265, 1991.
20. Puleo PR, Meyer D, Wathen C, et al: Use of a rapid assay of subforms of creatine kinase MB to diagnose or rule out acute myocardial infarction. *N Engl J Med* 331:561–566, 1994.
21. Lee TH, Goldman L: Serum enzyme assays in the diagnosis of acute myocardial infarction: Recommendations based on a quantitative analysis, in Sox HC Jr (ed): *Common Diagnostic Tests: Use and Interpretation,* ed 2. Philadelphia, American College of Physicians, 1990, pp 35–66.
22. Galen RS, Gambino RS: *Beyond Normality: The Predictive Value and Efficiency of Medical Diagnoses.* New York, John Wiley & Sons, 1975.
23. Sox HC Jr, Blatt MA, Higgins MC, et al (eds): *Medical Decision Making.* Boston, Butterworth, 1988.
24. Weinstein MC, Fineberg HV (eds): *Clinical Decision Analysis.* Philadelphia, WB Saunders, 1980.
25. Lundberg GD: Acting on significant laboratory results. *JAMA* 245:1762–1763, 1981.

26. Nosanchuk JS, Salvatore JD: Improved pneumatic tube system shortens stat turnaround time. *Lab Med* 8:21–25, 1977.
27. Handorf CR (ed): Alternate-site laboratory testing. *Clin Lab Med* 14:451–645, 1994.
28. Kiechle FL, Ingram-Main R: Bedside testing: Beyond glucose. *MLO* 25:65–68, 1993.
29. Travers EM, Wolke JC, Johnson R, et al: Changing the way lab medicine is practiced at the point of care. *MLO* 26:33–40, 1994.
30. Lundberg GD (ed): *Managing the Patient-Focused Laboratory.* Oradell, NJ, Medical Economics, 1975.
31. Kost GJ: Using critical limits to improve patient outcome. *MLO* 25:22–27, 1993.
32. Svirbely JR, Speicher CE: The importance of request and report forms in the interpretation of therapeutic drug monitoring data. *Ther Drug Monit* 2:211–216, 1980.
33. Grannis GF, Grümer H-D, Lott JA, et al: Proficiency evaluation of clinical chemistry laboratories. *Clin Chem* 18:222–236, 1972.
34. Kelley CR, Mamlin JJ: Ambulatory medical care quality: Determination by diagnostic outcome. *JAMA* 227:1155–1157, 1974.
35. Schneiderman LJ, DeSalvo L, Baylor S, et al: The "abnormal" screening laboratory results. *Arch Intern Med* 129:88–90, 1972.
36. Wheeler LA, Brecher G, Sheiner LB: Clinical laboratory use in the evaluation of anemia. *JAMA* 238:2709–2714, 1977.
37. Wigton RS, Zimmer JL, Wigton JH, et al: Chart reminders in the diagnosis of anemia. *JAMA* 245:1745–1747, 1981.
38. Williamson JW, Alexander M, Miller GE: Continuing education and patient care research. *JAMA* 201:938–942, 1967.
39. Kreisberg RA: Clinical problem solving: Stopping short of certainty. *N Engl J Med* 331:42–45, 1994.
40. Gambino SR: Poor clinical problem-solving: Failure to heed a critical test result. *Lab Rep Physicians* 16:69–70, 1994.
41. Barnett RN: *Clinical Laboratory Statistics,* ed 2. Boston, Little, Brown, 1979.
42. Copeland BE, Hoyt LH: Clinical chemistry, in Jones RJ, Palulonis RM (eds): *Laboratory Tests in Medical Practice.* Chicago, American Medical Association, 1980, pp 77–94.
43. Gambino SR: Laboratory services for intensive care units, in Kinney JM, Bendixen HH, Powers Jr SR (eds): *Manual of Surgical Intensive Care.* Philadelphia, WB Saunders, 1977, pp 143–149.
44. Jahn M: Turnaround time down sharply, yet clients want results faster. *MLO* 25:24–30, 1993.
45. Schiller L, Tiffany D: Reducing turnaround time for ABGs in the ICCU. *MLO* 26:43–45, 1994.
46. Fallon KD: Monitoring of metabolism, acid-base balance, and relevant laboratory considerations, in Shoemaker WC, Thompson WL (eds): *Critical Care, State of the Art,* vol 2. Fullerton, Calif, Society of Critical Care Medicine, 1981.
47. Gabel JC: Monitoring of body chemistry during anesthesia, in Saidman LJ, Smith NT (eds): *Monitoring in Anesthesia.* New York, John Wiley & Sons, 1978, pp 15–29.
48. Woo J, Treuting JJ, Cannon DC: Creatine and creatinine, in Henry JB (ed): *Clinical Diagnosis and Management by Laboratory Methods,* ed 16. Philadelphia, WB Saunders, 1979, pp 262–264.
49. Emmett M, Narins RG: Clinical use of the anion gap. *Medicine* 56:38–54, 1977.

50. Statland BE: *Clinical Decision Levels for Lab Tests.* Oradell, NJ, Medical Economics, 1983.
51. Speicher CE, Smith JW: Interpretive reporting in clinical pathology. *JAMA* 243:1556–1560, 1980.
52. Speicher CE, Smith JW: Interpretive reporting. *Clin Lab Med* 4:41–60, 1984.
53. Lundberg GD: Laboratory request forms (menus) that guide and teach. *JAMA* 249:3075, 1983.
54. Gambino R: The American College of Physicians and Blue Cross/Blue Shield guidelines. *Lab Rep Physicians* 10:44–48, 1988.
55. Speicher CE: Practice parameters: An opportunity for pathologists to take a leadership role in patient care. *Arch Pathol Lab Med* 114:823–824, 1990.
56. Woolf SH: Practice guidelines: A new reality in medicine. *Arch Intern Med* 153:2646–2655, 1993.
57. Grimshaw JM, Russell IT: Effect of clinical guidelines on medical practice: A systematic review of rigorous evaluations. *Lancet* 342:1317–1322, 1993.
58. McDonald CJ, Overhage JM: Guidelines you can follow and can trust: An ideal and an example. *JAMA* 271:872–873, 1994.
59. Expert Panel: Report of the National Cholesterol Education Program Expert Panel on detection, evaluation, and treatment of high blood cholesterol in adults. *Arch Intern Med* 148:36–69, 1988.
60. National Cholesterol Education Program: Detection, evaluation, and treatment of high blood cholesterol in adults (adult treatment panel II). *Circulation* 89:1329–1445, 1994.
61. Eddy DM (ed): *Common Screening Tests.* Philadelphia, American College of Physicians, 1991.
62. Sox HC Jr (ed): *Common Diagnostic Tests: Use and Interpretation,* ed 2. Philadelphia, American College of Physicians, 1990.
63. Panzer RJ, Black ER, Griner PF (eds): *Diagnostic Strategies for Common Medical Problems.* Philadelphia, American College of Physicians, 1991.
64. *Directory of Practice Parameters,* 1993 ed. Chicago, American Medical Association, 1993.
65. *Directory of Practice Parameters,* 1994 ed. Chicago, American Medical Association, 1994.
66. Phelps CE: The methodologic foundations of studies of the appropriateness of medical care. *N Engl J Med* 329:1241–1245, 1993.
67. Hyams AL, Brandenburg JA, Lipsitz SR, et al: Practice guidelines and malpractice litigation: A two-way street. *Ann Intern Med* 122:450–455, 1995.
68. Hayward RSA, Steinberg EP, Ford DE, et al: Preventive care guidelines: 1991. *Ann Intern Med* 114:758–783, 1991.
69. Czaja R, McFall SL, Warnecke RB, et al: Preferences of community physicians for cancer screening guidelines. *Ann Intern Med* 120:602–608, 1994.
70. Ohio State Faculty: Wellness screening and case finding, in *The Ohio State University Health Plan Clinical Notes,* vol 2, no 1. Columbus, Ohio State University, 1992.
71. Temple PC, DeCola D: Practice guidelines: Do they work? *Managed Care Medicine,* pp 27–30, May/June, 1994.
72. Ohio State Faculty: Diabetes mellitus, in *The Ohio State University Health Plan Clinical Notes,* vol 1, no 3. Columbus, Ohio State University, 1991.
73. Check WA: Changing how clinicians use the lab. *CAP Today,* 7:1, 1993.
74. Chodak GW: Screening for prostate cancer: The debate continues. *JAMA* 272:813–814, 1994.
75. Krahn MD, Mahoney JE, Eckman MH, et al: Screening for prostate cancer: A decision analytic view. *JAMA* 272:773–780, 1994.

76. Kolata G: Prostate cancer tests questioned. *New York Times*, p B7, June 23, 1993.
77. Wilson JD, Braunwald E, Isselbacher KJ, et al (eds): *Harrison's Principles of Internal Medicine*, ed 12. New York, McGraw-Hill, 1991.
78. Hamm CW: New serum markers for acute myocardial infarction. *N Engl J Med* 331:607–608, 1994.
79. Brook RH: Quality of care: Do we care? *Ann Intern Med* 115:486–490, 1991.
80. *A Guide to Establishing Programs for Assessing Outcomes in Clinical Settings*. Oakbrook Terrace, Ill, Joint Commission on Accreditation of Healthcare Organizations, 1994.
81. Southwick K: Labs step in to help map care. *CAP Today*, 8:1, 1994.
82. Dale JC, Pruett SK: Phlebotomy: A minimalist approach. *Mayo Clin Proc* 68:249–255, 1993.
83. Komaroff AL: Sore throat in adult patients, in Panzer RJ, Black ER, Griner PF (eds): *Diagnostic Strategies for Common Medical Problems*. Philadelphia, American College of Physicians, 1991, pp 186–195.
84. Centor RM, Meier FA, Dalton HP: Throat cultures and rapid tests for diagnosis of group A streptococcal pharyngitis in adults, in Sox HC Jr (ed): *Common Diagnostic Tests: Use and Interpretation*, ed 2. Philadelphia, American College of Physicians, 1990, pp 245–264.
85. Humphrey PA: Tissue sampling in the era of cost constraints. *Am J Clin Pathol* 101:247–248, 1994.
86. Cohen MB, Soloway MS, Murphy WM: Sampling of radical prostatectomy specimens: How much is adequate? *Am J Clin Pathol* 101:250–252, 1994.
87. Conn RB: Practice parameter—the lupus erythematosus cell test: An obsolete test now superseded by definitive immunologic tests. *Am J Clin Pathol* 101:65–66, 1994.
88. Greco PJ, Eisenberg JM: Changing physicians' practices. *N Engl J Med* 329:1271–1274, 1993.
89. Tierney WM, Miller ME: Physician inpatient order writing on microcomputer workstations. *JAMA* 269:379–383, 1993.
90. Wong ET, McCarron MM, Shaw ST Jr: Ordering of laboratory tests in a teaching hospital: Can it be improved? *JAMA* 249:3076–3080, 1983.
91. Durand-Zaleski I, Rymer JC, Roudot-Thoraval F, et al: Reducing unnecessary laboratory use with new test request form: Example of tumor markers. *Lancet* 342:150–153, 1993.
92. Finn Jr AF, Valenstein PN, Burke MD: Alteration of physicians' orders by non-physicians. *JAMA* 2549–2552, 1988.
93. Wilkinson DS: Clinical pathology: Practice, consultation, and management issues, in Weinstein RS, Graham AR (eds): *Advances in Pathology and Laboratory Medicine*, vol 6. St Louis, Mosby, 1993, pp 3–18.
94. Hart R, Musfeldt C: MD-directed critical pathways: It's time. *Hospital* 66:56, 1992.
95. Nardella A, Farrell M, Pechet L, et al: Continuous improvement, quality control, and cost containment in clinical laboratory testing. *Arch Pathol Lab Med* 118:965–968, 1994.
96. Blumenthal D: Total quality management and physicians' clinical decisions. *JAMA* 269:2775–2778, 1993.
97. Smith JW, Speicher CE: Computer workstations for pathologists. *Med Electronics*, pp 90–97, June 1985.
98. Mehler M: How hospitals are using software to guide patient care, trim costs. *Investor's Business Daily*, p 4, April 6, 1994.
99. Johnston ME, Langton KB, Haynes B, et al: Effects of computer-based clini-

cal decision support systems on clinician performance and patient outcome. *Ann Intern Med* 120:135–142, 1994.

100. Steiner JW, Root JM, Buck E: The regionalization of laboratory services. *MLO* 26:22–29, 1994.
101. Check W: Going the way of fewer, larger labs. *CAP Today* 8:1, 1994.
102. Barros A: Preparing for the lab of the 21st century. *MLO* 25:22–25, 1993.
103. Bucher WF, Brown JW: The impact of health care reform on the clinical lab. *MLO* 26:30–35, 1994.
104. Fattal GA, Frost Y, Winkelman JW: Operational and financial outcomes of shared laboratory services in a consolidated hospital system. *JAMA* 253:2076–2079, 1985.
105. Speicher CE: All laboratory tests are not created equal. *Arch Pathol Lab Med* 109:709–710, 1985.
106. Friedman BA, Mitchell W: Integrating information from decentralized laboratory testing sites: The creation of a value-added network. *Am J Clin Pathol* 99:637–642, 1993.
107. Friedman BA, Mitchell W: Horizontal and vertical integration in hospital laboratories and the laboratory information system. *Clin Lab Med* 10:627–641, 1990.
108. Elevitch FR: The fourth dimension: Management of the postmodern clinical laboratory. *Clin Lab Med* 12:849–859, 1992.

Benchmarking Laboratory Performance: Planning for the Future of Hospital Laboratory Services

Barry Portugal, M.B.A.

President, Health Care Development Services, Inc., Northbrook, Illinois

As the face of health care delivery systems began to significantly change in the late 1980s, hospital executives and laboratory directors sought new sources of information in order to plan how to decrease costs associated with operating hospital laboratories without having a negative impact on the quality of patient care. In the early 1980s, hospital administrators and laboratory directors had relied on the American Hospital Association Monitrends Program and the College of American Pathologists' (CAP) Workload Recording Program as sources of comparative information to evaluate financial performance and employee productivity.

Since both programs were limited in detail, each was terminated in the early 1990s. Other hospital laboratory benchmarking programs now provide hospital administrators and laboratory medical and administrative directors with comparative information by which to evaluate hospital laboratory operations. These programs include the LabTrends Hospital Laboratory Comparative Program, the CAP Laboratory Management Index Program, the Mecon Comparative Program, and a program sponsored by the Voluntary Hospitals of America (VHA). Information describing the extent of each program and their similarities/dissimilarities was presented at the 1994 annual meeting of the Clinical Laboratory Management Association (CLMA).[1]

The use of comparative information to benchmark operational and financial indicators as the basis for developing strategic plans for hospitals is acknowledged as an important part of the decision-making process. As Roger Kropf and James Greenberg noted in *Strategic Analysis for Hospital Management*, monitoring of internal and external data is a critical ingredient in the strategic planning process and "must be used to measure the attainment of strategic, managerial and operational objectives."[2]

Hospital-based laboratory medical directors today are faced with difficult choices on how to best deliver laboratory services. Together with hospital and laboratory administrative directors, pathologists must first

Advances in Pathology and Laboratory Medicine®, vol. 8
© 1995, Mosby–Year Book, Inc.

benchmark their laboratory operations in order to evaluate how they perform relative to other hospital laboratories with similar operating characteristics. They need to evaluate factors that have an impact on hospital laboratory financial performance, including test result turnaround time demands, employee productivity, medical staff utilization of laboratory tests, laboratory staff mix, and direct operating costs.[3]

HOSPITAL LABORATORY BENCHMARKING

The American Hospital Association acknowledged the importance of benchmarking financial and operational performance in its December 1993 Special Report.[4] In that report it was noted that there is a wide range of utilization rates for inpatient tests in hospitals with similar acuity levels. As shown in Table 1, the number of inpatient tests per discharge varies by almost 95% from hospital to hospital.

Although the inpatient case mix index for teaching hospitals is substantially higher than for nonteaching hospitals (1.241 vs. 0.973), patient acuity alone does not explain the substantial difference in the number of tests per discharge. Information presented in Table 2 indicates that inpatient laboratory utilization is markedly different in teaching hospitals and academic medical centers as compared with nonteaching hospitals. Inpatient test utilization is largely driven by the individual ordering the tests. In nonteaching hospitals, medical staff members order laboratory tests. In teaching hospitals and academic medical centers, medical residents are more likely to order laboratory tests. The process of training medical residents causes a greater number of laboratory tests to be ordered, notwithstanding the acuity of the inpatient population.

OUTCOMES MEASUREMENT STUDIES/TEST UTILIZATION

Many hospitals and health care systems are developing outcomes measurement studies in order to better evaluate how clinical laboratory tests affect inpatient length of stay and the diagnostic and therapeutic pro-

TABLE 1.

Case Mix Index Impact on the Average Length of Stay and Inpatient Tests per Discharge*

	ALOS† and Tests per Discharge					
	25th Quartile		Mean		75th Quartile	
Case Mix Index	ALOS	Tests/ Discharge	ALOS	Tests/ Discharge	ALOS	Tests/ Discharge
Less than 1.00	3.7	14.7	5.2	21.5	6.2	27.2
1.00–1.20	5.6	27.8	6.4	37.9	7.4	48.2
More than 1.20	5.9	29.8	6.5	43.7	7.6	58.1

*From Health Care Development Services, Inc., LabTrends Hospital Laboratory Comparative Program, Northbrook, Ill. Used by permission.
†ALOS = average length of stay.

TABLE 2.
Hospital Teaching Status and Laboratory Utilization*

Teaching Status	Inpatient Tests per Discharge		
	25th Quartile	Mean	75th Quartile
Nonteaching hospitals	15.5	18.4	20.2
Teaching hospitals and academic medical centers	24.0	33.5	43.3

*From Health Care Development Services, Inc., LabTrends Hospital Laboratory Comparative Program. Used by permission.

cesses. Since no one source of information is necessarily considered the "state of the art," many hospital-based laboratory medical directors are preparing their own studies to identify clinical pathways specific to their institutions. As Dr. Carl Speicher wrote in his book on laboratory test utilization, "It makes sense to organize the approach to laboratory testing in terms of a limited number of common and important clinical problems rather than an almost endless list of individual laboratory tests."[5] Dr. Speicher and others are contributing exceptional information that will help in making the decision-making model shown in Figure 1 a framework for laboratory testing.

TESTING PERSONNEL PRODUCTIVITY

Another important factor that should be considered in any benchmarking analysis is the effect that test result turnaround times have on em-

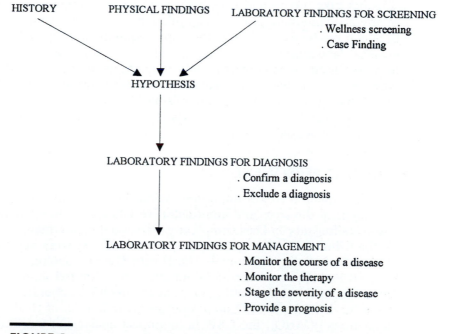

FIGURE 1.
A decision-making model that incorporates laboratory testing.

TABLE 3.
Testing Personnel Productivity and Turnaround Time
Demands*

Percentage of Testing Performed in Less Than 2 hr†	Tests per Testing FTE		
	25th Quartile	Mean	75th Quartile
40%–50%	6,521	8,108	9,772
51%–60%	6,872	8,625	10,155
More than 60%	7,955	9,737	10,129

*From Health Care Development Services, Inc., LabTrends Hospital Laboratory Comparative Program. Used by permission.
†Time that elapses from when a specimen arrives in the laboratory until the result is available to a nonlaboratorian.

ployee productivity. Historical perspectives should be re-examined, specifically the view that more testing, performed in shorter time frames, has a negative impact on productivity. Testing personnel productivity (shown in Table 3) reflects the impact that high-throughput, automated analyzers have had in hospital laboratory environments.

When greater proportions of hospital testing are performed in shorter time frames, testing personnel productivity increases. On the average, 20% more tests per testing full time equivalent (FTE) are performed when more than 60% of all testing results are provided within 2 hours of the time that the specimen arrives in the laboratory. Although that difference drops to only 4% at the database 75th quartile, it is clearly important to consider how turnaround time has an impact on employee productivity in any benchmarking process. The relationship of test result turnaround time and productivity reflects the scope of automation typically found in hospital laboratories. Many hospital laboratory directors and managers have replaced nonautomated and semiautomated testing instruments with automated "walkaway" equipment when requirements for fast test results have exceeded the laboratory's budget limits for additional labor. The result has been improved medical staff satisfaction, lowered labor costs, and increased productivity.

MIX OF TESTING PERSONNEL

Probably one of the most important aspects facing hospital-based laboratory medical directors and administrative laboratory directors is the issue of staffing mix and test complexity. Personnel requirements mandated by the Clinical Laboratory Improvement Act (CLIA) were hotly debated as they were being developed. The Health Care Financing Administration (HCFA) approved accreditation status to a limited number of state departments of public health, Commission on Office Laboratory Accreditation (COLA), the Joint Commission on Accreditation of Healthcare Organizations (JCAHO), and CAP. In its impact analysis of the CLIA rules, the American Hospital Association identified several issues that might seriously affect hospitals as a result of CLIA personnel standards.[6] Those issues included the following:

- Hospitals in which laboratory testing personnel do not have an associate's or higher degree or have not passed a Department of Health and Human Services (HHS; Health, Education and Welfare [HEW])-approved proficiency examination will be required to have a general supervisor *on site* whenever highly complex testing is performed until September 1, 1997. After that date, personnel performing high-complexity testing must have associate's degrees or have passed the HHS-approved proficiency examination. Since several blood banking procedures, including crossmatching and typing blood for transfusion, are now defined as highly complex, this provision could have a significantly negative impact on hospitals in which laboratory workers have modest educational credentials and/or have not been certified by passing HHS-approved program proficiency examinations.
- Some hospitals may have laboratory general supervisors who have not passed the HHS (HEW) proficiency examination or lack an associate's or higher degree in laboratory science or medical technology and 2 years of experience. To qualify as a general supervisor in a laboratory performing high-complexity testing, those individuals would have to return to college to earn at least an associate's degree. In the interim, the laboratory director or other qualified individuals would have to assume some general supervisor responsibilities.
- The proposed personnel requirement of a bachelor's degree plus 4 years' experience for a technical supervisor may force the temporary reclassification of individuals now in that position. Laboratory directors may also act as technical supervisors so that job responsibilities can be continued. Technical supervisors who do not currently have a bachelor's degree will have to return to college to earn the CLIA-mandated minimum educational requirement.
- Some hospitals may use blood gas test methodologies that fall in the highly complex category (four test systems have been categorized as highly complex). In these environments, only those respiratory therapists who have earned a bachelor's degree or pulmonary function personnel who have earned an associate's degree may perform highly complex blood gas testing.

More than 70% of all testing performed in hospital laboratories falls into the moderate-complexity category as defined by the HCFA,[7, 8] Although it is generally believed that the management of most hospital laboratories would not staff moderate-complexity testing positions proportionately to the number of moderate-complexity tests performed, many hospital laboratory directors are planning a gradual transition to moderate-complexity personnel into their organizations as attrition levels require the replacement of testing staff.

The financial impact of introducing moderate-complexity personnel into hospital laboratories has recently been studied.[8] Based on test volume and differences in salary per hour between high-complexity and moderate-complexity personnel, the study found that hospital laboratories might reduce direct labor costs (from $7,000 to $400,000 per year).

TABLE 4.
Laboratory Testing Personnel Annual Salary Differences According to Moderate-Complexity vs. High-Complexity Testing*

Billed Test Volume	Total Number of Testing FTEs	10% Moderate Complexity			20% Moderate Complexity			30% Moderate Complexity		
		FTEs	$2/hr Difference	$4/hr Difference	FTEs	$2/hr Difference	$4/hr Difference	FTEs	$2/hr Difference	$4/hr Difference
50,000– 250,000	16.5	1.7	$ 7,072	$ 14,144	3.3	$ 13,728	$ 27,456	5.0	$ 20,800	$ 41,600
250,000– 500,000	32.1	3.2	$13,312	$ 26,624	6.4	$ 26,624	$ 53,248	9.6	$ 39,936	$ 79,872
500,000– 750,000	46.6	4.7	$19,552	$ 39,104	9.3	$ 38,688	$ 77,376	14.0	$ 58,240	$116,480
750,000– 1,000,000	73.7	7.4	$30,784	$ 61,568	14.7	$ 61,152	$122,304	22.1	$ 91,936	$183,872
>1,000,000	158	15.8	$65,728	$131,456	31.5	$131,040	$262,080	47.3	$196,768	$393,536

*From Health Care Development Services, Inc. Used by permission.

TABLE 5.
Supply Costs per Test*

On-Site Performed Test vol/yr	Supply Cost per Test†		
	25th Quartile	Mean	75th Quartile
50,000–200,000	$2.79	$2.92	$3.28
200,001–400,000	$2.49	$2.90	$3.14
400,001–600,000	$2.46	$2.69	$2.92
More than 600,000	$2.16	$2.51	$2.94

*From Health Care Development Services, Inc., LabTrends Hospital Laboratory Comparative Program. Used by permission.
†Supply costs include phlebotomy, consumable testing, quality control/proficiency testing, office supplies, and noncapitalized equipment.

Given the significant pressures to reduce operating costs, hospital administrators are carefully reviewing how best to transition the laboratory workforce to include moderate complexity testing personnel. As presented in Table 4, transitions in staffing mix represent substantial opportunities to reduce labor costs.

SUPPLY COSTS ISSUES

When organizing benchmark analyses, it is also important to consider the supply cost per test. Since the supply cost per test represents about 15% to 22% of most hospital laboratories' direct costs,[4] evaluating instrument and manual methodology reagents, controls, and supplies is an integral component of any strategic planning process. As shown in Table 5, the supply cost per test can vary dramatically in hospital laboratories with a similar test volume and test mix.

Because the supply cost differs by about $0.60 per test on average—from the 25th quartile to the 75th quartile—a hospital laboratory whose costs are at the higher end of the scale might have significant opportuni-

TABLE 6.
Cost per Referred Test*

On-Site Performed Test vol/yr	Cost per Referred Test		
	25th Quartile	Mean	75th Quartile
50,000–200,000	$17.03	$22.36	$27.46
200,001–400,000	$25.71	$30.95	$35.39
400,001–600,000	$28.65	$36.30	$40.55
More than 600,000	$40.06	$47.69	$54.64

*From Health Care Development Services, Inc., LabTrends Hospital Laboratory Comparative Program. Used by permission.

TABLE 7.
Summary of Systematic Changes Due to Restructuring Within the Health Care System*

Observation	Forecast
Greater proportions of surgical procedures will be performed in outpatient settings. Many acute care beds will be replaced with subacute care beds.	Overall acute care hospital average length of stay will range from 3.0 to 4.0 days.
Benchmarks are being developed to measure patient outcomes based on the number and mix of tests per diagnosis-related grouping.	The number of inpatient tests per discharge will range between 15 and 20 with modest inpatient acuity levels and between 30 and 35 where more tertiary care is provided.
Large numbers of physician-hospital organizations, managed care plans, employer groups, and other constituencies will develop risk-sharing programs.	More than 80% of all inpatient and outpatient health care will be provided under some form of risk-sharing system.
Quality assurance plans that develop systems to monitor and track patient outcomes will become a significant part of administrative and medical director responsibilities.	Outcomes measurement will replace total quality management/continuing quality improvement as the major focus in hospitals and hospital laboratories.
The proliferation of managed care "exclusive" contracts for outpatient laboratory services will require extraordinary economies of scale in order to provide the competitive pricing found only in very large, highly automated laboratories.	A small number of commercial laboratories and hospital consortium-owned regional laboratories will control most of the outpatient and outreach markets.

Technology new to the United States (now in Japan) will automate a substantial portion of laboratory operational work flow from specimen accessioning to refrigerated storage.

Patient-focused model hospital delivery systems will incorporate emerging technology for use by caregivers to perform moderately complex testing at or near the patient's bedside.

Only urgent/stat testing will be performed in laboratories and near-patient sites located in hospitals.

More personnel with "moderate-complexity" testing training will work in laboratories. Medical technologists will take on new, expanded roles as managers of technology and of personnel who perform moderately complex tests.

Economics of physician-hospital organizations, managed care, etc., contracts will ultimately produce a "low-bidder" mentality. Care must be taken so that quality of care is not compromised.

There will be greater price competition for anatomic pathology services.

Hospital-based pathologist compensation arrangements will be based on the reimbursement received by the hospital.

Robotics and automated specimen-handling systems will reduce the hospital work force by 25% to 35% of current levels.

Point-of-care laboratory and other ancillary service testing will expand throughout hospitals.

On-site hospital laboratory test menus will include no more than 50 test names.

Personnel performing laboratory testing will more closely reflect a mix of moderately complex vs. highly complex testing.

Testing performed in physician office laboratories will be minimal. All other nonurgent testing will be referred to laboratories that control exclusive risk-sharing plans for outpatient laboratory services.

The majority of surgical pathology specimens will emanate from outpatients rather than inpatients.

Hospital-based pathologist administrative medical director compensation will be linked with capitation/reimbursement from integrated provider agreements.

*From Health Care Development Services, Inc. Used by permission.

ties for cost reduction. For example, a laboratory performing 500,000 tests per year and paying $2.90 per test for supplies could save approximately $105,000 per year if it were able to negotiate supply costs equivalent to the database mean of $2.69 per test.

REFERRED TESTING COSTS

Although expenses related to specimens referred to outside reference laboratories generally reflect only 1% to 4% of a hospital laboratory's operating costs,[4] it is important to evaluate the proportion of send-out tests and cost per send-out test. Table 6 shows that there is a strong relationship between on-site volume and the cost per referred test. Most likely this reflects the mix and type of tests referred out by different laboratories.

Usually, hospital laboratories with higher volume perform greater proportions of esoteric testing on site. Therefore tests that are sent out are most likely low-volume/high-cost tests. Laboratories with lower test volume tend to send out what larger-volume laboratories might consider "routine" tests, as well as esoteric tests to outside reference laboratories. As a result, their cost per referred test is much lower.

THE FUTURE OF HOSPITAL LABORATORIES

Many factors are expected to drastically influence how and where hospital laboratory testing is performed in the future and who will be responsible for delivering laboratory services in environments where much of the health care is provided under one form or another of managed care. Most health care industry analysts agree that restructuring the health care delivery system will result in systemwide changes in the hospital laboratory delivery system and other hospital-based ancillary services.[9] Although any crystal ball is no less cloudy than the next, the projected changes listed in Table 7 represent part of the analysis of the future of hospital laboratories.

WHERE WILL TESTING BE PERFORMED?

One of the significant changes that may occur is the *place* where laboratory testing is performed. In 1994, it was estimated that approximately 45% of all laboratory testing was performed in hospitals[9] (Fig 2). By 1997, the hospital-based proportion of testing might be as low as 35% or may increase to 60%, depending on the factors identified in Figures 3 to 5.[9]

STRATEGIC RESPONSES

In response to the critical nature of these important issues, hospital administrators, laboratory medical directors, and laboratory administrative directors are developing strategic responses to the challenges facing them. As part of their strategies, they are implementing significant changes in how and where laboratory services are delivered as part of their overall

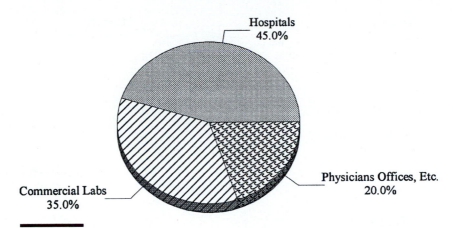

FIGURE 2.

Estimated test volume by site (1994). (Courtesy of Health Care Development Services, Inc., Northbrook, Ill.)

strategy to lower operating costs. Many of the re-engineering processes being implemented follow Hammer and Champy's notion of *discontinuous thinking*—identifying and abandoning the outdated rules and fundamental assumptions that underlie current laboratory operations.[12] They recognize that the old rules based on assumptions about technology, people, and organizational goals no longer hold. As the authors of *Re-engineering the Corporation* observe, unless companies change old rules, "any superficial reorganizations they perform will be no more effective than dusting the furniture in Pompeii."[10]

RE-ENGINEERING INTERNAL OPERATIONS

Since labor usually represents about half of a hospital laboratory's expenses, many re-engineering activities focus on improving work flow; how specimens are collected, accessioned, and tested; and how results are reported. For example, one of the growing trends in the hospital labo-

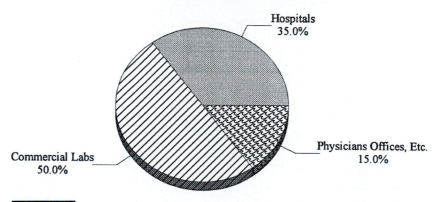

FIGURE 3.

Predicted 1997 test volume by heavy managed care site with no or few hospital laboratory networks in place and the Clinical Laboratory Improvement Act intact. (Courtesy of Health Care Development Services, Inc., Northbrook, Ill.)

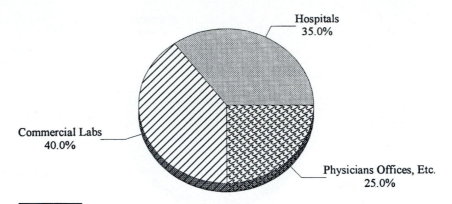

FIGURE 4.

Predicted 1997 test volume by heavy managed care site with the Clinical Laboratory Improvement Act gutted and no or few hospital laboratory networks in place. (Courtesy of Health Care Development Services, Inc., Northbrook, Ill.)

ratory services delivery system is using "patient care technicians" (PCTs) for specimen collection. Not just simply transferring phlebotomy responsibilities from the laboratory to nursing, the creation of PCT positions is more an extension of the movement toward the patient caregiver model. By putting responsibility for specimen collection closer to the patient, many hospitals have found that specimen collection costs are substantially reduced. Unlike most hospital phlebotomists, PCTs have a wider scope of responsibilities and contribute more to delivering a wide spectrum of health care services. Although finding and training good PCTs continue to be an arduous process, the elimination of laboratory-based phlebotomy services seems to be a worthwhile strategy to consider.

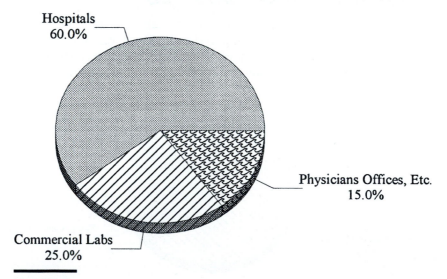

FIGURE 5.

Predicted 1997 test volume by heavy managed care site with a substantial number of hospital laboratory networks in place and the Clinical Laboratory Improvement Act mostly intact. (Courtesy of Health Care Development Services, Inc., Northbrook, Ill.)

Re-engineering work flow and the number and placement of workstations is another important aspect of many hospitals' strategies to better organize laboratory services. Since much of the high-throughput chemistry and hematology instrumentation today does not require constant operator intervention, laboratory directors are choosing technology based in part on "walkaway" features that allow technicians and technologists to manage the testing activities of more than one instrument at the same time.

Instrument manufacturers have acknowledged the need for lower labor input per performed test and have redesigned their products to perform more tests on fewer instruments. By arranging these instruments in "clusters," many hospitals have created small core laboratories within the main laboratory where specimen accessioning, processing, and testing are performed for 60% to 70% of *all* tests. Although it might surprise some laboratorians, approximately 500,000 tests per year are accessioned, processed, and performed in areas less than 5,000 ft^2 when properly designed and equipped.

Information systems also play a critical role in the re-engineering process. Laboratory information system vendors have recognized the need for autofax, result reporting algorithms, accommodation for instrument bidirectional interfaces, and other important information system features necessary to support the efforts to re-engineer hospital laboratory services. Although hard-wired remote printing of results is not a new aspect of most laboratory information systems, the introduction of "wireless" data transmission from point-of-care instruments to the laboratory information system and then back to handheld data receivers is expected to accelerate the use of point-of-care technology in selected hospital settings.

REORGANIZING REPORTING RELATIONSHIPS

In traditional stand-alone hospital laboratory environments, the relationships between managers, supervisors, testing personnel, and support personnel vary widely and are a major factor that drives organizational performance. As presented in Table 8, the proportion of managers, supervisors, testing personnel, and support personnel varies significantly based on the volume of testing performed on site. The proportion of managers appears to go up as on-site test volume increases, whereas the proportion of supervisors decreases and may reflect better use of middle managers in higher-volume laboratories. The proportion of testing personnel also reflects the level of automation. Hospitals need to evaluate whether supervisors or testing personnel are doing tasks that could be performed by lower-cost support personnel.

The relationship between the number of supervisors per manager, number of FTEs per supervisor, and number of testing personnel per technical supervisor is not necessarily linked to on-site test volume. Table 9 shows that there is little relationship between hospital laboratory test volume and organizational reporting relationships.

Although the tables of organization in hospital laboratories are undergoing close scrutiny today, most are organized along traditional lines of reporting relationships. As presented in Figure 6, historically most hos-

TABLE 8.

Proportion of Staff by Job Classification*

On-Site Performed Test vol/yr	Percentage of Staff (Mean Value)			
	Managers	Supervisors	Testing Personnel†	Support Personnel
50,000–200,000	1.6	14.5	55.3	28.6
200,001–400,000	1.8	13.7	47.8	36.7
400,001–600,000	1.9	11.3	47.2	39.6
More than 600,000	2.5	7.8	53.0	36.7

*From Health Care Development Services, Inc., LabTrends Hospital Laboratory Comparative Program. Used by permission.
†Does not include time spent by supervisors performing testing.

pital laboratories were organized with technical and nontechnical supervisors reporting directly to a laboratory manager/administrator. Given the changing mix of testing performed, increased utilization of highly automated technology, and diffusion of testing sites, hospital laboratory administrative and medical directors must consider how to best reorganize the structure of reporting relationships. Issues such as managing decentralized/near-patient testing sites, removing layers of historical supervisory management, and matching job responsibilities to meet new demands placed on the laboratory will challenge traditional hospital laboratory reporting relationships.

Hospital laboratory organizational relationships might change over the next few years. As more point-of-care/near-patient testing, regionalization of laboratory testing, and automated specimen handling/testing systems proliferate, new organizational reporting relationships in hospital laboratories may emerge. Figure 7 presents one version of an organizational structure that some hospitals have recently implemented.

TABLE 9.

Organizational Reporting Relationships*

On-Site Performed Test vol/yr	Average Number of FTEs		
	Supervisors per Manager	FTEs per Supervisor	Number of Technical Supervisors
50,000–200,000	3.7	7.9	5.5
200,001–400,000	6.6	6.7	4.8
400,001–600,000	8.5	8.3	6.0
More than 600,000	4.3	12.0	9.9

*From Health Care Development Services, Inc., LabTrends Hospital Laboratory Comparative Program. Used by permission.

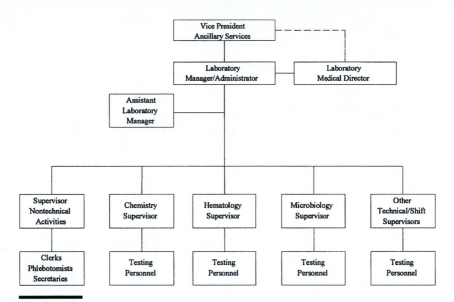

FIGURE 6.
Traditional hospital laboratory organization structure. (Courtesy of Health Care Development Services, Inc., Northbrook, Ill.)

DEVELOPING NETWORKS TO CAPTURE MANAGED CARE PLAN OUTPATIENT CONTRACTS

In early 1994, some managed care plans "carved out" contracts for outpatient laboratory services, and overnight some hospitals' outpatient laboratory testing decreased dramatically. Cigna, U.S. Healthcare, Blue Cross/Blue Shield, and other insurance companies with a wide range of managed care products negotiated "exclusive" contracts with commercial laboratories to provide capitated outpatient laboratory services. Hospitals, even those with active outreach programs, found themselves losing substantial market shares as a result of these exclusive contracts.

In mid-1994 and early 1995, some hospitals began to discuss the development of "networks" designed to compete for this segment of the outpatient managed care laboratory market. In California, Oregon, Washington, Michigan, and Ohio, for example, hospitals are investigating whether or not they can develop such networks.[11]

Although no statewide hospital laboratory network had been formed as of February 1995, it is expected that hospital-sponsored laboratory networks may be formed in the near future in order to compete for carved-out managed care plan contracts. The nature of such networks will require a delicate balancing act (Fig 8) to ensure that the letter of federal antitrust regulations is met. In order to help avoid any accusations of *per se* violations of Department of Justice/Federal Trade Commission regulations, hospital executives and laboratory directors should review the published analytic principles.[12]

No one model has emerged as a template for developing statewide hospital laboratory networks for bidding on managed care plan outpatient

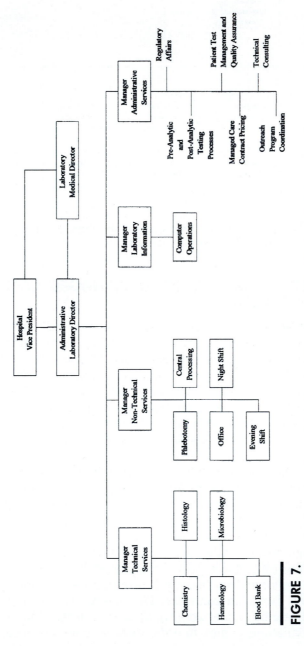

FIGURE 7.
Hospital laboratory organization of the future. (Courtesy of Health Care Development Services, Inc., Northbrook, Ill.)

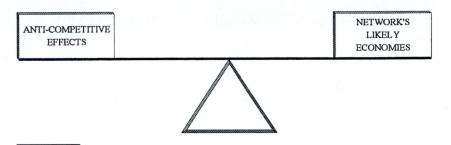

FIGURE 8.

Necessary delicate balance of anticompetitive effects and economies of scale.

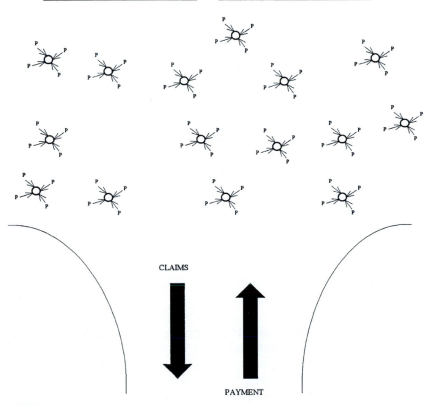

FIGURE 9.

Patients *(P)* directed to one of many specimen collection sites *(circles)*.

laboratory service contracts. As shown in Figures 9 to 11, patients may be directed to local/regional collection sites in a statewide model (Fig 9), to regional sites (Fig 10) in a one-network model, or to regional sites in a multiprovider, multinetwork model (Fig 11).

Many industry observers believe that in order to effectively develop single/multiple provider networks, it will be necessary to create a management services organization (MSO) to support the individual hospitals

56   B. Portugal

REGIONAL LAB TESTING MODEL - ONE STATE-WIDE NETWORK

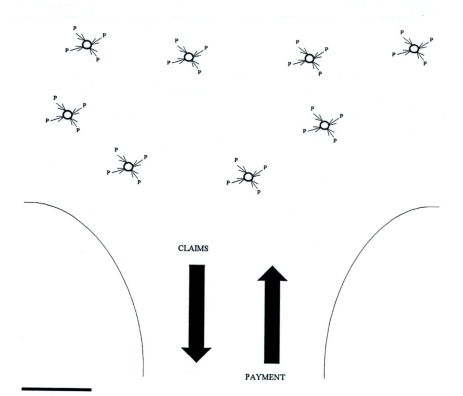

FIGURE 10.
Patients *(P)* and specimens directed to a limited number of specimen collection and testing sites *(circles)* in regional laboratory testing model.

in the network. Important aspects of an MSO include the following services:

- Communications and data processing software link individual practices into the MSO central office. Software supports the transmission of claims, referral requests, eligibility data, clinical information, patient credit applications, employee payroll data, and network messages.
- Marketing services contract with insurance agents and general agents to support local area sales of plans that use the MSO physicians. The MSO can develop custom-insured and self-funding plans exclusive to the MSO and consulting services for individual practice development.
- Individual practice association contracts and capitation can be administered and may include claims adjudication, payment of providers, withhold accounting, utilization review agendas, referral management, and protocol development.
- An MSO can provide business services that include patient and insurance billing, analysis of accounts receivable problems, bookkeeping, employee benefits, payroll processing, bulk purchasing, patient credit programs, legal services, and financial and management consulting services.

REGIONAL LAB TESTING MODEL - MULTI-PROVIDER NETWORKS

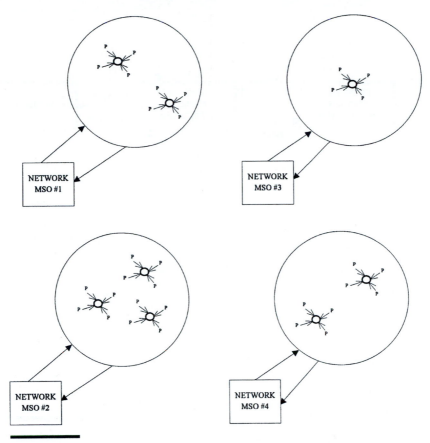

FIGURE 11.

The role of a management services organization (MSO) in supporting a regional, multiprovider network (P = patients; *circles* = testing sites).

Although MSOs can have many different types of business relationships with providers, insurers, and patients, Figure 12 presents a typical set of business arrangements that an MSO might develop.

LABORATORY CONSOLIDATION/REGIONALIZATION STRATEGIES

Among the alternative strategies hospital executives and laboratory directors are considering, laboratory consolidation and/or regionalization ranks close to the top.[13] Although it is generally believed that three different levels (Table 10) of strategies reflect the range of options available, no one strategy has emerged ahead of those involving laboratory consolidation and/or regionalization.

Each strategy is designed to decrease operating and capital costs and has resulted in differing rates of cost reduction. Figure 13 depicts cost savings ranging from 2% to 3% to almost 20%, depending on which strategy is implemented. In some cases—as with some contract management arrangements—the actual costs are higher than those of comparative hos-

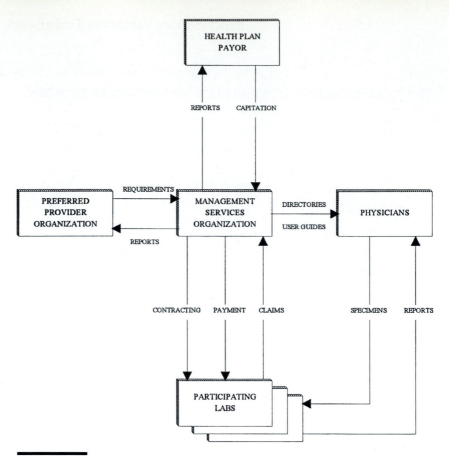

FIGURE 12.

Depiction of management services organizations as the hub of multiprovider regional laboratory systems.

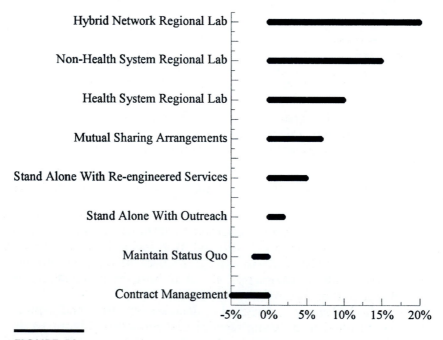

FIGURE 13.

Representation of strategic alternatives with respect to potential cost savings. (Courtesy of Health Care Development Services, Inc., Northbrook, Ill.)

TABLE 10.
Hospital Laboratory Strategic Planning Alternatives

Conservative Strategies	Moderate Strategies	Aggressive Strategies
Maintain status quo	Mutual sharing arrangements	Contract management
Stand-alone hospital laboratory with a re-engineered delivery system	Health care system regional laboratory	Competing hospital regional laboratory
Stand-alone hospital laboratory with an expanded outreach program		Hybrid health care network regional laboratory

TABLE 11.
Advantages and Disadvantages of Mutual Sharing Arrangements

Advantages
  Eliminates duplication of testing disciplines and creates areas of expertise
  Produces modest economic savings
Disadvantages
  Operationally difficult to manage
  Ineffective when more than 2 hospitals participate and when the outreach
    market volume exceeds 40%–50% of the total test volume
  Information system nightmare

pital laboratories. Occasionally, the "make/buy" decision results in higher referred testing costs.

Laboratory consolidation among hospitals may take several forms. Among the models being considered, the mutual sharing arrangement (Fig 14) is considered to be the least cost-effective. In this model, some of the previously referred testing is brought in-house; low-volume, non–time-dependent testing is consolidated at one site, and duplication of specialty testing among the participating hospitals is eliminated. The mutual sharing arrangement model offers certain advantages and includes other disadvantages (Table 11).

On the other end of the scale, the single-site off-campus regional laboratories formed by multiple hospitals, affiliated group practices/practice plans, physician-hospital organizations, and other providers/payers are thought to be positioned to best serve the needs in a managed care environment. Although no one model best depicts the regional laboratory, Figure 15 portrays how these organizations look in a stereotypic format.

The hybrid regional laboratory model probably presents the most cost-effective solution to developing laboratory services. Although the advantages of the regional model far outweigh the disadvantages, only a few health care systems have begun implementing it as of early 1995. As noted

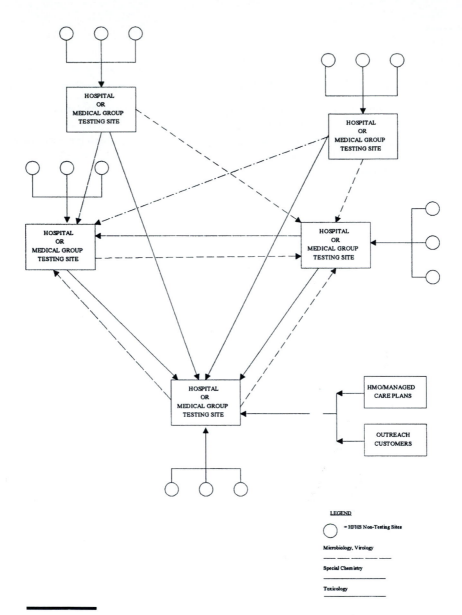

FIGURE 14.
Networking/regionalization strategies for a mutual sharing arrangement. (Courtesy of Health Care Development Services, Inc., Northbrook, Ill.)

in Table 12, health care system hospital test volume and differences in vision may prove to be obstacles to the development of regional laboratories.

SUMMARY

The hospital laboratory industry is adjusting to changing times. Administrators, laboratory medical directors, and administrative directors are making decisions that once and forever are changing the face of how and where laboratory services are provided. The decisions are based on comparative operational and financial performance indicators and evolve

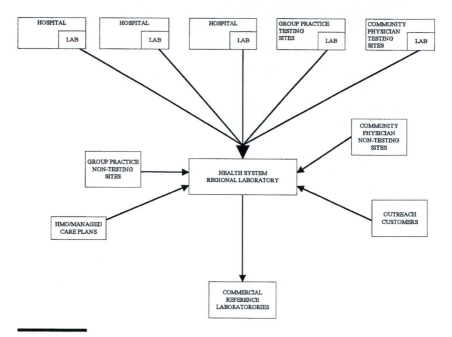

FIGURE 15.

Networking/regionalization strategies for a single-site regional laboratory. (Courtesy of Health Care Development Services, Inc., Northbrook, Ill.)

through re-engineering, reorganization, and the development of utilization review strategies.

Although benchmarking laboratory performance is the basis of the planning process, no real lasting change can take place without innovative leadership. Laboratory directors who acknowledge the four following basic postulates of innovation will be able to lead their organizations into the future:

1. Innovation means doing something different.
2. Innovation can only happen when people feel they are on a mission.
3. Organizations do not innovate—people do.
4. When innovation is encouraged, it flourishes.

TABLE 12.

Health System Regional Laboratories: Advantages and Disadvantages

---

Advantages
　Organizational obstacles are substantially reduced
　System hospitals and other health care providers may be geographically
　　proximate
　Affiliated physician-hospital organization management may be more sensitive
　　and patient to start-up problems
Disadvantages
　Health care system hospitals and affiliated providers may not have sufficient
　　test volume to produce significant economies of scale
　Individual members of the health care system may have different views on
　　laboratory services models

REFERENCES

1. Annual meeting of the Clinical Laboratory Management Association, Laboratory Benchmarking Programs, Orlando, Fla, 1994.
2. Kropf R, Greenberg J: *Strategic Analysis for Hospital Management.* Rockville, Md, Aspen, 1984.
3. Portugal B: Factors influencing relative financial performance of hospital laboratories. *Clin Lab Manage Rev* 3:81–87, 1989.
4. Portugal B: *Benchmarking Hospital Laboratory Financial and Operational Performance,* Hospital Technology Special Report, vol 12, no 17. Chicago, American Hospital Association, 1993.
5. Speicher C: *The Right Test.* Philadelphia, WB Saunders, 1993.
6. Mehl P, Portugal B: *The Clinical Laboratory Improvement Amendments and Final Regulations. An Impact Analysis for Hospital Executives and Laboratory Managers,* special AHA Member briefing. Chicago, American Hospital Association, June 1992.
7. Test complexity categorization, clinical laboratory improvement amendments. *Fed Register* 57:40258–40296, 1992.
8. Client alert. Northbrook, Ill, Health Care Development Services, February 1995.
9. Portugal B: The future of laboratory services. Presented at an American Hospital Association Seminar, San Francisco, Feb 2–3, 1995.
10. Hammer M, Champy J: *Reengineering the Corporation.* New York, Harper Business, 1993.
11. Nigon D: Initiating a regional laboratory network. *Clin Lab Manage Rev* 8:561–573, 1994.
12. Statements of Enforcement Policy and Analytical Principles Relating to Health Care and Anti-trust. Washington, DC, US Department of Justice and the Federal Trade Commission, Sept 27, 1994.
13. *Network Advantages/Scale of Economies and Cost Savings.* Washington, DC, Health Care Advisory Board, 1994.

Quality Assurance Issues and Problems Specific to Autopsies

Nancy A. Young, M.D.

Department of Pathology, Fox Chase Cancer Center, Clinical Associate Professor, Hahnemann University School of Medicine, Philadelphia, Pennsylvania

FINANCIAL DISINCENTIVES AND DECLINE OF AUTOPSIES: IMPACT ON QUALITY

The autopsy is the gold standard for measuring the quality of patient care; however, there are few guidelines for auditing the quality of the autopsy and autopsy report.[1] As autopsy rates have plummeted, the quality of the procedure is at risk *now* more than ever. Although most published autopsy quality assurance (QA) programs describe how to best use the autopsy for tracking and reporting missed diagnoses, unexpected findings, and errors in patient care,[2-6] this chapter will also focus on the often neglected aspects of improving quality at the pathology departmental level.

Beginning at least a decade before the deletion of the 20% autopsy rate required for accreditation by the Joint Commission on Accreditation of Healthcare Organizations (JCAHO) in 1971, there has been a steady decline in the percentage of autopsies done in the United States and elsewhere. In community hospitals, autopsy rates are now often less than 5% of hospital deaths.[7] Low rates have a direct impact on prosector experience and diagnostic skills. Furthermore, for the autopsy to provide a good index of the quality of patient care, an autopsy rate high enough for analysis is needed. An overall rate of about 35% of hospital deaths has been suggested as adequate.[8, 9]

There are a number of hypotheses as to why rates have dropped, including claims that pathologists just do not like to do autopsies.[10] However, a number of medical procedures including barium enemas and 8-hour surgeries might not be considered "pleasant" by some yet are still advocated and actively solicited by physicians performing these procedures. Much of the drop in enthusiasm for autopsies is due to the lack of direct reimbursement for this labor-intensive service.[6, 8, 9, 11]

Medicare and third-party payers have not been keen to reimburse for services performed in the morgue. Bureaucrats argue that because the deceased is not really a patient, the autopsy is not really a treatment and therefore no payment is justified.[10] The third-party payers who pay for health care in this country supposedly pay for autopsies, but not as a line

Advances in Pathology and Laboratory Medicine®, vol. 8

item that is visible on the budget, so hospital administrators often say that they do not have any money for autopsies.[12] The autopsy service is a cost center, not a revenue-generating center. In the new health care environment, as more procedures become capitated and are not directly reimbursed, it will be interesting to see whether enthusiasm and the number of perceived indications for other procedures decline as well.

Another change in the last two decades that has been blamed for the decline in the autopsy rate is the fear of litigation on the basis of what might be found at autopsy. Although autopsy findings may occasionally provide the foundation for a malpractice claim, a well-performed autopsy is more often likely to dispel the questions that prompt such action. In either event, a properly performed and documented autopsy provides factual and scientific evidence for resolving medical questions.[13]

To avoid autopsy, doctors rationalize that the scanners have told them everything they need to know, so the autopsy is unnecessary. Yet despite the advent of progressively more sophisticated investigative and imaging techniques, major discrepancies between clinical and autopsy diagnoses have remained between 10% and 30%.[2, 8, 10, 14-18] Often these studies show that the autopsies revealed findings that if detected before death, would have led to a change in management that might have resulted in a cure or prolonged survival.[19, 20] Ironically, the autopsy rate is the lowest in patients who receive the greatest amount of medical care—the elderly. Although we seem to be least curious about the cause of death in this age group, perhaps more autopsies could provide information about how to improve the quality of life with advancing age.[10]

Mortality statistics that are not supported by autopsy examinations should be viewed with caution. In autopsies performed on patients thought to have died of malignant disease, there was only a 75% agreement that the malignancy was the cause of death, and in only 56% was the primary site correctly identified. Doctors also tend to attribute most sudden unexpected deaths to heart disease, thus leading to a probable overestimation of cardiac causes of sudden death.[8, 21-23] Yet many pathologists are reluctant to promote autopsies or make them a highly visible educational instrument since it might mean performing more autopsies.

Hospitals for the most part are not eager to solicit or encourage autopsies unless minimal numbers are needed to maintain a residency program. In fact, some newer hospitals have been built without autopsy suites. The autopsy has become a low-priority, low-profile procedure that is delegated to the least experienced house staff and members of the department. However, malpractice can occur at the autopsy table as well as anywhere else in the hospital, with significant consequences in the courtroom not to mention the loss to our clinical knowledge base.

The situation is so bad that the College of American Pathologists (CAP) is looking into innovative solutions, including ways to restructure the whole autopsy practice. Ideas proposed include regionalized autopsy centers similar to the medical examiner system.[24] Bodies would be transported to these centers for an autopsy to be performed by experienced pathologists with an interest in autopsy pathology. Information would presumably be more reliable and centralized for epidemiologic studies. It is unlikely, however, that hospitals and pathology departments will readily relinquish their jurisdiction over autopsies. Since the cost of maintaining an autopsy service is factored into reimbursement, hospitals might fear that insurance companies could use this change as a justification for decreasing payments.

Survival of the autopsy and its role in QA programs depend on adequate compensation and accountability of funds intended to cover the autopsy service as well as voluntary and government regulation. It has been advocated that the Health Care Financing Administration and the principal other insurance companies should pay the expense for autopsies as a line item on the budget.[12] In addition, pathologists may have to change the standards for performing and reporting autopsies. Shorter report lengths and fewer histologic sections would cut down on costs and facilitate turnaround time.[10, 25] Some advocate studying the cost-effectiveness of limited goal-directed autopsies as well as evaluating for circumstances when the autopsy may have an especially high or low yield for new information.[26] However, in spite of financial pressures to do otherwise, we must maintain the quality of the autopsy and therefore its medical and scientific value to justify its cost within the hospital and our demands for adequate support and compensation.[27-29] To have an effective autopsy QA program in place not only fulfills the JCAHO and CAP requirements but is also in the best interests of pathologists and the entire medical community.

QUALITY ASSURANCE TERMINOLOGY AND APPROACHES

One thing confusing about QA is all the related terminology and jargon surrounding it that continues to grow every year. What is the difference between QA, quality control (QC), total quality management (TQM), and continuous quality improvement (CQI)? Quality control is one tool to promote QA.[30] Quality assurance is a comprehensive term that encompasses QC. *Quality assurance* has its origins in industry and refers to *all* the measures taken to produce a uniform, satisfactory product.[31] In anatomic pathology, specifically, autopsy pathology, our "product" is *service* consisting of the postmortem examination and delivery of the information obtained in the form of an autopsy report. Telephones and conferences are adjuvant means of relaying information to the appropriate "consumers." Therefore QA refers to those measures taken to ensure that the information from the autopsy is correct, reports are complete, and results are promptly and effectively communicated to the appropriate individuals.

Quality control, according to the CAP official definition, is "an integral component of quality assurance and is the aggregate of processes and techniques so derived to detect, reduce, and correct deficiencies in an analytical process."[32] In other words, QC measures accuracy and reproducibility. For instance, systematic inspection of the prosector's gross diagnoses and rereview of slides and microscopic diagnoses are all elements of quality control to detect and correct deficiencies in autopsy reports. On the other hand, QA encompasses the entire production/delivery system and emphasizes the satisfaction of client needs.[33] Quality assurance and not QC includes making sure that clinicians are routinely called about unexpected findings and that reports are issued within 30 working days.

Total quality management is a relatively recent concept that surfaced in health care about a decade ago. This style of QA has been popularized by the Japanese in their industries, and an effort has been made to try to apply it to hospital QA.[34] It is a global, systemwide program that recognizes the *interdependence* of processes throughout an organization. The goal is "customer satisfaction" as well as continual improvement of patient care by dealing with processes in the system from top management all the way down rather than focusing on a single event or individual.

Continuous quality improvement is another term often used interchangeably with TQM. It is the part of TQM that deals with seeking to continually improve.[34] Continuous quality improvement de-emphasizes "problem people" and focuses attention on continually improving the "processes" people use to achieve the objectives of the organization.

Most current quality management activity focuses on using inspection to find fault, usually with people. It gives no recognition to those who perform their job well or even display exceptional effort. This concept has been referred to as the theory of *bad apples*.[35] In other words, quality can be ensured by a vigorous search for persons who display deficient performance. This process can have an intimidating effect on well-meaning and competent workers. Continuous quality improvement is a change in organizational culture and uses statistical methods and multidisciplinary teams to analyze the underlying processes of care, diagnose problems, and seek continual improvement. The commitment must start at the top of the organization and involve everyone. *Supposedly*, fear will be driven out of the organization by convincing everyone that the system is the problem, not the bad apples.

For example, when I first became autopsy director, we had a tremendous problem complying with the CAP-recommended turnaround time of 30 working days for a routine final report. We had actually been cited on our CAP inspection for this deficiency. In response, I took the traditional approach of making staff and residents more accountable for their late cases and resorted to placing notification letters in the guilty residents' files when their cases were not completed in time.[1] Although there was an immediate improvement in autopsy turnaround time, I discovered that residents were under stress and resentful and were typing their own reports to avoid secretarial delays. Following the principles of TQM, I tried to analyze the whole system. For instance, how long does it take for slides to be cut and returned to the pathologist? What processes are occurring in the histology laboratory that might cause a delay? Has there been a recent increase in the surgical workload or an increase in the number of routine sections being taken? How long does it take for reports to be typed? If there is a delay, do the secretaries need more training in medical terminology, are the dictations or handwriting by staff clear, or is there a way to decrease the number of draft corrections? Is there a delay in transporting the autopsy report to the medical records or the clinician of record? One could look at the workload and see whether the administration is supplying enough funds for adequate professional and support staffing. Are residents or staff dictating their histories and gross descriptions right away and taking their sections promptly? Would some residents benefit from charting their cases to keep track of the progress of each case? Can the residency rotations be changed so that residents do not go off the autopsy service directly onto the surgical pathology service where they have no time to complete their autopsies and meet with the attending physicians? Is there the perception by residents and staff that the chairman and/or administration does not value the autopsy and that prompt completion of cases is not a priority?

I was able to identify problems in the system. Resident schedules were changed so that the autopsy rotation was followed by a relatively light service and residents would have a chance to finalize their cases. The inexperienced secretary typing autopsy reports was offered a course in medical terminology, and with time her skills improved. The number of rough drafts that were being typed was decreased.

The TQM approach to solving this one problem was performed only at the departmental level since we were not part of an organization-wide TQM program. If such a program were in place, one might also address the personnel policies that resulted in the placement of someone with minimal knowledge of medical terminology in the role of a medical secretary. It is difficult to correct some problems in a vacuum. The ideal situation is when the entire institution works cooperatively to address inefficiencies and errors in the system.

However, some of the early enthusiasm for TQM has fizzled as hospitals measure the return on their tremendous investments in time and money to implement it. A survey from Northwestern University's J.L. Kellogg Graduate School has found that except for some evidence of improved patient satisfaction and reduced cesarian section rates, TQM has made no discernible difference in most patient care outcomes despite the $400 million that the nation's hospitals pump into TQM projects each year.[36] Total quality management seems to be most successful when applied to procedure-based care and in those unusual institutions in which physicians work closely with administrators and get involved early and often in TQM projects. Therefore, many hospitals have yet to embrace TQM wholeheartedly.

ORGANIZATION OF AUTOPSY QUALITY ASSURANCE

The autopsy is unlike other areas of anatomic pathology practice in that it not only serves a direct patient care function but as itself also serves as a QA tool. Therefore a QA program in autopsy pathology must include indicators related to the autopsy itself and indicators that relate the autopsy to the quality of general medical practice.[37]

Figure 1 is a flow chart that summarizes the organizational structure of the types of QA activities that pertain to autopsy pathology. All of the items fall under either external or internal QA. *External QA* refers to the use of the autopsy to monitor clinician performance or hospital quality improvement. The JCAHO requires that autopsy findings be incorporated into an organization-wide quality improvement program. The structure of the quality improvement program should be individualized to suit the

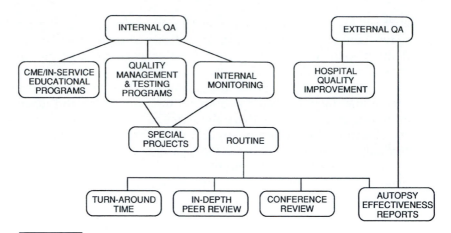

FIGURE 1.

Overview and organization of autopsy quality assurance. *QA* = quality assurance; *CME* = continuing medical education.

specific needs of the hospital. This can include routinely scheduled morbidity and mortality conferences, medical staff section review of deaths, and clinicopathologic conferences.[38] Autopsy monitoring activities presented at the departmental anatomic pathology quality improvement committee may be reported to the hospital quality improvement committee by the appointed representative from the department of pathology. Copies of meeting minutes or autopsy reports, particularly reports with significant discrepancies between the clinical and anatomic diagnoses, can be sent to risk management, hospital utilization review, or other appropriate committees when indicated. However, it is important that this information be used mainly as an educational tool. Clinician fears of punitive action have already been blamed as a major cause of dwindling autopsy rates. The institutional focus should be on improving the *system* and prevention, including better in-servicing, rather than focusing on a single event or individual.

Internal QA is monitoring the quality of the actual autopsy procedure and reports. There are few guidelines on how to accomplish this task. Figure 1 shows that internal QA or quality improvement encompasses three items[38]: (1) internal monitoring, (2) society-offered quality management and testing programs, and (3) continuing medical education (CME) and in-service educational programs.

INTERNAL MONITORING

Internal monitoring is an internally developed system of monitoring and evaluating cases, records, and systems. Internal monitoring can be categorized as either *routine* or *special*. In routine monitoring, one chooses the aspects of the autopsy service that should undergo ongoing monitoring such as completeness and accuracy of autopsy reports and turnaround time.

Special QA projects supplement the routine QA activities by picking a project to monitor for several months that is thereafter periodically followed. Participation in society-sponsored *quality management and testing programs* such as the CAP autopsy Q-Probe program is beneficial in that important parameters to study are identified and one can compare results with those of other laboratories. Q-Probe, a QA program for pathology and laboratory medicine, involves sending participants descriptive information and preprinted study input forms for data collection. On study completion, these forms are returned to the CAP computer center where the data are analyzed and an interinstitutional comparison is performed.[39] The autopsy Q-Probe has monitored such parameters as autopsy permit form adequacy, starting delays, and turnaround time. New QA parameters for study are periodically being developed.

One can tailor a special project to a perceived need in the institution. For instance, one might choose to monitor the gross photography files if photographs seem to be missing. One might choose to monitor communication of results back to the clinician or completeness of the face sheet if one does not routinely monitor these aspects of the service. The outcome may be that an excellent job is being done. On the other hand, if deficiencies are detected, action taken to correct them should be documented, along with monthly reports and monitors. Follow-up reviews will be maintained with those of the original studies.

Described in the following sections is the routine monitoring system developed for an academic pathology setting with a residency program.[1] This program is not a rigid structure and can be modified to fit other types of autopsy practices and departmental needs. Routine monitoring (see Fig 1) is divided into (1) in-depth peer review of autopsy reports, (2) review of autopsy reports at teaching conferences, and (3) monitoring turnaround times of provisional final autopsy reports.

IN-DEPTH PEER REVIEW

The members of the QC/QA Committee of the Association of Directors of Anatomic and Surgical Pathology recommend in their report dealing with QA and QC that 10% or two cases per month, whichever number is larger, be randomly selected for peer review.[40] If cases are being reviewed in conferences (see later), only one case may be required for review per month with this format. Each month a secretary chooses a report to be analyzed for in-depth peer review. The report is photocopied, with the prosector's and staff pathologist's names blocked out on the face sheet to maintain objectivity on the part of the reviewer. Autopsies are not chosen entirely at random, but with the intent that residents and staff members have equal turns at being reviewed and all staff members have a chance as a reviewer.

The autopsy report, slides, and review form (Fig 2) are given to the reviewer. After the form that contains many of the questions on the CAP checklist[41] is filled out and returned, the code is broken and the reviewer discusses the case with the resident and attending physician *before* the case is presented at the departmental QA conference. The word "before" is stressed since no one should ever be surprised by having one's case presented at a QA conference.

REVIEW AT CONFERENCES

If there are regularly scheduled autopsy conferences, one can use this opportunity to monitor the cases while they are being presented, although usually not in the same detail as in the in-depth peer review. At these

Autopsy Peer Review QA Form

Reviewer:_____

Month/year:_____

Case number: _____

Patient name:_____

1. Is clinical summary informative but concise? Yes___ No___

Comments: _____

2. Are the gross and microscopic descriptions of lesions clear
and concise?   Yes____ No____

Comments: _____

3. Are all pertinent findings adequately described? Yes___ No___

Comments: _____

4. Were the sections taken adequate to establish the extent of
major lesions? Yes___ No___

Comments: _____

5. Were special studies (cultures, special stains, EM, etc.) performed
to enhance the value of the autopsy? Yes___ No___

Comments: _____

6. Does the FAD and/or discussion explain the clinical problems
and correlate clinical signs, symptoms, and laboratory data with
the anatomic findings? Yes___ No___

Comments: _____

7. Are there significant discrepancies in anotmoic diagnoses by the
reviewer? Yes___ No___

Comments:_____

8. Other
comments?_____

_____

_____

FIGURE 2.

Autopsy peer review QA form. *QA* = quality assurance; *EM* = electron microscopy; *FAD* = final anatomic diagnosis.

conferences, the finalized reports are available, and as the history and
gross and microscopic findings are presented, any substantial errors are
documented on a conference QA form (Fig 3). Since much of QA involves
documentation, this approach is an efficient use of time by not increasing the number of staff responsibilities, but just documenting what is already being done. Frequently, clinicians also attend these conferences,
and one can get a better idea when there are unsuspected findings and
whether the clinicians had been promptly informed of them.

AUTOPSY EFFECTIVENESS REPORTS

Schned et al.[15] described a unique QA program that monitored both clinical and pathologic performance. Included in their monitoring program
was the clinical significance of the autopsy findings and the ability of the
autopsy to answer clinical questions. Some of the unanswered questions

Autopsy Conference QA Form

Month/year: _____

Case number: _____

Patient name: _____

Prosector/attending physician:

Clinical problems/questions: _____

_____

_____

Important gross findings presented: _____

_____

_____

Were appropriate photographs taken? Yes___ No___

Comments: _____

Any problems identified with the gross dissection shown? _____

_____

Important microscopic findings presented: _____

_____

_____

Were appropriate sections taken? Yes___ No___

_____

Were appropriate special studies done (cultures, special stains,
EM, etc.) to enhance the value of the autopsy? Yes___ No___

_____

Any discrepancies in gross or microscopic dianoses?
Yes___ No___   _____

Any significant discrepancies between clinical diagnoses and
autopsy findings? Yes___ No___

_____

Other problems identified? _____

_____

_____

FIGURE 3.

Autopsy conference QA form. *QA* = quality assurance; *EM* = electron microscopy.

reflected an inherent inability of the autopsy to solve certain kinds of
problems. Some questions were left unanswered, however, because of
performer deficiencies.

The utility of the autopsy in answering clinical questions can be followed by using an autopsy effectiveness report.[38] The autopsy effectiveness report monitors whether the autopsy clarifies the clinical diagnosis
or uncovers an unexpected or additional diagnosis.

Autopsy effectiveness reports combine some aspects of internal QA
as well as external QA. The report can be filled out by clinicians, by the
pathology staff, or ideally by both in consultation with each other. Identifying how often the autopsy uncovers disagreements in diagnoses or

confirms or clarifies diagnoses is an audit of the usefulness and overall quality of the autopsy as well as the clinical service.

Questions to be addressed are whether the autopsy uncovered a major disagreement in diagnosis or unexpected or additional diagnoses, clarified the differential diagnosis, and/or confirmed the major diagnosis. The report can also probe whether the autopsy provided information on radiologic or endoscopic procedures or confirmed or disagreed with previous pathology laboratory reports. Cases that should be reviewed by an institutional death review committee may be identified this way, and to do so is one way of satisfying the JCAHO requirement that autopsy findings be incorporated into an organization-wide quality improvement program.

AUTOPSY
INTERNAL AND EXTERNAL QUALITY ASSURANCE FORM
Quality Assurance of Month of_____ 19___

Reviewer:_____

Date: _____

Case number: _____

Patient name:_____

Turnaround time:

Preliminary report_____ Final report_____

1. Face sheet is complete with the patient's name, autopsy number, date of birth, sex, admission date, date and time of death, autopsy date and time, attending pathologist, prosector, clinician, medical record number, extent of autopsy.
Yes_____ No_____
Comments:_____
_____

2. Is it documented that the clinician of record was notified of the autopsy results?   Yes_____ No_____
Comments:_____
_____

3. Clinical summary informative but concise.   Yes_____ No_____
Comments:_____
_____

4. Gross and microscopic descriptions clear and concise.
Yes_____ No_____
Comments:_____
_____

5. All pertinent findings adequately described. Yes_____ No_____
Comments:_____
_____

6. Sections are adequate to establish the extent of major lesions.
Yes_____ No_____
Comments:_____
_____

FIGURE 4.
Internal and external quality assurance form. *FAD* = final anatomic diagnosis.

7. Special studies performed to enhance the value of the autopsy.
Yes ____ No ____ N/A ____
Comments: _____
_____

8. FAD/discussion examines the clinical problems and correlates clinical signs, symptoms, and laboratory data with the anatomic findings.   Yes ____ No ____
Comments: _____
_____

9. Did this autopsy uncover a major disagreement in diagnosis?
Yes ____ No ____
Comments: _____
_____

10. Did this autopsy establish an unexpected or additional diagnosis?   Yes ____ No ____
Comments: _____
_____

11. Did this autopsy provide clarification of the differential diagnosis?   Yes ____ No ____
Comments: _____
_____

12. Did this autopsy provide information that if known before death might have affected patient management of the patient's clinical course?   Yes ____ No ____
Comments: _____
_____

13. Were the appropriate clinicians notified of the autopsy results?
Yes ____ No ____
Comments: _____
_____

14. Did this autopsy provide information that warrants case review by the institutional death review committee?
Yes ____ No ____
Comments: _____
_____

FIGURE 4—(cont.).

Many of these parameters have been incorporated into one QA form (Fig 4) for departments in which autopsy auditing is exclusively by in-depth peer review. The one form audits the level of information provided in the autopsy report by the pathologist, turnaround time, and the autopsy's clinical value in confirming premortem diagnoses or identifying significant discrepancies between antemortem and postmortem diagnoses.

IN-SERVICE EDUCATIONAL PROGRAMS

Continuing medical education and in-service educational programs for pathologists and their staff are the third aspect of internal QA. Participation in these types of programs should be documented. For example, the CAP offers the APEX program that stands for Performance Improvement Program in Autopsy Pathology. Autopsy case studies and photographic slides are sent to the participants. A short quiz follows each case. The responses are mailed back to the CAP, and the participants receive a discussion of the correct answers. Other teaching exercises are available from major pathology organizations such as the American Society of Clinical Pathologists (which offers the Check Sample Program) and the Armed Forces Institute of Pathology (which provides assessment programs for military and Veterans Administration hospitals).

These programs should be regarded only as educational, self-assessment, and performance improvement activities and not considered or used as "proficiency" tests. Participants do not have access to the gross specimen or the opportunity to communicate directly with the referring physician and obtain all the pertinent clinical data that are an essential component of the consultative practice of pathology.[30]

Other examples of continuing education are instructional videotapes that cover topics ranging from performance of high-risk autopsies to autopsy technique. Attendance at clinicopathologic correlation conferences and morbidity and mortality conferences should be documented.

CAN QUALITY ASSURANCE IMPROVE QUALITY?

A good QA program for autopsies can improve turnaround time as well as the quality of performing and reporting autopsies by setting standards and monitoring for compliance.[1] A harder question to answer, however, is whether properly performed autopsies on sufficient percentages of hospital deaths with effective communication of findings to clinicians will improve patient care.

Although intuitively one might think that autopsies performed under the aforementioned conditions would over time improve patient care, it has never been proved that there is a direct correlation between an increase in the autopsy rate and a subsequent decrease in clinicopathologic discrepancies.[42] However, a direct correlation between improved patient care and QA activity of any type is difficult to prove, and this problem is not limited to autopsies.[36] A recent study from Sweden[43] compared the diagnostic discrepancy rates between clinical and autopsy diagnoses and the sensitivity and specificity of clinical diagnostics in 10 diseases from 1977 to 1978 and 1987 to 1988. The autopsy rate had decreased from 80% to 39%, which corresponded to an increased discrepancy rate from 22% to 27% regarding the diagnoses of major principal diseases. Certain diseases were more likely than others to be misdiagnosed. There are so many variables in such a study that it is difficult to prove that the decreased autopsy rate had a direct effect on the diagnostic discrepancies. However, if this direct effect were to be demonstrated, then the indispensability of the autopsy in the clinical audit would be beyond question.[10, 44]

What is known is that the autopsy is a valuable method of QA and many diseases have been and continue to be discovered solely at autopsy.[10] We can also learn whether it is the disease or our newly evolving treatments that are responsible for patient mortality, provided that we continue to do autopsies at meaningful rates. We must, however, maintain the quality of autopsies while at the same time lobby for fair reimbursement for the professional and institutional costs of performing them.

REFERENCES

1. Young NA, Naryshkin S: An implenentation plan for autopsy quality control and quality assurance. *Arch Pathol Lab Med* 117:531–534, 1993.
2. Anderson RE: The autopsy as an instrument of quality assessment. *Arch Pathol Lab Med* 108:490–493, 1994.
3. Anderson RE, Hill RB, Gorstein F: A model for the autopsy-based quality assessment of medical diagnostics. *Hum Pathol* 21:174–181, 1990.
4. Landefeld SC, Goldman L: The autopsy in quality assurance: History, current status, and future directions. *Q Rev Biol* 15:42–48, 1989.
5. Pelletier LL, Friedrich K, Lancaster H: The autopsy: Its role in the evaluation of patient care. *J Gen Intern Med* 4:300–303, 1989.
6. Yesner R: Quality assessment of the autopsy. *Am J Clin Pathol* 86:250, 1986.
7. Lundberg GD: Now is the time to emphasize the autopsy in quality assurance. *JAMA* 260:3488, 1988.
8. The autopsy and audit. Report of the Joint Working Party of the Royal College of Pathologists, the Royal College of Physicians of London and the Royal College of Surgeons of England, London, August 1991.
9. Yesner R, Robinson MJ, Goldman L, et al: A symposium on the autopsy. *Pathol Annu* 20:441–447, 1985.
10. Berlinger NT: A mortal science. *Discover*, 15:30–35, 1994.
11. Nemetz PN, Ludwig J, Kurland LT: Assessing the autopsy. *Am J Pathol* 128:362–379, 1987.
12. Lundberg G: One pathologist's thoughts on the declining autopsy rate. *IOM News*, p 3, March 1994.
13. Foley T, Bianco EA, Zimmerly JG: The autopsy in malpractice litigation, in Hutchins GM (ed): *Autopsy Performance & Reporting*. Northfield, Ill, College of American Pathologists, 1990, pp 193–200.
14. Goldman L, Sayson R, Robbins S, et al: The value of the autopsy in three medical eras. *N Engl J Med* 308:1000–1005, 1983.
15. Schned AR, Mogielnicki P, Stauffer ME: A comprehensive quality assessment program on the autopsy service. *Am J Clin Pathol* 86:133–138, 1986.
16. Schned AR, Mogielnicki RP, Stauffer MA: Universal discordance rate (letter). *Am J Clin Pathol* 87:789, 1986.
17. Peacock SJ, Machlin D, DuBoulay CE, et al: The autopsy: a useful tool or an old relic? *J Pathol* 156:9–14, 1988.
18. Stothert JC Jr, Gbaanador G: Autopsy in general surgery practice. *Am J Surg* 162:585–588, 1991.
19. Fernandez-Segoviano P, Lazaro A, Estaban A, et al: Autopsy as quality assurance in the intensive care unit. *Crit Care Med* 16:683–685, 1988.
20. Laissue J-A, Altermatt HJ, Zurcher B, et al: The significance of the autopsy: Evaluation of current autopsy results by the clinician. *Schweiz Med Wochenschr* 116:130–134, 1986.
21. Mollo F, Bertoldo E, Grandi G: Reliability of death certifications for different types of cancer. An autopsy survey. *Pathol Res Pract* 116:130–134, 1986.
22. Thomas AC, Knapman PA, Krikler DM: Community study of the causes of 'natural' sudden death. *BMJ* 297:1453–1456, 1988.
23. Russell GA, Berry PJ: Postmortem audit in a paediatric cardiology unit. *J Clin Pathol* 42:912–918, 1989.
24. Hutchins GM: The wave of the future is regional autopsy centers. *CAP Today* 6:44–45, 1992.
25. Reid WA: Cost effectiveness of routine postmortem histology. *J Clin Pathol* 40:459–461, 1987.
26. Landefeld CS, Goldman L: The autopsy in clinical medicine. *Mayo Clin Proc* 64:1185–1189, 1989.

27. Saldino AJ: The efficacy of the autopsy in medical quality assurance. *Clin Lab Med* 4:165–184, 1984.
28. Cameron HM: The autopsy-illusion and reality. *Pathol Annu* 18:333–345, 1983.
29. Travers H: Mortui vivos docent. *Kansas Med* 87:329–333, 1986.
30. Rickert RR: Quality assurance in anatomic pathology. *Clin Lab Med* 6:697–706, 1986.
31. Diamond I: Quality assurance and/or quality control. *Arch Pathol Lab Med* 110:875–878, 1986.
32. Gilmer PR: Understanding quality control. *CAP Today* 5:29–31, 1991.
33. Cowan DF: Quality assurance in anatomic pathology. An information system approach. *Arch Pathol Lab Med* 114:129–134, 1990.
34. Barlett RC: Trends in quality management. *Arch Pathol Lab Med* 114:1126–1130, 1990.
35. Berwick BM: Continuous improvement as an ideal in health care. *JAMA* 320:53–56, 1989.
36. Oberman L: Quality quandary: Little clinical impact yet. *AMA News*, April 25, 1994.
37. Travers H: Quality assurance indicators in anatomic pathology. *Arch Pathol Lab Med* 114:1149–1156, 1990.
38. Hutchins GM: Autopsy pathology, in Travers H (ed): *Quality Improvement Manual in Anatomic Pathology.* Northfield, Ill, College of American Pathologists, 1993, pp 99–110.
39. Howanitz PJ: Quality assurance measurements in departments of pathology and laboratory medicine. *Arch Pathol Lab Med* 114:1131–1135, 1990.
40. Association of Directors of Anatomic and Surgical Pathology: Recommendations on quality control and quality assurance in surgical and autopsy pathology. *Hum Pathol* 22:1099–1101, 1991.
41. College of American Pathologists Commission on Laboratory Accreditation: *Inspection Checklist VIII: Anatomic Pathology and Cytology.* Northfield, Ill, College of American Pathologists, 1991.
42. Battle RM, Pathak D, Humble CG, et al: Factors influencing the discrepancies between premortem and postmortem diagnoses. *JAMA* 258:339–344, 1987.
43. Veress B, Alafuzoff I: Clinical diagnostic accuracy audited by autopsy in a university hospital in two eras. *Qual Assur Health Care* 5:281–286, 1993.
44. Laissue JA, Altermatt HA, Gebbers J-O, et al: Quality assessment program on the autopsy service. *Am J Clin Pathol* 87:788–789, 1986.

PART II

Diagnostic Pathology

Kinetic-Mode, Automated Double-Labeled Immunohistochemistry and in situ Hybridization in Diagnostic Pathology

Thomas M. Grogan, M.D.
Department of Pathology, University of Arizona College of Medicine, Tucson, Arizona

Catherine Rangel, B.A., H.T.L. (A.S.C.P.)
Department of Pathology, University of Arizona, Tucson, Arizona

Lisa Rimsza, M.D.
Department of Pathology, University of Arizona, Tucson, Arizona

William Bellamy, M.D.
Department of Pathology, University of Arizona, Tucson, Arizona

Ralph Martel, Ph.D.
Ventana Medical Systems, Tucson, Arizona

Darin McDaniel, B.S.
Ventana Medical Systems, Tucson, Arizona

Brian McGraw, B.S.
Ventana Medical Systems, Tucson, Arizona

William Richards, B.S.E.E.
Ventana Medical Systems, Tucson, Arizona

Lynne Richter, B.A., M.T. (A.S.C.P.) S.H.
Department of Pathology, University of Arizona, Tucson, Arizona

Paula Rodgers, M.S.
Ventana Medical Systems, Tucson, Arizona

James Rybski, Ph.D.
Ventana Medical Systems, Tucson, Arizona

Wayne Showalter
Ventana Medical Systems, Tucson, Arizona

Elizabeth Vela, M.S.
Department of Pathology, University of Arizona, Tucson, Arizona

Ron Zeheb, Ph.D.
Ventana Medical Systems, Tucson, Arizona

Advances in Pathology and Laboratory Medicine, vol. 8
© 1995, Mosby–Year Book, Inc.

T he ability to detect more than one molecular species in a tissue sample by double labeling could greatly aid the practice of diagnostic pathology. Specifically, in clinical practice the advantages of double labeling could include (1) detection of unique, aberrantly coexpressed tumor antigens; (2) differentiation of tumor from host response cells; (3) delineation of viral antigens relative to tumor or host antigens; (4) judgment of tumor clonality; (5) judgment of oncogene status relative to proliferation; and (6) combining protein and nucleic acid assays to relate cell protein and message status. Combined immunohistochemistry (IHC) and in situ hybridization (ISH) assays could allow study of the relationship of genotype to phenotype. This combination might relate chromosomal status via fluorescent ISH (FISH), message via ISH, and protein via IHC in individual cells. By using intact biopsy sections, tissue topography would be preserved and genotype and phenotype could be determined in a microanatomic context. This would allow an analysis of simultaneous alterations in transcription, translation, and post-translational events in pathology tissue samples.

The problem with this wishful thinking is the practical matter of the extreme difficulties of daily producing double-labeled and combined IHC/ISH assays in a reproducible and timely manner. The number of reagent variables, the labor intensity, and the prolonged assay time (8 to 12 hours) all combine to preclude everyday, practical success, so the procedure to date serves only as an occasional adjunct for demonstration purposes.

Seeking to perform these complex double and combined IHC and ISH assays in a medically timely diagnostic manner and seeking to reduce labor intensity, the coauthors have developed a kinetically driven, automated IHC and ISH device. This electronically controlled device leads to rapidly equilibrated reactions and a reduction in labor intensity and can give combined assays within 2 to 3 hours, thereby facilitating same-day diagnosis.

In this chapter we describe our experience with the development and utilization of this state-of-the-art, second-generation, kinetic-mode automatic staining device that automates both IHC and ISH staining. We first describe the mechanical principles involved in kinetic-mode IHC and ISH. We detail the biochemical features of multicolor chromogenic labeling. We further describe the methods of tissue preparation that are the initial prelude to optimized IHC and ISH assays. Finally, we illustrate a series of clinical cases to emphasize the clinical applicability of double labeling and combined IHC/ISH in diagnostic pathology.

METHODS

KINETIC-MODE AUTOMATED ASSAYS

To facilitate double labeling, including both IHC antigen colocalization and combined nucleic acid ISH and IHC assays, we use a kinetic-mode instrument (Ventana 320ES, IS) developed by the coauthors. As previously described, this instrument mixes and heats reagents, bathing tissue samples on glass slides in an electronically controlled, bar code−driven manner. This kinetic approach ensures a rapid reaction and achievement of equilibrium quickly. This rapid achievement of equilibrium ensures both a uniform test result and a timely clinical result. The gain in time and reduction in labor, aided by a multichromogen detection system (described later), greatly facilitates double labeling.

Although the mechanics of kinetic-mode IHC are fully described elsewhere,[1] several of the principles involved are relevant to this discussion of double labeling. The relevant principles include (1) compressed air mixing to overcome the "unstirred" layer effect, (2) liquid coverslipping to control evaporation, and (3) automated washing and agitation. We also include a description of some of the added features to allow automated ISH.

With manual methods we are accustomed to manipulating two factors: antibody concentration and incubation time; we ignore temperature and mixing. Yet the single greatest constraint to rapidly optimized IHC and ISH staining is a phenomenon known as the "unstirred layer" effect, whereby the initial reactants to solid-phase antigens or nucleic acids impede the simple diffusion of subsequent reactants.[2, 3] One solution to this phenomenon with manual methods has been to make time infinite (e.g., overnight incubation). Another solution, that of kinetic-mode IHC/ISH (driven by a desire to do assays in patient-priority mode), uses mixing and heating to aid Brownian motion. This "shake-and-bake" approach is central to the Ventana Medical Systems (VMS) immunostainer design.[1] In particular, it uses a column of compressed air directed at the tissue-bearing slide to give a vortexing effect and thereby overcome the impedance of the unstirred layer, greatly speeding reaction times.

The second adjunct to Brownian motion involves heating. Heat, while driving assay reactants and largely controlling denaturation and hybridization, also has the unwanted effect of enhancing reagent evaporation. Evaporation results in the true enemy of immunoassays: drying. Dryness precludes immunoreactivity and chromogen precipitation. Evaporation is overcome by using a liquid "coverslip," a lighter-than-water oil that is floated over the buffers on the tissue-bearing glass slide. This inert oil allows antibodies, oligonucleotide probes, and chromogens to pass through by simple gravity while also giving a cozy "pigs-in-a-blanket" effect precluding evaporation. This allows temperature cycling and nucleic acid denaturations and hybridizations in a "walkaway, hands-off" mode.

Regarding automated washing to improve sensitivity, this entails electronically controlled wash stations that pulse buffer onto the slide to produce a standing-wave effect. This improves sensitivity by reducing nonspecific staining or background noise. In solid-phase immunoassays, sensitivity is the net consequence of the signal-to-noise ratio, which in turn is related to the amount of specific stain relative to nonspecific background staining.[2, 3] Background staining is affected by both chemical (e.g., salt concentration) and physical factors (e.g., washing and agitation). The ability to wash and scrub out noise (akin to an automated dishwasher) is a key gain of automation; again, it is "commotion" that is pivotal.[1]

To go beyond protein and sugar IHC assays to DNA and RNA and to combined protein and nucleic acid assays, additional attributes were added to the automation process. In particular, to optimize nucleic acid denaturation and hybridization, discrete heating in a cyclic manner became a necessary critical attribute. This took the form of an etched-foil infrared heater manufactured in the same way as electronic printed circuit boards. This method provides an exceptionally uniform heat source with a very rapid response rate. A proportional, integral, differential (PID) temperature controller is employed to ensure precise temperature control. Another pivotal feature was the development of an electronically controlled stringency wash station that draws from separate low- and high-stringency stock wash solutions and electronically mixes operator-selected washes to a working stringency. This feature allows the operator to employ different wash stringencies for each slide of a run. By controlling the wash stringency in this way, multiple in situ assays using different probes and different conditions can be performed during the same run. Similarly, there is also electronic control for the time and temperature for each wash.

Bar code–driven options also allow the user the choice of different tissue pretreatment steps such as proteolytic enzyme digestion or treatment with dilute acids and control of the multichromogen detection cascade (described later). In this bar code–driven, kinetically controlled, automated mode of ISH, the turnaround time can be 2 to 3 hours or less, greatly compressing the more usual overnight or multiple-day process. This rapid turnaround greatly favors the iterative optimization of ISH assay development. With 13 to 14 key variables, the current manual method may take 2 to 14 days, only to learn of an unsatisfactory result. Manual ISH experiments can be frustrating since any of the variables (i.e., protease digestion concentration temperature and time of incubation; probe concentration, type, and guanine/cytosine (GC) content; denaturation time and temperature; hybridization time and temperature; detection reagent concentration and time; substrate temperature and concentration) are at play and it seems that any one can be askew at any time. The time lag and the large number of ambient variables frequently defeat the iterative process. In the controlled environment of bar code–driven ISH, the iterative process is favored by a 2- to 3-hour turnaround and the ability to keep 13 of 14 variables constant in a given experiment.

Finally, the ability of kinetic-mode IHC and ISH to perform assays *rapidly* is critical to combined IHC/ISH determinations. Combined protein/nucleic acid assays are not practical and applicable to diagnostic medicine unless they are timely and easily and reproducibly performed. The hands-off, walkaway manner of kinetic-mode IHC/ISH presents this prospect. In the end, the ultimate design goal was to facilitate dual staining for both nucleic acids and protein targets in individual cells. We sought the ability to relate chromosomal status, message, and protein product for a single gene within single cells. The intent is to determine the relationship of genotype to phenotype and consider alterations in transcription, translation, or post-translational events in a microanatomic context and to do so in a medically timely, diagnostic mode.

CHROMOGENIC DETECTION METHODS

A great variety of detection reagents and methodologies are available for IHC analyses. As illustrated (Fig 1) we use a four-step multichromogen

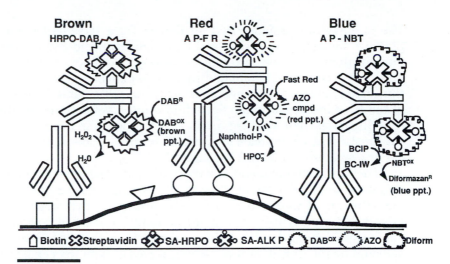

FIGURE 1.
Chromogenic detection cascade diagram (abbreviations in text).

detection method in a kinetic mode (VMS, Tucson, Arizona) that allows, as previously described, rapid and sensitive immunoassay in multiple colors (brown, red, blue).[1, 4, 5] The multichromogen capability facilitates antigen colocalization, as illustrated by the clinical examples in this chapter.

The Immunohistochemical Chromogen Detection Cascade
The first IHC detection step entails applying the primary antibody, which is either a monoclonal mouse antihuman hybridoma antibody or a polyclonal heteroserum from rabbits. If the primary antibody is directly linked to a chromogen or fluorochrome, specific detection is the result. However, sensitivity is limited. If, as in Figure 1, a secondary antibody and linked enzyme complex are added—the indirect method—then sensitivity is greatly increased. The specific signal is multiplied by both the added secondary antibody and the large size of the streptavidin-linked enzyme complex, which serves as a platform for chromogen dye precipitation and amplification.[4, 5]

The second step in our laboratory entails the use of a cocktail of secondary biotinylated (biotin- or vitamin B–labeled) antibodies. This cocktail, which includes two goat antimouse antibodies (anti-IgG and anti-IgM) and a goat antirabbit IgG,[1] ensures a broad spectrum of primary antibody detection. It allows the detection of both monoclonal and polyclonal primary antibodies in a single run. This broad detection also allows frozen sections, paraffin sections, and cytospin preparations to be run simulanteously—not frozen assays one day and paraffin runs the next. Thus in evaluating a lymphoma biopsy specimen (see Fig 10 later in this chapter), the pathologist may consider at once the findings related to monoclonal mouse antihuman IgG antibodies (e.g., pan-B and pan-T) and IgM antibodies (e.g., CD15) as well as polyclonal rabbit antihuman antibodies (e.g., CD3).

The third step entails the large streptavidin molecule linked to an enzyme—either horseradish peroxidase (HRPO) or alkaline phosphatase.

The streptavidin provides two attributes: (1) a large-molecular-weight platform for further reactivity and (2) a tight lock-and-key fit with the B vitamin (biotin) on the secondary antibody. The high affinity of the biotin–bacterial avidin (streptavidin) complex ensures that the IHC detection signal remains bound and does not diffuse. Incidentally, the strength of the B vitamin–avidin (an egg white protein very similar to streptavidin) link was first realized from a pathologic circumstance: feeding avidin-rich egg whites back to chickens resulted in beriberi from biological unavailability of bound B vitamin.[1]

The fourth step involves reactivity of the linked enzyme with a chromogen to produce a colored precipitated compound, or dye, that decorates the site of localization (e.g., cell surface). A chromogen is a compound that precipitates when oxidized/reduced or when combined with another compound.[4, 5] The oxidizing/reducing substance in this case is acted on by the linked enzyme, which serves as both the catalyst and the physical site of the oxidation:reduction process as shown in Figure 1. To produce a brown precipitate, we use a diaminobenzidine (DAB)-HRPO hydrogen peroxide (H_2O_2) solution. The H_2O_2 serves as the initial oxidizing substrate acted on by HRPO. To produce a red precipitate, naphthol serves as the substrate for the alkaline phosphatase enzyme, which reacts with the fast red chromogen to produce a stable red azo compound. To produce a blue precipitate, the nitroblue tetrazolium (NBT) chromogen is reduced by alkaline phosphatase acting on the 5-bromo-4-chloro-3-indolylphosphate (BCIP) substrate.[4, 5] These reactions in the chromogen cascade are illustrated in Figures 2, A and B, and 3. The reactants are also tabulated in Table 1.

The value of multiple chromogens is the ability to colocalize antigens (Figs 4 to 11). This reduces inferences from single-antigen analyses and allows the study of interactive molecules (e.g., p53 and BCL-2 (Figs 4 and 5) or allows the ability to differentiate lymphoid subpopulations (e.g., T-TIL vs. Ki67; Fig 6). The value of multiple enzyme systems also lies partly in the ability to avoid the periodic pitfall of confounding endogenous enzymes (neutrophilic peroxidase), pigments (e.g., melanin), or pseudoperoxidase (e.g., red blood cells).[1]

The In Situ Hybridization Chromogen Detection Cascade

The kinetic-mode ISH automated stainer uses either a chromogenic or fluorochrome system rather than a radioisotopic reporter system. This has the advantages of both reducing radiation-related risks and the need for waste disposal, and it also gives a permanent result that may be archived.

Although loss of sensitivity might be anticipated through the use of less sensitive chromogenic methods relative to radioactive systems, in practice there appears to be no loss of sensitivity because both the kinetic mechanics and built-in chromogen amplification favor the automated reaction. The speed of kinetic-mode ISH (2 to 3 hours) further favors the utility of automated ISH.

Regarding the chromogenic method, this entails the detection of specific cellular messenger RNA or DNA by using an appropriate complementary nucleic acid probe. This probe may be either double- or single-strand DNA, single-strand RNA, or an oligonucleotide. The probe is gen-

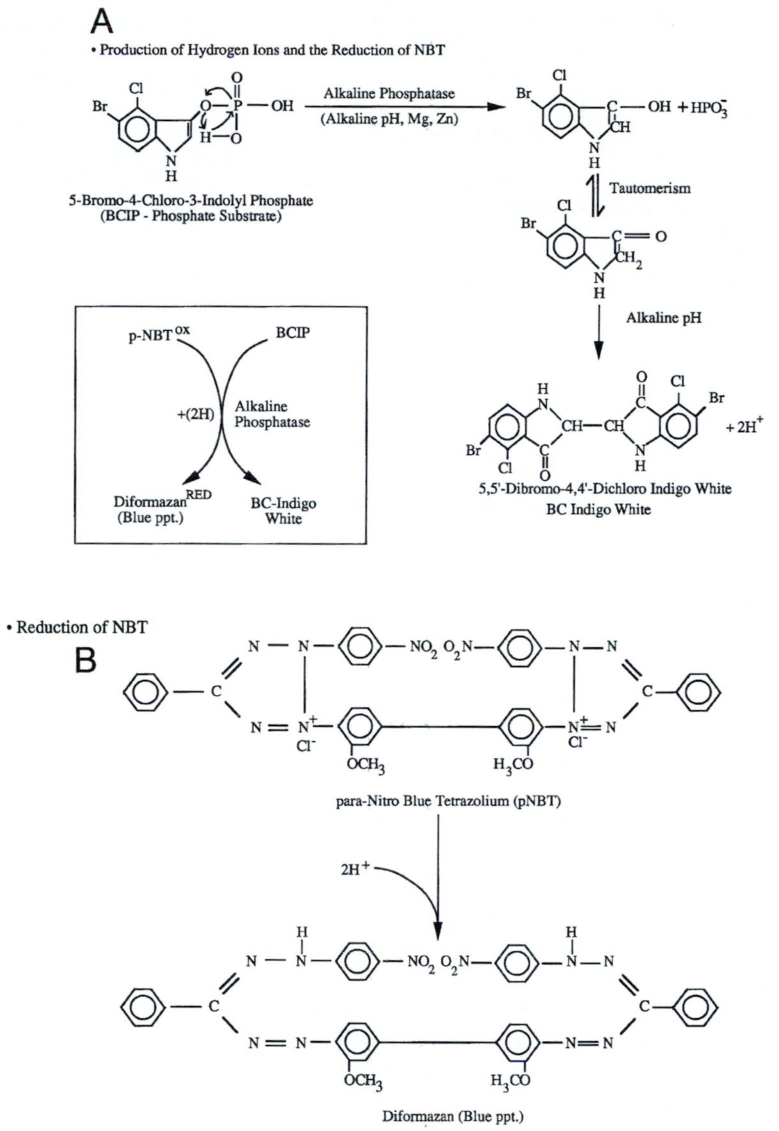
A
• Production of Hydrogen Ions and the Reduction of NBT
Alkaline Phosphatase
(Alkaline pH, Mg, Zn)
5-Bromo-4-Chloro-3-Indolyl Phosphate
(BCIP - Phosphate Substrate)
Tautomerism
Alkaline pH
5,5'-Dibromo-4,4'-Dichloro Indigo White
BC Indigo White
p-NBT ox
BCIP
+(2H)
Alkaline Phosphatase
Diformazan RED
(Blue ppt.)
BC-Indigo White
• Reduction of NBT
B
para-Nitro Blue Tetrazolium (pNBT)
2H+
Diformazan (Blue ppt.)

FIGURE 2.

A, fast blue alkaline phosphatase detection cascade, production of hydrogen ions. **B,** fast blue alkaline phosphatase detection cascade, reduction of nitroblue tetrazolium *(NBT)*.

erally labeled with immunogenic molecules (digoxigenin, dinitrophenol [DNP], fluorescein, or biotin). Bound probes are detected by using anti-digoxigenin or antibiotin antibodies covalently bound with an enzyme (e.g., alkaline phosphatase or HRPO) or a fluorescent molecule. In the example of the bound alkaline phosphatase, this reacts with a variety of substrates and results in a chromogenic reaction. Alternatively, if a biotin-labeled probe is used, either a streptavidin-conjugated enzyme complex or a free streptavidin:biotinylated enzyme detection cascade (similar to IHC) may be used. Ultimately, all these chromogen methodologies result

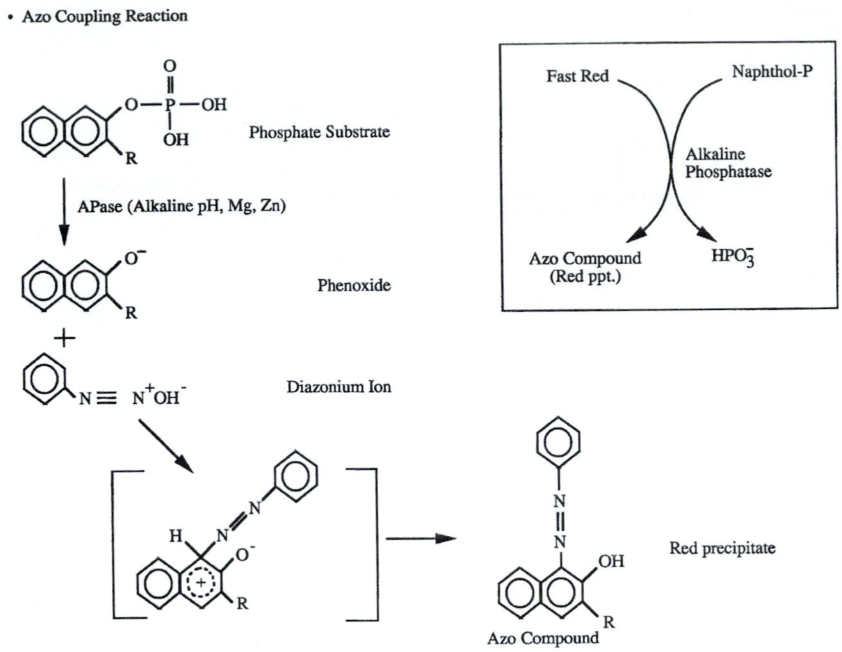

• Azo Coupling Reaction

FIGURE 3.
Fast red alkaline phosphatase detection cascade.

in a colored precipitate reaction product marking the location of probe incorporation into the specimen.

Regarding fluorochromes, these may be employed in the automated Ventana ISH device to perform chromosomal FISH assays. There are currently three types of probes available for FISH analysis: (1) probes for chromosome-specific repeat sequences (such as alpha satellite tanden repeats), (2) whole chromosome probes (also known as "paints"), and (3) probes for specific genes or loci. The probe or probe cocktail may be conjugated with a fluorochrome to effect direct immunofluorescence for subsequent visualization by any epifluorescence microscope. The clinical utility of FISH includes the detection of aneuploidy by centromeric FISH or chromosomal rearrangements (e.g., Philadelphia chromosome) relevant to a diagnosis of hematopoietic or lymphoreticular malignancies. With this method, single copies of the cellular oncogene c-*myc* have been detected in interphase lymphoid cell nuclei.

Combined Immunohistochemical/In Situ Hybridization Chromogen Detection

As illustrated in Figure 7, combined automated IHC protein and ISH RNA assays have been performed in an automated kinetic mode within 3.5 hours. This combined method runs the assays sequentially (e.g., first protein, then RNA) and takes advantage of the multicolored design of the tail-end chromogenic detection cascades (e.g., brown [DAB], red, and blue [NBT]).

TISSUE HANDLING AND PREPARATION

The quality of both the histologic and immunophenotypic data is highly dependent on the manner in which the tissue is handled and prepared.[1]

TABLE 1.
Key Components in the Detection Cascade

Chromogens
  DAB-HRPO*
    DAB solution: 3,3′-Diaminobenzidine tetrahydrochloride (DAB)
      When oxidized by HRPO in the presence of hydrogen peroxide, this
        chromogen produces a brown precipitate
    DAB—hydrogen peroxide solution: The substrate for HRPO
    Copper solution: Enhances the brown DAB precipitate
  Fast red—alkaline phosphatase
    Enhancer solution
      Magnesium chloride solution gives an enhanced signal-to-noise ratio
    Naphthol solution
      Solution for the alkaline phosphatase enzyme; dephosphorylation creates
        fluorescence
    Fast red A and B solutions
      A stabilized diazonium zinc salt results in a xylene-compatible precipitate
  Fast blue—alkaline phosphatase
    BCIP solution: 5-Bromo-4-chloro-3-indolylphosphate
      This substrate releases two hydrogen molecules when dephosphorylated
        by alkaline phosphatase
    NBT solution: p-Nitroblue tetrazolium
      A tetrazolium salt solution that yields a blue, xylene-compatible
        precipitate when reduced by the two hydrogen molecules
Inhibitors
  HRPO inhibitor solution
    Contains a mixture of hydrogen peroxide and sodium azide
    Inhibits red blood cell pseudoperoxidase and leukocyte myeloperoxidase
  Inhibitors of alkaline phosphate isoenzymes
    L-Homoarginine: Present in enzyme substrate solution and inhibits bone,
      liver, brain, and kidney isoenzyme; minimal effect on intestinal and
      placental isoenzymes
    Levamisole: Present in the enzyme substrate solution; a broad-spectrum
      inhibitor of nonintestinal isoenzyme

*HRPO = horseradish peroxidase.

In both histologic and tissue section IHC it is the technically poor slide
that defeats diagnosis. Quality slides begin with timely, adept gross tissue examination, appropriate tissue preservation (meaning both snap
freezing and fixation), followed by proper cutting and staining. Since absolutely fresh tissue is required for specialized procedures (like IHC,
genotyping, flow cytometry, or Northern blotting), we place a premium
on the pathologist going in the operating room or clinic to receive the
specimen within minutes of removal. This act alone may represent the
most difficult and important component of tissue diagnosis and IHC.[1]

After touch preparations are made, tissue preparation should include
fixation for histology. We fix "dime" thickness (2-mm) tissue slices in 10%
neutral buffered formalin for 4 hours and snap-freeze unfixed tissue for

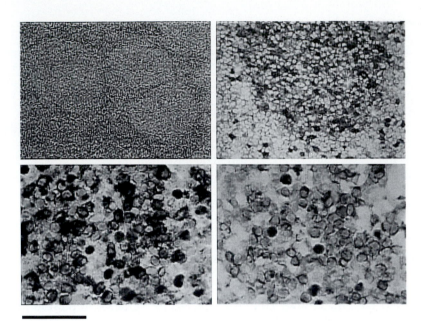

FIGURE 4.
Follicular lymphoma in clinical transformation. (See also color plate.)

IHC phenotyping. Since so many of the specialized procedures detailed earlier are needed for full tissue characterization, the habit of placing biopsy specimens entirely into formalin is no longer acceptable.

Snap freezing entails placing a pea- to almond-sized portion of tissue in OCT compound and freezing at −150°C for 10 seconds either in isopentane quenched in liquid nitrogen or in liquid nitrogen alone.[1] The tis-

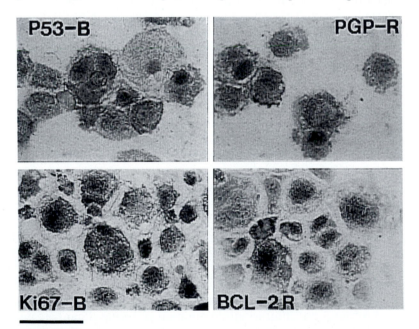

FIGURE 5.
Drug-resistant plasma cell myeloma. (See also color plate.)

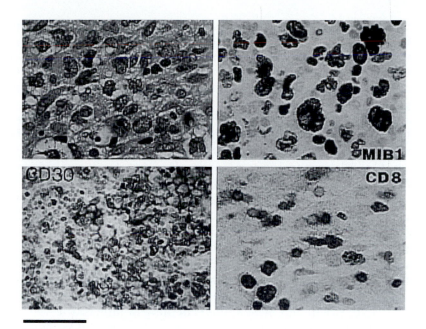

FIGURE 6.

Tumor and host response in anaplastic large cell lymphoma. (See also color plate.)

sue is then stored at −80°C in airtight containers. Sectioning tissue as thin as possible entails the use of sharp knives (e.g., disposable blades) to give 3-μm sections. For serial frozen section IHC, the sections are fixed in ice-cold (4°C) acetone for 10 minutes, air-dried, fixed again in 4°C acetone for another minute, and then air-dried again and stored in a dessicator

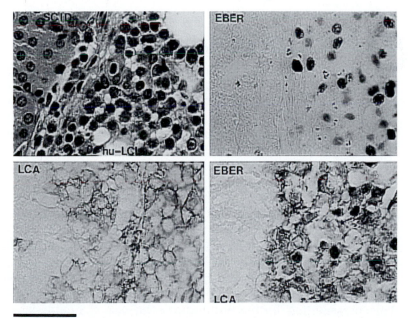

FIGURE 7.

Combined immunohistochemical assay for leukocyte common antigen and Ebstein-Barr virus transcripts in a human SCID mouse xenograft. (See also color plate.)

until stained and then stained. For most lymphoma typing, snap-frozen material is favored because it ensures maximum antigen preservation without epitope masking by cross-linking fixatives. Although it involves more time initially, snap freezing results in fewer antigen false-negative cases when compared with paraffin sections.[1] Full antigen preservation gives more reliable results.

Occasionally cytocentrifuge preparations are made to allow IHC or ISH analysis of body fluids. Typically this entails analysis of leukemia antigens in peripheral blood, cerebrospinal fluid, or marrow aspirate samples. These cytospin samples are also "double-dipped" in ice-cold acetone earlier.

In some instances, paraffin section IHC provides superior results. Certain antigens like cytoplasmic immunoglobulin in plasma cells benefit from the fixation process.[1] Paraffin IHC assays also benefit from superior morphologic detail, which may be critical in delineating single cells (e.g., CD15+ Reed-Sternberg cells). The major deficiency of paraffin IHC assays, the masking of epitopes by cross-linking fixatives, has been greatly obviated by the recent addition of new antibodies to fixative-resistant epitopes (e.g., L26, CD20) and new methods of antigen unmasking.[6]

Recently both tissue enzyme digests (e.g., trypsin or acid or alkaline proteinase digestions) and tissue acid hydrolysis via microwaving have greatly enhanced the detection of many antigens in paraffin sections, as illustrated later. Recent reviews suggest that specific combinations of enzyme and microwaving are relevant to specific epitopes and specific antibodies.[6] This arcane bit of immunoarcheology does afford the prospect of returning to stored banks of archival tissues and performing retrospective IHC analysis or allowing phenotyping of tissue fixed without additional frozen tissue.

CLINICAL AND RESEARCH APPLICATIONS

This section uses mainly patient cases and some human malignant cell lines to demonstrate the clinical value of double labeling. In the following case studies, double-labeling IHC and ISH assays are of benefit (1) in colocalizing interactive molecules relevant to pathogenesis, (2) in delineation of tumor and host response (immunosurveillance) phenotypes, (3) in localizing viral products, (4) in relating the RNA message to protein product, (5) in demonstrating unique diagnostic immunoarchitectural features, and (6) in demonstrating the clonality of tumor cells.

The cases are selected from one of the author's (T.M.G.) consultative hematopathology practice and lymphoma/myeloma research laboratory. The diagnoses were established within the rubric of the recently published Revised European American Lymphoma ("REAL") classification of lymphomas, of which the first author (T.M.G.) is a signatory.[7] The new "REAL" classification emphasizes integration of both morphologic and immunologic findings as pivotal to the proper diagnosis of lymphomas. This presentation further emphasizes the use of double-labeling multichromogen assays in tissue section to more fully integrate the immunologic, genetic, and morphologic features.

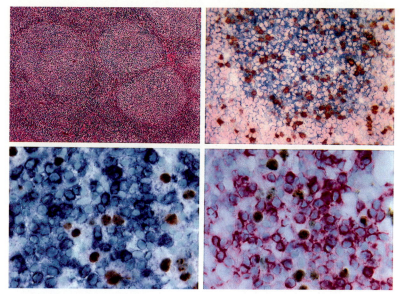

Plate I (see p. 88).

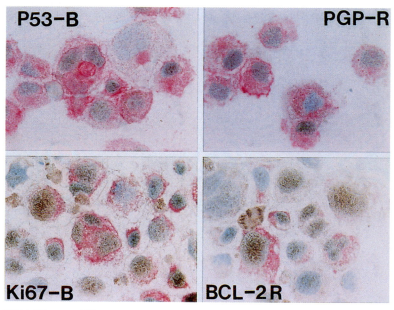

Plate II (see p. 88).

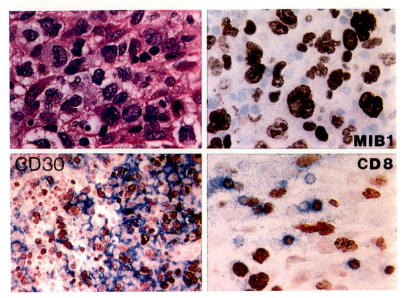

Plate III (see p. 89).

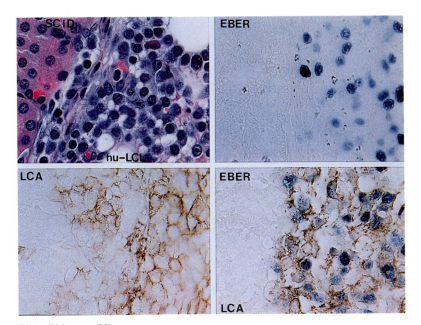

Plate IV (see p. 89).

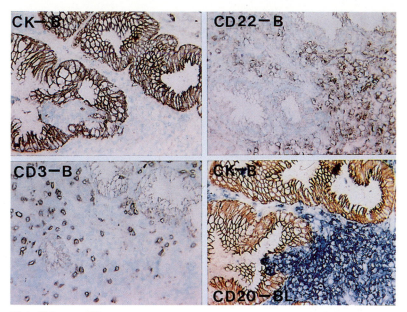

Plate V (see p. 95).

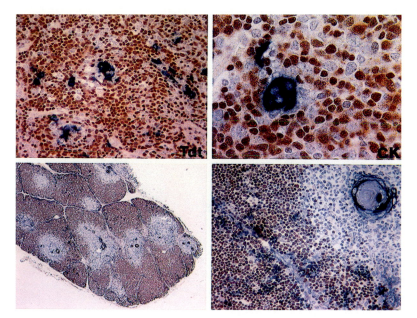

Plate VI (see p. 96).

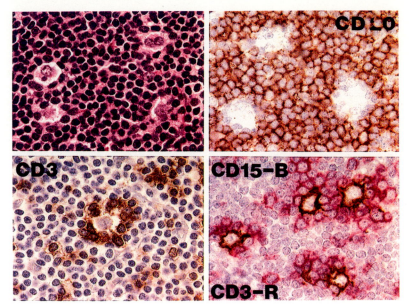

Plate VII (see p. 97).

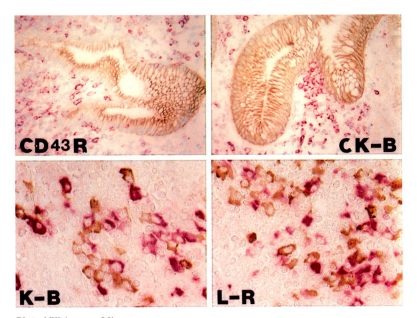

Plate VIII (see p. 98).

COLOCALIZATION OF INTERACTIVE MOLECULES

Figures 4 and 5 illustrate two pathologic circumstances in which oncogene interactions are revealed by double labeling: (1) follicular lymphoma in transformation and (2) drug-resistant plasma cell myeloma.

Follicular Lymphoma in Transformation

Figure 4 illustrates a lymph node biopsy specimen from a 44-year-old patient with a 10-year history of follicular small cleaved cell lymphoma (FSCL) in whom explosive disease developed. This double-labeled specimen reveals the key element of this transformation: p53 oncogene overexpression resulting in a loss of proliferative (Ki67) control. In the *upper left panel*, the histologic section reveals that the current lymphoma remains in a follicular pattern and retains a small cleaved cell type without evidence of histologic transformation to the large cell type. The histologic pattern then does not reflect the patient's altered clinical status. The *upper right panel* shows an immunophenotype finding relevant to clinical progression. In particular, the CD10+ follicular lymphoma cells have a high percentage of cells in the proliferative phase (Ki67-positive). The proportion of CD10+, Ki67+ cells is much higher than in the usual low-grade lymphoma (FSCL) and heralds a loss proliferative control.[8] The *lower left panel* shows that key oncogenes are at play. In particular, BCL-2 (blue)-expressive follicular lymphoma cells predominate. However, nuclear p53 staining (brown) reveals overexpressed, nonfunctional p53, which is not found in physiologic circumstances and has previously been noted in the pathologic circumstance of lymphoma.[9] In particular, p53 overexpression has been observed to characterize the clinical progression and transformation of follicular lymphomas.[9] The *lower right panel* colocalizes the nuclear proliferation antigen (Ki67) (nuclear brown) relative to the antiapoptotic oncogene BCL-2 (surface red). Notice that the BCL-2−bearing cells and Ki67-expressive cells appear to be mutually exclusive. This finding is consistent with the previous observation that BCL-2 generally confers resting, nonproliferative (Ki67-negative) status on lymphoid cells.[10] The Ki67+, BCL-2− lymphoma cells may be a newly emerged proliferative component heralding the patient's clinical progression of disease.[8]

This case illustrates the utility of IHC double labeling as an aid in the recognition of lymphoma progression and the scientific study of oncogene interactions as they may affect pathogenesis. Ultimately, the findings may also provide a therapeutic rationale for alternative therapy inasmuch as the finding of an increased component of cells in cycle suggests that cycle-specific therapy would be rational.

Drug-resistant Plasma Cell Myeloma

This example is chosen to illustrate the use of a cell line as a means to study oncogene interactions, including effects on nononcogenic molecules (e.g., p-glycoprotein).

The illustrative myeloma line (8226 Dox 40) was derived from a 61-year-old patient with plasma cell leukemia. It was selected with doxorubicin for permanent multidrug resistance (MDR)-associated p-glycoprotein overexpression by Dalton et al.[11] This cell line also coexpresses p53 and BCL-2. In Figure 5, the double labeling shows simultaneous expression of both p53 and p-glycoprotein. It also demonstrates BCL-2 overexpression in relation to the nuclear proliferative antigen (Ki67). The latter circumstance, in contrast with the preceding follicular lymphoma, suggests that the usually mutually exclusive BCL-2 and Ki67 may be coexpressed in some pathologic circumstances. The illustrated combined expression of p53 and p-glycoprotein is remarkable since p53 has been suggested as a transcriptional factor for activation of the *MDR1* gene, which leads to p-glycoprotein overexpression.[12] Although the 8226 Dox 40 cell line seems to confirm the link between p53 and p-glycoprotein, analysis of other myeloma cell lines (e.g., U226) and clinical samples indicates an inconsistent relationship with independent expression more common.[13, 14] Nonetheless, this myeloma line is a useful aid in the study of interactive oncogenic molecules, and this study is greatly facilitated by double labeling, as illustrated.

TUMOR AND HOST RESPONSE PHENOTYPES

A major advantage of tissue section IHC analysis is that the topography of the tissue is intact and morphologic and immunologic features can be integrated to allow microanatomic analysis of the immunoarchitecture. By this means, morphologically obvious neoplastic and antineoplastic immune reactive components (immunosurveillance) can be analyzed for their separate chemistries. In particular, a proliferative lymphoid immunosurveillance response may be measured directly within tumor biopsy samples. Specifically, the T-cytotoxic cells (CD8+) within the tumor, known as tumor-infiltrating lymphocytes (T-TILs), correlate with lymphoma containment, and an absence of CD8+ T-TILs has been associated with invariant lymphoma relapse.[15] As illustrated in Figure 6, a double-labeled T-TIL phenotype may specifically delineate whether T-TILs are proliferative (Ki67+) or not (Ki67−) and answer whether a proliferative immunosurveillance response is present. Ki67 is an antibody proliferation antigen found in proliferating cells in cycle (G_1 to G_5) and not resting cells (G_0). As shown, a strongly proliferative (MIB1+, a Ki67 antibody detecting a formalin-resistant epitope) CD8 population admixed within the CD30+ lymphoma cells is likely evidence of active immunosurveillance.

The case illustrated in Figure 6 is that of a 58-year-old physician with an anaplastic large cell lymphoma with a high proliferative rate (>80% MIB1+) who is alive and well 7 years after diagnosis and seemingly cured. As shown by double labeling, these CD30+ lymphoma cells were highly (>80%) proliferative (MIB1+), which predicted a poor outcome.[16] However, not all the proliferative cells are CD30+. As shown, double labeling for CD8 vs. the Ki67 paraffin active antibody (MIB1) reveals that many CD8+ (blue) T-TILs were also Ki67-positive (brown). As shown, many of these CD8 cells are in a proliferative phase, which is indicative of an intact immunosurveillance response. This case illustrates the efficacy of double labeling in characterizing the host response to neoplasia. Interestingly, prior studies of the poor prognosis of highly proliferative lymphoma note a high early death rate (82%) within 1 year. The 1-year survivors (18% of patients) may then experience a definitive cure, as in this patient.[16] A proliferative CD8+ T-TIL phenotype may be hypothesized as predicting this unusual favorable outcome.

RELATING THE RNA MESSAGE TO PROTEINS AND LOCALIZING THE VIRAL MESSAGE

The same principles of kinetic-mode immunoassay apply to tissue assay of DNA and RNA hybridizations. Furthermore, combined IHC and ISH assays are possible with the same mixing and heating device noted earlier with IHC. By dual staining for both nucleic acids and protein targets in individual cells and tissue biopsy specimens, we may gain the ability to relate chromosomal status, message, and protein product for a single gene within single cells. This delineates the relationship of genotype to phenotype and considers alterations in transcription, translation, or post-translational events in a microanatomic context. The speed of the automated kinetic mode may allow combined IHC and ISH assay very rapidly, as in 3.5 hours for the combined assay in the example that follows.

Figure 7 illustrates an example of combined automated IHC and ISH assay. This figure shows the presence of the Epstein Barr virus (EBV) in a human large cell lymphoma xenograft transplanted into a SCID mouse.[17] The EBV nuclear RNA transcript of EBER2 was hybridized with a 40-mer oligonucleotide digoxigenin-tailed antisense probe. The bound oligonucleotide probe was then detected by using an alkaline phosphatase–conjugated antidigoxigenin antibody with BCIP/NBT as the substrate (blue). In the *upper left panel*, as shown by standard histology, the mouse renal cells are pink (eosin rich) and the human lymphoma cells are purple (hematoxylin rich). In the *upper right*, the human cells, not mouse cells, are expressing EBER2 transcripts. In the *lower left*, the human cells express the CD45 glycoprotein (leukocyte common antigen [LCA]) not found on mouse cells. In the *lower right* we have combined protein IHC and EBER2 nucleic acid ISH showing single-cell localization of both products in human cells. The mouse cells not susceptible to the human EBV serve as the appropriate double-negative control. Lack of reactivity with a control sense strand EBER2 probe further ensured the specificity of EBER2 transcript detection. This combined IHC/ISH assay was performed sequentially on the kinetic-mode instrument in a total running time of 3.5 hours, with the LCA assay preceding the EBER2. This example highlights the power of combined nucleic acid/protein assays in a microanatomic context. The aforementioned multichromogen detection system is the basic building block behind this dual-assay capability.

The critical technical factors in extending automated IHC to combined ISH of nucleic acids was the addition of a discrete infrared cycling heater that facilitates nucleic acid denaturation at high temperatures (e.g., 95°C), RNA denaturation at 65 to 75°C, and nucleic acid hybridizations at 42 to 45°C. As illustrated, tissue section ISH for RNA transcripts is greatly facilitated by this means; however, with the addition of fluorochromes to increase sensitivity, the same instrumentation may allow rapid FISH assays of chromosomal DNA. By this means, interphase human cells may be assessed for chromosomal status. For example, separate fluorochromes may be used to tag respective cosmid probes to the X (female, green, fluorescein isothiocyanate [FITC]) and Y (male, red, Spectrum Orange, Uysis) chromosomes. In another example (not shown), a cosmid to the p53 gene may confirm the intactness of the p53 alleles in a follicular lymphoma or leukemia tissue sample. Contrariwise, it may delineate an allotypic deletion event with loss of one or both p53 genes. In the latter circumstance of p53 allotypic deletion, overexpression of mutant p53 without a contravailing normal p53 gene effect has been shown to herald a lethal clinical outcome.[18] As cited in this example, the marriage of p53 protein and chromosomal DNA data, as facilitated by rapid double labeling, is essential to full clinical understanding.

DEMONSTRATING UNIQUE MICROANATOMIC AND IMMUNOARCHITECTURAL FEATURES

This group of cases illustrates the use of double labeling to delineate unique microanatomic patterns that may be pathognomonic of specific diseases. The illustrative examples include (1) the clustered invasion by B cells within mucosa epithelium in mucosa-associated lymphoma (MALToma), (2) the presence of keratin-bearing epithelial islands admixed with immature (terminal deoxynucleotidyl [Tdt]-positive) T cells in lymphocytic thymoma, and (3) the distinctive T-cell rosettes surrounding Reed-Sternberg cells in Hodgkin's disease. In these instances, the diagnosis is not based on a single marker but on the microanatomic relationship of one cellular subpopulation relative to another.

Clustered B-cell Invasion of Epithelium in Mucosa-associated Lymphoma

Mature B-cell lymphoma (see Fig 8) characteristically involves epithelial-lined organs, especially the gastrointestinal tract, salivary glands, orbit, breasts, conjunctiva, and skin.[19] The pathogenic finding is the lympho-epithelial lesion representing invasion of the epithelial mucosa by a cluster of monoclonal B cells.[19] These epithelial lacunae of lymphocytes signal epithelial invasion highly analogous to the clustered cutaneous T cells (Pautrier's microabcesses) found in mycosis fungoides. In MALToma, the normal epithelial or glandular structures are focally disrupted, an observation made more obvious by keratin stains (see Fig 8). The invading B cells predominate over admixed T cells. Although each component (lymphoid and epithelial) is apparent in separate serial sections of the biopsy, the demonstration of clustered B-cell invasion of keratin-positive epithelium is most readily seen by double labeling, as shown in Figure 8. Clearly, the double-labeled colocalization of CD20 B-cell antigens and keratin in epithelial cells reduces the difficulty of using inferences from single-slide assays and adds to the assertion of the phenotypic diagnosis.

Assertive diagnosis of this entity has now taken on substantial clinical import since there are now reports of triple antibiotic therapy resulting in ablation and remission of gastric MALTomas.[20] Recent study suggests that gastric MALTomas may be antigen driven and related to the presence of *Helicobacter pylori* and that antibiotic therapy directed at the antigen may remove the antigenic stimulus with resolution of the lymphoproliferative process.[21]

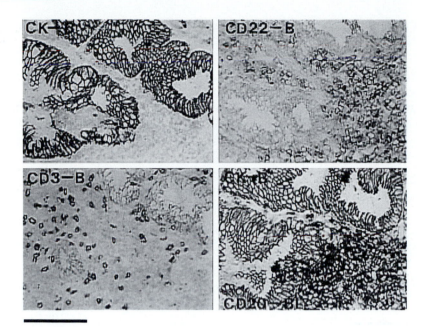

FIGURE 8.
Gastric mucosa—associated lymphoma. (See also color plate.)

Epithelial Islands in Lymphocytic Thymoma

A serious error in diagnosis may result when lymphocytic thymoma is confused with an immature T-cell lymphoblastic lymphoma. Since lymphocytic thymoma has a mediastinal location and a predominance of immature T cells expressing Tdt like lymphoblastic lymphoma, the prospect for confusion between the two is considerable on both a clinical and laboratory level. Because lymphoblastic lymphoma requires elaborate multidrug chemotherapy with central nervous system (CNS) prophylaxis and thymoma requires simple surgery, a mistake in diagnosis has profound therapeutic consequences and constitutes a serious error in medical judgment.[22]

As illustrated in Figure 9, the key to deciphering this difference is histologic and immunologic detection of the keratin-positive epithelioid cell component admixed within the Tdt-positive T cells. Figure 9 demonstrates with double labeling the simultaneous Tdt and cytokeratin expression in a lymphocytic thymoma. Double labeling with a single slide to illustrate both cellular components results in a visually more obvious diagnostic admixture. Also shown in the lower panel of the same figure is the same slide control of normal thymus, which shows the normal physiologic admixture of epithelium and Tdt-positive thymic cells. We consider same-slide controls as pivotal to quality control validation of double-labeled assays.

The case illustrated in Figure 9 is that of a 35-year-old male who had a large anterior mediastinal mass. The biopsy material obtained from mediastinoscopy was interpreted as a lymphoblastic lymphoma. A consulting hematopathologist concurred with this diagnosis, but only after confirming that cytokeratin staining on the formalin-fixed material was negative. Chemotherapy, including CNS prophylaxis, was initiated. However, since a thymoma was strongly suspected on radiologic grounds, use of

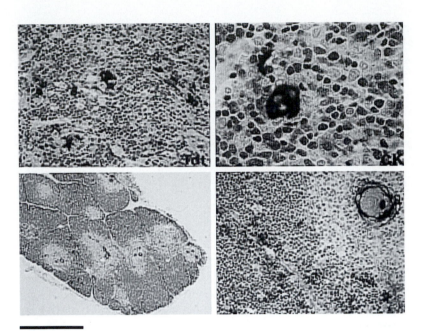

FIGURE 9.
Lymphocytic thymoma. (See also color plate.)

an antikeratin antibody following microwaving and antigen retrieval revealed the striking epithelial islands within Tdt-bearing lymphocytes mirroring the phenotype of a normal thymus and precluding the diagnosis of lymphoblastic lymphoma. This case emphasizes the importance of using more than one marker in immunophenotypic diagnosis. It also emphasizes the importance of antigen unmasking, particularly in the context of a negative finding.

T-Rosettes in Hodgkin's Disease
Another example of a distinctive immunoarchitectural feature that heralds a specific diagnosis is shown in Figure 10. In this instance of lymphocyte-predominant Hodgkin's disease, the CD15-positive Reed-Sternberg variant cells are characteristically surrounded by T-cell rosettes composed of CD57+, CD3+ natural killer (NK) cell–like T cells.[23] As shown by double labeling, these NK-like T cells occur preferentially as clusters surrounding Reed-Sternberg cells with surrounding B cells. This clustered CD57+ state differs conspicuously from the state in physiologic lymph nodes, where CD57+, CD3+ NK-like T cells occur as scattered single cells within B-cell germinal centers.[23] As revealed by double labeling, it is the presence of decidedly nonphysiologic CD57+ rosettes that suggests an altered immunosurveillance status in this form of Hodgkin's disease. T-rosetting of Reed-Sternberg cells suggests effective T-cell immunosurveillance or T-cell containment of neoplasia.[23] The operative word is containment, not elimination of Hodgkin's neoplasia, thus suggesting an element of aberrant neoplastic B- and T-cell symbiosis. Immunosurveillance aside, the large CD15+ polylobated cells surrounded by CD57+ T-cell rosettes present a pathognomonic IHC phenotypic pattern for lymphocyte-predominant Hodgkin's disease.[23] In particular, it is phe-

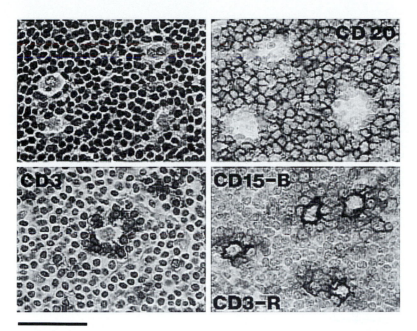

FIGURE 10.

T-rosettes in lymphocyte-predominant Hodgkin's disease. (See also color plate.)

notype merged with microanatomy (e.g., immunoarchitectural pattern) that is diagnostic.

DEMONSTRATING MONOCLONALITY

Fundamentally, lymphoma represents a single immortalized clone, and as such it is a paradigm of monoclonality.[24] In neoplastic B-cell lymphomas of a mid to late phase of differentiation, there is generally light- and heavy-chain immunoglobulin restriction, thus indicating monoclonal B-cell proliferation.[25] In normal tissue section assay for immunoglobulin it is the absence of one light and several heavy chains that heralds the light- and heavy-chain restriction of monoclonal B-cell proliferation. Usually this finding is inferred from single sections each separately stained for κ, λ, μ, γ, α, and δ immunoglobulin chains.[25] Double-labeled immunoglobulin assays greatly aid judgment of clonality by reducing inferences, as shown in Figure 11. As shown in the *lower panels*, the κ chains (brown) and λ light chains (red) occur in simultaneity, indicating polyclonality. This polyclonal cytoplasmic immunoglobulin determination was made in a group of submucosal plasma cells found in a case of chronic gastritis that (as shown in the *upper panels*) contained mainly T cells (CD43+, red) that rarely, singly invaded adjacent gastric mucosa (keratin-positive, brown). This case of chronic gastritis with its scattered T cells and admixed polyclonal plasma cells represents chronic gastritis found in the follow-up endoscopic gastric biopsy specimen of a triple-antibiotic–treated MALToma, as described in Figure 8. After 14 months of follow-up, although the MALToma has not returned, a low level of smoldering gastritis persists, as shown. Arguably this is a triple-antibiotic–"cured" gastric MALToma.[20, 21] Certainly in this instance, double-

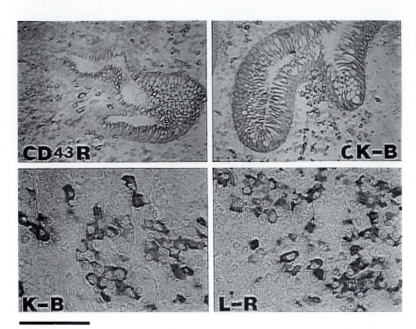

FIGURE 11.
Polyclonal plasma cells in chronic gastritis following antibiotic treatment for mucosa-associated lymphoma. (See also color plate.)

labeled immunoglobulin determination added to the assurance of a non-malignant polyclonal condition.

FUTURE CONSIDERATIONS

Combined kinetic-mode automated IHC and ISH/FISH assay heralds a new field of endeavor wherein genotype may be correlated with phenotype on a single-cell level. It anticipates the analysis of gene amplification relative to message and protein products in the microanatomic context. It anticipates a potential litany of aberrant discrepancies between gene, message, and protein. A case in point would be the recently reported discrepancies between BCL-2 message and protein. As revealed by Cleary et al.,[26] BCL message without BCL-2 protein may occur in some anatomic compartments (e.g., germinal center), whereas adjacent areas like the mantle zone may show the obverse (BCL-2 protein without BCL-2 message). These discordances are thought to reflect the sometime staggered, halting process of gene to protein expression. The ability to study comparable phenomena in an anatomic context and in a variety of both physiologic and pathologic circumstances suggests a new field of study uniquely open to pathologists.

REFERENCES

1. Grogan TM, Casey TT, Miller TP, et al: Automation of immunohistochemistry, In Weinstein RS (ed): *Advances in Pathology and Laboratory Medicine*, vol 6. St Louis, Mosby, 1993, pp 253–283.
2. Jackson TM, Ekins RP: Current practice and potential advantages of fluores-

cent Eu3+ chelates as non-radioisotopic tracers. *J Immunol Methods* 87:13–20, 1986.

3. Verkman AS, Dix JA: Effect of unstirred layers on binding and reaction kinetics at a membrane surface. *Anal Biochem* 142:109–116, 1984.

4. McGadey J: A terazolium method for non-specific alkaline phosphatase. *Histochemie* 23:180–184, 1970.

5. Eadie MJ, Tyrer JH, Kukums JR, et al: Aspects of tetrazolium salt reduction relevant to quantitative histochemistry. *Histochemie* 21:170–180, 1970.

6. Cattoretti G, Svurmeijer A: Antigen unmasking in formalin-fixed paraffin-embedded tissues using microwaves: A review. *Adv Anat Pathol* 2:2, 1995.

7. Harris NL, Jaffe ES, Stein H, et al: A revised European-American classification of lymphoid neoplasms: A proposal from the International Lymphoma Study Group. *Blood* 84:1361–1392, 1994.

8. Grogan TM, Miller TP: Immunobiologic correlates of prognosis in lymphoma. *Semin Oncol* 20:58–74, 1993.

9. Sander C, Yano T, Clark HM: P53 mutation is associated with progression in follicular lymphomas. *Blood* 82:1994, 1993.

10. Korsmeyer SJ: BCL-2 initiates a new category of oncogenes: Regulators of cell death. *Blood* 80:879, 1992.

11. Dalton WS, Grogan TM, Rybski J, et al: Immunohistochemical detection and quantitation of P-glycoprotein in multiple drug resistant human myeloma cells. Correlation with level of drug resistance and drug accumulation. *Blood* 73:747–752, 1989.

12. Chin KV, Ueda K, Pastan I, et al: Modulation of activity of the promoter of the human MDR1 gene by RAS and P53. *Science* 255:459–462, 1992.

13. van der Zee AGJ, Hollema H, Suurmeijer AJH, et al: Value of p-glycoprotein, glutathione s-transferase pi, c-erbB-2, and p53 as prognostic factors in ovarian carcinomas. *J Clin Oncol* 13:70–78, 1995.

14. Rouby SE, Thomas A, Costin D, et al: p53 gene mutation in B-cell chronic lymphocytic leukemia is associated with drug resistance and is independent of MDR1/MDR3 gene expression. *Blood* 82:3452–3459, 1993.

15. Lippman SM, Spier CM, Miller TP, et al: Tumor-infiltrating T-lymphocyte in B-cell diffuse large cell lymphoma. *Mod Pathol* 3:361–367, 1990.

16. Miller T, Grogan T, Dahlberg S, et al: Prognostic significance of the Ki67 associated proliferation antigen in aggressive non-Hodgkin's lymphomas: A prospective Southwest Oncology Group Trial. *Blood* 83:1460–1466, 1994.

17. Hersh EM, Grogan TM, Funk CY, et al: Suppression of human lymphoma development in the SCID mouse: Prevention by IMEXON therapy. *J Immunother* 13:77–83, 1993.

18. Döhner H, Fisher K, Bentz M, et al: P53 gene detection predicts for poor survival and non-response to therapy with purine analogs in chronic B-cell leukemias. *Blood* 85:1580–1589, 1995.

19. Isaacson P, Spencer J: Malignant lymphoma of mucosa-associated lymphoid tissue. *Histopathology* 11:445, 1987.

20. Wotherspoon A, Doglioni C, Diss T, et al: Regression of primary low-grade B-cell gastric lymphoma of mucosa-associated lymphoid tissue type after eradication of Helicobacter pylori. *Lancet* 342:575, 1993.

21. Hussell T, Isaacson P, Crabtree J, et al: The response of cells from low-grade B-cell gastric lymphomas of mucosa-associated lymphoid tissue to Helicobacter pylori. *Lancet* 342:571, 1993.

22. Grogan T, Spier C, Wirt DP, et al: The immunologic complexity of lymphoblastic lymphoma. *Diagn Immunol* 4:81–88, 1986.

23. Kamel OW, Gelb AB, Shibuya RB: Leu 7 (CD57) reactivity distinguishes nodular lymphocyte predominance Hodgkin's disease from nodular sclerosis

Hodgkin's disease, T-cell rich B-cell lymphoma and follicular lymphoma. *Am J Pathol* 142:541, 1993.

24. Tonegawa S: Somatic mutation of antibody diversity. *Nature* 302:575, 1983.
25. Stein H, Bank A, Tolksdorf G: Immunohistologic analysis of the organization of normal lymphoid tissue and non-Hodgkin's lymphomas. *J Histochem Cytochem* 28:746, 1980.
26. Chleq-Deschamps C, Le Brun D, Huie P, et al: Topographical dissociation of BCL-2 messenger RNA and protein expression in human lymphoid tissues. *Blood* 81:293–298, 1993.

Epitope Retrieval (Unmasking) in Immunohistochemistry

Hector Battifora, M.D.

Chairman, Division of Pathology, City of Hope National Medical Center, Duarte, California

Randa Alsabeh, M.D.

Division of Pathology, City of Hope National Medical Center, Duarte, California

Kay Ann Jenkins, H.T.(A.S.C.P.), H.L.T.

Division of Pathology, City of Hope National Medical Center, Duarte, California

Allen Gown, M.D.

Department of Pathology, University of Washington School of Medicine, Seattle, Washington

T he diminution or loss of immunoreactivity experienced by formalin-fixed tissues, a well-recognized obstacle to the clinical application of immunohistochemistry, was initially thought to be irreversible.[1] For this and other reasons, many replacement, formalin-free fixatives have been proposed, and some of these are now commercially available. Although these new fixatives often yield better antigen preservation, they do not seriously challenge formalin in terms of morphologic quality and low cost. Most histopathology laboratories continue to use formalin as their fixative of choice.

Digestion of formalin-fixed tissue sections with proteases enhances their immunostaining.[2] Although this finding provided evidence that the effect of formalin on antigens was reversible, its impact in diagnostic immunohistochemistry was tempered by the fact that few antigens appeared to benefit from the procedure.

Thanks to recent advances in "antigen" retrieval methodology, formalin fixation is enjoying a comeback as a reliable immunohistochemistry fixative. Shi et al. discovered that boiling tissue sections in a microwave oven in denaturing solutions containing metal salts[3] restored their immunoreactivity with several antibodies. Although initially met with skepticism,[4] their report gave rise to many publications claiming improvements in the heat-induced "antigen" retrieval method.[5–12] The advantages of heat-induced retrieval over protease digestion methods quickly became evident inasmuch as it improves the reactivity of a much larger proportion of antibodies than do enzyme-based methods. As a welcome bonus, heat-induced retrieval has made retrospective immunohis-

Advances in Pathology and Laboratory Medicine, vol. 8
© 1995, Mosby–Year Book, Inc.

tochemical studies based on formalin-fixed, paraffin-embedded archival tissues much more reliable than in the past. Although still in the process of evolution, the heat-induced retrieval method has now gained a strong foothold in many immunohistochemistry laboratories.

Without attempting a comprehensive review of the rapidly expanding heat-induced "antigen" retrieval literature, herein we endeavor to answer some relevant questions about fixation and "antigen" retrieval and offer useful technical hints gleaned from our daily experiences as well as ongoing experimentation.

WHY IS FORMALIN A PROBLEM?

Although the precise chemical reactions responsible for formalin fixation are not well understood, it is clear that formalin—as well as other aldehydes—fixes tissues by blocking amido groups and by forming methylene bridges between several amino acids in polypeptides. By this mechanism, formalin effects a variable number of chemical links not only within a protein molecule but also with adjacent proteins. Thus linked proteins are believed to block access of antibodies to their target epitopes, a process often called "masking" of antigens. Only loosely attached formaldehyde is dislodged by washing the fixed tissues; formaldehyde bound to amino acids is not removable by prolonged washing.[1] On the other hand, formaldehyde reacts with sugars by forming unstable hemiacetals, and these are readily broken down by washing. This may explain why polysaccharide-rich epitopes are generally resistant to formalin fixation.

Formaldehyde, a gaseous compound when pure, readily hydrates into methylene glycol and its polymers when diluted in water. Only a very small proportion of free formaldehyde remains available to react with amino acids.[1, 13] Although it quickly penetrates tissues, methylene glycol is not by itself a fixative. Once inside the tissue, it dehydrates to free formaldehyde by a slow process, measurable in hours, that has been termed "a clock reaction" by physical chemists.[13] This slow chemical process can be moderately accelerated only by high temperature, low pH, and high formalin concentrations. After 12 hours in formalin, only a few of the amino acid sites available to react have been bound by formalin. Saturation of all reactive sites requires at least 48 hours of immersion in neutral formalin at the standard 4% dilution and room temperature. Thus most tissues stated to be fixed in formalin are, in fact, only partially fixed by formalin. What occurs in daily practice is that the fixation begun in formalin is completed (via coagulation) in the alcohol solutions used to dehydrate the tissue before embedding. Thus hybrid fixation consisting of amino acid cross-linking and protein coagulation—in variable degrees—is the norm in most histopathology laboratories. Not surprisingly, tissues fixed in formalin for only a few hours reveal excellent preservation of antigenic sites since alcohol is an excellent immunohistochemical fixative. Conversely, tissues fixed for several days are more difficult to stain by immunohistochemistry (Fig 1). The success of some fixation protocols employing microwave ovens may be due to the fact that they use minimal exposure to formalin and maximal exposure to alcohol.[14] Because such hybrid fixation causes variable levels of antigen preserva-

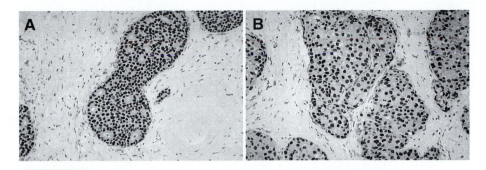

FIGURE 1.

Sections of breast containing ductal carcinoma in situ and stained with antibody to estrogen receptor (1D5). **A,** fixed for 6 hours in formalin; **B,** fixed for 72 hours in formalin. Both samples embedded in a single paraffin block and stained simultaneously in an automatic stainer (BioTek) after microwaving in 0.5M tris(hydroxymethyl)-aminomethane (TRIS) buffer at pH 10.0 for 10 minutes. Note the marked reduction in intensity of the reactivity that is entirely attributable to the excessive fixation time.

tion, it results in unreliable quantitative immunocytochemical assays. Fortunately, as we will discuss later, heat-induced retrieval has somewhat reduced this problem. Nonetheless, we strongly recommend standardizing fixation protocols for all specimens to diminish this source of variability of immunostains. In our laboratory we avoid fixation beyond 24 hours by modifying the cycling of the automatic processor so that the tissue cassettes initially placed in formalin move to the first alcohol bath before they reach the 24-hour limit and stay in alcohol until the processing restarts. This scheme is particularly important during weekends. It helps to know that prolonged exposure to ethanol (even for months) does not impair the immunoreactivity of most diagnostically important antigens.

WHAT ABOUT OTHER FIXATIVES AND ANTIGEN (EPITOPE) RETRIEVAL?

Coagulating fixatives such as absolute ethanol, Carnoy's, and methcarn excel in the preservation of most antigens and rarely benefit from any sort of epitope retrieval procedure. In fact, with most of these fixatives, the use of retrieval methods is often counterproductive because it tends to introduce serious morphologic artifacts. Nonetheless, we have observed that methcarn-fixed tissues will show enhanced immunoreactivity with antibody MIB-1 after brief exposure to heat-induced retrieval. Incidentally, this finding supports the idea that heat-induced retrieval does more than just break formaldehyde-induced cross-links.

Tissues fixed in fixatives that combine formalin and other coagulating agents (B5, Bouin's) are generally improved by the use of epitope retrieval. Frequently, with these fixatives the intensity of immunoreactivity is not greatly enhanced, but the amount of background staining is reduced by the retrieval procedure and interpretation of results is facilitated.

WHAT IS THE DIFFERENCE BETWEEN UNMASKING AND RETRIEVAL?

The term *unmasking* is used by some people to apply to protease-induced methods of immunoreactivity enhancement and the term *antigen retrieval* when denaturing or heat-based methods are used. This assumes that the two methods differ in mechanism of action, probably a valid assumption. Other terms such as "antigen rescue" or "tissue unfixing" may be considered satisfactory since the mechanisms by which such methods operate are not yet clearly understood.

Perhaps of greater importance is the fact that we now know that two monoclonal antibodies directed to different epitopes of the same molecule may differ substantially in their response to "antigen" retrieval procedures.[15] For example, immunostains with the monoclonal antibody to estrogen receptor H222 (Abbott Laboratories) are worsened by heat-induced retrieval and improved by protease digestion, whereas stains with the antibody ER-1D5 (Immunotech, Dako) to a different domain of the same molecule are greatly improved by the use of heat-induced retrieval and only marginally by enzyme-based methods. Thus it is probably more accurate to refer to the methods as *epitope* retrieval rather than as "antigen" retrieval. For the aforementioned reasons, we will use the terms *protease-induced epitope retrieval* (PIER) and *heat-induced epitope retrieveal* (HIER) henceforth in this text.

WHAT IS THE CURRENT ROLE OF PROTEASE-INDUCED EPITOPE RETRIEVAL?

Huang et al. in 1976 showed that protease digestion of formalin-fixed, paraffin-embedded tissue sections could be used to demonstrate immunoglobulins by immunofluorescence.[2] These studies were soon expanded to include other molecules and the immunoperoxidase method as well.[15] The enzyme-based retrieval method increased the range of useful antibodies that could be applied to routinely fixed paraffin-embedded tissue in diagnostic pathology and has since enjoyed wide acceptance.

Unfortunately, PIER has several drawbacks, the most important one being that only a limited number of antibodies benefit from it. Additionally, the method is difficult to reproduce because of, among other reasons, lot variation in the activity of commercially available enzymes. Moreover, adjustment of the digestion time to compensate for the length of exposure to fixative is critical for optimal results.[16] Another drawback of PIER is that briefly fixed tissues are easily overdigested, with resulting loss of morphologic detail.[16]

The choice of protease, its concentration, and its time of digestion is largely empirical. In our experience, it is more important to optimize the use of a couple of proteases rather than use a broad range of enzymes. In fact, many papers claiming advantage of one enzyme over another are often short in scientific rigor. We have found that nearly identical results can be obtained with many proteases, provided that each is used at their optimal concentration, pH, temperature, and incubation time.[16] For these reasons, it is not wise to strongly recommend any protease over another. Each laboratory must experiment with the smallest possible set of enzymes to identify their optimal conditions for application. Nonetheless, an epitope may be susceptible to the digestive action of one enzyme and may still benefit from the use of a different one, presumably incapable of cleaving it.

Since the advent of HIER, the need to use digestive enzymes for epitope retrieval in our laboratories has sharply decreased. This is because many antibodies that benefit from the use of a protease step are equally (or better) improved by HIER. Because HIER is simpler, less expensive, and easier to reproduce, we prefer it when either method works.

TABLE 1.
Antibodies for Which We Routinely Use Enzymatic Epitope Retrieval*

Antibodies to	Clone	Supplier	Enzyme	Time (min)	Temp, °C	Buffer/pH
Actin	HHF35	Dako†	BioTek	10	25	BioTek
CD21	1F8	Dako	Biotek	10	25	BioTek
CD40	B-B20	Serotec	BioTek	10	25	BioTek
Collagen type IV	CIV22	Dako	Pronase[1]	3	25	TRIS, 0.15%, 7.4
Factor VIII	F8/86	Dako	Trypsin[2]	12	37	PBS, 0.15%, 7.2
Factor XIII	N/A	Calbio	BioTek	10	25	BioTek
LMP	CS1-CS4	Dako	BioTek	10	25	BioTek
Neurofilament	2F11	Dako	Trypsin	5	37	PBS, 0.15%, 7.2
CD15	Leu-M1	B-D	Trypsin[1]	10	25	TRIS, 0.05%, 7.65
CMV	CCH2	Dako	Trypsin[1]	10	25	TRIS, 0.05%, 7.65
Neutrophil elastase	NP57	Dako	Trypsin[1]	10	25	TRIS, 0.05%, 7.65
Epithelial glycoprotein	Ber Ep4	Dako	Pronase[2]	20	25	PBS, 0.01%, 7.4
EGFR	31G7	Ciba	Pronase[2]	20	25	PBS, 0.01%, 7.4
CD3	Polyclonal	Dako	Pronase[2]	20	25	PBS, 0.01%, 7.4
Adenovirus	MAB805	Chem	Pronase[2]	20	25	PBS, 0.01%, 7.4
Melanoma	HMB45	Dako	Pronase[2]	10	25	PBS, 0.01%, 7.4
Melanoma	HMB50	Gown	Pronase[2]	15	25	PBS, 0.01%, 7.4
GCDFP-15	D6	Signet	Ficin	10	25	PBS 7.4

*Note: This table combines the preferences of two laboratories (A.G. and H.B.) at the time of writing this article.
†Dako = Dako Corp., Carpinteria, Calif; BioTek = Santa Barbara, Calif (proprietary protease cocktail and proprietary buffer, prediluted, for automated processors); Serotec = Serotec Ltd. (London) = Harlan Bioproducts (Indianapolis); Pronase[1] = Sigma no. P5147; TRIS = tris(hydroxymethyl)-aminomethane; Trypsin[2] = Cat. no. 103140, ICN Biochemicals, Aurora, Ohio; PBS = phosphate-buffered saline; Calbio = Calbiochem, San Diego; LMP = latent membrane protein; Trypsin[1] = type II, Sigma no. T8128 (St Louis); B-D = Becton Dickinson, Mountainview, Calif; CMV = cytomegalovirus; Pronase[2] = Calbiochem no. 53702; EGFR = epithelial growth factor; Ciba = Ciba Corning (formerly Triton Diagnostics, Alameda, Calif); Chem = Chemicon, Temecula, Calif; Gown = Dr. Allen Gown, University of Washington; Signet = Signet Laboratories, Dedham, Mass; Ficin = Sigma no. F4125.

Table 1 shows the antibodies for which we still use PIER in our laboratories, the type of enzyme used, and other technical details.

HEAT-INDUCED EPITOPE RETRIEVAL: A BRIEF HISTORY

Shi et al. reported that tissue sections of formalin-fixed tissues, when heated in a microwave oven in a lead thiocyanate solution for several minutes, showed improved immunoreactivity to a number of antibodies.[3] Concerns about the hazards of boiling toxic metallic salts spawned a search for less dangerous buffer solutions. Cattoretti et al. reported that excellent enhancement of reactivity could be obtained with the innocuous 0.01M citrate buffer at slightly acidic pH.[17] Although Cattoretti and associates' initial report was concerned only with retrieval of the Ki67 antigen with a new monoclonal antibody (MIB-1), it was soon determined that many other epitopes of a large proportion of clinically useful antibodies were also improved by the procedure.[5–7, 18]

In our laboratories we tested the efficacy of the modified microwave-based HIER on routinely processed, formalin-fixed tissues against a panel of 85 monoclonal and polyclonal antibodies.[6] The standard technique required the tissue sections to be immersed in a 0.01M citrate buffer, pH 6.0, and exposed for 8 to 12 minutes in a microwave oven. For most of the antibodies, this resulted in significantly improved immunostaining, often reducing nonspecific background and permitting the use of higher primary antibody dilutions. Where appropriate, the microwave technique was compared with standard digestion schemes (e.g., pronase or trypsin) and found to yield comparable or superior results in many cases (Fig 2). We found that a few of the monoclonal antibodies were reactive only when HIER was used (Fig 3). Table 2 summarizes our results and reflects the current use of HIER in our laboratories. For 7 antibodies, no consistent enhancement was seen with this technique (Table 3), and for 5 other antibodies, the technique either did not improve or gave worse immunostaining (Fig 4, Table 4).

Alternative methods of heating and different buffers were tried by sev-

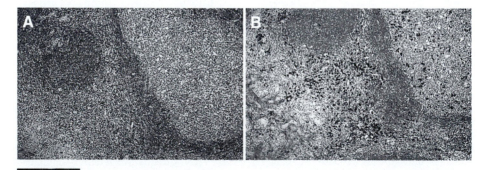

FIGURE 2.
Sections of normal tonsil fixed for 24 hours in formalin, embedded, and stained together for κ light chains (Dako, polyclonal). **A,** pretreated with trypsin; **B,** microwaved for 12 minutes in 0.01M citrate buffer, pH 6.0. Plasma cells stain with far greater intensity in the section treated by heat-induced epitope retrieval than in the enzyme-treated one.

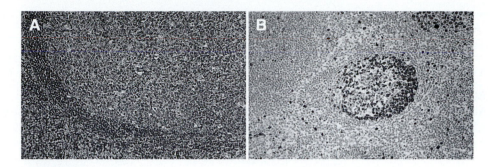

FIGURE 3.

Sections of normal tonsil fixed for 24 hours in formalin and stained with anti-body to Ki67 antigen MIB-1 (Immunotech). **A,** untreated slide; **B,** slide treated by heat-induced epitope retrieval (HIER) in citrate buffer. Note the strong staining of the proliferating compartment in the germinal center only in the HIER-treated slide.

eral researchers with results similar or better than those of previous studies.[8-11, 19-23] As a result, there is already quite a selection of HIER procedures, no doubt contributing to bewilderment among practicing pathologists.

EPITOPE RETRIEVAL USING MICROWAVE OVENS

The microwave oven, a convenient tool in the kitchen as well as in the laboratory, has to be used with caution. As anyone familiar with TV dinners knows, microwave ovens leave much to be desired in terms of uniformity of heat distribution. It is known that the volume of the load and the geometry of the container play a major role in heat distribution when using microwave ovens. An automatic rotating tray is recommended because it helps to reduce this problem. We use specially designed plastic slide carriers and containers (Tissue Tek slide holder, Cat. no. 4465-A, Miles, Inc., Elkhart, Ind) and use a uniform number of slides and amount of liquid. Moreover, the slide containers are always placed over marked spots on the rotating carousel for added reproducibility.

Two or three 4- to 6-minute cycles of microwaving are used by most laboratories. The optimal time period for normally fixed (24 hours or less) tissues should be determined by trial and error by every laboratory because there are many variables. It is important to replenish the level of the buffer solution in between cycles, preferably with distilled water. It is important to slowly cool the slides to room temperature while they are still in the buffer and never allow the slides to air-dry. Failure to observe these rules may introduce false-negative results. It is thought that the cooling period allows for restoration of the tertiary configuration of the heat-denatured proteins.

If we know that the specimen has been in formalin for over 48 hours, we add one or two more cycles to the normal time. The immunoreactivity of tissues fixed for long periods of time can be intensified to closely approximate that of optimally fixed tissues by this approach.

Although microwave ovens designed for the laboratory are capable of producing more uniform and better controlled temperature than com-

TABLE 2.
Antibodies for Which We Currently Use Heat-Induced Epitope Retrieval

Antibodies to	Supplier*	Clone	Dilution†
ACTH‡	Dako	Polyclonal	1:500
Actin, smooth muscle§	Gown	CGA7	1:1,000
Alpha heavy chains	Dako	Polyclonal	1:2,000
Androgen receptor	Monosan	F39.4.1	1:500
bcl-2	Dako	124	1:25
CD15	B-D	MMA	1:50
CD20	Dako	L26	1:200
CD30	Dako	BerH2	1:50
CD31	Dako	JC/70A	1:50
CD34	B-D	My10	1:50
CD45	Dako	PD7/26,2B11	1:50
CD45RA	Dako	4KB5	1:400
CD45RO	Dako	UCHL1	1:100
CD57	B-D	HNK1	1:20
CD99 (p30/32-MIC2)	Dako	12E7	1:200
CD99 (O13)	Signet	O13	1:50
CEA	B-M	CEJ065	1:3,500
CEA	Dako	A5B7	1:25
CEA	Dako	*Polyclonal*	1:2,000
c-erbB-2	Ciba	*Polyclonal*	1:200
Chromogranin A	B-D	LK2H10	1:1,200
Chromogranin A	Gown	PHE5	1:16,000
Cytokeratin, HMW	Dako	34βE12	1:75
Cytokeratin, LMW	B-D	CAM5.2	1:20
Cytokeratins, pan	Battifora	KC2 cocktail	1:300
Cytokeratins, pan	B-M	AE1/AE3 cocktail	1:50
Cytokeratins, pan	Sun	AE3	1:200
Cytokeratins, LMW	Sun	AE1	1:200
Desmin	Dako	D33	1:100
Epithelial membrane antigen	Dako	E29	1:50
Estrogen receptor	Dako, Immunotech	1D5	1:30
FSH	Biogenex	*Polyclonal*	1:40
Gamma heavy chains	Dako	*Polyclonal*	1:500
Gastrin	Dako	*Polyclonal*	1:6,400
Gross cystic disease fluid protein 15	Signet	D6	1:600
Growth hormone	Biogenex	*Polyclonal*	1:20
GFAP	Dako	6F2	1:100
GFAP§	Gown	GFP8	1:500
Hepatitis C	Immunotech	Tordjii-22	1:250

Continued.

TABLE 2 (cont.).

Antibodies to	Supplier*	Clone	Dilution†
Human chorionic gonadotropin	Dako	Polyclonal	1:2,400
Insulin	Dako	Polyclonal	1:3,200
Kappa light chains	Dako	Polyclonal	1:2,000
Ki67 antigen§	Immunotech	MIB-1	1:50
Ki67 antigen§	Dako	Ki67	1:40
Lambda light chains	Dako	Polyclonal	1:8,000
Luteinizing hormone	Biogenex	Polyclonal	1:20
Mu heavy chains	Dako	Polyclonal	1:500
Neuron specific enolase	Dako	BBS/NC/VI-H14	1:2,000
p53	Onc Sci	Pab1801	1:4,000
p53	Dako, Novocastra	D07	1:1,000
Placental alkaline phosphatase	Dako	Polyclonal	1:800
Progesterone receptor	Transbio	MPR1	1:500
Progesterone receptor	Transbio	MPR3	1:500
Progesterone receptor	Abbott	PgR-ICA	1:40
Progesterone receptor	Novocastra	PgR1A6	1:50
Prolactin	Biogenex	Polyclonal	1:40
Prostatic acid phosphatase	Dako	Polyclonal	1:8,000
Prostatic-specific antigen	Biogenex	8	1:5
Retinoblastoma gene product	UBI	3H9	1:200
S100 protein	Dako	Polyclonal	1:2,000
Somatostatin	Dako	Polyclonal	1:1,000
Synaptophysin	Dako	Polyclonal	1:100
Synaptophysin	B-M	SY38	1:10
Thyroglobulin	Dako	Polyclonal	1:5,000
TSH	Dako	Polyclonal	1:1,000
Villin§	Immunotech	BDID$_2$C3	1:20
Vimentin	Dako	V9	1:20
VIP	Dako	Polyclonal	1:1,000

*Vendors: Abbott = Abbott Laboratories, Abbott Park, Ill; B-D = Becton Dickinson, Mountainview, Calif; B-M = Boehringer-Mannheim, Indianapolis; Biogenex = Biogenex Laboratories, San Ramon, Calif; Ciba = Ciba-Corning, formerly Triton Diagnostics, Alameda, Calif; Dako = Dako Corporation, Carpinteria, Calif; Gown = antibody obtained from Dr. Gown, University of Washington; Immunotech = Immunotech, Inc., formerly AMAC, Westbrook, Me; Monosan = Monosan Laboratories, Uden, The Netherlands; Novocastra = Novocastra Laboratories, Newcastle-upon-Tyne, UK; Onc Sci = Oncogene Science, Uniondale, NY; Oxoid = Oxoid Laboratories, Ogdenburg, NY; Signet = Signet Laboratories, Dedham, Mass; Sun = Antibody supplied by Dr. Henry Sun, Department of Dermatology, SUNY, New York; Transbio = Transbio Laboratories, Paris; UBI = Upstate Biotechnology, Waltham, Mass.

†As supplied by the vendor. For antibodies designated from Gown, this represents dilution of ascites fluid. The anti-pan cytokeratin antibody KC2 is a cocktail of the following clones: AE1, CAM5.2, UCD/PR 10.11, and 35βH11; this represents dilution of a working solution that consists of mixed ascites, supernatants, and purified antibodies. For antibodies showing Dr. Sun as supplier, this represents dilution of hybridoma supernatant.

‡ACTH = adrenocorticotropic hormone; CEA = carcinoembryonic antigen; HMW = high molecular weight; LMW = low molecular weight; GFAP = glial fibrillary acidic protein; TSH = thyroid-stimulating hormone; VIP = vasoactive intestinal polypeptide.

§This antibody works well only with heat-induced epitope retrieval.

TABLE 3.
Antibodies Inconsistently Enhanced by Heat-Induced Epitope
Retrieval

Antibodies to	Supplier*	Clone	Working Dilution
Actin, muscle specific	Dako	HHF35	1:2,000
Calcitonin	Dako	polyclonal	1:800
CD68	Dako	KP1	1:500
Cytokeratin 20	Dako	K_s20.8	1:100
Cytokeratin, LMW	Dako	35βH11	1:200
Epithelial glycoprotein	Dako	BerEp4	1:50
Collagen, type IV	Dako	CIV22	1:25

*See the vendor listing at the bottom of Table 2.

mercial ovens, they are expensive and are not considered to be essential for HIER applications. It is more important to observe the aforementioned precautions and find the optimal microwaving time for each oven. We recommend that the oven be used at its maximum wattage for better reproducibility of results. It is probably better to use a microwave oven with a magnetron capable of operating at 700 to 800 W. The addition of a water load as a heat sink has been suggested as a means to obtain more consistent temperatures within the oven. For an erudite discussion of the mechanisms of microwave heating, the reader is directed to a paper by Boon and Kok.[24]

It must be emphasized that as is also the case with protease-mediated epitope retrieval, one must use very clean slides coated with a strong adhesive such as silane to prevent tissue sections from peeling off the slide during the heating step.

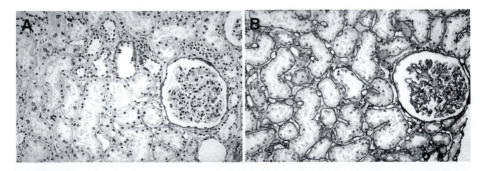

FIGURE 4.
Sections of normal kidney fixed in formalin for 72 hours and stained simultaneously with a monoclonal antibody to collagen type IV (Dako, CIV22). **A,** section pretreated with heat-induced epitope retrieval in citrate buffer, standard procedure; **B,** section digested with pronase by our usual procedure (see Table 1). Note the superior definition and intensity of basal lamina in the protease-treated slide.

TABLE 4.

Antibodies Not Enhanced or Worsened by Heat-Induced Epitope Retrieval

Antibodies to	Supplier*	Clone	Working Dilution	Comments
Lewis[y]	Signet	Bg8	1:5,000	No effect
Estrogen receptor	Abbott	H222	1:10	Worsened
GCDFP-15	Signet	D6	1:600	No effect
Melanoma antigen	Dako	HMB-45	1:750	No effect
Neutrophil elastase	Dako	NP57	1:200	Worsened

*See the vendor listing at the bottom of Table 2.

HOW ABOUT USING OTHER SOURCES OF HEATING?

Does the microwave radiation per se influence the results of HIER, or is it solely a function of heat in a hydrated solution? Data from our laboratories and others seem to indicate that the radiation itself does not significantly add to the results. Although much remains to be learned about the mechanisms involved in HIER, it seems evident that other sources of heating may be used with equal or better results. Alternate sources of heating that have been used are hot plates, dry ovens, autoclaves, and pressure cookers.[8–10] Ongoing experimentation with all of these allows us to offer the following preliminary findings.

REGULAR SOURCES OF HEAT

Hot plates and dry ovens are capable of giving results closely approximating those of microwave ovens, but only with some antibodies. It seems clear from the literature and our own experimentation that the conditions produced by this source of heating cannot match those of microwave ovens. Because microwave ovens heat the tissues directly by molecular agitation, it is likely that temperatures higher than boiling are developed at the tissue section level. Further support for this explanation is provided by the excellent results of HIER with systems such as pressure cookers that raise temperatures above the boiling point.

AUTOCLAVES AND PRESSURE COOKERS

These are largely interchangeable inasmuch as both work by raising temperatures above the boiling point. Thus in theory, they could approximate the effect of microwave oven HIER. Indeed, performing HIER with pressure cookers and wet autoclaves has been reported to give identical or superior results to microwave oven HIER.[8, 10] Our own experimentation supports these results (see later). Autoclaves and pressure cookers offer the following advantages over microwave ovens: (1) they are unaffected by the number of slides or the shape or size of the container; (2) they provide uniform heating, regardless of placement; (3) because there is no evaporation, a single heating-cooling period can be used; (4) when automated immunostainers are used, the slides can be placed directly in their metal racks, thus reducing steps and saving time. They have the following disadvantages: (1) handling of the hot pressure cookers has some hazards and may not be readily accepted by laboratory personnel; (2) cooling of slides takes more time than in the microwave oven unless, as some recommend, the pressure cooker is cooled in running water, thus increasing the hazards[9]; and (3) autoclaves, although easier to use, are considerably more expensive than household microwave ovens.

We have compared, over a large range of antibodies, microwave HIER with autoclave HIER in citrate buffer (unpublished data). For the latter, we used a standard laboratory autoclave set at humid heat, 120° C for 10 minutes, with an additional 20 minutes for cooling. Under these conditions, most of the antibodies tested gave superior results in terms of morphologic preservation, intensity of immunoreactivity, freedom from background, and reproducibility with autoclave HIER. In these experiments we compared autoclave HIER with our standard microwave oven HIER protocol. Thus for those immunohistochemical laboratories with easy access to an autoclave, this modification is a good, even preferable alternative to microwaving.

STEAMERS

The use of steamers has recently been proposed as a convenient HIER source with advantages over the microwave method.[24a] We have tested a large series of antibodies comparing the results of conventional microwave HIER with steaming HIER and autoclave HIER. We used a household Black & Decker steamer, model #HS90/HS10, in these experiments. The slides were steamed in citrate buffer solution, pH 6.0, for 20 minutes and allowed to cool off for 5 minutes before proceeding with the immunostaining. The results—which were read by an observer (H.B.) blinded to the method used—were entirely comparable with those of the autoclaved and microwaved slides. In fact, with some antibodies (TdT, myeloperoxidase, L26, Bc12, and CD30), the steamer epitope retrieval was judged to be slightly superior to those of the microwave HIER. Thus these results suggest that steamers offer a convenient and inexpensive approach to HIER, without the drawbacks of other methods.

WHAT BUFFER SHOULD WE USE FOR HEAT-INDUCED EPITOPE RETRIEVAL?

Many substitute solutions to avoid the toxic salts employed by Shi et al. in their original communication have been proposed. Many of these not only solve the toxicity problem but also offer better retrieval with a broader set of antibodies. Selection of the ideal solution (like the ideal protease) still rests upon the eye of the beholder. Nonetheless, although the search goes on, some clear winners have emerged. In a previously published study[6] we compared the now popular 0.01M citrate at pH 6.0 with (1) distilled water, (2) 0.01M sodium bicarbonate at pH 7.8, (3) 0.05M tris(hydroxymethyl)-aminomethanol (TRIS) buffer at pH 7.49, (4) 0.02M magnesium chloride at pH 5.51, and (5) 0.02M sodium chloride at pH 4.37. In these experiments we found citrate buffer to be superior, although all buffers, even distilled water, were better than no treatment at all. We then concluded that 0.01M citrate at pH 6.0 was the recommended buffer for routine HIER.

Recent publications have shown that at least for some antibodies, other buffer solutions may be more effective than citrate buffer in restoring the immunoreactivity of formalin-fixed tissues.[19, 21, 22, 25, 26] Among these solutions are high-molar urea, TRIS buffer at pH 10.0, and periodic acid. In view of these recent developments, we conducted additional experiments comparing the 0.01M citrate buffer at pH 6.0 with (1) 3M urea, (2) 4M urea, (3) 0.5M TRIS buffer at pH 10.0, and (4) periodic acid. As in previous studies, an assortment of tissues each fixed in neutral buffered formalin for 6, 12, 24, 48, and 72 hours and for 1 week were used in the study. All tissue samples were embedded in a single paraffin block to ensure uniform comparison. Triplicate sections were subjected to epitope retrieval for periods of 5, 10, and 15 minutes each in the same microwave oven and stained together in an automatic tissue stainer (Techmate 1000, BioTek Solutions, Santa Barbara, Calif). When appropriate, a section was treated with the protease giving optimal immunoreactivity for the particular antibody. We tested 17 commonly used antibodies in diagnostic immunohistochemistry and evaluated the results for intensity of immunoreactivity, specificity, background staining, and morphologic preservation. Particular attention was placed on assessing the capability of each buffer to recover immunostaining in overfixed tissues as well as on quality of morphology and the freedom from excessive background staining.

Citrate buffer gave the best overall results with the majority of the antibodies used in the study. Periodic acid gave poor morphologic preservation and was not further investigated. However, both molar urea solutions and TRIS buffer gave superior results with some of the antibodies in terms of intensity of the immunoreaction or freedom from background staining (Fig 5, Table 5). Yet the differences were not large enough to be considered a potential source of false-negative results when compared with citrate buffer. These results suggest that for most ordinary diagnostic uses, at the present time citrate buffer is the most convenient and saf-

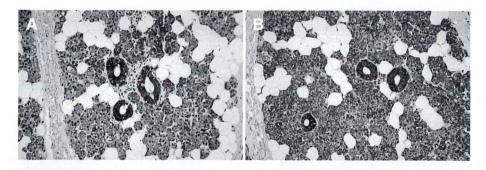

FIGURE 5.

Sections of normal salivary gland fixed in formalin for 24 hours and stained with antibody CAM-5.2 to low-molecular-weight cytokeratins. **A,** pretreated with heat-induced epitope retrieval (HIER) in citrate buffer; **B,** pretreated with HIER in 3M urea. Notice the moderately higher intensity of reactivity in the urea-treated section.

TABLE 5.
Comparison of Three Buffers*

Antibody†	Clone	Supplier	3M Urea‡	0.01M Citrate, pH 6.0	TRIS, pH 10.0
Estrogen receptor	1D5	Dako, Immunotech		Superior	
Progesterone receptor	PgR1A6	Novocastra		Superior	
CD20 (L26)	L26	Dako		Superior	
Prostate-specific antigen	8	Biogenex		Superior	
Prostatic acid phosphatase	Polyclonal	Dako		Superior	
CD45RO	UCHL1	Dako		Superior	
CD45 (LCA)	PD7/26,2B11	Dako	Superior§		Superior§
Cytokeratin	AE1	Dr. Sun	Superior§		Superior§
Cytokeratin	CAM5.2	B-D			Superior
Vimentin	V9	Dako			Superior
Leu-22			Superior§		Superior§
Bcl-2	124	Dako	Superior§		Superior§
S100 protein	Polyclonal	Dako			Superior
Smooth muscle actin			Superior§		Superior§
Neurofilament	2F11	Dako	Superior		

*A result was interpreted as superior when the intensity of the immunoreactivity was higher or the background lower (or both).
†Same antibodies and dilutions as shown in Table 2.
‡Urea, 4M, gave similar results.
§Indicates that results were judged equivalent and interchangeable and better than citrate buffer.

est buffer solution to employ. Nonetheless, for highest enhancement of immunostaining and thus sensitivity, it may be necessary to use alternative buffers in specific circumstances.

WHAT ARE THE ADVERSE EFFECTS OF HEAT-INDUCED EPITOPE RETRIEVAL?

There are a number of adverse effects that can result from HIER treatment of tissue. For example, for many antibodies there is a narrow window of heat application time that can be used effectively; prolonged heat application can result in destroyed antigenicity. Most forms of HIER treatment result in "burn-like" alterations in the appearances of tissue, especially in areas of loose connective tissue and fat. In addition, there may also be problems of tissue adherence to the slide following HIER; indeed, the "rate-limiting step" in optimizing HIER may be the "chewing up" of the tissue rather than the loss of immunoreactivity. A further consequence of HIER can be a loss of uptake by tissues of various counterstains (e.g., methyl green). Finally, there is evidence that HIER application, particularly in buffers at low pH, may induce false-positive immunostaining. For example, we frequently observe intense nucleolar staining when using HIER and antibody to CD20. Since the expected pattern of immunoreactivity with this antibody is predominantly one of cytoplasmic membrane staining, this HIER-caused artifact is inconsequential.

Perhaps a more important concern is that the sensitivity of the immunostaining may be raised by HIER to a point where biologically (or diagnostically) insignificant levels of antigen are being detected. In our experience, this has not been a problem for most of the antibodies currently used for diagnostic purposes in our laboratories. For example, the use of HIER for estrogen receptor immunohistochemical assay leads to approximately 10% more positive cases than enzyme-based immunohistochemical methods or the cytosol-based dextran-coated charcoal assay. However, a more robust correlation with overall survival is noted in the HIER-assayed group, which suggests that the extra positive cases are of biological significance.[27, 28] Chromogranin A is now detectable in a much larger proportion of high-grade neuroendocrine carcinoma such as oat cell carcinoma than before the use of HIER. We consider this to be advantageous inasmuch as recognition of high grade neuroendocrine carcinoma is facilitated. Nonetheless, an upward adjustment of the threshold of interpretation of what constitutes a positive result may become necessary in some instances. In a way we have been doing this all along since we usually adjust thresholds to compensate for the quality of antigen preservation. For example, it is not unusual to see positive immunostaining for cytokeratins in reticular cells in lymph nodes when methcarn-fixed frozen sections are studied.[29, 30] On the other hand, one rarely sees positivity in these cells in formalin-fixed tissues unless the fixation time is quite short or HIER is employed. In a sense HIER is bringing the level of detectability of many antigens to that observable in optimally treated, i.e., alcohol-fixed, specimens.

WHAT ABOUT COMBINING PROTEASE- AND HEAT-INDUCED EPITOPE RETRIEVAL?

In general, it is not a good idea to mix these two methods. Although we have found some synergism when combining methods, this applied to only a few antibodies and particularly with overfixed tissues. Major drawbacks of this approach are that the morphologic preservation is often poor (Fig 6) and keeping the sections attached to the slide is difficult.

CONCLUSIONS

Clearly the search for ideal conditions for HIER will continue. Until a clear winner is discovered, we recommend the use of citrate buffer as the routine buffer and either microwave ovens, autoclaves, or pressure cookers as heating sources.

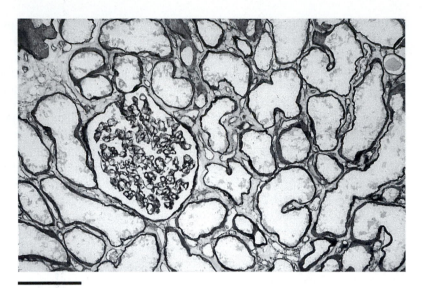

FIGURE 6.

Section of normal kidney, the same one shown in Figure 4, pretreated first with heat-induced epitope retrieval in 3M urea and then with pronase, thus combining the treatment in Figure 4, A and B. Although some enhancement of immunoreactivity is gained, it occurs at the expense of harm to morphologic preservation of the renal epithelium.

REFERENCES

1. Puchtler H, Meloan SN: On the chemistry of formaldehyde fixation and its effects on immunohistochemical reactions. *Histochemistry* 82:201–204, 1985.
2. Huang SN, Minassian H, Moore JD: Application of immunofluorescent staining on paraffin sections improved by trypsin digestion. *Lab Invest* 35:383–390, 1976.
3. Shi SR, Key ME, Kalra KL: Antigen retrieval in formalin-fixed paraffin-embedded tissues: An enhancement method for immunohistochemical staining based on microwave oven heating of tissue sections. *J Histochem Cytochem* 39:741–748, 1991.
4. Momose H, Mehta P, Battifora H: Antigen retrieval by microwave irradiation in lead thiocyanate. A comparison with protease digestion retrieval. *Appl Immunohistochem* 1:77–82, 1993.
5. Cattoretti G, Pileri S, Parravicini C, et al: Antigen unmasking on formalin-fixed, paraffin-embedded tissue sections. *J Pathol* 171:83–98, 1993.
6. Gown AM, De Wever N, Battifora H: Microwave-based antigenic unmasking: A revolutionary new technique for routine immunohistochemistry. *Appl Immunohistochem* 1:256–266, 1993.
7. Cattoretti G, Suurmeijer AJH: Antigen unmasking on formalin-fixed paraffin-embedded tissues using microwaves: A review. *Adv Anat Pathol* 2:2–9, 1994.
8. Miller K, Auld J, Jessup E, et al: Antigen unmasking in formalin-fixed routinely processed paraffin wax–embedded sections by pressure cooking: A comparison with microwave oven heating and traditional methods. *Adv Anat Pathol* 2:60–64, 1994.
9. Norton AJ, Jordan S, Yeomans P: Brief, high-temperature heat denaturation (pressure cooking): A simple and effective method of antigen retrieval for routinely processed tissues. *J Pathol* 173:371–379, 1994.

10. Bankfalvi A, Navabi H, Bier B, et al: Wet autoclave pretreatment for antigen retrieval in diagnostic immunohistochemistry. *J Pathol* 174:223–228, 1994.

11. Taylor CR, Shi S-R, Chaiwun B, et al: Strategies for improving the immunohistochemical staining of various intranuclear prognostic markers in formalin-paraffin sections: Androgen receptor, estrogen receptor, progesterone receptor, p53 protein, proliferating cell nuclear antigen, and Ki-67 antigen revealed by antigen retrieval techniques. *Hum Pathol* 25:263–270, 1994.

12. Dookhan DB, Kovatich AJ, Miettinen M: Non-enzymatic antigen retrieval in immunohistochemistry. Comparison between different antigen retrieval modalities and proteolytic digestion. *Appl Immunohistochem* 1:149–155, 1993.

13. Fox CH, Johnson FB, Whiting J, et al: Formaldehyde fixation. *J Histochem Cytochem* 33:845–853, 1985.

14. Azumi N, Joyce J, Battifora H: Does rapid microwave fixation improve immunohistochemistry? *Mod Pathol* 3:368–372, 1990.

15. Ordóñez NG, Manning JT, Brooks TE: Effect of trypsinization on the immunostaining of formalin-fixed, paraffin-embedded tissues. *Am J Surg Pathol* 12:121–129, 1988.

16. Battifora H, Kopinski M: The influence of protease digestion and duration of fixation on the immunostaining of keratins. A comparison of formalin and ethanol fixation. *J Histochem Cytochem* 34:1095–1100, 1986.

17. Cattoretti G, Becker MHG, Key G, et al: Monoclonal antibodies against recombinant parts of the Ki-67 antigen (MIB 1 and MIB 3) detect proliferating cells in microwave-processed formalin-fixed paraffin sections. *J Pathol* 168:357–363, 1992.

18. Cuevas EC, Bateman AC, Wilkins BS, et al: Microwave antigen retrieval in immunocytochemistry: A study of 80 antibodies. *J Clin Pathol* 47:448–452, 1994.

19. Shi S-R, Chaiwun B, Young L, et al: Antigen retrieval using pH 3.5 glycine-HCl buffer or urea solution for immunohistochemical localization of Ki-67. *Biotech Histochem* 69:213–215, 1994.

20. Beckstead JH: Improved antigen retrieval in formalin-fixed, paraffin-embedded tissues. *Appl Immunohistochem* 2:274–281, 1994.

21. Ho J, Shintaku IP, Preston M, et al: Can microwave antigen retrieval replace frozen section immunohistochemistry in the phenotyping of lymphoid neoplasms? A comparative study of kappa and lambda light chain staining in frozen sections, B5 fixed paraffin sections, and microwave urea antigen retrieval. *Appl Immunohistochem* 1994, in press.

22. Kwaspen F, Smedts F, Blom F, et al: Periodic acid as a non-enzymatic enhancement technique for the detection of cytokeratin immunoreactivity in routinely processed carcinomas. *Appl Immunohistochem* 1994, in press.

23. Suurmeijer AJH, Boon ME: Optimizing keratin and vimentin retrieval in formalin-fixed, paraffin-embedded tissue with the use of heat and metal salts. *Appl Immunohistochem* 1:143–148, 1993.

24. Boon ME, Kok LP: Microwaves for immunohistochemistry. *Micron* 25:151–170, 1994.

24a. Pasha T, Montone KT, Tomaszewski JE: Nuclear antigen retrieval utilizing steam heat. *Mod Pathol* 8:167(a), 1995.

25. Shi SR, Chaiwun B, Young L, et al: Antigen retrieval technique utilizing citrate buffer or urea solution for immunohistochemical demonstration of androgen receptor in formalin-fixed paraffin sections. *J Histochem Cytochem* 41:1599–1604, 1993.

26. Van den Berg FM, Baas IO, Polak MM, et al: Detection of p53 overexpression in routinely paraffin-embedded tissue of human carcinomas using a novel target unmasking fluid. *Am J Pathol* 142:381–385, 1993.

27. Esteban JM, Ahn C, Mehta P, et al: Biologic significance of quantitative estrogen receptor immunohistochemical assay by image analysis in breast cancer. *Am J Clin Pathol* 102:158–162, 1994.

28. Battifora H, Mehta P, Ahn C, et al: Estrogen receptor immunohistochemical assay in paraffin-embedded tissue: A better gold standard? *Appl Immunohistochem* 1:39–45, 1993.

29. Franke WW, Moll R: Cytoskeletal components of lymphoid organs. Synthesis of cytokeratin 8 and 18 and desmin in subpopulation of extrafollicular reticulum cells of human lymph nodes, tonsils, and spleen. *Differentiation* 36:145–163, 1987.

30. Doglioni C, Dell'Orto O, Zanetti G, et al: Cytokeratin-immunoreactive cells of human lymph nodes and spleen in normal and pathological conditions. An immunocytochemical study. *Virchows Arch A Pathol Anat Histopathol* 416:479–490, 1990.

The Role of Human Papillomavirus in Gynecologic Diseases

Gerard J. Nuovo, M.D.

Associate Professor of Pathology and Obstetrics and Gynecology, Director of Cytopathology, State University of New York at Stony Brook, Health Sciences Center School of Medicine, Stony Brook, New York

T he field of molecular diagnostics has become increasingly important to surgical pathologists and cytopathologists. Advances in the field have led to many commercially available kits for the detection of a wide variety of DNA and RNA viruses and DNA sequences of clinical importance, such as gene rearrangements and oncogene amplifications. It can be argued that testing for human papillomavirus (HPV) has been at the forefront of diagnostic molecular pathology. As of this writing, no fewer than *seven* companies offer kits for the detection of HPV DNA or RNA in clinical samples. Recent advances in molecular diagnostics, especially improved nonisotopic detection systems, were made possible in large part by HPV research. There are several reasons that so much attention has been focused on HPV in molecular diagnostics. First, it is a very common disease. It is estimated that clinically evident HPV infection of the genital tract develops in over 1 million people per year in the United States.[1-3] This makes HPV the most common of the sexually transmitted viral diseases. The fact that genital tract HPV is transmitted sexually is another important impetus behind the availability of diagnostic molecular tests for this family of viruses. Like many sexually transmitted infectious agents, HPV is highly fastidious and difficult to grow in the laboratory, much like *Treponema pallidum*, the causative agent of syphilis. Indeed, the great difficulty in propagating HPV in the laboratory setting, either in an animal model or in tissue culture, was a critical factor in developing molecular diagnostics in HPV disease. While at Columbia University College of Physicians and Surgeons, this author had the good fortune to practice colposcopy under the guidance of Dr. Daniel Smith. Direct contact with patients made especially clear to me the magnitude of the emotional implications of a diagnosis of "cervical HPV disease." The patients are understandably distraught and concerned as to the source of their venereal disease. It is not an overstatement to say that an important role for molecular diagnostics in HPV testing is to reassure women (and men) who have either clinical and/or pathologic findings suggestive but not diagnostic of the viral infection and do not have the virus. Finally,

Advances in Pathology and Laboratory Medicine, vol. 8

the clear-cut association of HPV and cervical cancer has increased the importance of detecting this virus in the genital tract.

Our discussion will begin with a brief review of the virology of HPV and the various molecular tests that can be used to detect it. This will be followed by an analysis of the role of the virus in diseases of the cervix, vagina, vulva, endometrium, and the ovary.

VIROLOGY OF HUMAN PAPILLOMAVIRUS

The papillomaviruses have the ability to induce lesions, usually of the skin or mucosal surfaces, in a wide variety of animals.[4-7] The rabbit papillomavirus was one of the first viruses implicated in the "malignant transformation" of a wart. The bovine papillomavirus has been extensively studied because it, unlike HPV, is readily grown in the laboratory; it has been associated with benign and malignant fibroepithelial lesions in cattle. Human papillomavirus is actually a group of viruses. Although the members of this group share certain genomic sequences in common, by definition each different type has, overall, less than 50% homology with the other identified types. As of this writing, at least 70 distinct HPV types have been cloned and characterized. About 25 of these types have been found in lesions of the lower genital tract.[1-3, 7] Although most of these 25 types have been detected in the cervix, it has been observed that HPVs 6, 11, and 16 by far predominate in the vagina, vulva, rectum, and penis.[8-16] Other "genital tract" HPV types are rarely found at these sites. The 55 "nongenital" HPV types are associated with a wide variety of benign and malignant conditions, primarily on the skin. These include the common finger and plantar verruca (warts), where HPVs 1 and 2 are often detected, and uncommon conditions such as epidermodysplasia verruciformis.[17, 18] The latter is a congenital condition marked by the presence of many verrucae planae (flat warts), and invasive squamous cell cancers develop in about 20% of these patients. Human papillomavirus types 5, 8, 26, and others have been associated with this disease.[17, 18]

Each HPV type contains about 7,900 base pairs. They are DNA viruses, and certain types such as HPVs 16 and 18 have a propensity to integrate into the host genome. The genome of HPV can be divided into certain regions called open reading frames (ORFs) that correspond to a variety of transcripts. Two ORFs related to the protein coat that are expressed relatively late in the infection are called L (late) 1 and L2. At least 7 early ORFs have been identified in HPV. Of these, ORFs E2, E6, and E7 have been the most studied. E2 dictates the synthesis of a variety of regulatory proteins, some of which have direct effects on expression of the E6 and E7 ORFs.[5, 19] The E6 and E7 products are oncoproteins because transfection of the corresponding DNA segment can transform cells. Several groups have shown that either by long-term passage or cotransfection with, for example, the *ras* oncogene, the E6 or E7 ORF can induce invasive and metastatic behavior in the previously benign squamous cell line.[20-23] Disruption of the E2 ORF, as often occurs during integration of HPV into the host genome, can lead to increased expression of E6 and E7. This process probably plays an important role in the evolution of cervical cancer. The E6 and E7 oncoproteins can inactivate host antioncogenes, including p53 and the retinoblastoma gene product, respectively.[19-24] The resultant increased proliferation most likely predisposes the transformed cell to other molecular events that ultimately lead to an invasive tumor.

An important observation with regard to the different genital HPV types is that some, such as HPVs 6 and 11, were rarely associated with invasive cervical cancer whereas other types, such as HPVs 16 and 18, were commonly detected in these invasive tumors.[1-3] This finding provides a unique and important opportunity to study the role of viral infection in oncogenesis. An obvious question that has received much attention is what molecular differences between HPVs 6/11 and HPVs 16/18 are related to their dramatic difference in potential clinical behavior. Although more work needs to be done, it has been shown that the HPV 6/11 E6 and E7 proteins have much less avidity for the p53 and retinoblastoma gene products, respectively, than do the corresponding proteins for HPVs 16 and 18.[20, 24]

As noted earlier, at least 50% of the DNA sequence of a given HPV must be different from all the other identified types before it can be classified as a new HPV type. However, it is important to remember that certain regions of the genome will be similar for most of the 70 HPV types that have been characterized. Other regions will be relatively homologous among the oncogenic types and poorly homologous with the so-called benign types. Still other regions, such as those that correspond to some of the antigenic determinants of the different types, will be different among the various HPV types. The practical implications of these observations relate to consensus probes/primers, cross-hybridization, and determination of the specific HPV type.

CONSENSUS PROBES/PRIMERS

By choosing nucleotide sequences from regions of strong homology between the different HPV types, one can generate primers or probes that can be used to determine whether a given lesion contains HPV regardless of the specific type. This concept has been successfully employed in polymerase chain reaction (PCR) testing, where a variety of consensus primers have been described. One set, called MY9 and MY11, can detect at least 40 of the HPV types, including virtually all that have been found in the genital tract.[25-27] Several companies market consensus probes for HPV testing. Examples include the wide-spectrum HPV probe from Oncor (Gaithersburg, Md) and the Omniprobe from Digene Diagnostics (Silver Spring, Md). These probes can detect nearly 100% of the HPV types found in genital warts of the vagina, vulva, and penis and over 90% of the HPV types found in cervical lesions. Consensus probes are very useful when one is dealing with a histologically equivocal lesion and the issue is whether HPV is present or not.

CROSS-HYBRIDIZATION

Cross-hybridization occurs when a probe used to detect one HPV type also detects another related but distinct HPV type. As expected, this occurs more commonly between types associated with similar clinical conditions. For example, cross-hybridization is common for the two HPV types associated with "benign" vulvar and penile warts, HPVs 6 and 11, and is also common between HPVs 16 and 31, which are both associated with cervical precancers and cancers.[1-3, 28-31] However, HPV 45, another genital virus type that can be associated with cervical precancers and cancers, rarely cross-hybridizes with HPV 16 but commonly cross-hybridizes with HPV 18. The key practical implications of cross-hybridization are twofold: (1) the presence of a signal, especially at low stringency with a given HPV probe, does *not* prove that a *specific* type of HPV is present in that lesion, and (2) a tissue sample may demonstrate a hybridization signal with more than one HPV probe. In over 90% of cases, a signal obtained with multiple probes is due to cross-hybridization and *not* to infection by more than one HPV type. True productive infection of a given tissue by more than one HPV type is a rare event that occurs in only 2% of cases (Figs 1 and 2).

DETERMINATION OF THE HUMAN PAPILLOMAVIRUS TYPE

On theoretical grounds, a determination of the specific HPV type should be possible by choosing a region of the viral genome from a given type that has poor homology with the other known types. Most biotechnological companies and researchers have not taken this approach for HPV

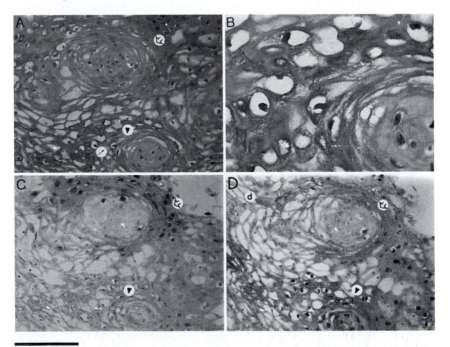

FIGURE 1.
Dual infection by HPV. A low-grade squamous intraepithelial lesion was evident on biopsy. Note the variable cell density and perinuclear halos that vary in size and shape (**A** and, at higher magnification of area marked by small arrow, **B**); nuclear atypia is minor. HPV 6 was detected in the cells toward the upper part of the figure (**C**, *open arrow*); note how the cells toward the bottom are negative (*closed arrow*). HPV 16 was detected in these cells (*closed arrow*) but not in the cells toward the upper part of the figure (**D**).

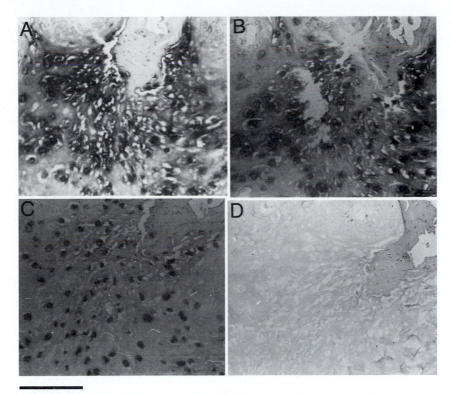

FIGURE 2.

Cross-hybridization by HPV. This vulvar biopsy specimen contained HPV 6. Note how a signal is evident in the same groups of cells if genomic probes against HPV 6 **(A)** and HPV 11 **(B)** are used; the latter represents cross-hybridization between the closely related HPVs 6 and 11. If subgenomic probes (from Oncor) are employed that are from regions where these types share little homology, then a signal is evident with the HPV 6 probe **(C)** but not the HPV 11 probe **(D)**.

probes. Rather, they use genomic probes and then use varying stringencies to ascertain the specific HPV type present in a lesion. One company, Oncor, has developed a series of type-specific probes that do not cross-hybridize with other types even at low stringency. An example of this type-specific subgenomic probe system is presented in Figure 2. Note that one can differentiate even the closely related HPV types 6 and 11 at low stringency, but only if these subgenomic probes are employed. The determination of a specific HPV type with individual DNA sequences is well suited to PCR. Here one can take advantage of 3' mismatches to prevent amplification even if there is some homology in the other part of the oligoprimer. As early as 1990, type-specific HPV primers were generated that could distinguish between HPV types 6, 11, 16, 18, 31, 33, and 35.[32] Many such sequences have been published and are often directed to parts of the E6 or E7 ORF.

MOLECULAR TESTS FOR HUMAN PAPILLOMAVIRUS

The principles just described for the use of consensus probes/primers, for cross-hybridization, and for the determination of specific HPV types are applied in molecular testing. The major principle for the different molecular tests is that a specific sequence of DNA or RNA that is typically labeled, called the *probe,* is used to detect a homologous sequence in the sample. This is achieved by the process of selective hybridization; hence these tests are sometimes called molecular hybridization assays. The reader is referred to several references that describe molecular hybridization tests.[1-3] A brief review will be given here to assist inexperienced readers.

HYBRIDIZATION ASSAYS

Each of the hybridization tests employs a known *probe* that is usually labeled. Although radioactive labels can be used, most laboratories employ nonisotopic tagged nucleotides that may be detected by fluorescence or colorimetric changes. A common colorimetric reaction is based on biotin-labeled nucleotides that avidly bind streptavidin, which in turn is conjugated to alkaline phosphatase. This enzyme can then catalyze the precipitation of a substrate that can easily be seen with light microscopy. The sensitivity of the nonisotopic systems is equivalent to that of the radioactive labels.[1, 29, 33] A strand of nucleic acid in the sample being analyzed that is homologous to the labeled probe is called the *target.*

Several techniques have evolved on the basis of the ability of a labeled probe to bind to and thus permit detection of the target nucleic acid sequence of interest. One approach is to extract the DNA, both target and nontarget, from a sample and bind it to a filter where it can then be hybridized with the labeled probe. This is called *filter hybridization.* Oftentimes the sample DNA is directly placed on the filter with the aid of a vacuum manifold that has slot-like spaces for each sample, hence the term *slot blot* (or dot blot) hybridization. Alternatively, for *Southern blot* hybridization, the sample DNA is first separated according to size and configuration by electrophoresis on a gel and then transferred to a filter (Fig 3). In both of these techniques the tissue is destroyed, thus precluding direct histologic correlation. A third methodology based on hybridization of a target and the probe allows this correlation because the target DNA is not extracted from the tissue or cell source, but rather kept inside the intact cell where it may bind to the probe. This, of course, is in situ hybridization. Finally, PCR is based on the ability of a small sequence of DNA, called a *primer,* to selectively hybridize to the desired target and thus initiate synthesis of the target by a DNA polymerase.

A discussion comparing filter hybridization, PCR, and in situ hybridization is in order so that the reader may better appreciate the advantages and limitations of these different methodologies. An important difference among these techniques is their detection thresholds. Detection of a DNA sequence by in situ hybridization requires about 10 to 20 copies per cell. This occurs when there is a selective increase in the amount of that sequence because of, for example, oncogene amplification or viral proliferation. On the other hand, only one virus need be present per every 100 cells for detection with the filter hybridization test. In the case of this low copy number of the target, the in situ test would be scored as negative. Of course, in PCR there is a selective increase in the amount of tar-

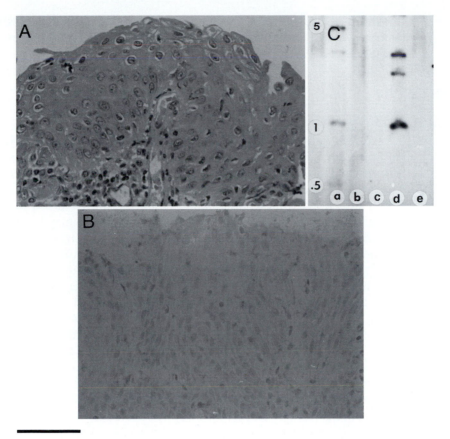

FIGURE 3.

Different detection thresholds of filter vs. in situ hybridization. This cervical bi-opsy sample from a woman with a Papanicolaou smear of squamous atypia shows well-ordered cells with uniform halos and nuclei consistent with reactive, inflam-matory changes **(A)**. Note the nucleoli, which are typical of reactive change; there is no evidence of dysplasia. As expected, HPV DNA was not detected by in situ hybridization **(B)**. However, HPV DNA was detected by Southern blot analysis from the subjacent tissue section **(C**, lane *d;* the numbers refer to kilobases). An explanation for this common finding is that the virus is present in the tissue but is not actively proliferating.

get because of its synthesis, which enhances one's ability to detect it. However, it is essential to realize that during the PCR the primers may also hybridize to nontarget sequences. When HPV-specific primers are used, this nonspecific binding may be either to human DNA or to them-selves. The consequence of this binding is that the detection threshold of the assay will be increased. Under standard conditions and with 1 μg of background nontarget DNA, the detection threshold of PCR is about 1,000 to 3,000 copies per sample, which is similar to that in filter hybridiza-tion.[34–36] However, if primer extension (i.e., hybridization) is prevented until a temperature is reached whereby the primer-nontarget complexes mostly denature, these nonspecific pathways can be inhibited to cause a concomitant decrease in the detection threshold. This technique for con-trolling hybridization is the basis for "hot-start" PCR. It has been shown that withholding the Taq polymerase until 55°C decreases the detection threshold of PCR to an extraordinary 1 copy per tissue.[34-36] With this background preparation, let us begin a discussion of HPV and the female genital tract.

THE CERVIX

NORMAL EPITHELIUM

It has been well documented that HPV can be detected in normal cervical epithelium. "Normal" usually refers to a woman with no prior history of an HPV-related lesion and a concurrent normal Papanicolaou smear. It is important to realize that the detection rates in this so-called occult infection will vary markedly depending on the test and the specific probe/primers used. In most investigators' experience, including our own, HPV DNA will not be detected by in situ hybridization in the cells of a normal Papanicolaou smear or in histologically normal cervical tissue.[37, 38] However, filter hybridization analyses have reported occult HPV infection rates of 5% to 15%.[11, 37-44] The higher rates are usually from those groups using at least six distinct HPV probes at low stringency to optimize cross-hybridization with other HPV types. Detection rates with PCR will be as low as 5% when primers specific for HPVs 6, 11, 16, and 18 are employed and as high as 25% to 30% when the consensus primers from Perkin-Elmer are used.[27] One of the initial PCR studies of occult HPV infection reported a detection rate of about 90% for HPV 16 alone! It soon became clear that other groups could not reproduce this result, and the paper was retracted when the authors realized that crossover contamination by HPV 16 had led to many false-positive results.[45, 46]

Because HPV can be detected in occult infection only by the PCR and filter hybridization, it has not been possible to determine which cells contain the virus. Recently, we attempted to address this issue by using PCR in situ hybridization. Our preliminary results suggest that occult infection occurs primarily in normal-appearing metaplastic cells in the transformation zone of the cervix (Nuovo GJ, unpublished observations).

The clinical outcome of occult infection is likewise poorly understood. As of this writing, I am not aware that any large-scale study of occult infection has been published. A small study involved 13 women who had HPV detected in the setting of a normal Papanicolaou smear and negative colposcopic examination. After following these patients for 1 year, repeat testing did not reveal the development of biopsy-proven HPV-related lesions.[47] Confirmation of such findings will require much larger prospective studies.

PRECANCER

Human papillomavirus–related disease has been extensively studied in cervical precancers. These lesions are very common and represent a major health care issue because of the costs of diagnosis and treatment. Further, because they can evolve into malignant lesions, study of HPV-related cervical disease has provided important insight into molecular events that can presage an invasive carcinoma. Surgical pathologists and cytopathologists have recognized cervical precancers for decades, and many different terms have been used to describe them. At the present, cervical squamous intraepithelial lesion (SIL) is commonly used. Other terms that have been used extensively in the past include dysplasia (mild to severe), carcinoma in situ, condyloma, and cervical intraepithelial neoplasia (CIN). It is important to appreciate that these terms are describing different stages in the process of development of the same disease, i.e., HPV-related disease in the cervix. This author will use the SIL nomenclature.

To describe the association of HPV with SILs, a brief description of the microscopic appearance of the cervix is in order. Two different types of epithelium meet in the cervix: glandular and squamous epithelium. They meet in an area called the transformation zone because, over time, the squamous cells gradually replace the glandular epithelium. Normal cervical epithelium is easily recognized by the orderly arrangement of the squamous epithelium, as seen in Figure 4. Also note that perinuclear clearings or, as they are more commonly called, halos are evident. These represent glycogen deposition. These halos are also well ordered and are similar to each other in size and shape. Finally, note that the nuclei are similar from one to the next in their size, shape, and chromaticity.

The most important histologic feature that marks HPV-related SILs is a disorganized growth pattern. As can be seen in Figure 5, the cells are crowded and show a disorganized variable cell density pattern. This reflects the hyperplasia induced by the HPV infection. Figure 5 also shows nuclear variability, the other histologic diagnostic feature of an SIL. The cell nuclei shown in the figure vary in size, shape, and chromaticity.

Squamous intraepithelial lesions are subdivided into two categories: low-grade and high-grade. Both grades show the two features described in the preceding paragraph. In low-grade SILs, these changes are most evident in the middle and superficial areas of the epithelium. The cells in deep areas of the epithelium may show minimal atypia, but the well-ordered "picket-fence" arrangement of this layer is usually maintained. Also, perinuclear halos that differ in size and shape are prominent, especially toward the surface squamous cells. In contrast, high-grade SILs are characterized by marked nuclear atypia and many mitotic figures in the basal zone. Perinuclear halos are less evident (Fig 5). The changes of a high-grade SIL are directly comparable to what is seen in cell culture when normal squamous epithelium is transfected with an oncogenic HPV type and can thus be considered equivalent to the process of transformation. The histologic changes of a low-grade SIL were reproduced in an animal model by Krieder et al.[48] Squamous cells that had been infected with HPV 11 were implanted under the renal capsule of nude mice. Productive infection was demonstrated in cells in which the features of a "low-grade" SIL had developed.

Tissue analyses using filter hybridization and PCR have shown that most cervical SILs contain HPV.[1-3] It is important to realize that the detection rates in these studies are highly dependent on the number of probes (for filter hybridization) or type specificity of the primers (for PCR). Because over 20 types of HPV are present in cervical SILs, detection rates of only about 70% will be expected if filter hybridization is employed with probes for HPVs 6, 11, 16, 18, and 31, as was typical of earlier studies. However, if one analyzes the apparently "HPV-negative" cases with,

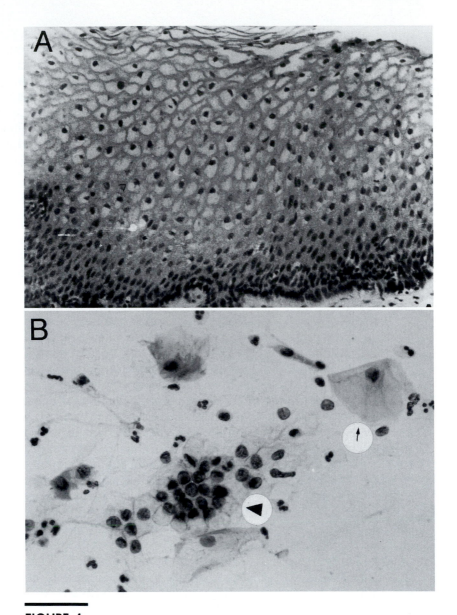

FIGURE 4.
Pathology of a normal cervix. Note the well-ordered appearance of the squamous cells adjacent to the transformation zone in a woman with a normal Papanicolaou smear. The halos are uniform in size and the nuclei are uniform in their chromaticity, shape, and size **(A)**. The corresponding Papanicolaou smear shows normal superficial squamous cells *(arrow)* and endocervical cells *(arrowhead)* **(B)**.

for example, HPV consensus primers and PCR or filter hybridization with additional probes, detection rates of 100% can be obtained.[15, 31, 49, 50]

Although PCR and filter hybridization have documented that in effect, all cervical SILs contain HPV, the DNA extraction that is a prerequisite for these molecular analyses precludes identification of the histologic distribution of the virus in cervical SILs. In situ hybridization has

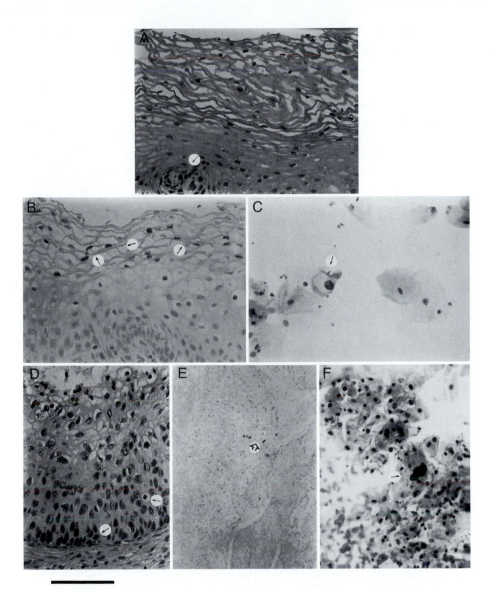

FIGURE 5.

Pathology and virology of cervical squamous intraepithelial lesions (SILs). Note the disorganized, crowded, variable cell density growth pattern toward the superficial part of this cervical tissue **(A)**. The halos and nuclei vary in size and shape, and the nuclei also vary in chromaticity. The cells toward the basal epithelium are minimally altered (an *arrow* marks the basal layer). These are the features of a low-grade SIL. The intense signal toward the surface cells when an HPV 51 probe is used demonstrates that the virus is actively proliferating in these cells **(B)**. The corresponding Papanicolaou smear is seen in **C**; note the distinct, large perinuclear halo with a condensed cytoplasmic rim and the nuclear hyperchromaticity. Compare this with the tissue that shows similar features toward the surface but where there is marked nuclear atypia and disorganization toward the epithelial base **(D)**; also note the mitotic figures toward the base *(arrows)*. HPV 16 is present but is detectable in far fewer cells **(E, lower magnification)**. The corresponding Papanicolaou smear is seen in **F**; note the intense hyperchromaticity, which is the most reliable diagnostic feature of a high-grade SIL, and the nuclear indentations *(arrow)* **(F)**.

provided invaluable information about the histologic distribution of HPV in cervical SILs that can be summarized in two main points:

1. The copy number of HPV DNA, i.e., the number of viral particles per infected cell, tends to be much greater in low-grade SILs relative to high-grade lesions.
2. The viral copy number is most abundant in the middle and superficial layers of the epithelium, being especially abundant in cells that show perinuclear halos. In contrast, HPV DNA is rarely detected in the cells of the basal epithelium (see Fig 5).

An obvious question with regard to point 2 is whether the viral DNA is present in the basal epithelium but in numbers below the detection threshold for in situ hybridization analysis (about 10 copies per cell). This problem can be addressed by combining the extreme sensitivity of PCR with the cell localizing ability of in situ hybridization in a technique called PCR in situ hybridization. This technique has shown that viral DNA is detectable in the basal cells of a cervical SIL.[51]

The aforementioned observations indicate that HPV infection is most productive in low-grade lesions. Viral protein capsid antigens are similarly much more abundant in low-grade SILs relative to high-grade lesions. This strongly suggests that the low-grade SILs are probably much more infectious than the high-grade lesions. The ability of the virus to increase its nucleic acid synthesis in the more superficial cells seems to be to its advantage in that it can easily enter the cervical mucus and thus be more readily transmitted during sexual intercourse. In high-grade SILs, viral nucleic acid patterns change. There is less DNA synthesis, capsid proteins are difficult to detect, and transcripts corresponding to the E6 and E7 ORFs become more evident.[1–3] These events presage the pattern that has been documented in cervical cancers.[1–3]

Determination of the HPV type in a cervical SIL by molecular hybridization has yielded some important results. These data, presented in Table 1, can be summarized in 3 main points:

1. There is a much greater diversity of HPV types in low-grade SILs than in high-grade SILs.
2. Human papillomavirus types 6, 11, 42, 43, and 44 are very rarely detected in high-grade SILs. These types are much more common in low-grade SILs, where they are found in about 20% of such lesions.
3. On histologic grounds one cannot differentiate low-grade SILs that contain the so-called benign HPV types such as HPV 6 or 11 from the oncogenic types.

It is not clear why such a great diversity of HPV types may be found in low-grade cervical SILs. However, the lesser number of types found in high-grade SILs certainly reflects a selection process for the oncogenic HPV types. In the cervix it appears that most early HPV lesions represent productive infections that are recognized by pathologists as a low-grade SIL. This low-grade SIL is probably the end point for lesions associated with HPV 6 or 11 because these will most likely regress. However, for those low-grade SILs associated with an oncogenic HPV type, although

TABLE 1.

Segregation of Human Papillomavirus Types in Lower Genital Tract Lesions

	HPV 6/11	HPV 16	HPV 18	HPV 31/33/35	Others*
Cervix: SIL†					
Low-grade	20‡	35	1	30	14
High-grade	<1	75	1	19	5
Vulva/penis: SIL					
Low-grade	95	<1	0	3	2
High-grade	<1	90	0	10	0
Cervix: cancer					
Squamous cell	<1	65	20	10	5
Adenocarcinoma	<1	35	60	5	<1

*Human papillomavirus types 42, 43, 44, 45, 51, 52, and 56.
†SIL = squamous intraepithelial lesion.
‡Values are percentages.

regression still occurs in about 30% of cases, the potential for progression to a high-grade lesion is clearly present.

Determination of HPV types in cervical SILs by in situ hybridization has also provided information about viral recurrence after ablative therapy. It has been shown that in over 90% of cases the HPV type present in an SIL pretreatment will be *different* from the HPV type present in an SIL that occurs after ablative therapy in the same woman. Interestingly, this is not the case for immunocompromised women, where recurrence is associated with the same HPV type.[52-54] These findings suggest that a type-specific immunity may be induced by ablative therapy. That ablation in immunocompetent women may result in type-specific immunity is supported by HPV analyses on recurrence of cervical SILs after cone biopsy in which the lesion is removed by a scalpel. In such cases, recurrence in immunocompetent women is associated with infection by the same HPV type.[54] Clearly, the study of HPV in recurrence of SILs requires much additional research and may yield information that would be of use in the development of HPV vaccines. This would be of particular interest in countries where routine Papanicolaou smear screening is not done. In many of these countries, such as Columbia and Brazil, cervical cancer is the leading cause of cancer-related death in women.[1-3]

CERVICAL CANCER

Given the strong association of HPV and cervical SILs, it is to be expected that there would be an equally strong relationship between the virus and cervical cancer. This is indeed the case. Over 90% of cervical cancers contain HPV, and it is thought that the patients testing negative for HPV probably contain rare, uncharacterized types.[1-3] This hypothesis has been supported by PCR studies using consensus primers. In a study of adenocarcinomas and squamous cell carcinomas of the cervix, it was demonstrated that viral RNA was detectable in almost all cases when the consensus MY9 and MY11 primers were used. The one interesting exception was clear cell carcinoma of the cervix, a rare tumor that has been associated with exposure to diethlystilbestrol (Nuovo GJ, unpublished observations).

Just as the copy number of HPV decreases from low-grade to high-grade SILs, the trend continues in cervical cancers, where the average copy number decreases to that below the level in high-grade SILs. The low-grade lesions can be viewed as the acute productive infectious form of the disease, whereas in high-grade lesions, viral nucleic synthesis shifts from high levels and intact virion production to more subtle dysregulation of the host cell. The viral copy number in cervical cancers is usually between 1 to 20 copies. As would be expected, most HPV-positive cervical cancers would be scored negative by in situ hybridization. More sensitive tests such as filter hybridization and, as indicated earlier, PCR are needed to detect the virus in such tissues.

As described before, PCR in situ hybridization demonstrated that most of the cells of an SIL, even the basal cells, contain viral DNA. We have also performed this analysis on tissue samples from cervical cancers. Human papillomavirus DNA was detected by PCR in situ hybridization in at least 90% of the cancer cells. Interestingly, viral RNA was detectable in a far smaller percentage of cells. Viral expression of the E2 ORF was found in about 20% of HPV 18−positive cancers, whereas E6 and E7 transcripts were found in 30% to 50% of cancer cells (Nuovo GJ, unpublished observations). This is in keeping with in vitro data demonstrating that viral integration, which is invariably present in cervical cancers, is associated with interruption of the E2 ORF and a concomitant upregulation of the E6 and E7 ORF.

The distribution pattern of HPV types in cervical cancers reveals a very interesting difference when compared with the pattern in high-grade SILs. Although HPV 16 is common in cervical cancers, accounting for about 65% of cases, HPV 18 is also commonly found in these lesions. About 30% of cervical squamous cell cancers contain HPV 18; the rate is often over 50% for cervical adenocarcinomas.[1−3, 55−58] Recall that only about 1% of high-grade cervical SILs contain HPV 18 (see Table 1). The basis for this finding is not known. It may reflect the poor ability of many of the so-called oncogenic HPV types such as HPVs 31, 33, 35, and 51 to promote progression to invasive lesions. That is, although HPV 18−containing SILs may be rare, they may have a greater incidence of progression to cervical cancer than SILs containing these other types, with the exception of HPV 16. Indeed, HPV 18 is far more efficient at inducing transformation and immortalization in vitro than are those other oncogenic types. For these reasons, HPV 18 is sometimes referred to as a type with "high oncogenic potential." Human papillomavirus types 31, 33, 35, 51, and some others are described as having "intermediate oncogenic potential." It should be appreciated, however, that in some studies HPV 18 has been detected in over 10% of occult infections, which implies that its presence may not always indicate a strong likelihood of cancer (Groff D, personal communication, 1993).

Cervical cancers have been extensively studied with regard to clinical correlates of the histologic features of the tumor. Specifically, it has been shown that tumors confined to the cervix that invade less than 3 mm into the stroma and do not invade the microvasculature have a cure rate of nearly 100% with surgery. However, even when confined to the cervix, the 5-year survival rate decreases to about 50% if the tumor invades more than 3 mm and is associated with microvasculature invasion.[1-3] What is the molecular basis for this marked disparity in clinical behavior? Several groups have correlated these and other histologic features with the detection of specific HPV types. One group reported that HPV 18–positive cancers had a worse prognosis, another stated that the HPV-negative tumors (by Southern blot hybridization) had a worse prognosis, whereas another study did not find any correlation between HPV type and prognosis.[1, 55, 59]

If HPV type does not appear to correlate with prognosis in cervical cancer, perhaps certain host factors do. One such variable that has received much attention in cancer prognosis is breakdown of the stromal and basement membrane matrix. In order for a cancer to invade these tissues barriers, gelatinases are needed. Two commonly studied gelatinases are referred to as metalloproteinase 92 and 72 (MMP-9 and MMP-2, respectively), and their presence in tissue samples has been correlated with the processes of tumor cell invasion and metastasis.[60] Cancer cell invasion is the result of complex, multifactorial processes that include transcriptional control of the genes encoding proteinases, activation of degradative enzymes, and production of their natural inhibitors, TIMP-1 and TIMP-2. We have studied the relationship of cervical cancer invasion and the expression of these key molecules by reverse transcriptase in situ PCR. These analyses have shown that in cancers with a good prognosis, the MMP-to-TIMP ratio is about 1. One might envision that this balance allows for a controlled breakdown of the basement membrane. In cervical cancers with a poor prognosis, the MMP-to-TIMP ratio is much higher (e.g., greater than 15:1 in areas of vascular invasion), perhaps resulting in a more uncontrolled and rapid breakdown of the tissue compartments by the invasive tumor cells. We are now investigating whether either MMP or TIMP expression relates to the presence of various HPV transcripts in an attempt to see whether, for example, E6 and E7 may exert their oncogenic activity by influencing the key balance between the MMPs and the TIMPs.

EQUIVOCAL TISSUE

Thus far we have discussed the features associated with unequivocal cervical pathology, including normal tissue, SILs, and cancer. It is important to appreciate that in many instances the clinical and pathologic findings may be not be straightforward. A common scenario is one in which the Papanicolaou smear shows atypical squamous cells of undetermined significance (squamous atypia). This author uses the term "squamous atypia" to refer to cells in a Papanicolaou smear with features that could represent reactive changes but could also be indicative of dysplasia. The inability to make this distinction is due in part to the nature of the spectrum of reactive squamous cell changes and SILs, which show some overlap. Many clinicians will do a colposcopic examination when the Papanicolaou smear shows squamous atypia. In such cases, areas of increased whitening may be evident on the cervix, often at the transformation zone, where most SILs arise. Because these white patches are seen after the application of a 3% acetic acid solution, they are commonly referred to as acetowhite lesions. These acetowhite lesions reflect a focal increase in cell density masking the underlying blood vessels. It is important to understand that although SILs are associated with a focally increased squamous cell density, many other common conditions can produce a focal increase in cell density. For example, an acetowhite lesion may be seen in areas of squamous metaplasia and localized inflammation.

To summarize, a Papanicolaou smear showing squamous atypia may lead to a colposcopic examination in which an acetowhite lesion may be seen. The tissue will not be normal on histologic examination. In about 30% of cases there will be an unequivocal SIL. In this author's experience, 50% of such cases show clear-cut squamous metaplasia and inflammation with no suggestion of an SIL on histologic examination. The remaining 20% of cases show histologic features suggestive but not diagnostic of an SIL (Fig 6). This last 20% of cases is a very important category that presents problems to the pathologist, the clinician, and most importantly, the woman. Pathologists may use terms such as "borderline changes" or "suggestive of an SIL." Although this ambiguity reflects the problems inherent in the histologic findings, it may understandably lead to uncertainty for the clinician on the proper treatment. I have observed that many clinicians treat these lesions as SILs and either ablate or remove the lesion by loop excision electrocautery procedure (LEEP). This aggressive therapy involves considerable cost for the patient and emotional stress because of the implication that she has a sexually transmitted disease.

Given the strong association of HPV with cervical SILs, it is easy to realize that viral testing may have considerable benefit in these equivocal cases. Detection of HPV strongly suggests that the lesion is indeed an SIL. More important, the absence of HPV in conjunction with equivocal findings raises the strong possibility that the lesion is *nonspecific*, i.e., not an SIL. We have performed in situ hybridization analysis on hundreds of such equivocal cervical tissues from women who, for the most part, had squamous atypia on Papanicolaou smears. When consensus HPV probes were used that can detect nearly all of the 20 viral types found in the cervix, about 2% of the these equivocal cases were positive. This compares with a rate of 92% for low-grade SILs and 0% for normal cervical tissue taken from areas where there is no lesion. In the event that the in situ test is HPV-negative, this author reports the case as "negative for SIL"; if positive, it is called an SIL (Fig 6).

The use of filter hybridization and the development of PCR have led to more sensitive testing. What is the viral detection rate in equivocal tissue with these techniques? If one uses many probes and low-stringency (for filter hybridization) and consensus primers for PCR, then one obtains detection rates of about 25% to 35% in such cases. This author does *not* call such cases SILs. One may recall that given the high sensitivity of these assays, about 10% of woman with a normal Papanicolaou smear have HPV

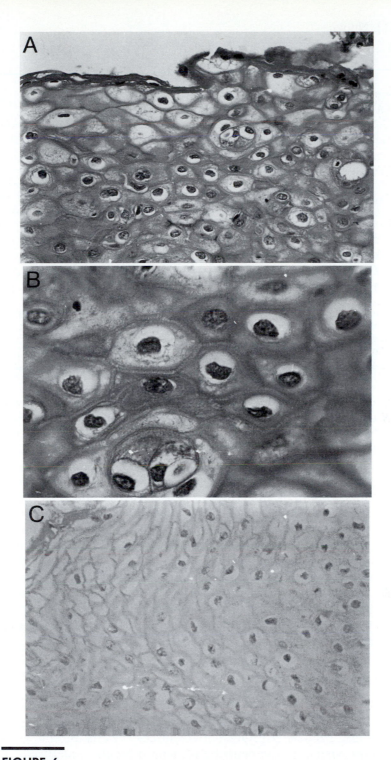

FIGURE 6.
Utility of HPV testing in equivocal cervical biopsy tissue. There is some cellular disorganization in this cervical biopsy sample from a woman with a history of squamous atypia on Papincolaou smears. However, the halos do not show marked variability, and the nuclei atypia is judged inadequate to be classified as a squamous intraepithelial lesion. The uniform nuclear chromaticity is evident at higher magnification **(B).** HPV DNA was not detected by in situ hybridization **(C)** or polymerase chain reaction (not shown). Thus this lesion is interpreted as representing reactive and nondysplastic types of changes.

TABLE 2.
Correlation of the Papanicolaou Smear and Human Papillomavirus
Detection by Slot Blot Hybridization on the Rate of Biopsy-Proven
Squamous Intraepithelial Lesions After a 1-Year Follow-Up in
Women With an Indeterminate Colposcopic Examination*

Correlation	Normal	Squamous Atypia	SIL†
Concurrent Papanicolaou Smear Diagnosis			
HPV DNA–positive	6/49 (12%)	16/41 (39%)	9/19 (47%)
Rate of biopsy-proven SIL in follow-up examination			
HPV DNA–positive	0/6	10/16 (63%)	7/9 (78%)
HPV DNA–negative	2/43 (5%)	3/25 (12%)	4/10 (40%)

*Indeterminate colposcopic examination refers to women who were referred to colposcopy because of an abnormal Papanicolaou smear, usually squamous atypia, and where no SIL was evident after biopsy.
†SIL = squamous intraepithelial lesion.

detected by filter hybridization. We have followed a group of women with abnormal Papanicolaou smears and indeterminate colposcopic examinations (i.e., negative for SILs) for at least 1 year to determine whether the detection of HPV was related to an increased risk of a biopsy-proven SIL.[47, 61] These data are presented in Table 2. Note that if the concurrent Papanicolaou smear shows squamous atypia *and* HPV is detected, then there is a high risk of an SIL over the 1-year period. The risk appears to be much lower for women with squamous atypia when HPV is not detected in the cervix. This leads to a decision-making flowchart based on the Papanicolaou smear and HPV result that is recommended by this author (Fig 7). Note that this scheme includes *only* women with a previous abnormal Papanicolaou smear; I do not believe that HPV testing has clinical utility in women with no history of abnormal Papanicolaou smears. It must be stressed that this proposed patient management plan is based on preliminary findings and awaits additional, larger studies to determine its usefulness.

THE VULVA AND VAGINA

Although it is true that HPV-related disease is by far most common in the cervix, infections of the vulva and vagina are important for several reasons. Human papillomavirus–induced warts of the vulva are, of course, visible to the patient and more difficult to eradicate. The recurrence rate after treatment with keratinolytic agents is about 60% vs. about 10% for cervical SILs treated with ablative therapy.[1–3] Vulvar (and penile) warts may become very large. Most contain large amounts of HPV and thus represent an overt source of potential infection to the sexual partner.

Despite some important differences, one crucial feature is shared by the vulva and cervix when considering HPV lesions: mimics of the infection are common. As previously discussed, squamous metaplasia with in-

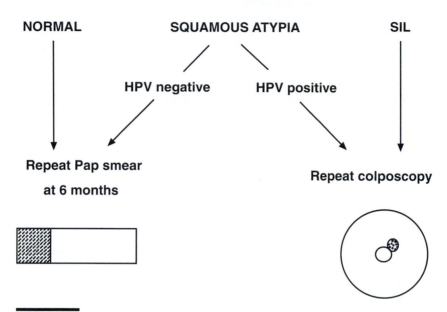

FIGURE 7.

A proposed management scheme for women with indeterminate colposcopic examinations. This scheme emphasizes the importance of the concurrent Papanicoloau smear and HPV DNA analysis in the treatment plan for women with indeterminate colposcopic examinations.

flammation can mimic a cervical SIL on cytologic, histologic, and/or colposcopic examination. Similarly, many common conditions of the vulva and vagina can produce papillary lesions that appear to be HPV-related warts on gross examination. Histologic analysis of such tissues may demonstrate features suggestive but not diagnostic of a low-grade SIL. The potential for overdiagnosis and the implications for the woman are, of course, just as important for vulvar and vaginal lesions as for cervical lesions. In my experience, in situ hybridization and PCR in situ hybridization for HPV have provided essential information to the clinician and pathologist in dealing with this very difficult area. It is not overstating the point to note that HPV testing in equivocal vulvar/vaginal biopsy tissue has spared many women the high costs of therapy and the emotional "costs" of the diagnosis of a sexually transmitted disease when no such disease was present.

NORMAL TISSUE

As noted in the discussion on the cervix, about 10% of women with a normal Papanicolaou smear have HPV present in the cervix if filter hybridization analyses are employed. Similar detection rates have been obtained by analyzing scrapings of the vulva (or penis) for HPV DNA with filter hybridization. However, the detection rate, in my experience, is 0% if standard in situ hybridization is used on vulvar tissue taken from an area where no lesion is evident. As was true for the cervix, this again suggests that the virus in such conditions is not actively proliferating. It is unclear but seems unlikely that such people are infectious given the inability to detect cells, especially toward the surface, with more than 10 viral genomes in them. The 0% detection rate by in situ hybridization offers a very high specificity when analyzing vulvar and vaginal lesions for HPV.

HUMAN PAPILLOMAVIRUS–RELATED LESIONS (CONDYLOMA AND HIGH-GRADE SQUAMOUS INTRAEPITHELIAL LESIONS)

As in the cervix, one can divide HPV-related lesions of the vulva and vagina into two groups: low-grade and high-grade lesions. In this discussion, we will use the synonymous term condyloma for low-grade SILs because it is more commonly used when referring to vulvar or penile lesions.

Before discussing the histologic features of vulvar and vaginal HPV-related lesions, a brief description of the microscopic appearance of the normal vulva and vagina is in order. The vulva is lined by a keratinizing squamous epithelium. The cells mature in an orderly fashion through different strata in the epithelium. The most immature basal cells are arranged in a "picket-fence" pattern and rarely show mitotic activity. The next layer, which is the thickest, consists of a five- to ten-cell thickness of squamous cells that are very well ordered. This leads to the granular cell layer, where dark blue keratohyaline granules are evident. It is important to realize that in the normal vulva, this layer is uniformly from one to two cell layers in thickness. Above the granular cell layer is the keratin layer, where anucleated squamous cells are organized in a "basket-weave" pattern of usually two to three cells thick.

It is important to realize that vulvar skin is not of uniform thickness. Rather, small skin folds, more evident on the labia majora, are often evident. These folds are also evident on the vagina, especially near the introitus. When these folds are exaggerated, a micropapillary lesion may be evident and can look like a condyloma. Vaginal epithelium has the appearance of the ectocervical aspect of the cervix on histologic examination; no granular cell layer or keratin is present. As in a normal vulva, there are key histologic features with regard to normal vaginal epithelium:

1. The cells are well organized.
2. The nuclei are similar in size, shape, and chromaticity.
3. Perinuclear halos are common in vaginal epithelium. As in the cervix, when they are of similar size and shape, this usually represents glycogen deposition and not HPV "koilocytes." Perinuclear halos are less commonly seen in normal vulvar epithelium.

The most important histologic feature that marks vulvar or vaginal condyloma is a disorganized growth pattern. The cells are crowded and show a variable cell density pattern of growth. In the vulva (or penile epithelium), these changes are most evident in the granular cell layer. Note in Figure 8 the perinuclear halos in cells in the granular layer that are invariably seen in unequivocal vulvar condylomas. Vaginal condylomas demonstrate variably sized and shaped perinuclear halos, similar to

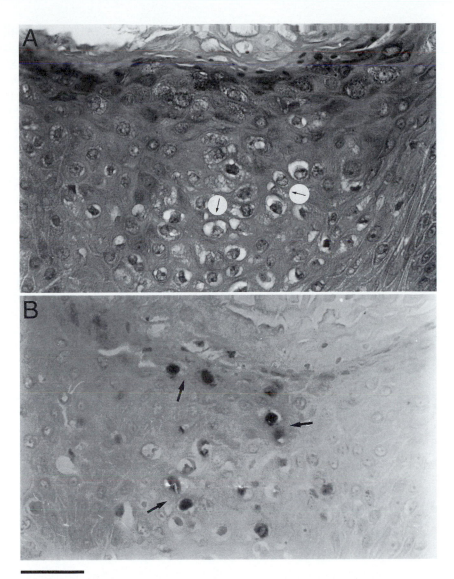

FIGURE 8.
Pathology and virology of vulvar condyloma. The perinuclear halos of variable size and shape just beneath the granular cell layer are diagnostic of condyloma **(A)**. Many of these cells contain large numbers of HPV 6 as determined by in situ hybridization **(B)**.

their counterpart in the cervix. The basal epithelium shows minimal changes in condyloma. However, the epithelium is usually irregularly thickened with overt acanthosis and an exaggeration of the size of the rete ridges, which often have an "inward" slant. In high-grade lesions, marked atypia is present in the basal zone, which also shows a large number of mitotic figures. The perinuclear halos are less evident. Many high-grade SILs of the vulva also show prominent parakeratosis, which is an unusual feature in condylomas.

As in cervical SILs, filter hybridization analyses and PCR have shown that basically all of these lesions contain HPV. The detection rate with in situ hybridization in my experience is 100% for condylomas and about 75% for high-grade SILs.[3] The lower percentage for high-grade SILs reflects the decreased copy number per cell typical of the higher-grade lesions, as was noted in the cervix. In situ hybridization analysis has revealed some interesting similarities and differences between vulvar/vaginal and cervical HPV-related lesions. The similar findings are as follows:

1. The viral copy number is most abundant in the middle and superficial layer of the epithelium, being especially abundant in cells that show perinuclear halos. Alternatively, HPV DNA is rarely detected in the cells of the basal epithelium. Clearly, this orientation facilitates venereal spread of the virus.
2. Human papillomavirus types 6 and 11 are rarely found in high-grade SILs (or vulvar cancers).

The following differences are noted:

1. Human papillomavirus types 6, 11, and 16 are found in over 90% of vulvar/vaginal HPV-related lesions, whereas, as you will recall, they account for only about 50% of the HPVs that are found in cervical SILs.
2. Human papillomavirus type 16 is rarely found in vulvar condyloma, although it is found in about 30% of the equivalent lesion of the cervix. However, HPV 16 is commonly found in high-grade vulvar/vaginal SILs, as expected from the cervical data.
3. Polymerase chain reaction in situ hybridization analysis has shown that HPV DNA is rarely present in the basal cells of a vulvar (or penile) condyloma.[62, 63]

Before leaving the topic of vulvar condyloma, one more important issue should be discussed. This concerns sexual abuse in children. Genital "warts" are relatively common in children and, when found, raise the obvious concern of sexual abuse. Analyses of such lesions in children have shown the following:

1. About 80% of such lesions are due to HPV 6 or 11.
2. Most of the other cases are due to HPV 2.[15, 64]

These observations are significant because HPVs 6 and 11 are very rarely detected on the skin at nongenital sites, even by PCR, whereas HPV 2 is the most common type in nongenital warts but is very rarely if ever detected in the genital tract of adults. It follows that the detection of HPV 2 in a genital wart in a child implies a nongenital source for the infection. Alternatively, detection of HPV 6 or 11 implies genital tract–to–genital tract transmission. This is not to say that HPV detection per se in genital warts in children can prove (HPV 6 or 11) or disprove (HPV 2) sexual abuse, but taken in the context of the total picture, including the social and psychological findings, it can provide very useful information in this most difficult area.

CANCER

Relative to carcinoma of the cervix, vulvar cancer is rare. This is probably a reflection of the much greater incidence of precancers of the cer-

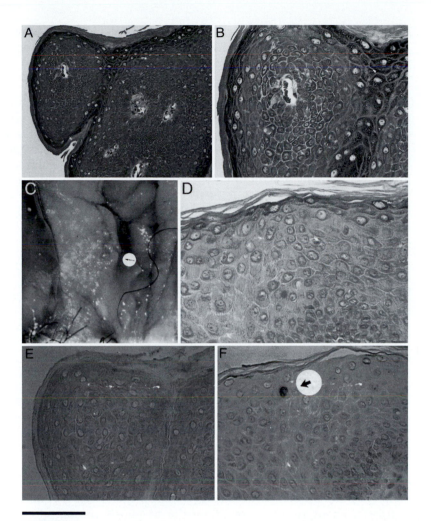

FIGURE 9.

Utility of HPV testing in equivocal vulvar biopsy tissue. These two biopsy specimens came from papillary vulvar lesions suggestive of condyloma. The first specimen (**A** and, at higher magnification, **B**) shows acanthosis and papillomatosis as would be expected from its clinical appearance (**C**). Similar histologic findings are evident in the other specimen (**D**). Neither sample showed halos and nuclear variability in the granular cell layer and were thus initially termed "suggestive but not diagnostic of condyloma." Human papillomavirus was not detected in the first specimen by in situ hybridization (**E**) or in situ polymerase chain reaction (not shown) but was detected by in situ hybridization in the specimen from the other woman (**F**). It was concluded that the first lesion represented a nonspecific mimic of a condyloma whereas the second specimen is best interpreted as a condyloma, even though only a few cells were positive (see Fig 10).

vix as compared with the vulva and vagina. There are two other interesting points to consider when comparing carcinoma of the cervix with vulvar cancer:

1.   Vulvar cancers have two distinct histologic forms—highly keratinizing, with the adjacent epithelium showing nonspecific acanthosis, and less keratinizing, with a high-grade SIL evident toward the periphery of the invasive cancer.

2. Epidemiologic data suggest two distinct risk factor categories for vulvar cancer—one category related to venereal risk factors, as for cervical cancer, and the other not apparently related to the patient's sexual history.[14, 65]

About 3 years ago, several groups working independently showed that unlike cervical cancer, which was strongly HPV related, most vulvar cancers were HPV-negative, even when highly sensitive techniques such as PCR were used. When the viral findings were correlated with the histologic and epidemiologic data, it became clear that the more common highly keratinizing variant of vulvar cancer was HPV-negative. It is of interest that this histologic type is very rare in the cervix. It was the less keratinized squamous cell cancer of the vulva that often showed areas of high-grade SILs that were HPV-positive and related to a history of multiple sexual partners.[14, 65]

EQUIVOCAL TISSUE

In this author's experience, the site where the surgical pathologist is most likely to analyze a lesion suggestive but not diagnostic of HPV infection is the vulva (and penis). When one considers that HPV-related lesions and their mimics are common, it is not surprising that the histologic features of vulvar condyloma tend to be less overt than those in the cervix, and that vulvar and penile lesions will be visible to the patient. A common scenario is a patient who is concerned that she (or he) may have been exposed to HPV via sexual relations and, because of this concern, notices an oftentimes small lesion on the vulva (or penis). It is in these cases of uncertainty that this author believes that HPV testing has the greatest utility for patient care. When probes for HPVs 6, 11, and 16 and in situ hybridization are used, a papillary vulvar lesion equivocal for condyloma on histology that is negative for HPV is best considered a mimic and not a condyloma. If the lesion contains HPV, as is true in about 10% of cases, then the diagnosis of condyloma should be used.

Because in situ hybridization may not detect the virus due to its relatively high detection threshold, there is the potential for a false-negative result. We have studied both vulvar and penile lesions for HPV by using PCR in situ hybridization. The major findings were as follows:

1. Most equivocal vulvar (and penile) lesions negative for HPV by in situ hybridization will also be negative by PCR in situ hybridization.

2. For those equivocal tissues positive by PCR in situ hybridization, the histologic marker of viral infection was a focally thickened granular

---

FIGURE 10.

Utility of in situ polymerase chain reaction (PCR) analysis of a difficult vulvar lesion. This papillary vulvar lesion lacked the diagnostic features of a condyloma **(A)**. HPV 6 DNA was rarely detected in a few cells by in situ analysis **(B)**. An intense hybridization signal was observed in many more cells in these areas after amplification by PCR **(C)**. The signal localized to areas where a focally thickened granular layer was noted in the epithelial crevices. These histologic features are a useful marker of HPV infection in these equivocal cases.

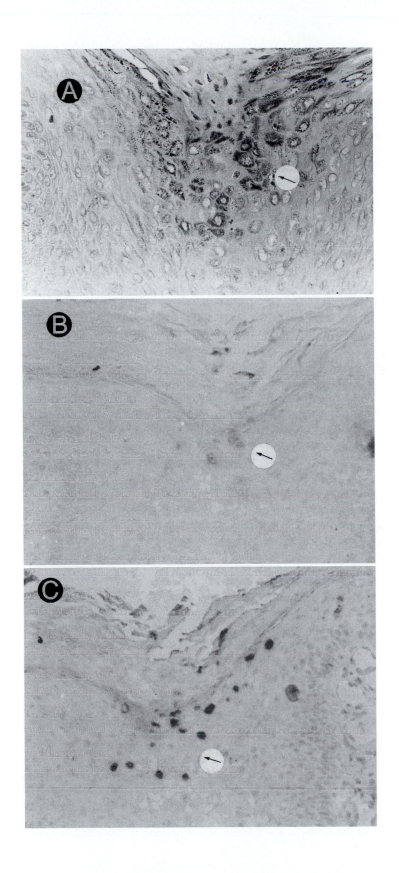

layer, oftentimes in association with an epithelial crevice and parakeratosis or hyperkeratosis (Figs 9 and 10).

It is evident that most vulvar tissues that are equivocal for condyloma and lack a focally thickened granular cell layer in areas of epithelial crevices will be HPV-negative and are best considered mimics of condyloma. This author still recommends HPV testing in such cases because it provides reassurance to many patients. In addition, there have been rare cases in which the tissue did not show a focally thickened granular cell layer and was still HPV-positive (see Figure 9).

What is the etiology of HPV-negative papillary vulvar lesions? These areas are often micropapillary and probably represent exaggerated skin folds or nonspecific changes caused by chronic inflammation, which can develop from conditions such as candidiasis, eczema, or tinea.

THE ENDOMETRIUM AND OVARY

Over the past 10 years, there have been scattered but persistent attempts to link HPV with endometrial and ovarian pathology. Papillary lesions of the ovary are very common and include papillary serous tumors and surface papillomatosis. Reports of HPV detection in such tumors have been published. However, many other groups with extensive experience in HPV testing have not been able to detect HPV in a wide variety of tissues, including papillary tumors in the ovary and endometrium.[66, 67] This has been my experience as well. Indeed, I have used this observation in studying adenocarcinomas that are in the endocervix and endometrial cavity. It may not be possible to determine, on histologic grounds, the site of origin when an adenocarcinoma has invaded both the endocervix and endometrium. This distinction has important clinical implications with regard to treatment. We have used HPV testing in such cases to distinguish an HPV-positive endocervical primary tumor from an HPV-negative endometrial primary tumor.

ACKNOWLEDGMENT

The author is deeply indebted to Ms. Phyllis MacConnell for expert editorial advice and to Dr. Christopher Crum and Mr. S.B. Lewis for their support. Data from studies reported in this paper were supported by grants to G.J.N. from the Lewis Foundation, the Perkin-Elmer Corporation, Roche Molecular Systems, and the Center for Biotechnology of the State of New York.

REFERENCES

1. Nuovo GJ: *Cytopathology of the Lower Female Genital Tract: An Integrated Approach.* Baltimore, Williams & Wilkins, 1993.
2. Ehrmann R: *Benign to Malignant Progression in Cervical Squamous Epithelium.* New York, Igaku-Shoin, 1993.
3. Crum CP, Nuovo GJ: *Genital Papillomaviruses and Related Neoplasms.* New York, Raven Press, 1991.
4. O'Banion MK, Reichmann ME, Sundberg JP: Cloning and characterization of

a papillomavirus associated with papillomas and carcinomas in the European harvest mouse (Micromys minutus). *J Virol* 62:226–233, 1988.

5. McBride AA, Byrne JC, Howley PM: E2 polypeptides encoded by bovine papillomavirus type 1 form dimers through the common carboxyl-terminal domain: Transactivation is mediated by the conserved amino-terminal domain. *Proc Natl Acad Sci U S A* 86:510–514, 1989.

6. Cowsert LM, Pilacinski WP, Jenson AB: Identification of the bovine papillomavirus L1 gene product using monoclonal antibodies. *Virology* 165:613–615, 1988.

7. deVilliers EM: Heterogeneity of the human papillomavirus group. *J Virol* 63:4898–4903, 1989.

8. Bergeron C, Naghashfar Z, Canaan C, et al: Human papillomavirus type 16 in intraepithelial neoplasia (bowenoid papulosis) and coexistent invasive carcinoma of the vulva. *Int J Gynecol Pathol* 6:1–11, 1987.

9. Buscema J, Naghashfar Z, Sowada E, et al: The predominance of human papillomavirus type 16 in vulvar neoplasia. *Obstet Gynecol* 71:601–605, 1988.

10. Nuovo GJ, Blanco JB, Silverstein SJ, et al: Histologic correlates of papillomavirus infection of the vagina. *Obstet Gynecol* 72:770–774, 1988.

11. Reid R, Greenberg M, Jenson AB, et al: Sexually transmitted papillomaviral infections I. The anatomic distribution and pathologic grade of neoplastic lesions associated with different viral types. *Am J Obstet Gynecol* 156:212–222, 1987.

12. Nuovo GJ, O'Connell M, Blanco JB, et al: Correlation of histology and human papillomavirus DNA detection in condyloma acuminatum and condyloma-like vulvar lesions. *Am J Surg Pathol* 13:700–706, 1989.

13. Crum CP, Burkett BJ: Papillomavirus and vulvovaginal neoplasia. *J Reprod Med* 34:566–571, 1989.

14. Nuovo GJ, Delvenne P, MacConnell P, et al: Correlation of histology and detection of human papillomavirus DNA in vulvar cancers. *Gynecol Oncol*, 43:275–280, 1991.

15. Nuovo GJ, Lastarria D, Smith S, et al: Human papillomavirus segregation patterns in genital and non-genital warts in prepubertal children and adults. *Am J Clin Pathol* 95:467–472, 1991.

16. Nuovo GJ, Hochman H, Eliezri YD, et al: Detection of human papillomavirus DNA in penile lesions histologically negative for condylomata: Analysis by in situ hybridization and the polymerase chain reaction. *Am J Surg Pathol* 14:829–836, 1990.

17. Ensser A, Pfister H: Epidermodysplasia verruciformis associated human papillomaviruses present a subgenus-specific organization of the regulatory genome region. *Nucleic Acids Res* 18:3919–3922, 1990.

18. Orth G: Epidermodysplasia verruciformis: A model for understanding the oncogenicity of human papillomavirus. *Ciba Found Symp* 120:157–174, 1986.

19. Burnett S, Strom AC, Jareborg N, et al: Induction of bovine papillomavirus E2 gene expression and early region transcription by cell growth arrest: Correlation with viral DNA amplification and evidence for differential promoter induction. *J Virol* 64:5529–5541, 1990.

20. Dyson N, Howley PM, Munger K, et al: The human papilloma virus-16 E7 oncoprotein is able to bind to the retinoblastoma gene product. *Science* 243:934–936, 1989.

21. DiPaolo JA, Woodworth CD, Popescu NC, et al: Induction of human cervical squamous cell carcinoma by sequential transfection with human papillomavirus 16 DNA and viral Harvey ras. *Oncogene* 4:395–399, 1989.

22. Pecoraro G, Lee M, Morgan D, et al: Evolution of in vitro transformation and tumorigenesis of HPV 16 and HPV 18 immortalized primary cervical epithelial cells. *Am J Pathol* 138:1–8, 1991.

23. Tindle RW, Fernando GJP, Sterling JC, et al: A "public" T-helper epitope of the E7 transforming protein of human papillomavirus 16 provides cognate help for several E7 B-cell epitopes from cervical cancer–associated human papillomavirus genotypes. *Proc Natl Acad Sci U S A* 88:5887–5891, 1991.

24. Munger K, Yee CL, Phelps WC, et al: Biochemical and biological differences between E7 oncoproteins of the high- and low-risk human papillomavirus types are determined by amino-terminal sequences. *J Virol* 65:3943–3948, 1991.

25. Schiffman MH, Bauer HM, Lorincz AT, et al: A comparison of Southern blot hybridization and polymerase chain reaction methods for the detection of human papillomavirus DNA. *J Clin Microbiol* 29:573–579, 1991.

26. Greer CE, Peterson SL, Kiviat NB, et al: PCR amplification from paraffin-embedded tissues. Effects of fixative and fixation times. *Am J Clin Pathol* 95:117–124, 1991.

27. Bauer HM, Ting Y, Greer CE, et al: Genital human papillomavirus infection in female university students as determined by a PCR-based method. *JAMA* 265:472–477, 1991.

28. Nuovo GJ: Buffered formalin is the superior fixative for the detection of human papillomavirus DNA by in situ hybridization analysis. *Am J Pathol* 134:837–842, 1989.

29. Nuovo GJ: A comparison of slot blot, Southern blot and in situ hybridization analyses for human papillomavirus DNA in genital tract lesions. *Obstet Gynecol* 74:673–677, 1989.

30. Nuovo GJ, Richart RM: Human papillomavirus: A review, in Mishell DR, Kirschbaum TH, Morrow CP (eds): *Year Book of Obstetrics and Gynecology.* St Louis, Mosby, 1989, pp 297–313.

31. Nuovo GJ: Determination of HPV type by in situ hybridization analysis: A comparative study with Southern blot hybridization and the polymerase chain reaction. *J Histotech* 15:99–104, 1992.

32. Nuovo GJ, Darfler MM, Impraim CC, et al: Occurrence of multiple types of human papillomavirus in genital tract lesions: Analysis by in situ hybridization and the polymerase chain reaction. *Am J Pathol* 58:518–523, 1991.

33. Nuovo GJ: A comparison of different methodologies (biotin based and 35S based) for the detection of human papillomavirus DNA. *Lab Invest* 61:471–476, 1989.

34. Chou Q, Russell M, Birch DE, et al: Prevention of pre-PCR mis-priming and primer dimerization improves low copy number amplifications. *Nucleic Acids Res* 20:1717–1723, 1992.

35. Nuovo GJ, Gallery F, Hom R, et al: Importance of different variables for optimizing in situ detection of PCR-amplified DNA. *PCR Methods Appl* 2:305–312, 1993.

36. Erlich HA, Gelfand D, Sninsky JJ: Recent advances in the polymerase chain reaction. *Science* 252:1643–1650, 1991.

37. Nuovo GJ, Cottral S, Richart RM: Occult infection of the uterine cervix by human papillomavirus in postmenopausal women. *Am J Obstet Gynecol* 160:340–344, 1989.

38. Nuovo GJ, Nuovo MA, Cottral S, et al: Histological correlates of clinically occult human papillomavirus infection of the uterine cervix. *Am J Surg Pathol* 12:198–204, 1988.

39. Myerson D, Hackman RC, Nelson JA: Widespread presence of histologically occult cytomegalovirus. *Hum Pathol* 15:430–439, 1984.

40. Schneider A, Meinhardt G, Kirchmayr R, et al: Prevalence of human papillomavirus genomes in tissues from the lower genital tract as detected by molecular in situ by hybridization. *Int J Gynecol Pathol* 10:1–14, 1991.

41. Shibata D, Fu YS, Gupta JW, et al: Detection of human papillomavirus in nor-

mal and dysplastic tissue by the polymerase chain reaction. *Lab Invest* 59:555–559, 1988.

42. Syrjanen S, Saastamoinen J, Chang F, et al: Colposcopy, punch biopsy, in situ DNA hybridization, and the polymerase chain reaction in searching for genital human papillomavirus infections in women with normal Pap smears. *J Med Virol* 31:259–266, 1990.

43. deVilliers EM, Schneider A, Miklaw H, et al: Human papillomavirus infections in women with and without abnormal cervical cytology. *Lancet* 1:703–706, 1987.

44. Colgan TJ, Percy ME, Suri M, et al: Human papillomavirus infection of morphologically normal cervical epithelium adjacent to squamous dysplasia and invasive carcinoma. *Hum Pathol* 20:316–319, 1989.

45. Tidy JA, Parry GCN, Ward P, et al: High rate of human papillomavirus type 16 infection in cytologically normal cervices. *Lancet* 1:434, 1989.

46. Tidy JA, Vousden KH, Farrell PJ: Relation between infection with a subtype of HPV 16 and cervical neoplasia. *Lancet* 1:1225–1227, 1989.

47. Nuovo GJ, Walsh LL, Gentile J, et al: Correlation of the Papanicolaou smear and human papillomavirus type in women with biopsy proven cervical intraepithelial lesions. *Am J Clin Pathol* 96:544–548, 1991.

48. Kreider JW, Howett MK, Leure-Dupree AE, et al: Laboratory production in vivo of infectious human papillomavirus type 11. *J Virol* 61:590–593, 1987.

49. Nuovo GJ, Friedman D: In situ hybridization analysis of HPV DNA segregation patterns in lesions of the female genital tract. *Gynecol Oncol* 36:256–262, 1990.

50. Delvenne P, Engellenner W, Nuovo GJ: Detection of human papillomavirus DNA in biopsy proven cervical intraepithelial lesions in pregnant women. *J Reprod Med* 37:829–833, 1992.

51. Nuovo GJ, MacConnell P, Forde A, et al: Detection of human papillomavirus DNA in formalin fixed tissues by in situ hybridization after amplification by PCR. *Am J Pathol* 139:847–854, 1991.

52. Nuovo GJ, Babury R, Calayag P: Human papillomavirus types and recurrent cervical warts in immunocompromised women. *Mod Pathol* 4:632–636, 1991.

53. Nuovo GJ, Pedemonte BA: Human papillomavirus types and recurrent genital warts. *JAMA* 263:1223–1226, 1990.

54. Nuovo GJ, Moritz J, Mann W: Human papillomavirus types and recurrent genital warts after conization. *Gynecol Oncol* 46:304–308, 1992.

55. Walker J, Bloss JD, Liao S-Y, et al: Human papillomavirus genotype as a prognostic indicator in carcinoma of the uterine cervix. *Obstet Gynecol* 74:781–785, 1989.

56. Wilczynski SP, Bergen S, Walker J, et al: Human papillomaviruses and cervical cancer: Analysis of histopathologic features associated with different viral types. *Hum Pathol* 19:697–704, 1988.

57. Lorincz AT, Temple GF, Kurman RJ, et al: Oncogenic association of specific human papillomavirus types with cervical neoplasia. *J Natl Cancer Inst* 79:671–677, 1987.

58. Cullen AP, Reid R, Champion M, et al: Analysis of the physical state of different human papillomavirus DNAs in intraepithelial and invasive cervical neoplasia. *J Virol* 65:606–612, 1991.

59. Riou G, Favre M, Jeannel D, et al: Association between poor prognosis in early stage invasive cervical carcinomas and non-detection of HPV DNA. *Lancet* 169:1171–1174, 1990.

60. Liotta LA, Steeg PS, Stetler-Stevenson WG: Cancer metastasis and angiogenesis: An imbalance of positive and negative regulation. *Cell* 64:327–336, 1991.

61. Nuovo GJ, Blanco JS, Leipzig S, et al: Human papillomavirus detection in cervical lesions histologically negative for cervical intraepithelial neoplasia: Correlation with Pap smear, colposcopy, and occurrence of cervical intraepithelial neoplasia. *Obstet Gynecol* 75:1006–1011, 1990.

62. Nuovo GJ, Gallery F, MacConnell P: Analysis of the distribution pattern of PCR-amplified HPV 6 DNA in vulvar warts by in situ hybridization. *Mod Pathol* 5:444–448, 1992.

63. Nuovo GJ, Becker J, MacConnell P, et al: Histological distribution of PCR-amplified HPV 6 and 11 DNA in penile lesions. *Am J Surg Pathol* 16:269–275, 1992.

64. Obalek S, Jablonska S, Favre L, et al: Condylomata acuminata in children: Frequent association with human papillomaviruses responsible for cutaneous warts. *J Am Acad Dermatol* 23:205–213, 1990.

65. Park JS, Jones RW, McLean MR, et al: Possible etiologic heterogeneity of vulvar intraepithelial neoplasia. *Cancer* 67:1599–1607, 1991.

66. deVilliers EM, Schneider A, Gross G, et al: Analysis of benign and malignant urogenital tumors for human papillomavirus infection by labelling cellular DNA. *Med Microbiol Immunol* 174:281–286, 1986.

67. Ostrow RS, Manias DA, Fong WJ, et al: A survey of human cancers for human papillomavirus DNA by filter hybridization. *Cancer* 59:429–434, 1987.

Legionella*

Paul H. Edelstein

Clinical Microbiology Laboratory, Departments of Pathology and Laboratory Medicine, Department of Medicine, Hospital of the University of Pennsylvania, University of Pennsylvania School of Medicine, Philadelphia, Pennsylvania

Richard D. Meyer

Department of Medicine, University of California, Los Angeles, UCLA School of Medicine, Los Angeles, California

L egionnaires' disease was first recognized as a distinct entity during the summer of 1976, when pneumonia developed in some 200 people attending an American Legion convention in Philadelphia.[1] About 35 people died despite what was thought to be appropriate treatment for pneumonia. The cause of the epidemic eluded city, state, and federal investigators for months. The disease was called legionnaires' disease after the American Legion. Senator Kennedy initiated Senate hearings, and multiple scientists and critics put forth hypotheses regarding the etiology of the epidemic; these ranged from toxic fumes generated by photocopy machines to biological warfare experiments conducted by the Central Intelligence Agency. Some even suggested that the epidemic was a hoax promulgated by the U.S. Centers for Disease Control (CDC) to "cover up" mass immunization for influenza that proved to be unneeded. However, Joseph McDade of the CDC discovered in January 1977 that the etiology was a "novel" bacterium that did not grow on conventional bacteriologic media. Poor staining of the bacterium by conventional staining techniques and its fastidious growth characteristics had resulted in delay of its detection. This bacterium was named *Legionella pneumophila*. It is now known that *L. pneumophila* was responsible for an outbreak of pneumonia in the 1950s and that *Legionella* bacteria had been isolated as long ago as the 1940s.[2-4] Thus neither the disease nor the causative bacterium was new; rather they were simply rediscovered.

Another disease attributed to *Legionella* bacteria is Pontiac fever.[4-6] This is named after an outbreak of a nonfatal influenza-like illness that caused disease in most occupants of a health department in Pontiac, Michigan, in 1968. In 1977 it was discovered that serum obtained from victims of this disease contained antibodies to *L. pneumophila* and that the building's malfunctioning air-conditioning system contained *L. pneumophila*.

*Modified with permission from Edelstein PH, Meyer RD: *Legionella* pneumonias, in Pennington JE (ed): *Respiratory Infections. Diagnosis and Management*, ed 3. New York, Raven Press, 1994, pp 455–484.

Advances in Pathology and Laboratory Medicine, vol. 8
© 1995, Mosby–Year Book, Inc.

ETIOLOGY

The *Legionella* spp. (Table 1) are fastidious gram-negative bacilli that are strict aerobes.[7] There is a nutritional requirement for L-cysteine and in most cases iron. Because of these nutritional requirements, they do not grow on routine bacteriologic media such as MacConkey or blood agar. The optimal growth medium, called buffered charcoal yeast extract (BCYEα), contains L-cysteine, iron, yeast extract, an organic buffer, and α-ketoglutarate, which serves as a growth supplement.[8] All species grow

TABLE 1.
Legionella Species and Serogroups

Species	No. of Serogroups	Clinical Isolates?
L. adelaidensis	1	No
L. anisa	1	Yes
L. birminghamensis	1	Yes
L. bozemanii	2	Yes
L. brunensis	1	No
L. cherrii	1	No
L. cincinnatiensis	1	Yes
L. dumoffii	1	Yes
L. erythra	1	No
L. fairfieldensis	1	No
L. feeleii	2	Yes
L. gormanii	1	Yes
L. gratiana	1	No
L. hackeliae	2	Yes
L. israelensis	1	No
L. jamestowniensis	1	No
L. jordanis	1	Yes
L. lansingensis	1	Yes
L. longbeachae	2	Yes
L. micdadei	1	Yes
L. moravica	1	No
L. oakridgensis	1	Yes*
L. parisiensis	1	No
L. pneumophila	15	Yes
L. quinlivanii	1	No
L. rubrilucens	1	No
L. sainthelensi	2	Yes
L. santicrucis	1	No
L. shakespearei	1	No
L. spiritensis	2	No
L. steigerwaltii	1	No
L. tucsonensis	1	Yes
L. wadsworthii	1	Yes

*By DFA test only.

well in humidified air at 35°C; some species grow better in 2.5% to 3.0% CO_2. The average incubation time required for first growth is 3 days, with a range of 1 to 10 days.

At least 15 serogroups and several subserogroups have been identified for *L. pneumophila;* 33 other *Legionella* species have been characterized.[9, 10] The nomenclature is confusing because some strains are named after cities, some after states, and others from initials of patients. *Legionella pneumophila* serogroups 1, 4, and 6 appear to be the most common causes of infection, with about 80% of cases caused by serogroup 1 and 5% to 10% caused by each of the other two groups. Infections caused by legionellae other than *L. pneumophila* are uncommon, constituting perhaps 20% to 30% of infections, and occur almost exclusively in immunosuppressed patients. Of these, infections caused by *L. micdadei, L. longbeachae, L. dumoffii,* and *L. bozemanii* appear to be the most common in that order.

The natural reservoir for legionellae is fresh water, where they are ubiquitous, especially in warm water.[9, 11] There is substantial evidence that these bacteria exist in nature by growing in free-living amebas such as *Acanthamoeba, Hartmannella,* and *Naegleria;* unsettled is whether legionellae are facultative or obligate parasites of these protozoa.[12] *Legionella pneumophila* within amebas is protected from high levels of chlorine, which makes eradication of the organism from the environment difficult and fosters its presence in treated water.[13, 14]

PATHOGENESIS AND IMMUNITY

Legionnaires' disease is caused by inhalation or perhaps aspiration of virulent *Legionella* spp.[9, 15–17] Rarely, disease is caused by direct inoculation of *Legionella* spp. into a wound or the skin.[18, 19] Devices that aerosolize *Legionella*-contaminated water serve as disseminators of the disease. Such devices have included cooling towers, humidifiers, respiratory therapy equipment, an ultrasonic nebulizer used to mist vegetables, shower heads, faucets, and industrial cooling sprays. The actual bacterial form that causes infection is uncertain; some hypothesize that *Legionella* bacteria contained within amebas cause disease.

Once the bacteria gain entrance to the lung, whether by aerosol or aspiration, they are phagocytosed by alveolar macrophages.[20, 21] Because of their ability to grow and survive in macrophages, the *Legionella* bacteria multiply in the lung. The bacteria are toxic to macrophages, eventually causing their death and resulting in the release of large numbers of extracellular bacteria. This cycle starts again in other uninfected macrophages, which serves to greatly amplify bacterial concentrations within the lungs. In a guinea pig model of Legionnaires' disease, *L. pneumophila* attains concentrations in the lung as high as 10^{11} bacteria per gram. Extrapulmonary spread of bacteria occurs experimentally and in at least some humans with Legionnaires' disease; it is probable that hematogenous spread is facilitated by the circulation of *Legionella*-infected monocytes.[22, 23] Activation of alveolar macrophages by interferon-γ, and probably other cytokines greatly slows bacterial growth in vitro and probably has a similar effect in humans.[24, 25]

Several important *L. pneumophila* virulence determinants have been described, although the molecular pathogenesis of infection is still incompletely understood.[20, 21, 26] A bacterial protein called MIP (macrophage infectivity potentiator) is important for bacterial entry into cells.[27] The product of a gene called DOT (defect in organelle trafficking) is responsible for phagolysosomal fusion inhibition and allowing intracellular growth.[28] Macrophage complement receptors may serve as receptors for *L. pneumophila,* although this is controversial, as is the role of serum complement in uptake of the bacterium into the macrophage.[29-31] Several different exotoxins as well as a weakly active endotoxin have been described for *L. pneumophila.* One of the most interesting is a protease that may be important in the pathogenesis of *L. pneumophila* infections, at least in animals.[32, 33] Several toxins that inhibit white blood cell function or integrity have been characterized, including a cytotoxin, a phospholipase, an inhibitor of oxidative metabolism and intracellular killing, and an inhibitor of chemotaxis.[34-38] Similar findings have been made for *L. micdadei.* Virtually nothing is known about the virulence factors of the other *Legionella* species.

The systemic manifestations of the disease are likely caused by toxin elaboration by the bacterium rather than by extrapulmonary infection. Host inflammatory mediators doubtless play a major role in producing the manifestations of Legionnaires' disease. However, extrapulmonary infection involving the brain, intestine, lymph nodes, kidneys, liver, spleen, peritoneum, bone marrow, myocardium, pericardium, and the bloodstream itself has been documented.[19, 39-42]

The cellular immune system is most important for immunity to Legionnaires' disease, most particularly macrophages, monocytes, and probably lymphocytes.[9, 21] Cellular rather than humoral immunity appears to play the major role in host defenses against Legionnaires' disease. Animals can be protected from lethal challenge by immunization with several bacterial components such as an outer membrane protein and a protease; vaccination with these proteins induces cellular immunity and to a lesser extent humoral immunity.[43, 44] Immunization with a bacterial heat shock protein (HSP 60) induces very strong humoral immunity and weak cellular immunity and is variably protective in animals.[45, 46] Both animals and humans may recover from this disease without antibody formation. Finally, those at greatest risk of disease have defects in cellular immune function, pulmonary clearance mechanisms, or both. Polymorphonuclear leukocytes appear to play little role in protective immunity, as evidenced by the paucity of Legionnaires' disease cases in patients with neutropenia but intact macrophage function. The implications of this are that medical therapies or underlying diseases that reduce systemic or local cellular immunity greatly increase the risk of Legionnaires' disease. Because of the ability of *Legionella* spp. to evade extracellular host defenses, relapses of disease are seen after short courses of antimicrobials or with renewed immunosuppression.

The pathogenesis of Pontiac fever is not understood and has not been studied thoroughly. The leading hypotheses include intoxication caused by inhalation of *Legionella* and other bacterial toxins, self-limited pulmonary infection caused by *Legionella* strains that are able to infect macrophages but not multiply within them, and an infectious or toxic disease caused by microorganisms coexisting with *Legionella* in contaminated waters.

PATHOLOGY

Consistent pathologic findings are usually limited to the chest cavity. Lobar or, less commonly, segmental consolidations are constant findings. Abnormalities are usually confined to the alveoli and respiratory bronchioles, with dense infiltration of intra-alveolar polymorphonuclear leukocytes and macrophages; microabscesses are not uncommon. The larger airways and alveolar septa are spared. Pleural inflammation may occur. Organisms have rarely been seen in hilar lymph nodes.[47-49]

Extrapulmonary *L. pneumophila* has been detected in the kidney, lymph nodes, muscle, skin, brain, spleen, bone marrow, liver, blood, peritoneum, intestine, pericardium, and myocardium. Pathologic findings in large series do not, however, reveal consistent changes in these organs.[47] It can only be concluded that in extraordinary cases, particularly in immunosuppressed patients, extrapulmonary dissemination can occur. Microabscess formation has been demonstrated in association with *L. pneumophila* infection of multiple extrapulmonary organs of a severely immunosuppressed child.[39] Infection of nonpulmonary organs, in the absence of pneumonia, has been documented to occur in prosthetic heart valves, respiratory sinuses, the pleural space, skin and muscle, and wounds. These extrapulmonary infections are caused either by bacteremia during open heart surgery without subsequent pneumonia or by direct seeding of susceptible tissues by *Legionella*-contaminated water.

The usual tissue stains do not show bacteria. These include hematoxylin and eosin, Brown-Brenn, and methenamine silver stains. Mycobacterial stains do not show organisms, except for the Kinyoun acid-fast stain, which demonstrates the presence of a minority of *L. micdadei* organisms.[48] The best nonimmunologic method of demonstrating bacilli from the lung is a Giménez stain of a tissue imprint; this can be either fresh or fixed tissue. Once the tissue is embedded in paraffin, the Dieterle silver impregnation stain or a modified Giménez stain can be used.[7] These methods are nonspecific and probably relatively insensitive. Direct immunofluorescence examination is the most specific and sensitive means of visualizing *Legionella* organisms in tissues and body fluids and is also suitable for formalinized specimens.[7, 50] A monoclonal antibody (Genetic Systems, Seattle), widely used for examination of nonfixed clinical specimens, cannot be used for formalin-fixed tissues; commercially available polyvalent reagents should be used instead. All of the immunologic techniques have the major drawback of being species and serogroup specific and may therefore lead to a false-negative diagnosis if the wrong serogroup or species conjugate is used. *Legionella*-specific DNA probes have been used to visualize the bacteria in tissues.[51] Culture of tissue and respiratory secretions is a sensitive and specific method (see later).

EPIDEMIOLOGY

Legionnaires' disease exists both in outbreaks and as sporadic cases.[9] Over 30 nosocomial outbreaks and a smaller number of building-associated outbreaks have been reported. Sporadic cases greatly outnumber cases associated with defined outbreaks. It is estimated that Legionnaires' disease occurs in about 6 per 100,000 U.S. adults per year, which is roughly 10,000 cases per year. This constitutes about 0.5% to 5% of all causes of adult pneumonias. In the United States there is apparent tremendous geographic variation in the frequency of Legionnaires' disease, although differences in the vigor of case finding may account for some of these differences.[52] Legionnaires' disease has been reported worldwide, with the bulk of cases reported in western Europe and North America.

Risk factors for Legionnaires' disease include glucocorticosteroid administration or its endogenous production, cigarette smoking, age greater than 50 years, male gender, chronic obstructive lung disease, and congestive heart failure; of these, glucocorticosteroid administration and cigarette smoking are the principal risk factors.[9] Organ transplant patients are at high risk because of the administration of glucocorticosteroids and other immunosuppressive therapy. Infection caused by human immunodeficiency virus (HIV) also appears to be a risk factor, although Legionnaires' disease is an unusual cause of pneumonia in HIV-infected patients.[53] Cytotoxic chemotherapy has also been shown to be a risk factor for nosocomial legionnaires' disease.[54] Working with or around water does not appear to be a major risk factor. The proximity of residence to a cooling tower is a risk factor for Legionnaires' disease in Glasgow, Scotland.[52, 55, 56]

The sources of *Legionella* spp. causing disease have been principally either cooling towers or potable water systems, although many other warm water–containing sites have been linked to cases of Legionnaires' disease. Transmission usually results from the inhalation of aerosols.[9, 15, 57] Aspiration is a possible mode of transmission in hospitalized patients.[16] Rarely, wound infections follow irrigation with contaminated water, as has been reported for sternal wound and pleural infections.[19]

CLINICAL FEATURES

After the usual incubation period of 2 to 10 days, pneumonia usually develops and may be severe. Infection with L. *pneumophila* may, however, cause many different diseases, some of which could be asymptomatic.[58] The finding of elevated antibody levels in the general healthy population indicates that Legionnaires' disease could occur as an asymptomatic infection. However, cross-reacting antibodies could also partly account for these findings.[59] Several prospective studies have demonstrated that neither community-acquired nor nosocomial Legionnaires' disease can be differentiated from other common causes of pneumonia by clinical, radiographic, or nonspecific laboratory findings.[60–63] We describe the classic manifestation of Legionnaires' disease because we believe that a subset of patients with this disease do have distinctive symptoms and signs.

PNEUMONIA

The disease usually has a gradual onset, but it may be more abrupt, especially in immunosuppressed patients. The first symptoms are often malaise, lethargy, headache, weakness, myalgia, and anorexia; the headache may be severe. Complaints of sore throat or rhinitis are usually absent. The majority of patients have a dry nonproductive cough. In about one half to one fourth of patients, the sputum may be purulent or bloody; this usually occurs after the illness has progressed for several days. About 75% of patients have recurrent rigor.[58, 64, 65]

Complaints of a systemic nature are common. These include diarrhea, nausea, vomiting, and headache. One fourth to one third of patients complain of pleuritic pain, which in association with hemoptysis often makes one think of pulmonary infarction. Myalgia and arthralgia may be prominent and lead one to a consideration of collagen vascular disease. Diaphoresis is sometimes seen.[64, 65]

EXTRAPULMONARY MANIFESTATIONS

Abnormalities of mental status are common and are found in about one fourth of the patients with pneumonia. Findings noted include disorientation, agitation, stupor, confusion, obtundation, coma, hallucinations, ataxia, grand mal seizure, and focal neurologic findings.[64, 66, 67] Focal visceral abscesses, pancreatitis, peritonitis, pericarditis, myocarditis, leukoencephalitis, cellulitis with myositis, myositis with motor neuropathy, and Henoch-Schönlein purpura have also been separately described.[18, 47, 48, 68–72]

Disease caused by *Legionella* not involving the lung concurrently has been rarely noted. Aside from Pontiac fever, there have been relatively few well documented cases of *Legionella* not involving the lung. Prosthetic valve endocarditis, peritonitis, and infections of wounds and paranasal sinuses with *Legionella* have been well documented.[19]

Abnormalities of other systems, including the hepatic, renal, and musculoskeletal systems, e.g., myositis or rhabdomyolysis, occur but are usually noted only on laboratory examination. The spectrum of associated renal disease includes interstitial nephritis and less commonly acute tubular necrosis, myoglobinuria, or perhaps glomerulonephritis.[73, 74]

Radiographic findings are variable but may include alveolar filling patterns with lobar, nodular, patchy, or subsegmental consolidation.[75, 76] Interstitial pulmonary infiltrates are very rare but may be seen very early in the disease. Pulmonary cavitation may occur in immunosuppressed patients.[77]

PONTIAC FEVER

Pontiac fever is manifested by fever, chills, myalgia, and headache. Diarrhea, cough, and neurasthenia may also occur. Pneumonia has not been documented. Most symptoms are short-lived and generally do not require medical care.

LABORATORY DIAGNOSIS

NONSPECIFIC FINDINGS

A number of nonspecific laboratory abnormalities may occur in Legionnaires' disease. These include abnormal urinalysis with proteinuria and hyaline or granular casts, hypophosphatemia, hyponatremia, and less commonly, elevations in aldolase or creatine kinase levels.[64] Extreme electrolyte abnormalities related to massive diarrhea occur rarely.[78] Renal failure has also been reported rarely. The renal failure may occur in conjunction with myositis and/or marked elevations in creatine kinase and aldolase concentrations or with myoglobinuria and may represent rhabdomyolysis.[79, 80] In addition, interstitial nephritis and mesangial proliferative and progressive glomerulonephritis have all been reported.[73] The white blood cell count is elevated ($>10,000/mm^3$), often with a left shift in about one half to three fourths of patients. Leukopenia and thrombocytopenia are observed in severe disease. Serum cold agglutinins and even cold agglutinin disease have also been observed in several cases.[58] Disseminated intravascular coagulation is observed rarely. Elevations in lactic dehydrogenase, alkaline phosphatase, and aspartate aminotransferase levels are also common.[1, 58, 64, 79] Bilirubin elevation is less common. Hypoxemia is usually in proportion to the degree of pulmonary involvement seen on radiography.[64] None of the nonspecific laboratory findings predict with reasonable certainty whether a patient has legionnaires' disease or another cause of pneumonia.

SPECIFIC FINDINGS

There are four currently used methods for the specific laboratory diagnosis of *Legionella* infections (Table 2): determination of antibody level, demonstration of the bacterium in tissues or body fluids by using immunofluorescent microscopy, actual isolation of the organism on culture media, and detection of antigenuria.[7, 47, 81–84] Polymerase chain reaction amplification of *Legionella* DNA is being used experimentally.[85–88]

Estimation of serum antibody to *L. pneumophila* is the most commonly used means of diagnosing Legionnaires' disease.[59] The vast majority of laboratories use an indirect immunofluorescent assay (IFA) technique to determine antibody concentrations. Antibody to a variety of *Legionella* antigens is measured by different laboratories. In about three quarters of the patients with culture-proven Legionnaires' disease caused by *L. pneumophila* serogroup 1, a fourfold rise in titer develops 1 to 9 weeks after the onset of illness. The mean time required for demonstration of seroconversion is about 2 weeks; however, up to 25% of seroconversions are missed unless serum is collected up to 8 weeks after the onset of illness. Since between 5% and 30% of healthy populations sampled have *L. pneumophila* serogroup 1 antibody titers of 1:128 or greater when using a heat-fixed antigen, only a fourfold rise in titer to 1:128 or greater can be considered significant; significant titers for formalin-fixed antigen are a rise in titer to 1:32 or greater. In the face of an outbreak of Legionnaires' disease, a single titer of greater than 1:256 (heat-fixed antigen) in a patient with a compatible clinical illness has been considered significant. However, in sporadic cases such single high titers cannot be interpreted. The specificity of the IFA test in a hospitalized population is not well known; this probably approximates 90% for a fourfold titer rise, although in an epidemic situation in nonhospitalized patients the specificity is close to 100%. Cross-reactions have been reported in patients with

TABLE 2.
Laboratory Diagnosis of Legionnaires' Disease

Test Type	Sensitivity* (%)	Specificity (%)	Comments
Antibody estimation			Optimal sensitivity requires parallel testing of specimens collected acutely and 6 to 9 wks later. Highest specificity is for *L. pneumophila* serogroup 1; testing for antibodies to other species and serogroups is strongly discouraged.
Seroconversion	75	95 to 99	
Single specimen	Unknown	50 to 70	
Immunofluorescent detection of antigen			Highest specificity is for a *L. pneumophila*–specific monoclonal antibody. Use of non–*L. pneumophila* antibodies is strongly discouraged. Often positive for several days after the start of antibiotic therapy.
Sputum or BAL†	25 to 75	95 to 99	
Lung biopsy	80 to 90	99	
Culture			Special media and selective techniques are needed for optimal yield. Culture is more sensitive than all other methods. Often positive after the start of antibiotic therapy, although less sensitive. Therapy with third-generation cephalosporins appears to decrease the yield.
Sputum or BAL	?80 to 90	100	
Lung biopsy	?90 to 99	100	
Blood	10 to 30	100	
Urinary antigen	80 to 99	99.9	Specific for *L. pneumophila* serogroup 1. May be positive for weeks to months after the completion of therapy and when culture is negative.

*The sensitivity given for all methods except culture is on the basis of the use of culture positivity as a gold standard. The question mark preceding the sensitivity estimates for sputum, BAL, and lung cultures denotes that this is a best-guess estimate of the absolute sensitivities; the figure given for blood culture gives the sensitivity relative to respiratory tract cultures.
†BAL = bronchoalveolar lavage; TTA = transtracheal aspiration.

tuberculosis, pneumococcal pneumonia, *Pseudomonas* pneumonia, exacerbations of cystic fibrosis, tularemia, plague, *Bacteroides fragilis* bacteremia, and leptospirosis.[89, 90] Up to 20% of patients with *Campylobacter* enteritis have been reported to have cross-reactive antibody to *L. pneumophila*.[91, 92] Antibody testing is most specific when using *L. pneumophila* serogroup 1 antigen, especially when a formalin-fixed antigen is used. The specificity of a fourfold antibody rise to the serogroup 1 antigen is at least 99%, whereas test specificity is considerably lower when using antigens from other *L. pneumophila* serogroups or from other species. Aside from variability in antibody test results caused by the type and numbers of antigens tested, other methodologic variables may affect the results.[59] None of the commercially available kits for determination of antibody status use exactly the same methods that were used for the determination of test performance. In addition, a valid study of the clinical specificity and sensitivity of kits using multiple antigens or antigens other than *L. pneumophila* serogroup 1 has never been conducted. Thus it is improper to use cutoff values determined for *L. pneumophila* serogroup 1 antibodies when interpreting the meaning of antibodies to other antigens. Because of this, it is better to not test for antibody to antigens other than *L. pneumophila* serogroup 1, except for epidemiologic studies. In addition to the fact that serologic testing is retrospective in nature (and does not influence the choice of therapy) and that a possibility of cross-reactions exists, the other major drawback of diagnosing *Legionella* infections by serologic means is that if a patient has infection with a serotype that is not tested for, the test may be negative. Thus serologic testing in the diagnosis of this disease is much more helpful to epidemiologists than to clinicians caring for individual patients.

Immunofluorescent microscopy of respiratory tract secretions, lung, and pleural fluid is one of the rapid test methods available to establish a laboratory diagnosis of Legionnaires' disease (Fig 1).[7, 50] When this technique is used with an antibody conjugated with a fluorochrome, it is termed a direct immunofluorescence assay (DFA). About 2 to 3 hours is required to complete this test. This technique has been used very successfully with expectorated sputum, endotracheal suction aspirates, lung biopsy tissue, and transtracheal aspirates. The use of secretions or biopsy

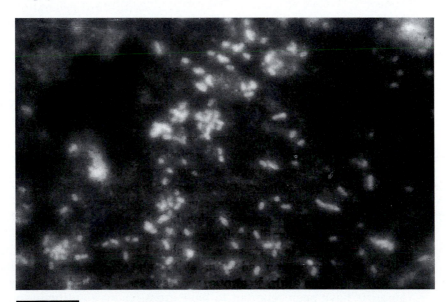

FIGURE 1.
Positive direct immunofluorescence of the lung of a patient with legionnaires' disease (magnification × 250).

specimens obtained by bronchoscopy has not resulted in high yield in our experience, although others have had more success. Pleural fluid examination in patients with Legionnaires' disease is usually unproductive, both in terms of culture and DFA positivity, but has occasionally been helpful.[58] The true sensitivity of the DFA test is unknown. About 25% to 70% of patients with culture-proven Legionnaires' disease have positive sputum DFA tests for L. pneumophila. The test specificity is greater than 99.9%; therefore a negative result does not rule out disease and a positive result is almost always diagnostic of it.[50] Antisera used to detect infection caused by L. pneumophila, especially L. pneumophila serogroups 1 to 4, are more specific than other antisera; the use of antibodies other than these is problematic because of cross-reactions, and testing should be confined to normally sterile tissues and fluids (e.g., lung biopsy specimens) if at all possible. A monoclonal antibody DFA reagent that reacts with all serogroups of L. pneumophila provides optimal specificity and eliminates the need to use multiple antisera to detect this species (Genetic Systems, Seattle).[93] Unlike polyvalent reagents, it does not cross-react with some Pseudomonas, Flavobacterium-Xanthomonas, and Bacteroides strains; however it cannot be used to stain tissues fixed in formalin for prolonged periods.[94] When antibodies other than the monoclonal antiserum are used, it is wise to use extreme caution when interpreting positive smears of tissues or fluids containing large quantities of known cross-reacting bacteria. Exceptional skill is needed to read DFA test slides properly. Direct immunofluorescence tests of sputum remain positive for 2 to 4 days after the initiation of specific antibiotic therapy for legionnaires' disease and often much longer in cases of cavitary pulmonary disease.

Isolation of Legionella from clinical specimens is routinely performed in many laboratories. The medium used, BCYEα, is easily prepared by any large clinical microbiology laboratory and can be made in a selective form.[8, 82] Use of selective media and specimen decontamination with acid are obligatory for optimal culture yield from normally nonsterile tissue and fluid. Optimal yield is obtained by plating specimens treated with and without pretreatment acidification on three different media (total of six plates): BCYEα (nonselective), buffered charcoal yeast extract medium supplemented with cephamandole, polymyxin B; and anisomycin (BMPA, selective, also called CAP* or PAC), and Modified Wadowsky Yee medium with anisomycin (MYEA selective, also called PAV or VAP).* The use of two different selective media is required because some Legionella spp. and some strains of L. pneumophila serogroup 1 will not grow on BMPA medium, which is the most selective medium.[95] Use of multiple media also increases the chances of detecting very small numbers of Legionella bacteria present in the specimen. Specimen dilution before plating is also important because Legionella growth may be inhibited by certain cations, by other bacteria, and by tissue factors. BCYEα, BMPA, and MYEA media are all commercially available. The organism has been

---

*CAP = cephamandole, anisomycin, polymyxin B; PAC = polymyxin B, anisomycin, cephamandole; PAV = polymxin E, anisomycin, vansomycin; VAP = vansomycin, anisomycin, polymyxin E.

successfully isolated from sputum, transtracheal aspirates, endotracheal suction specimens, blood, lung biopsy tissue, pleural fluid, bronchial lavage fluid, pericardial fluid, peritoneal fluid, wounds, bowel abscesses, prosthetic heart valves, brain abscesses, myocardium, kidney, liver, vascular grafts, and respiratory sinuses.[19, 50, 64, 96] Cultures generally remain positive for several days after the initiation of antimicrobial therapy and may remain positive for weeks or months from pulmonary abscesses. Broad-spectrum antimicrobial therapy decreases culture yield. Like all other tests for Legionnaires' disease, the absolute sensitivity of culturing is unknown; however, in comparative studies of test yield, culture has been more sensitive than other types of testing.

Once isolated on a culture medium, *Legionella* spp. are relatively easy to identify to the genus level. This is based on characteristic colonial morphology, growth requirement for L-cysteine, and serotyping.[7, 82, 97] Also helpful in differentiation are characteristic branched-chain cellular fatty acid and ubiquinone compositions and failure to produce acid from carbohydrates. Because of the antigenic complexity of legionellae, it is impossible to serologically distinguish several of the species. When combined with a paucity of other useful phenotypic characteristics, this means that identification to the species level can be very difficult, except for extremely sophisticated research laboratories. However, all laboratories should be able to identify *L. pneumophila* and other legionellae to the genus level.

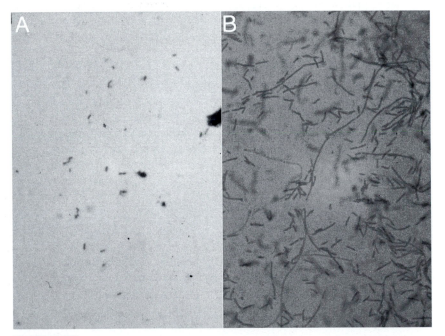

FIGURE 2.

A, Gram stain of Legionella pneumophila taken from a BCYEα culture plate (magnification × 1,200). **B,** Giménez stain of *L. pneumophila* in the lung of patient with legionnaires' disease (same magnification as **A**). Note that *L. pneumophila* in the lung is much smaller than when it grows on a culture plate.

Microscopic morphology of the organisms depends on growth conditions. They are usually very faintly staining small coccobacilli in lung specimens and sputum and are often long and filamentous bacilli when taken from a culture plate (Fig 2). Although colonies growing on artificial media stain well with Gram stain (especially if basic fuchsin rather than safranin is used as the counterstain), the bacteria are exceptionally difficult to visualize when this stain is used on fixed lung specimens and often on fresh tissues and fluids as well. The Giménez stain is a more effective method to examine tissues and is much simpler and more sensitive than the previously touted Dieterle silver impregnation stain.[7] In addition, the polymerase chain reaction has been used to diagnose Legionnaires' disease, but this test is still regarded as a research tool.[85, 88]

Legionella pneumophila serogroup 1 antigenuria can be detected by using a commercial radioimmunoassay (Binax, Portland, Me).[81, 99] Cross-reactions between serogroups are uncommon, which somewhat limits the usefulness of this test. This is a rapid test with extraordinary specificity; we have never documented a false-positive test. Test sensitivity has been 95% in culture-proven disease and about 80% in serologically proven disease. We have observed many instances of positive urine antigen tests with negative sputum cultures, probably because testing has been done after more than 5 days of specific antibiotic therapy. One minor drawback of this test is that it may remain positive for weeks to months after recovery from pneumonia. Recently, an enzyme immunoassay format of the same test has been marketed by the same company; its performance is not as yet well studied.

THERAPY

Erythromycin is the drug of choice in the treatment of Legionella infections.[1, 64, 100, 101] This is based chiefly on retrospective reviews of therapy for legionnaires' disease because unfortunately no prospective comparative study of antimicrobial therapy for the disease has been performed. Case fatality rates vary widely and are generally lower for community-acquired disease in otherwise healthy persons than for nosocomial legionnaires' disease, which often occurs in immunocompromised patients. Untreated fatality rates range from 0% to 80%, with the average being about 15% for community-acquired pneumonia. Prompt treatment with erythromycin lowers fatality rates by about twofold. Other antimicrobials also appear to be active, including tetracyclines, fluoroquinolones, and the newer macrolides and azalides. Penicillin, cephalosporin, and aminoglycoside therapies are ineffective.

The use of in vitro susceptibility testing to predict clinical response in Legionnaires' disease can be very misleading. For example, all aminoglycosides and cefoxitin inhibit Legionella at low concentrations. However, these drugs do not work clinically. The reason for this is in part the ability of only some antimicrobials to enter the alveolar macrophage. Erythromycin, other macrolides, and tetracycline enter the alveolar macrophage quite readily and in fact are concentrated in it, whereas the penicillin drugs do not achieve significant levels within macrophages.[102] The fluoroquinolones also penetrate monocyte-derived cells well. Use of animal models of infection may lead to a better prediction of the efficacy of antimicrobials in therapy for Legionnaires' disease.[103]

REFERENCES

1. Fraser DW, Tsai TR, Orenstein W, et al: Legionnaires' disease: Description of an epidemic of pneumonia. *N Engl J Med* 297:1189–1197, 1977.
2. Osterholm MT, Chin TD, Osborne DO, et al: A 1957 outbreak of legionnaires' disease associated with a meat packing plant. *Am J Epidemiol* 117:60–67, 1983.
3. Tatlock H: Clarification of the cause of Fort Bragg fever (pretibial fever)—January 1982. *Rev Infect Dis* 4:157–158, 1982.
4. Broome CV, Fraser DW: Epidemiologic aspects of legionellosis. *Epidemiol Rev* 1:1–16, 1979.
5. Kaufmann AF, McDade JE, Patton CM, et al: Pontiac fever: Isolation of the etiologic agent *(Legionella pneumophila)* and demonstration of its mode of transmission. *Am J Epidemiol* 114:337–347, 1981.
6. Glick TH, Gregg MB, Berman B, et al: Pontiac fever. An epidemic of unknown etiology in a health department: I. Clinical and epidemiologic aspects. *Am J Epidemiol* 107:149–160, 1978.
7. Jones GL, Hebert GA: *"Legionnaires': The Disease, the Bacterium, and Methodology.* Atlanta, US Department of Health, Education, and Welfare, Public Health Service, Centers for Disease Control, Bureau of Laboratories, 1978.
8. Edelstein PH: Improved semiselective medium for isolation of *Legionella pneumophila* from contaminated clinical and environmental specimens. *J Clin Microbiol* 14:298–303, 1981.
9. Barbaree JM, Breiman RF, Dufour AP: *Legionella,* Washington, DC, American Society for Microbiology, 1993.
10. Dennis PJ, Brenner DJ, Thacker WL, et al: Five new *Legionella* species isolated from water. *Int J Syst Bacteriol* 43:329–337, 1993.
11. Fliermans CB, Cherry WB, Orrison LH, et al: Ecological distribution of *Legionella pneumophila*. *Appl Environ Microbiol* 41:9–16, 1981.
12. Rowbotham TJ: Current views on the relationships between amoebae, legionellae and man. *Isr J Med Sci* 22:678–689, 1986.
13. Barker J, Brown MR, Collier PJ, et al: Relationship between *Legionella pneumophila* and *Acanthamoeba polyphaga*: Physiological status and susceptibility to chemical inactivation. *Appl Environ Microbiol* 58:2420–2425, 1992.
14. Kilvington S, Price J: Survival of *Legionella pneumophila* within cysts of *Acanthamoeba polyphaga* following chlorine exposure. *J Appl Bacteriol* 68:519–525, 1990.
15. Bartlett CLR, Macrae AD, Macfarlane JT: *Legionella Infections.* Baltimore, E Arnold, 1986, pp 1–163.
16. Marrie TJ, Haldane D, MacDonald S, et al: Control of endemic nosocomial legionnaires' disease by using sterile potable water for high risk patients. *Epidemiol Infect* 107:591–605, 1991.
17. Marrie TJ, MacDonald S, Clarke K, et al: Nosocomial legionnaires' disease: Lessons from a four-year prospective study. *Am J Infect Control* 19:79–85, 1991.
18. Waldor MK, Wilson B, Swartz M: Cellulitis caused by *Legionella pneumophila*. *Clin Infect Dis* 16:51–53, 1993.
19. Lowry PW, Tompkins LS: Nosocomial legionellosis: A review of pulmonary and extrapulmonary syndromes. *Am J Infect Control* 21:21–27, 1993.

20. Dowling JN, Saha AK, Glew RH: Virulence factors of the family Legionellaceae. *Microbiol Rev* 56:32–60, 1992.
21. Horwitz MA: Interactions between macrophages and *Legionella pneumophila*. *Curr Top Microbiol Immunol* 181:265–282, 1992.
22. Davis GS, Winn WC Jr, Gump DW, et al: The kinetics of early inflammatory events during experimental pneumonia due to *Legionella pneumophila* in guinea pigs. *J Infect Dis* 148:823–835, 1983.
23. Davis GS, Winn WC Jr, Gump DW, et al: Legionnaires' pneumonia after aerosol exposure in guinea pigs and rats. *Am Rev Respir Dis* 126:1050–1057, 1982.
24. Byrd TF, Horwitz MA: Lactoferrin inhibits or promotes *Legionella pneumophila* intracellular multiplication in nonactivated and interferon gamma–activated human monocytes depending upon its degree of iron saturation. Iron-lactoferrin and nonphysiologic iron chelates reverse monocyte activation against *Legionella pneumophila*. *J Clin Invest* 88:1103–1112, 1991.
25. Byrd TF, Horwitz MA: Interferon gamma–activated human monocytes downregulate transferrin receptors and inhibit the intracellular multiplication of *Legionella pneumophila* by limiting the availability of iron. *J Clin Invest* 83:1457–1465, 1989.
26. Cianciotto N, Eisenstein BI, Engleberg NC, et al: Genetics and molecular pathogenesis of *Legionella pneumophila*, an intracellular parasite of macrophages. *Mol Biol Med* 6:409–424, 1989.
27. Cianciotto NP, Eisenstein BI, Mody CH, et al: A mutation in the mip gene results in an attenuation of *Legionella pneumophila* virulence. *J Infect Dis* 162:121–126, 1990.
28. Isberg RR, Rankin S, Roy CR, et al: *Legionella pneumophila*: Factors involved in the route and response to an intracellular niche. *Infect Agents Dis* 2:220–223, 1993.
29. Mintz CS, Schultz DR, Arnold PI, et al: *Legionella pneumophila* lipopolysaccharide activates the classical complement pathway. *Infect Immun* 60:2769–2776, 1992.
30. Husmann LK, Johnson W: Adherence of *Legionella pneumophila* to guinea pig peritoneal macrophages, J774 mouse macrophages, and undifferentiated U937 human monocytes: Role of Fc and complement receptors. *Infect Immun* 60:5212–5218, 1992.
31. Rodgers FG, Gibson FC: Opsonin-independent adherence and intracellular development of *Legionella pneumophila* within U-937 cells. *Can J Microbiol* 39:718–722, 1993.
32. Baskerville A, Conlan JW, Ashworth LA, et al: Pulmonary damage caused by a protease from *Legionella pneumophila*. *Br J Exp Pathol* 67:527–536, 1986.
33. Moffat JF, Edelstein PH, Regula DP Jr, et al: Effects of an isogenic Zn-metalloprotease–deficient mutant of *Legionella pneumophila* in a guinea-pig pneumonia model. *Mol Microbiol* 12:693–705, 1994.
34. Rechnitzer C, Bangsborg JM, Shand GH: Effect of *Legionella pneumophila* sonicate on killing of *Listeria monocytogenes* by human polymorphonuclear neutrophils and monocytes. *APMIS* 101:249–256, 1993.
35. Rechnitzer C, Kharazmi A: Effect of *Legionella pneumophila* cytotoxic protease on human neutrophil and monocyte function. *Microb Pathog* 12:115–125, 1992.
36. Lochner JE, Bigley RH, Iglewski BH: Defective triggering of polymorphonuclear leukocyte oxidative metabolism by *Legionella pneumophila* toxin. *J Infect Dis* 151:42–46, 1985.
37. Baine WB: Cytolytic and phospholipase C activity in *Legionella* species. *J Gen Microbiol* 131:1383–1391, 1985.

38. Husmann LK, Johnson W: Cytotoxicity of extracellular *Legionella pneumophila. Infect Immun* 62:2111–2114, 1994.
39. Cutz E, Thorner PS, Rao CP, et al: Disseminated *Legionella pneumophila* infection in an infant with severe combined immunodeficiency. *J Pediatr* 100:760–762, 1982.
40. Dournon E, Bure A, Kemeny JL, et al: *Legionella pneumophila* peritonitis (letter). *Lancet* 1:1363, 1982.
41. Fogliani J, Domenget JF, Hohn B, et al: Maladie des légionnaires avec localisation digestive. Une observation. *Nouv Presse Med* 11:2699–2702, 1982.
42. Nelson DP, Rensimer ER, Raffin TA: *Legionella pneumophila* pericarditis without pneumonia. *Arch Intern Med* 145:926, 1985.
43. Blander SJ, Horwitz MA: Vaccination with the major secretory protein of *Legionella* induces humoral and cell-mediated immune responses and protective immunity across different serogroups of *Legionella pneumophila* and different species of *Legionella. J Immunol* 147:285–291, 1991.
44. Blander SJ, Horwitz MA: Vaccination with *Legionella pneumophila* membranes induces cell-mediated and protective immunity in a guinea pig model of legionnaires' disease. Protective immunity independent of the major secretory protein of *Legionella pneumophila. J Clin Invest* 87:1054–1059, 1991.
45. Weeratna R, Stamler DA, Edelstein PH, et al: Human and guinea pig immune responses to *Legionella pneumophila* protein antigens OmpS and Hsp60. *Infect Immun* 62:3454–3462, 1994.
46. Blander SJ, Horwitz MA: Major cytoplasmic membrane protein of *Legionella pneumophila,* a genus common antigen and member of the hsp 60 family of heat shock proteins, induces protective immunity in a guinea pig model of legionnaires' disease. *J Clin Invest* 91:717–723, 1993.
47. Winn WC JR: *Legionella* and Legionnaires' disease: A review with emphasis on environmental studies and laboratory diagnosis. *Crit Rev Clin Lab Sci* 21:323–381, 1985.
48. Winn WC Jr, Myerowitz RL: The pathology of the *Legionella* pneumonias. A review of 74 cases and the literature. *Hum Pathol* 12:401–422, 1981.
49. Pendlebury WW, Perl DP, Winn WC Jr, et al: Neuropathologic evaluation of 40 confirmed cases of *Legionella* pneumonia. *Neurology* 33:1340–1344, 1983.
50. Edelstein PH, Meyer RD, Finegold SM: Laboratory diagnosis of legionnaires' disease. *Am Rev Respir Dis* 121:317–327, 1980.
51. Fain JS, Bryan RN, Cheng L, et al: Rapid diagnosis of *Legionella* infection by a nonisotopic in situ hybridization method. *Am J Clin Pathol* 95:719–724, 1991.
52. Bhopal RS: Geographical variation of legionnaires' disease: A critique and guide to future research. *Int J Epidemiol* 22:1127–1136, 1993.
53. Blatt SP, Dolan MJ, Hendrix CW, et al: Legionnaires' disease in human immunodeficiency virus–infected patients: Eight cases and review. *Clin Infect Dis* 18:227–232, 1994.
54. Carratala J, Gudiol F, Pallares R, et al: Risk factors for nosocomial *Legionella pneumophila* pneumonia. *Am J Respir Crit Care Med* 149:625–629, 1994.
55. Bhopal RS, Fallon RJ, Buist EC, et al: Proximity of the home to a cooling tower and risk of non-outbreak legionnaires' disease. *BMJ* 302:378–383, 1991.
56. Bhopal RS, Fallon RJ: Variation in time and space of non-outbreak legionnaires' disease in Scotland. *Epidemiol Infect* 106:45–61, 1991.
57. Brundrett GW: *Legionella and Building Services.* Oxford, England, Butterworth-Heinemann, 1992, pp 1–410.

58. Balows A, Fraser DW: International symposium on legionnaires' disease. *Ann Intern Med* 90:481–714, 1979.

59. Edelstein PH: Detection of antibodies to *Legionella*, in Rose NR, de Macario EC, Fahey JL, et al: (eds): *Manual of Clinical Laboratory Immunology*, ed 4. Washington, DC, American Society for Microbiology, 1992, pp 459–466.

60. Fang GD, Fine M, Orloff J, et al: New and emerging etiologies for community-acquired pneumonia with implications for therapy. A prospective multi-center study of 359 cases. *Medicine (Baltimore)* 69:307–316, 1990.

61. Granados A, Podzamczer D, Gudiol F, et al: Pneumonia due to *Legionella pneumophila* and pneumococcal pneumonia: Similarities and differences on presentation. *Eur Respir J* 2:130–134, 1989.

62. Roig J, Aguilar X, Ruiz J, et al: Comparative study of *Legionella pneumophila* and other nosocomial-acquired pneumonias. *Chest* 99:344–350, 1991.

63. Yu VL, Kroboth FJ, Shonnard J, et al: Legionnaires' disease: New clinical perspective from a prospective pneumonia study. *Am J Med* 73:357–361, 1982.

64. Kirby BD, Snyder KM, Meyer RD, et al: Legionnaires' disease: Report of sixty-five nosocomially acquired cases of review of the literature. *Medicine (Baltimore)* 59:188–205, 1980.

65. Woodhead MA, Macfarlane JT: Legionnaires' disease: A review of 79 community acquired cases in Nottingham. *Thorax* 41:635–640, 1986.

66. Falcó V, Fernández de Sevilla T, Alegre J, et al: *Legionella pneumophila*. A cause of severe community-acquired pneumonia. *Chest* 100:1007–1011, 1991.

67. Harris LF: Legionnaires' disease associated with acute encephalomyelitis. *Arch Neurol* 38:462–463, 1981.

68. Bull PW, Scott JT, Breathnach SM: Henoch-Schönlein purpura associated with legionnaires' disease. *BMJ* 294:220, 1987.

69. Lück PC, Helbig JH, Wunderlich E, et al: Isolation of *Legionella pneumophila* serogroup 3 from pericardial fluid in a case of pericarditis. *Infection* 17:388–390, 1989.

70. Nomura S, Hatta K, Iwata T, et al: *Legionella pneumophila* isolated in pure culture from the ascites of a patient with systemic lupus erythematosus. *Am J Med* 86:833–834, 1989.

71. Warner CL, Fayad PB, Heffner RR Jr: *Legionella* myositis. *Neurology* 41:750–752, 1991.

72. Tokunaga Y, Concepcion W, Berquist WE, et al: Graft involvement by *Legionella* in a liver transplant recipient. *Arch Surg* 127:475–477, 1992.

73. Fenves AZ: Legionnaires' disease associated with acute renal failure: A report of two cases and review of the literature. *Clin Nephrol* 23:96–100, 1985.

74. Wegmüller E, Weidmann P, Hess T, et al: Rapidly progressive glomerulonephritis accompanying legionnaires' disease. *Arch Intern Med* 145:1711–1713, 1985.

75. Kirby BD, Peck H, Meyer RD: Radiographic features of legionnaires' disease. *Chest* 76:562–565, 1979.

76. Fairbank JT, Mamourian AC, Dietrich PA, et al: The chest radiograph in legionnaires' disease. Further observations. *Radiology* 147:33–34, 1983.

77. Edelstein PH, Meyer RD, Finegold SM: Long-term followup of two patients with pulmonary cavitation caused by *Legionella pneumophila*. *Am Rev Respir Dis* 124:90–93, 1981.

78. Foltzer MA, Reese RE: Massive diarrhea in *Legionella micdadei* pneumonitis. *J Clin Gastroenterol* 7:525–527, 1985.

79. Friedman HM: Legionnaires' disease in non-legionnaires. A report of five cases. *Ann Intern Med* 88:294–302, 1978.

80. Meyer RD, Edelstein PH, Kirby BD, et al: Legionnaires' disease: Unusual clinical and laboratory features. *Ann Intern Med* 93:240–243, 1980.

81. Aguero-Rosenfeld ME, Edelstein PH: Retrospective evaluation of the Du Pont radioimmunoassay kit for detection of *Legionella pneumophila* serogroup 1 antigenuria in humans. *J Clin Microbiol* 26:1775–1778, 1988.

82. Edelstein PH: The laboratory diagnosis of legionnaires' disease. *Semin Respir Infect* 2:235–241, 1987.

83. Edelstein PH: Use of DNA probes for the diagnosis of infections caused by *Mycoplasma pneumoniae* and legionellae—a review. *Adv Exp Med Biol* 263:57–69, 1990.

84. Edelstein PH, Bryan RN, Enns RK, et al: Retrospective study of Gen-Probe rapid diagnostic system for detection of legionellae in frozen clinical respiratory tract samples. *J Clin Microbiol* 25:1022–1026, 1987.

85. Lisby G, Dessau R: Construction of a DNA amplification assay for detection of *Legionella* species in clinical samples. *Eur J Clin Microbiol Infect Dis* 13:225–231, 1994.

86. Matsiota-Bernard P, Pitsouni E, Legakis N, et al: Evaluation of commercial amplification kit for detection of *Legionella pneumophila* in clinical specimens. *J Clin Microbiol* 32:1503–1505, 1994.

87. Kessler HH, Reinthaler FF, Pschaid A, et al: Rapid detection of *Legionella* species in bronchoalveolar lavage fluids with the EnviroAmp *Legionella* PCR amplification and detection kit. *J Clin Microbiol* 31:3325–3328, 1993.

88. Jaulhac B, Nowicki M, Bornstein N, et al: Detection of *Legionella* spp. in bronchoalveolar lavage fluids by DNA amplification. *J Clin Microbiol* 30:920–924, 1992.

89. Bornstein N, Janin N, Bourguignon G, et al: Prevalence of anti-*Legionella* antibodies in a healthy population and in patients with tuberculosis or pneumonia. *Pathol Biol (Paris)* 35:353–356, 1987.

90. Edelstein PH, McKinney RM, Meyer RD, et al: Immunologic diagnosis of legionnaires' disease: Cross-reactions with anaerobic and microaerophilic organisms and infections caused by them. *J Infect Dis* 141:652–655, 1980.

91. Marshall LE, Boswell TC, Kudesia G: False positive Legionella serology in Campylobacter infection: Campylobacter serotypes, duration of antibody response and elimination of cross-reactions in the indirect fluorescent antibody test. *Epidemiol Infect* 112:347–357, 1994.

92. Boswell TC, Kudesia G: Serological cross-reaction between *Legionella pneumophila* and *Campylobacter* in the indirect fluorescent antibody test. *Epidemiol Infect* 109:291–295, 1992.

93. Edelstein PH, Beer KB, Sturge JC, et al: Clinical utility of a monoclonal direct fluorescent reagent specific for *Legionella pneumophila*: Comparative study with other reagents. *J Clin Microbiol* 22:419–421, 1985.

94. Tenover FC, Edelstein PH, Goldstein LC, et al: Comparison of cross-staining reactions by *Pseudomonas* spp. and fluorescein-labeled polyclonal and monoclonal antibodies directed against *Legionella pneumophila*. *J Clin Microbiol* 23:647–649, 1986.

95. Lee TC, Vickers RM, Yu VL, et al: Growth of 28 *Legionella* species on selective culture media: A comparative study. *J Clin Microbiol* 31:2764–2768, 1993.

96. Schlanger G, Lutwick LI, Kurzman M, et al: Sinusitis caused by *Legionella pneumophila* in a patient with the acquired immune deficiency syndrome. *Am J Med* 77:957–960, 1984.

97. Edelstein PH: *Legionnaires' Disease Laboratory Manual*, ed 3. Springfield, Va, National Technical Information Service, 1985.

98. Pasculle AW, Veto GE, Krystofiak S, et al: Laboratory and clinical evalua-

tion of a commercial DNA probe for the detection of *Legionella* spp. *J Clin Microbiol* 27:2350–2358, 1989.

99. Sathapatayavongs B, Kohler RB, Wheat LJ, et al: Rapid diagnosis of legionnaires' disease by urinary antigen detection. Comparison of ELISA and radioimmunoassay. *Am J Med* 72:576–582, 1982.

100. Edelstein PH: Macrolides in legionellosis, in Bryskier AJ, Butzler JP, Neu HC, et al (eds): *Macrolides: Chemistry, Pharmacology, and Clinical Uses.* Paris, Arnette Blackwell, 1993, pp 235–239.

101. Edelstein PH: Legionnaires' disease. *Clin Infect Dis* 16:741–747, 1993.

102. Johnson JD, Hand WL, Francis JB, et al: Antibiotic uptake by alveolar macrophages. *J Lab Clin Med* 95:429–439, 1980.

103. Edelstein PH, Calarco K, Yasui VK: Antimicrobial therapy of experimentally induced legionnaires' disease in guinea pigs. *Am Rev Respir Dis* 130:849–856, 1984.

Muscle Pathology for the General Pathologist

Reid R. Heffner, Jr., M.D.

Professor and Associate Chairman, Department of Pathology, School of Medicine and Biomedical Sciences, State University of New York at Buffalo, Buffalo, New York

MUSCLE BIOPSY: PROCEDURES AND TECHNIQUES

With much greater frequency than in years past, the pathologist is expected to process and interpret muscle biopsy specimens that are submitted for diagnosis in clinics and hospitals of all sizes, from smaller community hospitals to large academic medical centers.

Since neuromuscular diseases are medical rather than surgical conditions, the pathologic examination of muscle tissue becomes only one part of the entire diagnostic evaluation of the patient and cannot be isolated from the patient's history, physical examination, and laboratory tests. In the discussions of individual neuromuscular diseases, the impact of clinical data will become evident. For example, the progress of disease is often revealing. Rapidly developing weakness is suggestive of an inflammatory myopathy, whereas an insidious onset and steady progression favor muscular dystrophy. The location where the weakness begins frequently indicates whether the neuromuscular disorder is a primary myopathy, in which case the weakness tends to be proximal in location, or a denervating disease, in which case the weakness occurs in distal muscle groups. A carefully obtained medical history may disclose familial muscle disease suggesting a diagnosis of one of the congenital myopathies or other hereditary disorders. Selected laboratory data can reinforce the clinical or pathologic impression. Elevated serum levels of creatine kinase (CK) are seen in active muscle disease, most notably in myopathic rather than atrophic processes. Electromyography (EMG) can be indispensable in demonstrating myotonia or myasthenia and helpful in discriminating between myopathic and denervating disorders.

When collecting a biopsy specimen, several routine aspects are important.[1, 2] It is necessary that the biopsy sample be representative of the disease process. To illustrate, a patient may have weakness confined to the legs. A biopsy of the upper extremity is not likely to accurately portray this disease process. Also, the biopsy sample should be removed from a muscle in which the disease is still active rather than from a chronically affected wasted muscle in which there is considerable weakness or atrophy. The second sample will reveal end-stage disease that is difficult to interpret. Muscle that has withstood previous trauma from needle EMG or intramuscular injections of medications should never be selected for biopsy. The lesions of trauma—fiber necrosis, regeneration, inflammation, endomysial fibrosis—simulate the features of various neuromuscular diseases and will confuse even the most experienced pathologist.

In most laboratories that process biopsy tissue, two separate specimens, one fixed and one fresh (unfixed), are routinely collected. The first specimen is submitted in an isometric muscle clamp to prevent the contraction artifact that results from excision of the tissue and immersion into fixative. With vigorous and undisciplined contraction, the muscle fibers begin to shear apart. This common artifact is more obvious in longitudinal sections in which dark perpendicular contraction bands and lucent tears appear within the sarcoplasm. In transverse sections, these tears are seen as irregular cracks within the fibers. Contraction artifact particularly damages resin-embedded tissue since the sarcoplasm is visualized in greater detail than in paraffin sections. In our experience the isometric clamp has several other advantages over any alternative method designed to prevent contraction. Because the muscle is always placed into the clamp in the longitudinal plane, the specimen is thus properly oriented for processing. The use of a clamp also ensures that an adequate sample size is submitted since the specimen must span the width of the instrument. When a clamp is used, the fixed specimen will measure a minimum of 1 cm in length and 0.5 cm in width. The fixed sample is versatile and amenable to the preparation of paraffin, 1-μm resin-embedded, and ultrathin sections for electron microscopy as well as immunohistochemical procedures. A second specimen measuring at least $1 \times 0.5 \times 0.5$ cm is retained in the unfixed state for the preparation of frozen sections. Several techniques are available for tissue freezing. The essential condition governing the procedure is that it permit almost instant freezing. Most laboratories successfully use liquid nitrogen as the primary freezing medium, either by coating the specimen with the talc first or by freezing directly in isopentane cooled in liquid nitrogen. Serial frozen sections are then subjected to a standard panel of stains. Routine stains in our laboratory are hematoxylin-eosin (HE), rapid Gomori trichrome (RTC), adenosine triphosphatase (ATPase), and a representative oxidative enzyme reaction, NADH-TR. As required by the diagnostic workup, additional stains such as periodic acid–Schiff (PAS) for glycogen, oil red O or another suitable method for fat, phosphorylase, and supplementary histochemical reactions may be performed. Frozen tissue may also be used in selected cases for immunohistochemical or biochemical analysis and immunofluorescence microscopy.

NORMAL STRUCTURE

Striated muscles are divided into fascicles, fiber bundles separated from each other by a connective tissue sheath, the perimysium, through which the intramuscular nerves and blood vessels are routed. The epimysium encircles groups of fascicles and the entire muscle as it merges with the overlying fascia. Every muscle fiber is invested with a thin, unobtrusive endomysium that supports the rich capillary bed within the muscle. The muscle fiber is a multinucleated, syncytial-like cell with a shape corresponding to a cylinder. In cross section, a normal mature fiber is polygonal rather than perfectly rounded in configuration. The diameter of fibers measured in the transverse plane depends on several factors. Proximal muscles are composed of fibers with larger mean diameters (85 to 90 μm) than those of distal or ocular muscles (20 μm). In general, muscles designed for precisely coordinated movement have smaller fibers than muscles involved in less refined or postural activity. Muscle fibers in infants (mean diameter, 12 μm) and children are smaller than those in healthy young adults. Some reduction in fiber size also occurs with advancing age. In longitudinal paraffin sections, striations within the sarcoplasm are faintly visible and reflect the arrangement of the myofibrils, which is seen better in PAS than in HE stains. In HE-stained cross sections, the sarcoplasm has an unstructured appearance without evidence of striations. The sarcolemmal nuclei are peripherally located and number four to six per fiber.

A portion of the fixed specimen can be embedded in resin and examined in 1-μm-thick sections as well as ultrastructurally. Any disruption of the orderly striated architecture is more easily visualized in longitudinal sections than in transverse sections. Each muscle fiber comprises a series of parallel myofibrils, which are minute, linear contractile elements with an average diameter of 1 μm. A myofibril is a repetition of identical subunits known as sarcomeres. The sarcomeres of each myofibril are of equal length and are aligned in register with others in the fiber. The cross-striations of the muscle fiber are a function of the periodicity of the sarcomeres. The length of the sarcomeres is 2.5 to 3 μm and is measured between consecutive Z bands, which are the lateral boundaries of the sarcomere. The Z band (Zwischenscheibe or intermediate disk) is an extremely dense line perpendicular to the long axis of the myofibril. The Z band bisects the I (isotropic) bands of adjacent sarcomeres. Within the sarcomere, the I bands are lateral to, more lightly stained, and shorter in length than the central A (anisotropic) band. Inside the sarcomere are thick filaments composed of myosin that measure 15 nm in diameter and thin filaments that contain predominantly actin with a diameter of 8 nm. The thick filaments stretch across the A band whereas the thin filaments extend from the Z band and traverse the I band, where only thin filaments are present. They enter the A band to interdigitate with the thick filaments. The organelles of the myofiber tend to be located around the nuclei and between the myofibrils. Glycogen granules are found in greater concentration in type 2 fibers. Lipid vacuoles and mitochondria are more prevalent in type 1 fibers.

Certain physical and biochemical differences exist among skeletal muscle fibers, insight into some of which can be gained in histochemical preparations. Red fibers, which have a higher myoglobin content, have a larger mitochondrial population and are more specialized for aerobic respiration and slow contraction. White fibers, which are endowed with fewer mitochondria, have abundant glycogen stores and are more suited to anaerobic respiration and fast contraction. In lower vertebrates a muscle may be composed entirely of either red or white fibers, but human muscles contain both fiber types arranged in a pattern like that of a checkerboard. A typical muscle contains approximately 35% to 40% type

1 (red) fibers and 60% to 65% type 2 (white) fibers. Fiber typing is not evident in routine HE-stained sections. Our laboratory and most others use two complementary histochemical reactions performed on fresh frozen sections to demonstrate the histochemical properties of muscle fibers. Oxidative enzyme reactions such as NADH-TR reflect the mitochondrial content of the muscle fiber. Darkly stained fibers are designated as type 1 (oxidative) and lighter fibers as type 2 (Fig 1). Most oxidative enzyme reactions further subdivide type 2 fibers into two populations, type 2B fibers being most lightly stained and type 2A fibers being intermediately stained. In the ATPase reaction, the staining reaction can be altered by varying the pH of the incubating solution during the staining procedure. When the alkaline ATPase reaction is run at a pH of 9.4, type 1 fibers are light and type 2 fibers are dark. Fibers with intermediate staining properties are not apparent in this reaction. To reverse the staining reaction, the incubation is done at an acidic pH, usually 4.6. In the reverse ATPase reaction, type 1 fibers are most darkly stained, type 2A fibers are almost unstained, and type 2B fibers are intermediate in their staining intensity between the two. Histochemical reactions for phosphorylase, which is more abundant in type 2 (glycolytic) fibers, can be employed as a means of fiber typing. Type 2 fibers appear dark and type 1 fibers appear light in this staining reaction, which is not as reliable as the ATPase reaction. In frozen sections, glycolytic, phosphorylase-rich, type 2 fibers may stain more intensely than type 1 fibers with PAS stains owing to their greater glycogen content. Although not ideal, PAS stains can be used as

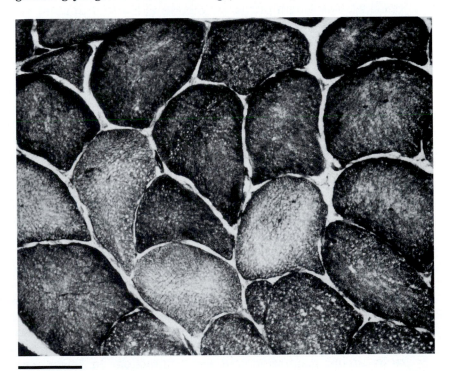

FIGURE 1.
Normal muscle. Fibers are polygonal in shape, and there are two fiber populations: dark fibers are designated type 1, and light fibers are type 2 (NADH-TR).

an alternative method for fiber typing when frozen tissue and enzyme histochemistry are not available. It is now possible to determine fiber types in paraffin sections by immunohistochemical analysis. The procedure involves monoclonal antibodies to fast myosin so that type 2 fibers are labeled with more reaction product (dark) than type 1 fibers (light).[3] A similar procedure exists for antibodies to slow myosin.

DENERVATING DISEASES

In our experience, more than 50% of muscle biopsies are performed on patients with denervating conditions, so it is appropriate to begin the discussion of individual neuromuscular diseases with this group of disorders. Normal structure and function of the muscle fiber are closely related to the preservation of its nerve supply and a variety of neural trophic influences. Neurogenic atrophy may arise from disease of the motor end plate, the anterior horn cell, as exemplified by amyotrophic lateral sclerosis and Werdnig-Hoffmann disease, or the motor axon. More than 80% of cases of neurogenic atrophy are attributable to some form of peripheral neuropathy. A detailed account of the motor neuron diseases and peripheral neuropathies is a complex undertaking well beyond the scope of this chapter.

With the exception of motor end-plate disorders and Werdnig-Hoffmann disease, the pathologic findings in all denervating diseases are essentially the same. In early denervation there is fiber atrophy and randomly scattered, small fibers. Atrophic fibers are angular when cut transversely, with tapered or pointed rather than blunt ends. Atrophic fibers appear fusiform, with the longer diameter often reaching that of a normal fiber while the shorter diameter is markedly reduced. At this stage of denervation, many or all of the atrophic fibers are type 2 (Fig 2). Inasmuch as the most common manifestation of muscle disease is a random variation in fiber size secondary to atrophy, this pattern of pathologic change is not specific for denervation. The size of the muscle fiber is contingent not only on intact innervation but also on other trophic influences. Any disturbance of these influences may lead to fiber atrophy. The maintenance of normal fiber volume depends on regular muscular activity. Confinement to bed or restricted movement such as in orthopedic casting or splinting, which reduces or prevents normal muscle contraction, results in disuse atrophy. A reduction in fiber size may also result from poor nutrition or aging. For unexplained reasons, disuse, malnutrition, and aging, like denervation, cause selective atrophy of type 2 fibers. The same selective atrophy is associated with corticosteroid therapy and Cushing syndrome, connective tissue diseases, particularly rheumatoid arthritis, and systemic malignancy.[4] Staining frozen sections for esterase may be useful in that denervated fibers can be distinguished from fiber atrophy in most other conditions by a positive esterase reaction. It has recently been discovered that denervated fibers also express neural cell adhesion molecule (N-CAM), which can be demonstrated by immunohistochemical methods.[5] As denervation progresses, the number of atrophic type 1 and type 2 fibers is equalized. Chronic denervation exhibits a pattern of atrophy that has evolved from one that is random to one in which there

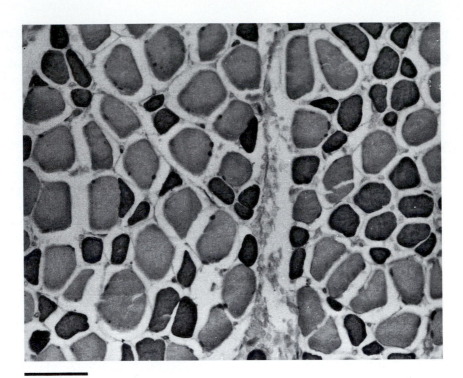

FIGURE 2.

Type 2 fiber atrophy. Small fibers are darkly stained (immunohistochemical analysis with anti–fast myosin antibody).

is grouping of affected fibers. Grouped atrophy is typified by multiple groups of five or more small, fusiform fibers in the biopsy sample (Fig 3). In long-standing neurogenic disease, the normal checkerboard profile is replaced by type grouping, defined as abnormally large aggregates of muscle fibers with similar staining reactions (Fig 4). Type grouping occurs when surviving intramuscular nerve fibers undergo collateral sprouting to reinnervate denervated, atrophic fibers. In human biopsy samples, target fibers are diagnostic of chronic denervation. It is regrettable that such an important criterion is absent in more than half of the cases of neurogenic atrophy. The target fiber has a distinctive architecture with three zones (Fig 5). The central zone, which resembles an unstructured core (see the section on central core disease), is surrounded by an intermediate zone, a thin ring that is darkly stained in oxidative enzyme reactions, which creates the appearance of a bull's-eye. The intermediate zone is one of transition between the disrupted center and the third zone, which is the subsarcolemmal portion of the fiber and is composed of normal sarcoplasm.

In contrast to the atrophic pattern encountered in adult denervation, the atrophy has a different pathologic appearance in Werdnig-Hoffman disease or infantile spinal muscular atrophy. Fiber atrophy in young infants tends to be severe and extensive. Numerous atrophic fibers are observed within most fascicles, a pattern known as panfascicular atrophy. This pattern presumably represents the infantile counterpart of grouped atrophy in adult patients. Rather than an angular shape, atrophic fibers

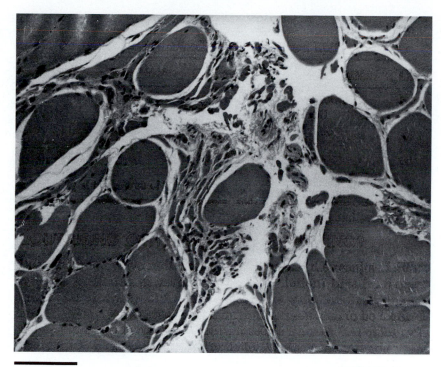

FIGURE 3.

Chronic neurogenic atrophy. Atrophic fibers are found in groups. Note that they are also angular, which is typical of denervated fibers (hematoxylin-eosin).

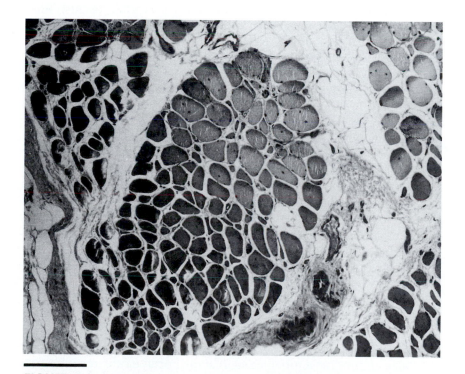

FIGURE 4.

Denervation with reinnervation. Type grouping has replaced the normal checkerboard pattern (periodic acid–Schiff).

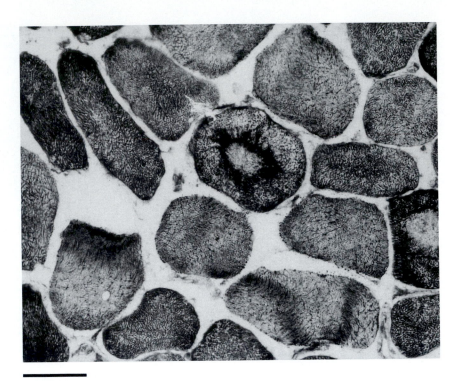

FIGURE 5.
Chronic denervation: target fiber with a pale center and a rim of intense staining (NADH-TR).

are rounded, a potentially confusing observation because fibers that are round are more suggestive of myopathies. Hypertrophic fibers are more frequently present in Werdnig-Hoffmann disease than in denervating diseases in older individuals. The hypertrophic process only affects type 1 fibers in many cases. Unlike typical denervation, for obscure reasons Werdnig-Hoffmann disease is not associated with type grouping or the formation of target fibers.

DISORDERS OF THE NEUROMUSCULAR JUNCTION

Motor end-plate disease produces functional denervation of the muscle, but the pathologic changes are not the stereotyped abnormalities of typical denervation atrophy. In routine muscle biopsies, examination of the motor end-plate region by electron microscopy is impractical since the end plates are localized at the innervation zone of the muscle, which can only be accurately identified by electrical stimulation during the biopsy procedure. The definitive diagnosis of motor end-plate disease is challenging even for the most sophisticated laboratories, and this group of disorders will be only briefly considered.

MYASTHENIA GRAVIS

Myasthenia gravis is an autoimmune disease in which patients synthesize circulating antibodies against the postsynaptic receptor protein at the motor end plate. These autoantibodies bind to the postsynaptic membrane of the motor end plate and interfere with neuromuscular transmission. Antibody attachment to postsynaptic sites activates the complement system and initiates complement-dependent destruction of the end-plate region.[6] The ultrastructural findings in this disease are a simplification of the normally complex junctional folds and a widening of the synaptic clefts of the motor end plate.[7]

Myasthenia gravis is more common in young women, with onset usually before 40 years of age. Easy fatigability and muscular weakness that is worse in the late afternoon and evening are typical. At first, symptoms predominate in the extraocular and facial muscles, and patients complain of diplopia, dysphagia, and dysarthria. In most institutions, the diagnosis depends on a beneficial response to anticholinesterase drugs like edrophonium and an EMG examination during which there is a decrement in motor action potentials during repetitive stimulation. The muscle biopsy is frequently unremarkable or characterized by mild nonspecific atrophy. The well-known finding of moderate to severe type 2 fiber atrophy is present in fewer than 50% of cases. Despite its immune-mediated pathogenesis, myasthenia gravis is not a typical inflammatory myopathy. Tiny focal lymphocytic infiltrates are seen in muscle biopsy samples in about 25% of cases.

LAMBERT-EATON SYNDROME

The Lambert-Eaton myasthenic syndrome (LEMS) is a dysimmune presynaptic disorder of neuromuscular transmission.[8] Myasthenic symptoms involve proximal limb muscles more than ocular and bulbar groups. Dry mouth, constipation, and impotence indicate coexisting autonomic nervous system disease in many patients. Neuromuscular transmission is slow at lower frequencies of electrical stimulation but paradoxically recovers at higher frequencies. Abnormal neuromuscular transmission in LEMS is due to inadequate acetylcholine discharge from the motor nerve terminal. Freeze-fracture electron microscopy has shown a reduction in active-zone particles where the calcium channels are located in the presynaptic membrane. The defect in quantal release of acetylcholine is related to impaired calcium entry into the nerve terminal. Both non-neoplastic and paraneoplastic LEMS, 60% of which in the latter type of disease are discovered in patients with small cell pulmonary carcinoma, are mediated by IgG autoantibody. The particles in the active zones are now known to be the targets of the autoimmune reaction.[9]

CONGENITAL MYASTHENIC SYNDROMES

Several of these genetic diseases have been described. They may be due to impaired acetylcholine synthesis, a deficiency of acetylcholinesterase, an insufficiency of acetylcholine receptors, or retarded closure of ion channels. The syndrome of congenital paucity of secondary synaptic clefts (CPSC) and the slow channel syndrome have been studied most intensively. The CPSC syndrome is a familial condition occurring in children or younger adults. It is characterized by ptosis and extraocular muscular weakness and is not progressive. Pathologically, the ratio of motor end plates to muscle fibers is increased perhaps as a compensatory response. Ultrastructurally, the secondary synaptic clefts are poorly developed and resemble those of fetal muscle.[10, 11] Slow channel syndrome is also familial, with onset in adulthood. Weakness and fatigability are noted in the neck, shoulders, and arms.[12] Histochemical analysis of muscle reveals a predominance of type 1 fibers and fiber atrophy involving type 1 and type 2 fibers. Electron microscopic studies show damage to the junctional folds, loss of acetylcholine receptor, and thickening of the motor end-plate basal lamina. In this syndrome, the acetylcholine-induced ion channels remain open for an abnormally lengthy period so that there is increased influx of calcium into the neuromuscular junction.

CONGENITAL MYOPATHIES

The congenital myopathies are often diagnosed in childhood, but many cases are not truly congenital since symptoms are not appreciated until long after birth. In very young patients there are signs of the floppy infant syndrome with weakness, hypotonia, and little spontaneous movement.[13] Being genetic diseases, the congenital myopathies usually display a familial inheritance pattern. Unlike the muscular dystrophies, the clinical course is benign and either static or progressive at a slow rate. Metabolic myopathies such as lipid and glycogen storage diseases, which are also congenital, are conventionally excluded from this disease category. Although the congenital myopathies are similar from a clinical standpoint, each is characterized by a distinct morphologic feature. Hence the muscle biopsy is extremely valuable in the diagnostic evaluation of patients with these neuromuscular diseases.

CENTRAL CORE DISEASE

Central core disease is a myopathy of infants and children, in whom there is a delay in motor development. Muscle involvement is seldom severe, mainly proximal, and nonprogressive. When a sufficient number of family members can be evaluated, an autosomal dominant pattern of inheritance usually prevails. The abnormal gene in some cases appears to be located on chromosome 19.[14] In frozen sections, cores are visualized as regions of depleted or absent oxidative enzyme activity (Fig 6). They may be pale in PAS-stained paraffin sections. If viewed in resin sections, cores are either structured, in which case the cross-banding pattern is maintained, or unstructured as a result of myofibrillar disorganization and a loss of cross-striations.[15] Structured and unstructured cores may coexist in the same biopsy specimen. Ultrastructurally, within the core there are abnormalities of the organelles, including a depletion of glycogen and mitochondria. In congenital disease, cores are numerous, usually solitary, and centrally positioned in the fiber. Cores cannot be relied on as a specific pathologic observation in light of their presence in other diseases, particularly in chronic denervation. When they are nonspecific, cores are seen in only a few fibers, and they tend to be large and eccentric.

NEMALINE (ROD) MYOPATHY

Nemaline myopathy may be inherited as a mendelian dominant or recessive trait. When seen by the physician, the child, more often a girl, will

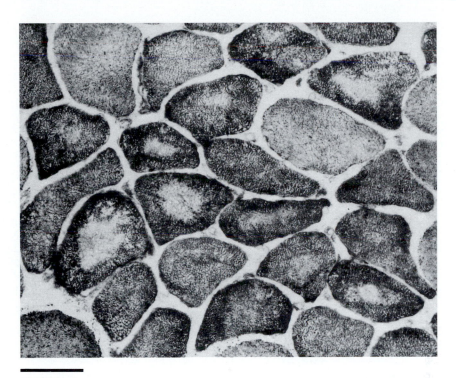

FIGURE 6.

Central core disease. Areas of reduced enzyme activity (cores) are seen in the fibers (NADH-TR).

list as the chief complaint an inability to physically keep up with peers. During neurologic examination, motor performance is noted to be impaired in the facial and proximal muscles. The diagnosis should be entertained in children in whom there is craniofacial dysmorphism with mandibular prognathism and a high arched palate. The term *nemaline*, derived from the Greek word meaning "thread," refers to the sine qua non of this disease.[16] These threads or rods are very difficult to identify in HE-stained sections and are best detected with RTC stains on frozen sections (Fig 7) and in resin sections. Rods may be haphazardly arranged in the sarcoplasm or form focal subsarcolemmal collections. They are osmiophilic and rectangular to cylindrical. In continuity with the Z bands, they are believed to arise as replications of Z-band material. Immunohistochemical stains demonstrate that rods, like normal Z disks, are composed of α-actinin.[17] They have a lattice-like ultrastructure, similar to that of a normal Z band.[18] It has become increasingly clear that rods are not a unique pathologic finding since they have been reported in many conditions such as muscular dystrophy and polymyositis. However, nonspecific rods are few in number and found in only occasional fibers.

MYOTUBULAR MYOPATHY

Centronuclear or myotubular myopathy is genetically diverse and may be transmitted as a dominant, recessive, or X-linked abnormality. The onset varies from very young to middle age. There is a progression of weakness in some cases, but the prognosis is difficult to predict. Extraocular

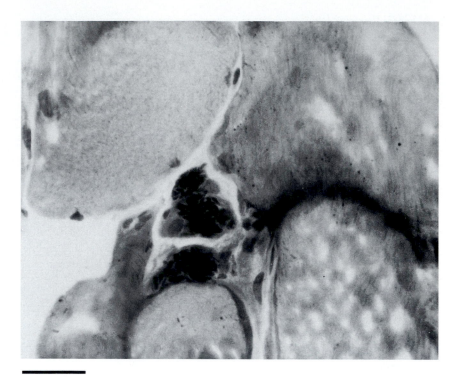

FIGURE 7.
Nemaline myopathy. Many darkly stained rods are seen. Rods cluster in subsarcolemmal regions (rapid Gomori trichrome).

and facial muscle weakness occur along with loss of strength in the axial muscles.

In transverse microscopic sections, a central or off-center nucleus is visible within most muscle fibers. These abnormally situated nuclei have a larger than normal diameter and vesicular chromatin. The sarcoplasm around the central nucleus is clear with a halo that is poorly stained in paraffin sections. In some cases type 1 fiber hypertrophy has been reported. Myotubular myopathy is considered to represent an arrest of muscle maturation because of the resemblance of the muscle biopsy tissue to the fetal myotube stage of muscle development.[19] This embryologic explanation is conceptually useful but has not been proved.

CONGENITAL FIBER-TYPE DISPROPORTION

Congenital fiber-type disproportion has two defining pathologic features, type 1 fiber atrophy and type 2 fiber hypertrophy. A predominance of type 1 fibers has been described in some cases. The genetic mechanisms in this condition have not been established, but congenital fiber-type disproportion is apparently inherited in certain families. Both autosomal recessive and dominant modes of inheritance are probable. The clinical picture ranges from a fatal disease of infants to an indolent myopathy of adults in middle age. Osseous deformities including kyphoscoliosis, hip dislocation, joint contractures, and a high arched palate occur in over 50% of patients.[20]

THE MUSCULAR DYSTROPHIES

The muscular dystrophies are each somewhat distinct both clinically and pathologically. In general, these diseases become symptomatic in childhood or early adulthood. A major symptom is muscular weakness that progresses steadily and unremittingly. Not only are almost all types of dystrophy genetically inherited, but a family history of neuromuscular disease is also likely to be discovered in several members of a family. Pathologically, each of the dystrophies is characterized not by a single morphologic feature but by a set of several features that taken together are diagnostic.

DUCHENNE MUSCULAR DYSTROPHY

With a prevalence rate of 1 per 7,000 births, Duchenne muscular dystrophy (DMD) is the most common form of dystrophy. It is inherited as an X-linked recessive defect, and genetic mapping techniques have placed the *DMD* gene in band xp21 of the short arm of the X chromosome.[21] Molecular biologists have shown the gene to be a 2,500-kb sequence comprising over 70 exons.[22] The high mutation rate in DMD, accounting for 30% to 40% of new cases, is presumably related to the size of the *DMD* gene, the largest known in humans.[23] Studies using cDNA probes indicate that 65% of patients with Duchenne dystrophy have delections in the *DMD* gene.[24] The rest appear to have frameshift and point mutations. Molecular investigations have demonstrated that patients with Duchenne dystrophy lack the normal *DMD* gene product, dystrophin.[25] This 427-kD rod-shaped protein molecule contains 3,685 amino acids and is composed of four domains.[26] The N-terminal domain has homology with the calcium binding region of α-actinin. The central domain is similar to spectrin and has 24 repeats, each consisting of 109 amino acids arranged in a triple helix. Dystrophin is a cytoskeletal protein that attaches the sarcomeres at the I bands and M lines to the sarcolemma. Dystrophin is not directly joined to the membrane but attaches by means of a dystrophin-glycoprotein complex composed of four subunits.[27] The extracellular glycoprotein, 156 DAG, is bound to the matrix protein laminin. Within the muscle cell, the N-terminal of dystrophin is bound to F-actin, whereas the C-terminal is bound to a cytoskeletal protein, 59 DAP. Of uncertain importance is the fact that in DMD there is not only a loss of dystrophin but also a reduction in dystrophin-associated proteins. Dystrophin is most abundant in skeletal muscle, although it is not unique to myocytes. Isoforms of dystrophin are found in brain, smooth muscle, myocardium, and Schwann cells in smaller amounts. The association of dystrophin with the sarcolemmal membrane in skeletal muscle is presumed to stabilize the sarcolemma during muscular contraction.[28] The absence of dystrophin causes membrane destabilization, which allows an excessive influx of calcium ions into the cell. This calcium shift activates endogenous proteases that initiate cell necrosis.[29] In biopsy specimens from nondystrophic patients, monoclonal antibodies to various portions of the dystrophin molecule can be used to demonstrate a positive reaction at the normal sarcolemmal membrane (Fig 8). The sarcolemma of fibers in patients with DMD is nonreactive for dystrophin.

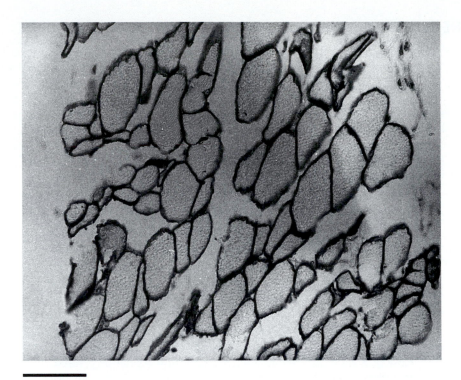

FIGURE 8.

Normal staining reaction for dystrophin at the sarcolemma of fibers (immunohistochemical with antidystrophin antibody, rod portion of the molecule).

Duchenne muscular dystrophy occurs in young males, the onset in most children being before the age of 5. Affected boys shows no clinical signs of disease at birth, but by the time they start to walk, awkwardness and frequent falling have become a reason to seek medical attention. Weakness beginning in the shoulder, pelvic, and proximal appendicular muscles is inexorably progressive and soon becomes generalized. For unknown reasons, the extraocular, facial, and pharyngeal muscles tend to be spared. Pseudohypertrophy, particularly in the calves and glutei, is highly suggestive of DMD. The enlarged muscles are actually weak and are replaced by fat and fibrous tissue. Myocardial along with striated muscle disease is common and results in tachycardia and cardiac arrhythmias. Mild mental retardation (mean IQ of 80) is not as yet well understood but is a consistent associated finding. The most informative laboratory test is the serum CK, which rises to high levels before detectable pathologic changes in the muscle.

Pathologically, the most striking features of DMD are necrotic and regenerating muscle fibers, which are often observed in groups. The acutely necrotic fiber assumes a bright eosinophilic color that gradually turns to a pale shade of pink. The sarcoplasm soon becomes coarsely granular, vacuolated, and finally fragmented. Necrosis stimulates phagocytosis of the dead cellular contents, and the sarcoplasm is invaded by macrophages. Regenerating fibers are rapidly identified in HE-stained sections because of the basophilia of their sarcoplasm. Ultrastructurally, the regen-

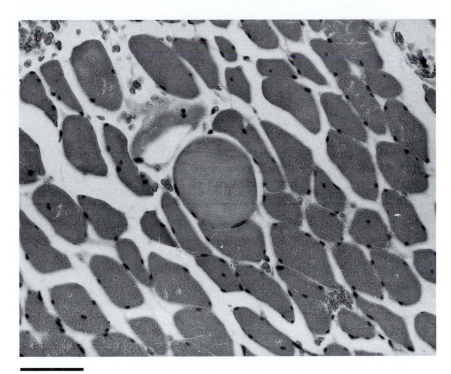

FIGURE 9.
Duchenne dystrophy. Hyaline fiber is rounded and opaque (hematoxylin-eosin).

erating fiber is full of ribosomes, which accounts for the sarcoplasmic basophilia under the light microscope. The nuclei of regenerating fibers are often internalized and enlarged, with vesicular chromatin and prominent nucleoli. The expression of vimentin and desmin appears to be a marker of fiber regeneration in immunohistochemical preparations. Hyaline or opaque fibers are also conspicuous. These fibers are named for their darkly stained sarcoplasm in both paraffin and frozen sections (Fig 9). They tend to be rounded, hypercontracted, and increased in diameter with smudged cytoplasm. Focal endomysial fibrosis, a predictable nonspecific reaction to injury in chronic, long-standing neuromuscular disease, ensues almost from the outset and is disproportionately early and severe when compared with the necrosis of muscle fibers.

BECKER MUSCULAR DYSTROPHY

This muscular dystrophy is also a sex-linked dystrophinopathy with an incidence that is 10% of that of DMD. When compared with DMD, Becker muscular dystrophy (BMD) is later in onset, less severe clinically, and slower in progression. Myocardial involvement is rare in these patients. The histologic findings resemble those in DMD but are less aggressive. Hyaline fibers, fiber necrosis, and regenerating fibers are not as numerous in the early stages of disease. The gene for Becker dystrophy is on the short arm of the X-chromosome and is allelic with the locus for *DMD*. Approximately 60% of patients with BMD have deletions of one or multiple exons in the dystrophin gene. Usually these deletions maintain the translational reading frame of mRNA and result in an abnormal, but partially functional dystrophin molecule.[30] Dystrophin is not significantly reduced in muscle, but its molecular weight is abnormal. Immunohistochemical techniques demonstrate that unlike DMD, where muscle fibers are unreactive with antibodies against dystrophin, in BMD fibers exhibit patchy or faint staining.

FACIOSCAPULOHUMERAL DYSTROPHY

Facioscapulohumeral (FSH) dystrophy has a reported prevalence of 5 per 100,000. It is a somewhat benign disorder chiefly involving the muscles of the neck, shoulders, upper part of the back, and arms with onset in the second or third decade. Facioscapulohumeral dystrophy follows an autosomal dominant mode of inheritance and is equally expressed in both genders. Genetic linkage analysis has localized the gene to the 4q35 region of the long arm of chromosome 4.[31] Muscle specimens reveal numerous atrophic and hypertrophic muscle fibers as well as moth-eaten or mottled fibers, which are best demonstrated in oxidative enzyme reactions (Fig 10). The appearance of these fibers is due to zones of diminished enzyme activity that are randomly dispersed in the sarcoplasm. The presence of inflammatory cells, almost exclusively mature lymphocytes, suggests that FSH dystrophy may be immune mediated. Lymphocytic infiltrates within the endomysium and surrounding perimysial blood vessels are usually only encountered during the early stages of the illness.

LIMB-GIRDLE DYSTROPHY

The first manifestations of this myopathy are in adolescence and early adulthood. The hallmark of disease is a decline in strength in the shoulder and pelvic girdles and in the proximal limb muscles.[32] The clinical course is one of steady, but slow deterioration. The majority of cases are inherited through an autosomal recessive mechanism. Muscular pseudohypertrophy similar to DMD is a significant clinical finding in about one third of patients. The pathologic features in this disorder are prominent internalization of sarcolemmal nuclei, fiber atrophy, and striking fiber hypertrophy followed by widespread fiber splitting of enlarged fibers (Fig 11). Lobulated fibers resembling moth-eaten fibers with irregular margins or borders may be present. Fiber necrosis and regeneration tend to occur in chronic disease.

DISTAL MYOPATHY

Distal myopathy in many ways violates the definition of muscular dystrophy because of its atypical clinical features. Disease onset is later in life, between ages 40 and 60. Most patients are males. Weakness and wasting affect primarily the distal rather than the proximal muscles of the arms and legs. The largest geographic cluster of cases has been reported in Scandinavia, where distal myopathy is a dominantly transmitted infirmity. Pathologic examination of muscle shows increased numbers of internal nuclei and selective atrophy of type 1 fibers. In many cases, so-

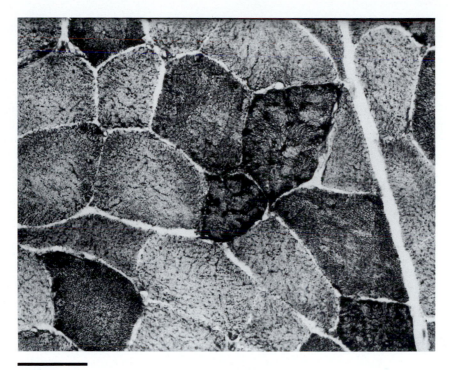

FIGURE 10.
Facioscapulohumeral dystrophy. Moth-eaten fibers are darkly stained with multiple, small unreactive sarcoplasmic areas (NADH-TR).

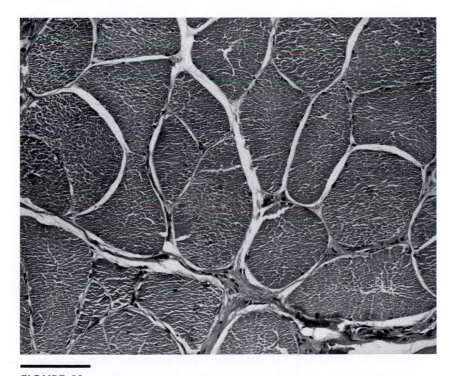

FIGURE 11.
Limb-girdle dystrophy. Hypertrophic fiber at the center has split into three smaller segments (hematoxylin-eosin).

called rimmed vacuoles, which ultrastructurally appear to be autophagic vacuoles, have been described[33] (see the section on inclusion body myositis).

MYOTONIC MUSCULAR DYSTROPHY

Myotonic muscular dystrophy (MyD) is comparable to DMD in incidence in the United States, about 1 per 8,000 population. It is therefore the most common dystrophy in adults and the most noteworthy of the myotonic disorders, other examples of which are myotonia congenita, paramyotonia, chondrodystrophic myotonia (Schwart-Jampel syndrome), and acquired myotonia, which may be drug induced or paraneoplastic. Myotonic muscular dystrophy is dominantly inherited with variable penetrance. Hence the age of onset and clinical expression are highly variable. Symptoms bring the average patient to a physician during the third or fourth decade. Muscular weakness and atrophy are noted in the face and distal portions of the extremities. Ptosis, a vacant stare, a slack transverse smile, and difficulty swallowing are early signs. Myotonia, a prerequisite for the diagnosis of MyD, is an inability of muscle to relax after contraction. It is a consequence of muscle membrane instability and may be elicited during vigorous voluntary muscle contraction or by percussion of the muscle. Electromyography is often needed to verify or detect myotonia, especially when clinically silent. Myotonic muscular dystrophy is a systemic disease in which ocular cataracts, testicular atrophy, endocrine dis-

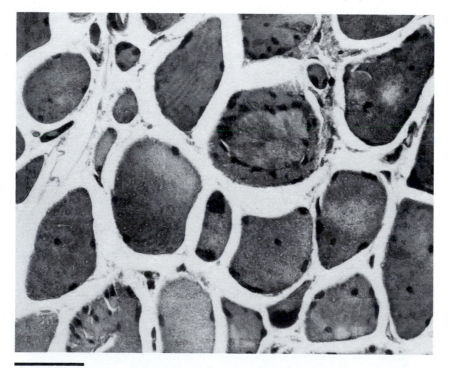

FIGURE 12.

Myotonic dystrophy. A ring fiber at the center of the photograph has its central portion enclosed by a ring of myofibrils that are oriented longitudinally. Internal nuclei separate the outer ring from the normal center (periodic acid–Schiff).

turbances such as hyperinsulinism, cardiomyopathy, and dementia are common. There may also be smooth muscle dysfunction in the esophagus, colon, urinary bladder, and uterus.

Linkage analysis has established that the *MyD* gene, a 200-kb segment, is located on the proximal long arm of chromosome 19 (19q13.2–13.3).[34] The genetic basis for MyD is a mutation involving the insertion of trinucleotide (CTG) repeats. The number of repeats ranges from 50 to several thousand; a normal gene has only 5 to 40 repeats. Phenotypic expression is governed by expansion of this region of the gene such that longer CTG repeat sequences are associated with earlier onset and more severe disease. This mutation interrupts the 3' untranslated region that codes for myotonin protein kinase. Low levels of this enzyme may explain the clinical and pathologic findings in MyD since certain protein kinases modulate channel proteins.[35] In muscle biopsy specimens numerous internal nuclei and selective atrophy of type 1 fibers are found initially. Ring fibers, in which a group of external myofibrils are circumferentially oriented and encircle the normal internal portion of the fiber, are frequently identified in MyD (Fig 12). Sometimes they are best seen in PAS stains, which reveal the cross-striations within the ring. In muscle samples from patients with long-standing disease, the classic dystrophic changes, including fiber necrosis, regeneration, and reactive fibrosis, are observed.

INFLAMMATORY MYOPATHIES

POLYMYOSITIS

Polymyositis is the most frequently biopsied inflammatory myopathy occurring in adults. Data from epidemiologic studies indicates that polymyositis has a mean annual incidence of 5 to 10 cases per million population. The peak age of onset is 35 to 40 years, and the disease is more prevalent (2:1) in females. Muscular weakness often escalates abruptly over a few weeks. Proximal muscles are the most severely involved, although weakness is generalized, except for the facial and extraocular muscles, which are seldom affected. Ancillary symptoms such as fever, malaise, and myalgias are common. The clinical course is one of remissions and exacerbations, not steady progression. During the acute phase there is an elevation of the erythrocyte sedimentation rate and a significant rise in plasma CK levels, typically to 500 to 1,000. Electromyographic recordings register small, short-duration, low-amplitude motor units with increased insertional activity. A number of antinuclear antibodies have been associated with polymyositis, such as anti–PM-1, an extractable nuclear antigen. This autoantibody is present in more than 50% of patients with polymyositis. Antibodies reactive to Jo-1 antigen, a subunit of histidine tRNA synthetase, are observed in patients with polymyositis who have interstitial lung disease. Diffuse, chronic pulmonary disease is about twice as common in polymyositis (70% of patients) as in dermatomyositis.

Polymyositis is an autoimmune disease in which a cell-mediated mechanism of tissue damage is basic.[36] Immunologic studies have shown that lymphocytes, specifically T cells, become sensitized to muscle antigens and invoke a cell-mediated attack on muscle fibers that leads to cell necrosis. Humoral mechanisms may also play a role in polymyositis, but the nature of their participation in the pathogenesis is unknown. Although deposits of immunoglobulins and complement have been reported in cases of polymyositis,[37] studies in our laboratory and several others have concluded that deposits cannot be visualized by immunofluorescence microscopy.[38] Lytic C5b-9 complement components or membrane attack complexes have been localized to necrotic fibers. However, the presence of membrane attack complexes is a consequence of complement activation and probably represents a nonspecific epiphenomenon in a variety of diseases.[39] The inflammatory cells in polymyositis encircle necrotic fibers and, to a lesser extent, the intramuscular blood vessels. The inflammatory response consists mainly of mature lymphocytes and is usually devoid of plasma cells, neutrophils, and eosinophils. A minority of mononuclear cells are macrophages and the remainder are T cells. Most of the T cells are CD8+ cytotoxic cells, many of which exhibit Ia markers indicating activation. Major histocompatibility complex class I (MHC-I) expression is considered obligatory for antigen-specific, T cell–directed cytotoxicity. In immunohistochemical preparations, fibers under attack by CD8+ cytotoxic lymphocytes express MHC-I antigen, which is not detectable in normal muscle tissue.[40] During active phases of disease, many inflammatory cells and necrotic fibers are encountered. Soon thereafter, regenerating fibers become prominent. Small, often angulated fibers are increasingly numerous with time and represent immature regenerating cells. In recurrent polymyositis, inflammatory infiltrates are less abundant. Fibrosis of the endomysium and widespread atrophy of fibers dominate the findings.

DERMATOMYOSITIS

Adult dermatomyositis is seen more often in women than in men (3:2). The muscular manifestations are very similar to those in polymyositis. In 90% to 95% of patients, cutaneous lesions are the first sign of disease. The dermatologic findings are often diagnostic and start as dusky erythematous eruptions in a butterfly pattern on the face or as a purple discoloration on the eyelids with surrounding periorbital edema. A rash is also frequently present on the neck, chest, and extensor surfaces of the fingers and toes. Many cases of childhood dermatomyositis are actually a systemic vasculopathy involving, in addition to skin and muscle, the intestine, peripheral nerves, and subcutaneous tissues.[41] Angiitis of the bowel may be complicated by mucosal ulcerations, gastrointestinal hemorrhage, and perforation.

Regarding its pathogenesis, the humoral rather than the cellular arm of the immune system is more influential than in polymyositis. Many of the findings in dermatopolymyositis can be explained on the basis of an immune complex–mediated vascular disease. By direct immunofluorescence microscopy, deposits of immunoglobulin (IgG, IgM) and complement, particularly C3, can be localized to intramuscular vessels in most children and in many adults with dermatomyositis. Moreover, C5b-9 complement components or membrane attack complexes can be immunolocalized to the same blood vessels.[42] The granularity of the deposits by electron microscopy is consistent with the presence of immune complexes, although the antigenic portion of the immune complexes has not been determined.

Lymphocytic inflammation tends to surround blood vessels and, to some extent, muscle fibers as well. Many of the lymphocytes are T cells, but more CD4+ and B lymphocytes are present than in polymyositis. Ultrastructural examination of intramuscular blood vessels reveals viral-like undulating tubular profiles in endothelial cells and pericytes.[43] Despite this observation, molecular studies have not shown enteroviral or other viral nucleic acid sequences in dermatomyositis.[44] As a result of vascular damage, there is a loss of capillaries in the muscle.[45] The capillary loss is greater in children than in adults with dermatomyositis. Atrophy of fibers at the periphery of the fascicles becomes extensive in advanced disease and occurs more frequently in younger individuals (Fig 13). Perifascicular atrophy is thought to be due to ischemia that is secondary to vasculopathy and more intense in the distal vascular bed, presumably located at the fascicular margins.

Dermatomyositis and, less often, polymyositis are paraneoplastic manifestations of cancer. The incidence of malignancy in patients with dermatomyositis and polymyositis is probably 10% to 15%, but it is about 25% to 30% in those over 55 years of age. The most common malignancies are carcinomas of the lung, breast, and gastrointestinal tract. The tumor may be occult and be preceded by a myositis, or the development of inflammatory myopathy may be an early sign of recurrent cancer.

INCLUSION BODY MYOSITIS

Patients with inclusion body myositis (IBM) are usually males 50 to 70 years of age. Inclusion body myositis is typically indolent in its course, but progressive and resistant to therapy with corticosteroids.[46] However, there is reason to believe that IBM may respond to treatment with intravenous immunoglobulin.[47] The muscle disease is painless, and weakness is considered to be greater distally. Serum CK levels are minimally elevated and sometimes normal. Histologic examination of muscle tissue often does not immediately suggest inflammatory myopathy. Inflammation, fiber necrosis, and regeneration are present in a minority (40%) of cases. Hypertrophic fibers, which are rare in polymyositis and dermatomyositis, are more frequently seen. Cryostat sections are best suited to identify the diagnostic rimmed vacuoles filled with numerous granules, which are basophilic in HE and red in RTC stains (Fig 14). Sometimes rimmed vacuoles appear to be lined by tiny granules at the rim or margin of the vacuolar space. Ultrastructurally, the basophilic granules are whorls of membranous profiles usually located in aggregates beneath the sarcolemma and within the vacuoles. Masses of viral-like tubular filaments measuring 15 to 18 nm in diameter (inclusions) are visible within muscle fiber nuclei and in the sarcoplasm, often inside rimmed vacuoles. The nature of the filaments is controversial, but a viral origin has been strongly considered, yet never verified.[48] Recent reports suggest that the filaments may be amyloid, but they tend to be refractory to Congo red

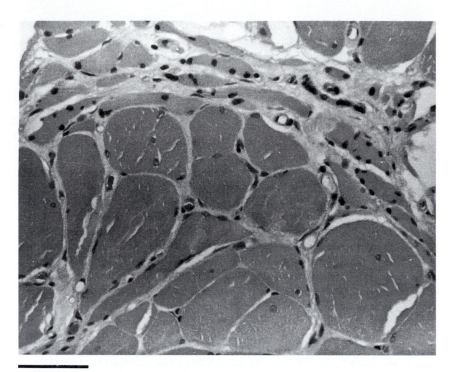

FIGURE 13.

Dermatomyositis. At the top of the picture can be seen perifascicular atrophy (hematoxylin-eosin).

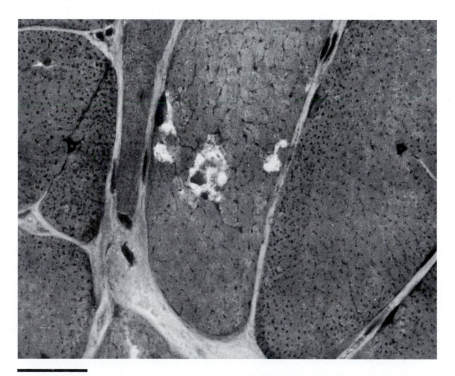

FIGURE 14.

Inclusion body myositis with a rimmed vacuole containing numerous small dark red granules (cryostat section, rapid Gomori trichrome).

staining.[49] Ubiquitin has been found in the rimmed vacuoles in immunohistochemical preparations, thus supporting the idea that there is intracellular degradation of the abnormal tubular filaments.[50]

METABOLIC MYOPATHIES

CARBOHYDRATE STORAGE DISEASES

Acid Maltase Deficiency

Acid maltase (α-glucosidase) is a lysosomal enzyme functioning optimally at pH 4 to 5 that cleaves glycogen, oligosaccharides, and maltose into glucose. Enzyme deficiency is an autosomal recessive disease that occurs in two clinical forms. Pompe's disease is a fatal systemic glycogenosis with onset in infancy. The course is rapidly progressive, usually resulting in death by 2 years of age and characterized by progressive weakness, hypotonia, macroglossia, and organomegaly. Massive accumulations of glycogen, up to 15% of the wet weight of affected tissue, develop in skeletal muscle, cardiac muscle, and the liver. Late-onset acid maltase deficiency begins in young or middle-aged adults. It is slowly progressive and more limited to skeletal muscle.[51] Patients generally exhibit proximal muscle weakness, so the initial diagnosis is often misdirected toward limb-girdle dystrophy, late-onset congenital myopathy, or polymyositis. Nearly half of adult patients seek out a physician because of respiratory difficulty and typically complain of fatigue, dyspnea, and orthopnea. Respiratory failure is frequently a cause of death in adult patients. Accumulations of glycogen in skeletal muscle do not exceed 5% of the wet tissue weight.

Muscle biopsy specimens have numerous vacuoles of various sizes within the muscle fibers. Vacuoles are more extensive in infants and replace much of the sarcoplasm. In paraffin sections vacuoles are clear, whereas in frozen sections stained with HE they are filled with blue granular material that is almost diagnostic of glycogen deposits. Vacuoles are PAS-positive, particularly in frozen sections where tissue processing has not dissolved much of the glycogen. Vacuoles are secondary lysosomes and react strongly in histochemical stains for acid phosphatase. Ultrastructurally, vacuoles are surrounded by a membrane and contain glycogen granules of normal size or reduced diameter, indicative of partial degradation. Autophagic vacuoles containing heterogeneous debris from the breakdown of sarcoplasm and glycogen granules are also encountered. Membrane-bound vacuoles are presumptive evidence of acid maltase deficiency, but they are sometimes found in other glycogen storage diseases. Since acid maltase activity cannot be demonstrated histochemically, a definitive diagnosis is based on a biochemical analysis of muscle or other tissue.

McArdle's Disease

Myophosphorylase deficiency is a recessively inherited, often familial disease in which the diagnosis is seldom suspected before the patient is 10 years of age and often not until early adulthood. The disease is characterized by myalgias, stiffness, and muscle cramps, frequently during or after physical exertion.[52] Symptoms are classically relieved by rest. Many patients do not appreciate the significance of their exercise intolerance and avoid activities that result in pain or cramps. Their condition may remain undiagnosed because symptoms are episodic and a problem only during strenuous activity. Sustained weakness is reported in fewer than one third of patients. Vigorous exercise is followed by myoglobinuria in some individuals, and renal failure is a risk in such patients.

The ischemic exercise test is a useful procedure in the diagnosis of McArdle's disease. The test is not specific since any defect in the glycolytic pathway can reduce lactate production under ischemic conditions. Positive tests are also obtained in patients with phosphofructokinase (PFK) and debrancher deficiencies. The basis for the test is the inability of affected patients to generate adequate lactate since they cannot properly break down α-1,4-glucosidic linkages. On histologic examination, numerous crescent-shaped vacuoles or blebs are seen in the subsarcolemmal portions of the muscle fibers (Fig 15). These vacuoles stain intensely with the PAS reagent. However, in some cases no vacuoles are visible, even in PAS stains. Under the electron microscope, large numbers of β-glycogen particles are seen within the vacuoles and to a lesser extent between myofibrils. Histochemical reactions for phosphorylase are used to confirm an absence of enzyme.

Phosphofructokinase Deficiency

This glycogenosis is an inherited disorder that resembles McArdle's disease clinically and pathologically. For unexplained reasons, PFK defi-

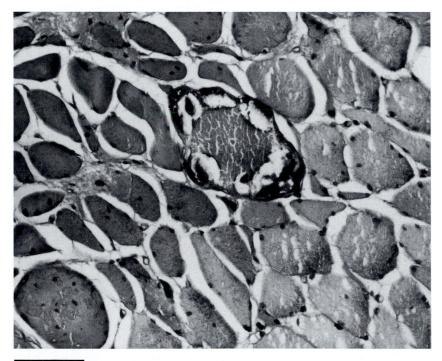

FIGURE 15.
McArdle's disease. Several darkly stained, glycogen-filled vacuoles are seen (periodic acid–Schiff).

ciency is more common in males and seems to obey a recessive pattern of inheritance in most families. Fixed weakness is far less common than in McArdle's disease. LIke McArdle's disease, a normal rise in venous lactate fails to occur during the ischemic exercise test. On microscopic examination, the muscle biopsy specimens are indistinguishable from those of patients with McArdle's disease. Numerous subsarcolemmal PAS-positive crescents are shown to contain glycogen particles by electron microscopy. It is possible, but often difficult to demonstrate PFK deficiency histochemically. Histochemical stains for the enzyme are somewhat unreliable, and the diagnosis should be confirmed by biochemical analysis of muscle tissue.

LIPID STORAGE DISEASES

The lipid storage diseases are characterized by abnormal accumulations of fat within muscle fibers and, in some cases, by lipid storage in other organs as well. Like the glycogen storage diseases, this group of storage diseases is often suspected in routine microscopic sections because of vacuolar change within cells. The lipid content of the vacuoles is revealed in frozen sections stained with oil red O or other suitable fat stains. In resin-embedded tissue, lipid vacuoles have a very distinctive light green color in toluidine blue−stained sections.

Carnitine Deficiency

Carnitine is necessary for the transport of long-chain fatty acids into the mitochondria and as a regulator of coenzyme A (CoA). Carnitine deficiency renders long-chain fatty acids, a major substrate of β oxidation, unavailable for mitochondrial metabolism. Carnitine deficiency may be manifested as a myopathy in which the disease remains confined to skeletal muscle[53] or as a systemic disease, either primary or secondary. Carnitine deficiency myopathy is a slowly progressive disease with myalgia and mild muscle weakness. The onset of disease ranges from infancy to middle age. Primary systemic carnitine deficiency is rare. Secondary carnitine deficiency has many causes, the most common underlying conditions being acyl-CoA dehydrogenase deficiency, a variety of organic acidurias, Reye syndrome, chronic renal failure, liver cirrhosis, and myxedema. Systemic carnitine deficiency is recognized by the presence of acute encephalopathy, cardiac failure, hepatic dysfunction, and hypoglycemia. As a reflection of systemic disease, serum carnitine is below normal levels. The essential pathologic change in the muscle biopsy sample is widespread vacuolization of muscle fibers in which vacuoles are multiple and variable in size within the sarcoplasm. In oil red O stains and in resin sections vacuoles are identified as lipid containing. Ultrastructural examination of muscle may reveal mitochondria of abnormal size and shape like those seen in the mitochondrial myopathies. None of the pathologic alterations are specific, and a reliable diagnosis of carnitine deficiency depends on biochemical analysis of tissue.

Carnitine Palmitoyltransferase Deficiency

The first symptom in many patients is myoglobinuria, which is precipitated by exercise, fasting, infection, or stress.[54] Myoglobinuria is frequently episodic, and patients usually experience several episodes before contacting a physician. Additional clinical findings are muscular weakness, cramps, and tenderness when the muscle is palpated. Carnitine palmitoyltransferase (CPT) deficiency appears to be inherited as an autosomal recessive disease, and the predominance in male patients (85%) is unexplained. If a muscle specimen is harvested between episodes of myoglobinuria, usually no significant morphologic changes are observed. Excessive lipid deposits are a variable finding and are not mandatory for diagnosis. A deficiency of CPT must be demonstrated by biochemical means. The function of CPT is to facilitate the transfer of long-chain fatty acids into the mitochondria. Long-chain fatty acids that are converted to acyl-CoA cannot cross the inner mitochondrial membrane. They must first be transferred to carnitine by the enzyme CPT-I. Once across the inner mitochondrial membrane, a second CPT (CPT-II) catalyzes the formation of acyl-CoA from acylcarnitine, thereby making acyl-CoA compounds available for β oxidation.

MITOCHONDRIAL MYOPATHIES

The mitochondrial myopathies are a heterogeneous group of diseases from a clinical, pathologic, molecular, and biochemical point of view.[55-57] Some cases appear to be sporadic, yet others are genetically inherited by means of either nuclear or mitochondrial DNA. The onset of symptoms ranges from infancy to adulthood, and the distribution of weakness is typically proximal, although there is also a high incidence of ptosis and ophthalmoplegia. Mitochondrial dysfunction may be largely confined to skeletal muscle or may be more generalized. In the primary mitochondrial disorders the dominant pathologic changes affect the mitochondria in which there is a biochemical disturbance related to one or more defects in mitochondrial metabolism. The morphologic changes appear to be secondary rather than primary in some cases. Mitochondrial abnormalities have been described in Canavan's disease, Zellweger syndrome, myotonic dystrophy, acid maltase deficiency, hyperthyroidism, and ischemia and after treatment with such agents such as corticosteroids and zidovudine. In these secondary disorders a pre-existing clinical condition causes the mitochondrial changes, but they are not a major part of the overall pathologic picture.

The structural abnormalities of mitochondria are very much the same in all the mitochondrial myopathies, differing only in the severity and complexity of the abnormalities. Therefore, specific mitochondrial diseases defy classification or definitive diagnosis purely on the basis of morphologic criteria. Most mitochondrial myopathies are recognized in RTC-stained frozen sections by the presence of ragged-red fibers, which have bright red, subsarcolemmal protrusions from the cell surface. Hence the involved fibers are irregular and ragged in their outlines. These fibers are also visible in oxidative enzyme reactions, in which large collections of mitochondria are revealed as intensely stained, coarsely granular deposits that are subsarcolemmal and also diffusely distributed throughout the fiber (Fig 16). In resin sections, mitochondrial aggregates form clusters of osmiophilic granules associated with numerous capillaries that prolifer-

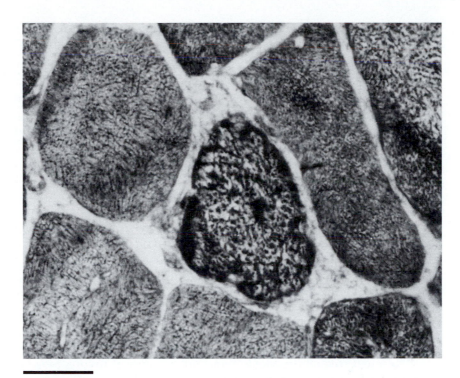

FIGURE 16.
Mitochondrial myopathy. Fiber with abnormal mitochondria is darkly stained.
(NADH-TR)

ate around and often indent involved fibers. Viewed ultrastructurally, ragged-red fibers contain numerous mitochondria that are enlarged and bizarre in shape. The mitochondrial cristae may be excessive or deficient in number, disorganized, or abnormally formed, at times resembling concentric whorling in membranes. Various matrix inclusions such as glycogen aggregates, floccular densities, myelin figures, and paracrystalline bodies that have a rectangular, grid-like structure are seen.

The central role of mitochondrial function involves energy metabolism. There are potential defects at numerous points along several of these energy-producing metabolic pathways. Transport of substrates into the mitochondria, substrate utilization, oxidation and phosphorylation coupling, respiratory chain function, and ATP synthesis represent defects that are the criteria for the metabolic classification of mitochondrial myopathies.

Defective Energy Conservation

A rare example of this type of mitochondrial myopathy is Luft's disease. Oxidative phosphorylation studies in muscle mitochondria reveal a maximum respiratory rate in the absence of adenosine diphosphate (ADP), which normally stimulates respiration. There is a loss of respiratory control, so oxidation proceeds at a furious rate independently from phosphorylation. The inefficient conversion of excess energy to heat leads to hypermetabolism and clinical hyperthermia. Following these earlier reports, it has become evident that many mitochondrial myopathies are associated with an uncoupling of oxidative phosphorylation. This common metabolic abnormality is considered to be an epiphenomenon and not a primary defect of mitochondrial function.

Impaired Substrate Utilization

Diseases in this category are carnitine deficiency and CPT deficiency, which were discussed previously, pyruvate decarboxylase deficiency, and pyruvate dehydrogenase (PDH) deficiency. Aside from the lipid storage diseases, defects in the PDH complex are the most important. The PDH complex regulates the conversion of pyruvate to acetyl-CoA, which in turn is involved in the citric acid cycle and the synthesis of fatty acids and acetylcholine. Defects in the PDH complex lead to a number of different clinical syndromes. The diagnosis should always be considered when the patient has lactic acidosis, with or without elevations in blood pyruvate levels. Among the well-known syndromes with PDH deficiency is Leigh syndrome, which is inherited as an autosomal recessive trait manifested during infancy or early childhood. Neurologic symptoms such as somnolence, blindness, deafness, ataxia, and neuropathy predominate. The lesions in the central nervous system closely resemble those seen in Wernicke's encephalopathy.

Respiratory Chain Defects

The most frequently encountered mitochondrial myopathies are due to defects in the respiratory chain, a series of five functional complexes (I to V) located within the inner mitochondrial membrane. Mitochondria are the only known source of extranuclear DNA. Each mitochondrion has multiple copies of an identical circular genome, 16,569 base pairs in length, that encodes 13 polypeptides. Seven subunits in complex I, one subunit in complex III (cytochrome b), and three subunits in complex IV (cytochrome c oxidase) represent the gene products. Diseases in which there is dysfunction of the respiratory chain components encoded by mitochondrial DNA (mtDNA) often result from mutations in the mitochondrial genome. Since mtDNA is inherited from the mother, these diseases tend to show a maternal pattern of inheritance. Point mutations in mtDNA are thought to be responsible for MELAS and MERRF (see later) and for Leber's hereditary optic neuropathy. Deletions of varying size have also been described in the Kearns-Sayre syndrome.

Several clinical syndromes have been reported in association with complex I (NADH-coenzyme Q reductase) deficiency. The most common manifestation is that of a multisystem disease designated as mitochondrial myopathy, encephalopathy, lactic acidosis, and stroke-like episodes (MELAS), which may be familial with maternal inheritance. Molecular studies have shown that MELAS is caused by a point mutation in the tRNA$^{Leu(UUR)}$ gene.[58] Most patients experience an abrupt onset of stroke-like episodes before 15 years of age accompanied by lactic acidosis. Encephalopathy and dementia are progressive, and neurologic deficits may worsen after repeated stroke-like episodes. Computed tomography reveals multiple low densities in the cerebral cortex and calcifications within the basal ganglia. Muscle weakness is often overshadowed by the central nervous system symptoms. In addition to the presence of ragged-red fibers in muscle biopsy specimens, intramuscular arteries have granular deposits with high succinate dehydrogenase activity. Electron microscopic examination of blood vessels reveals numerous enlarged and atypical mitochondria within endothelial and smooth muscle cells.

Cases of complex II and complex III deficiency are uncommon. A deficiency of complex IV (cytochrome c oxidase) is observed in a variety of disorders, including Alper syndrome, Leigh syndrome, Menkes' disease, and Lowe syndrome. Apart from these, two distinct forms of myopathy have been extensively studied. Myoclonic epilepsy with ragged-red fibers (MERRF) is a hereditary encephalomyopathy that is presumably transmitted by nonmendelian maternal inheritance. The typical clinical syndrome is characterized by myoclonus, seizures, ataxia, dementia, muscular weakness, and short stature with onset before adulthood. A complex IV defect in MERRF is due to a mutation in the mitochondrial tRNA^{Lys} gene.[59] A second condition associated with a defect in the cytochrome oxidase system is the Kearns-Sayre syndrome.[60] This syndrome is usually recognized before the age of 21 by the combination of progressive external ophthalmoplegia, pigmentary retinal degeneration, and cardiac conduction abnormalities. Ataxia, sensorineural hearing loss, insulin-dependent diabetes mellitus, and hypoparathyroidism are seen in some patients.

REFERENCES

1. Bossen EH: Collection and preparation of the muscle biopsy, in Heffner RR (ed): *Muscle Pathology*. New York, 1984, Churchill Livingstone, pp 11-14.
2. Pamphlett R: Muscle biopsy, in Mastaglia FL, Walton JN (eds): *Skeletal Muscle Pathology*. New York, 1992, Churchill Livingstone, pp 95-121.
3. Jay V, Becker LE: Fiber-type differentiation by myosin immunohistochemistry on paraffin-embedded skeletal muscle. *Arch Pathol Lab Med* 118:917–918, 1994.
4. Barron SA, Heffner RR: Weakness in malignancy: Evidence for a remote effect of tumor on distal axons. *Ann Neurol* 4:268, 1978.
5. Illa I, Leon-Monzon M, Dalakas MC: Regenerating and denervated human muscle fibers and satellite cells express neural cell adhesion molecule recognized by monoclonal antibodies to natural killer cells. *Ann Neurol* 31:46, 1992.
6. Engel AG, Lambert EH, Howard FM: Immune complexes (IgG and C3) at the motor end-plate in myasthenia gravis: Ultrastructural and light microscopic localization and electrophysiologic correlations. *Mayo Clin Proc* 52:267, 1977.
7. Santa T, Engel AG, Lambert EH: Histometric study of neuromuscular junction ultrastructure. I. Myasthenia gravis. *Neurology* 22:71, 1972.
8. Eaton LM, Lambert EH: Electromyography and electrical stimulation of nerves in diseases of the motor unit: Observations on a myasthenic syndrome associated with malignant tumors. *JAMA* 163:1117, 1957.
9. Nagel A, Engel AG, Lang B, et al: Lambert-Eaton myasthenic syndrome IgG depletes presynaptic membrane active zone particles by antigenic modulation. *Ann Neurol* 24:552, 1988.
10. Wokke JHJ, Jennekens FGI, Molenaar PC, et al: Congenital paucity of secondary synaptic clefts (CPSC) syndrome in 2 adult sibs. *Neurology* 39:648, 1989.
11. Smit LME, Hageman G, Veldman H, et al: A myasthenic syndrome with congenital paucity of secondary synaptic clefts: CPSC syndrome. *Muscle Nerve* 11:337, 1988.
12. Engel AG, Lambert EH, Mulder DM, et al: A newly recognized congenital my-

asthenic syndrome attributed to a prolonged open time of the acetylcholine-induced ion channel. *Ann Neurol* 11:553, 1982.

13. Greenfield JG, Cornman T, Shy GM: The prognostic value of the muscle biopsy in the "floppy infant." *Brain* 81:461, 1958.

14. Haan EA, Freemantle CJ, McCure JA, et al: Assignment of the gene for central core disease to chromosome 19. *Hum Genet* 86:187, 1990.

15. Neville HE, Brooke MH: Central core fibers structured and unstructured, in Kakulas BA (ed): *Basic Research in Myology. Proceedings of the Second International Congress on Muscle Diseases, Perth, Australia.* Amsterdam, Exerpta Medica, 1973, p 497.

16. Shy GM, Engel WK, Somers JE: Nemaline myopathy: A new congenital myopathy. *Brain* 86:793, 1963.

17. Hashimoto K, Shimizu T, Nonaka I, et al: Immunochemical analysis of alpha-actinin of nemaline myopathy after two-dimensional electrophoresis. *J Neurol Sci* 93:199, 1989.

18. Heffner RR: Electron microscopy of disorders of skeletal muscle. *Ann Clin Lab Sci* 5:338, 1975.

19. Spiro AJ, Shy GM, Gonatas NK: Myotubular myopathy: Persistence of fetal muscle in an adolescent boy. *Arch Neurol* 14:1, 1966.

20. Clancy RR, Kelts KA, Oehlert JW: Clinical variability in congenital fiber type disproportion. *J Neurol Sci* 46:257, 1980.

21. Hejtnancik JF, Harris SG, Tsao CC: Carrier diagnosis of Duchenne muscular dystrophy using restriction fragment length polymorphisms. *Neurology* 36:1553, 1986.

22. Koenig M, Hoffman EP, Bertelson CJ: Complete cloning of the Duchenne muscular dystrophy (DMD) CDNA and preliminary genomic organization of the DMD gene in normal and affected individuals. *Cell* 50:509, 1987.

23. Prior TW: Genetic analysis of the Duchenne muscular dystrophy gene. *Arch Pathol Lab Med* 115:984, 1991.

24. Liechti-Gallati S, Koenig M, Kunkel LM: Molecular detection patterns in Duchenne and Becker type muscular dystrophy. *Hum Genet* 81:343, 1989.

25. Hoffman EP, Fischbeck KH, Brown RH, et al: Characterization of dystrophin in muscle-biopsy specimens from patients with Duchenne's or Becker's muscular dystrophy. *N Engl J Med* 318:1363–1368, 1988.

26. Emery AEH: *Duchenne Muscular Dystrophy.* New York, Oxford University Press, 1993.

27. Ohlendieck K, Matsumura K, Ionasescu VV, et al: Duchenne muscular dystrophy: Deficiency of dystrophin-associated proteins in the sarcolemma. *Neurology* 43:795, 1993.

28. Uchino M, Araki S, Miike T, et al: Localization and characterization of dystrophin in muscle biopsy specimens from Duchenne muscular dystrophy and various neuromuscular disorders. *Muscle Nerve* 12:1009, 1989.

29. Fong P, Turner PR, Denetclaw WF, et al: Increased activity of calcium leak channels in myotubes of Duchenne human and mdx mouse origin. *Science* 250:673, 1990.

30. Gangopadhyay SB, Sherratt TG, Heckmatt JZ, et al: Dystrophin in frameshift deletion patients with Becker muscular dystrophy. *Am J Hum Genet* 51:562, 1992.

31. Sarfarzi M, Wijmenga C, Upadhyaya M, et al: Regional mapping of facioscapulohumeral muscular dystrophy gene on 4q35. *Am J Hum Genet* 51:396, 1992.

32. Chutkow JG, Heffner RR, Kramer AA, et al: Adult-onset autosomal dominant limb-girdle muscular dystrophy. *Ann Neurol* 20:240, 1986.

33. Markesbery WR, Griggs RC, Herr B: Distal myopathy: Electron microscopic and histochemical studies. *Neurology* 27:727–735, 1977.

34. Shelbourne P, Davies J, Buxton J, et al: Direct diagnosis of myotonic dystrophy with a disease-specific DNA marker. *N Engl J Med* 328:471, 1993.

35. Fu YH, Friedman DL, Richards S, et al: Decreased expression of myotonin-protein kinase messenger RNA and protein in adult form of myotonic dystrophy. *Science* 260:235, 1993.

36. Heffner RR: Inflammatory myopathies. A review. *J Neuropathol Exp Neurol* 52:339, 1993.

37. Oxenhandler R, Adelstein EH, Hart MN: Immunopathology of skeletal muscle: The value of direct immunofluorescence in the diagnosis of connective tissue disease. *Hum Pathol* 8:321, 1977.

38. Heffner RR, Barron SA, Jenis EH, et al: Skeletal muscle in polymyositis: Immunohistochemical study. *Arch Pathol Lab Med* 103:310–313, 1979.

39. Engel AG, Biesecker G: Complement activation in muscle fiber necrosis: Demonstration of the membrane attack complex of complement in necrotic fibers. *Ann Neurol* 12:289, 1982.

40. Emslie-Smith AM, Arahata K, Engel AG: Major histocompatibility complex class I antigen expression, immunolocalization of interferon subtypes, and T cell–mediated cytotoxicity in myopathies. *Hum Pathol* 20:224–231, 1989.

41. Banker BQ, Victor M: Dermatomyositis (systemic angiopathy) of childhood. *Medicine (Baltimore)* 45:261, 1966.

42. Kissel TJ, Mendell JR, Rammohan K, et al: Microvascular deposition of complement membrane attack complex in dermatomyositis. *N Engl J Med* 314:329, 1986.

43. Banker BQ: Dermatomyositis of childhood: Ultrastructural alterations of muscle and intramuscular blood vessels. *J Neuropathol Exp Neurol* 34:46, 1975.

44. Leon-Monzon M, Dalakas MC: Absence of persistent infection with enteroviruses in muscles of patients with inflammatory myopathies. *Ann Neurol* 32:219, 1992.

45. Carpenter S, Karpati G, Rothman S, et al: The childhood type of dermatomyositis. *Neurology* 26:952, 1976.

46. Carpenter S, Karpati G, Heller I, et al: Inclusion body myositis: A distinct variety of idiopathic inflammatory myopathy. *Neurology* 28:8, 1978.

47. Soueidan SA, Dalakas MC: Treatment of inclusion-body myositis with high-dose intravenous immunoglobulin. *Neurology* 43:876, 1993.

48. Chou SM: Inclusion body myositis: A chronic persistent mumps myositis? *Hum Pathol* 17:765, 1986.

49. Mendell JR, Sahenk Z, Gales T, et al: Amyloid filaments in inclusion body myositis: Novel findings provide insight into nature of filaments. *Arch Neurol* 48:1229, 1991.

50. Askanas, V, Serdaroglu P, Engel WK, et al: Immunocytochemical localization of ubiquitin in inclusion body myositis allows its light-microscopic distinction from polymyositis. *Neurology* 42:460, 1992.

51. DiMauro S, Bonilla E, Hays AP, et al: Skeletal muscle storage diseases: Myopathies resulting from errors in carbohydrate and fatty acid metabolism, in Mastaglia FL, Walton JN (eds): *Skeletal Muscle Pathology,* ed 2. New York, Churchill Livingstone, 1992, p 425.

52. DiMauro S, Tonin P, Servidei S: Metabolic myopathies, in Rowland LP, DiMauro S (eds): *Handbook of Clinical Neurology,* vol 18. Amsterdam, Elsevier, 1992.

53. Engel AG: Carnitine deficiency syndromes and lipid storage myopathies, in Engel AG, Banker BQ (eds): *Myology: Basic and Clinical.* New York, 1986, McGraw-Hill, pp 1663–1696.

54. DiMauro S, Papadimitriou A: Carnitine palmitoyltransferase deficiency, in

Engel AG, Banker BQ (eds): *Myology: Basic and Clinical.* New York, 1986, McGraw-Hill, pp 1697–1708.

55. DiMauro S, Bonilla E, Zeviani M, et al: Mitochondrial myopathies. *Ann Neurol* 17:521, 1985.

56. Morgan-Hughes JA: Mitochondrial diseases, in Mastaglia FL, Walton JN (eds): *Skeletal Muscle Pathology*, ed 2. New York, 1992, Churchill Livingstone, pp 367–424.

57. Sparaco M, Bonilla E, DiMauro S, et al: Neuropathology of mitochondrial encephalomyopathies due to mitochondrial DNA defects. *J Neuropathol Exp Neurol* 52:1, 1993.

58. Remes AM, Majamaa K, Herva R, et al: Adult-onset diabetes mellitus and neurosensory hearing loss in maternal relatives of MELAS patients in a family with the$^{Leu(UUR)}$ mutation. *Neurology* 43:1015, 1993.

59. DiMauro S, Moraes CT: Mitochondrial encephalomyopathies. *Arch Neurol* 50:1197, 1993.

60. Moraes CT, DiMauro S, Zeviani M, et al: Mitochondrial DNA deletions in progressive external ophthalmoplegia and Kearns-Sayre syndrome. *N Engl J Med* 320:1293, 1989.

Hirschsprung Disease: Pathology and Molecular Pathogenesis

Raj P. Kapur, M.D., Ph.D.

Assistant Professor, Department of Pathology, University of Washington School of Medicine, Children's Hospital and Medical Center, Seattle, Washington

The Danish pediatrician Harald Hirschsprung (1830–1916) is credited with the first published description in 1887 of the disease that bears his name. Ideas about the pathogenesis of Hirschsprung disease (HSCR) remained controversial until the 1940s, when a series of papers unequivocally indicated that ganglion cells were absent from the distal portion of the intestinal tract of such patients (see Cass[1] for a historical review of this subject). Since then the term *aganglionosis coli* has been used interchangeably with HSCR, and absence of ganglion cells is considered the essential diagnostic feature of this congenital defect.

"True" HSCR is a congenital condition. The incidence of HSCR is estimated to be 1 per 5,000 live births.[2, 3] If prenatal or perinatal demises are included, the frequency may be significantly higher since HSCR is often seen in the context of multiple malformations but is not clinically apparent prenatally. Acquired HSCR has been reported as a rare condition in which some antecedent neurodestructive process can usually be identified such as cytomegalovirus infection, Chagas disease, or enteric ischemia.

The percentage of patients with HSCR who are seen as neonates ranges widely in reported series.[4] A survey by the American Academy of Pediatrics included 1,196 patients and found that HSCR was diagnosed in the first month in only 15%.[5] However, in other published series, neonatal diagnosis was much more common.[4] In neonates, HSCR is characterized by signs of obstruction, including abdominal distension, vomiting, and occasionally gastrointestinal bleeding. In addition, 50% to 95% of neonates with HSCR fail to pass meconium during the first 48 hours of life.[4, 6] Occasionally, perforation will occur proximal to the aganglionic segment, but this is uncommon. In older individuals, HSCR can be manifested by similar symptoms or by chronic constipation or toxic enterocolitis.

With the advent of surgical therapy for HSCR, much of the mortality associated with HSCR is due to delayed recognition of the birth defect and subsequent enterocolitis. Enterocolitis is attributed to stasis and bacterial overgrowth in the intestinal tract proximal to the aganglionic zone. Since most patients with HSCR are obstructed but enterocolitis develops

Advances in Pathology and Laboratory Medicine, vol. 8
© 1995, Mosby–Year Book, Inc.

in only a subset, additional factors may be involved. Specifically, coexistent immunologic defects or infections have been hypothesized.[2, 7, 8] *Clostridium difficile* has been implicated in a subset of patients.[7] The earliest sign of enterocolitis is diarrhea, which may progress to abdominal distension, vomiting, fever, and sepsis. Mortality from enterocolitis is high (33% to 50%).[2]

ORGANIZATION OF THE ENTERIC NERVOUS SYSTEM

The enteric nervous system (ENS) is a complex network of neurons and glia that has been broadly divided into two components. The first part is projections from extrinsic neurons, the cell bodies of which are located outside the gut in parasympathetic (vagal and sacral), sympathetic (paravertebral and prevertebral), and sensory (dorsal root) ganglia.[9, 10] The second part of the ENS is intrinsic to the gut wall and includes neurons and glia located in two types of enteric ganglia, myenteric (Auerbach's) and submucosal (Meissner's). Although some authors consider the ENS to be only a part of the peripheral or autonomic nervous systems, enteric neurobiologists have emphasized unique features of the intrinsic component of the ENS, including biochemical and morphologic properties that are similar to the central nervous system (CNS). Particular emphasis has been given to the lack of collagen in enteric ganglia and the properties of enteric glial cells.[11]

Extrinsic nerves contain both myelinated and unmyelinated fibers and use a variety of neurotransmitters.[10, 12] Although many of these neurotransmitters are also synthesized and secreted by intrinsic neurons, the only noradrenergic fibers in the gut are projections from extrinsic neurons. Large extrinsic nerve fascicles can be distinguished morphologically from intrinsic neurons because the former resemble peripheral nerves found elsewhere in the body. In the colon, extrinsic nerve fascicles run along the surface of the intrinsic myenteric plexus rather than through ganglia.[9] Unfortunately, detailed information about the intramural distribution of extrinsic innervation is not available. Small branches from extrinsic fascicles enter the intrinsic enteric neural plexus and ganglia and acquire morphologic features indistinguishable from those of intrinsic neurons.

The intrinsic ENS runs throughout the entire length of the gastrointestinal tract. It has been estimated that 10^8 neurons are present in the myenteric and submucosal ganglia, a number comparable to the number of neurons in the spinal cord.[13] Although both submucosal and myenteric ganglia are found in all parts of the gut, myenteric ganglia are considerably larger and more closely spaced and outnumber submucosal ganglia. The myenteric ganglia are somewhat irregularly distributed in a complex plexus of nerve fibers. These arrays are best appreciated in whole mounts stained with vital dyes or *en face* "maceration-microdissection" preparations of gut wall.[14] In most portions of the gut, the myenteric ganglia are located around the entire circumference between the outer longitudinal and inner circular layers. However, in the appendix, the arrangement of muscle fibers is less orderly, and myenteric ganglia are interspersed between the muscle fascicles and occasionally on the serosal surface of the muscularis propria. Within the plexus, myenteric ganglia exist as both discrete collections of cell bodies and poorly defined groups that merge inconspicuously with one another. Maximal separation of ganglia is generally less than 5 mm.[15]

Accurate quantitation of ganglion cells is difficult. Measurements of neuronal density in the myenteric plexuses have yielded widely disparate results that range from 7 to 756 per millimeter of colon (reviewed by Smith[15]). In all studies, a broad variation of neuronal density was found between "normal" individuals even at the same age. Submucosal ganglia are less densely clustered and typically contain 3 or fewer neuron cell bodies. In addition to circumferential myenteric and submucosal plexuses, radial plexuses communicate between the two types of ganglia. Innervation of the lamina propria exists but is generally inconspicuous by light microscopy or acetylcholinesterase (AChE) histochemistry.

The relative density of enteric ganglia and the total number of intrinsic neurons vary in different portions of the gut and between normal individuals in the same region of gut.[15–17] These facts have clinical significance in two respects. First, a well-documented hypoganglionic zone exists in the terminal portion of the rectum just above the anal valve.[18] In this segment, submucosal and myenteric ganglia are often absent and hypertrophic nerve fibers may be present, even in normal individuals. Therefore, biopsy specimens (submucosal or myenteric) to rule out HSCR should be taken at least 2 cm above the anal valve. Second, a diagnosis of hypoganglionosis or hyperganglionosis (intestinal neuronal dysplasia), conditions that may mimic HSCR, requires experience and/or careful comparison with appropriate samples from the same site in normal individuals.[15, 17, 19]

INTERSTITIAL CELLS OF CAJAL

Small projections from enteric ganglia infiltrate the muscularis propria and muscularis mucosa. As in other sites of smooth muscle innervation, discrete synaptic connections analogous to those observed in skeletal muscle are not present. However, interposed between some of these neuronal processes and the smooth muscle are morphologically distinctive cells termed *interstitial cells of Cajal* (ICC).[20, 21] The latter cannot be distinguished in routine histologic specimens but have characteristic ultrastructural and staining characteristics that facilitate their identification. Historically, they have been interpreted as either specialized neurons, glia, or smooth muscle cells. Ultrastructural properties support the latter, and it is generally believed that ICC function as "pacemaker" cells for the smooth muscle in the intestines. Potential pathology involving ICC in disorders of intestinal motility has yet to be adequately investigated in patients with HSCR or other disorders of intestinal motility, although alterations in lower esophageal ICC have been described in patients with achalasia.[22]

DEVELOPMENT OF THE ENTERIC NERVOUS SYSTEM

Much of our understanding about the embryology of the ENS is based on studies of avian, rodent, and amphibian embryos[23–26] (Fig 1). Intrinsic

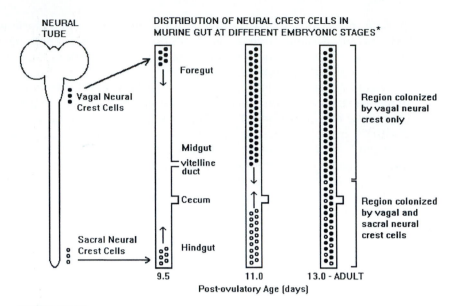

FIGURE 1.

Origin of enteric ganglion cells from the vagal and sacral portions of the neural crest based on combined evidence from avian, rodent, and human embryos. The gut is colonized from its cranial and caudal ends by cells derived from the vagal and sacral neural crest, respectively. Vagal neural crest cells (solid circles) colonize the entire length of the gut. Sacral neural crest cells (open circles) populate only the "postumbilical" gut. Survival and/or neural differentiation of sacral enteric neural crest cells is dependent on successful colonization of the caudal gut by vagal neural crest cells. Ages shown correspond to murine embryos.

ganglion cells and associated glial cells are derived from the vagal and sacral portions of the neural crest. Vagal neural crest cells colonize the entire length of the gut, whereas sacral crest cells colonize only the post-umbilical gut (distal portion of the ileum and large intestine). Vagal crest cells migrate along the course of the vagus nerves into the foregut and then caudal through the gut wall until the entire length of the gut is colonized. Sacral crest cells colonize in the opposite direction beginning in the terminal portion of the hindgut. Myenteric ganglia are formed first and submucosal ganglia appear later.

Colonization by vagal enteric neural crest cells has been studied intensively, in part because immunohistochemical and transgenic markers are available to identify these cells.[27–29] The distribution of vagal neural crest cells, as established during embryogenesis, appears to determine the permanent distribution of ganglion cells. Mutations or experimental manipulations that impair complete colonization of the entire length of the gut by vagal enteric neural crest cells lead to aganglionosis.[30, 31] By contrast, it appears that neural differentiation and/or survival of sacral neural crest cells depends on the presence of vagal neural crest cells. Thus although sacral neural crest cells are present in the hindgut and contribute to normal development of the ENS, successful cranial-to-caudal colonization of the entire gut by vagal neural crest cells appears to be a necessary event to avoid congenital aganglionosis coli (discussed by Gershon et al.[24]).

Colonization of the gut by vagal neural crest cells is generally a smooth cranial-to-caudal process that takes place around the entire circumference of the gut wall.[29] As the gut is colonized, ganglion cell precursors replicate, migrate, and eventually differentiate. According to contemporary models, aganglionosis coli is a congenital malformation related to incomplete colonization of the gut by vagal enteric neural crest cells. This theory explains the fact that aganglionosis is almost invariably a continuous lesion that extends to the anorectal junction.

ANATOMIC PATHOLOGY

In classic HSCR, the terminal portion of the large intestine and a variable amount of more proximal contiguous intestinal tract is devoid of ganglion cells. The aganglionic segment is generally nondistended, lacks fecal content, and is often described as "narrow" in contrast with the proximal portion of the intestinal tract. The aganglionic segment shows other microscopic changes in addition to an absence of ganglion cells.[32] These include hypertrophy of nerve fibers in the myenteric and submucosal plexuses. The aganglionic nerve plexuses, which are normally paucicellular accumulations of "neuropil" reminiscent of CNS white matter, are replaced by thick nerve fibers similar histologically to peripheral nerves elsewhere in the body. The hypertrophic plexuses are more cellular and contain parallel arrays of wavy Schwann cell nuclei. Ultrastructurally or immunohistochemically, thickened basal lamina and excess extracellular matrix components have been demonstrated in this zone as well[33-38] (see later).

Immediately proximal to the aganglionic segment is usually a "transitional zone" of hypoganglionic gut.[32] This zone generally corresponds to a relatively short, funnel-shaped segment where the normal intestine tapers to the narrow diameter of the aganglionic gut. However, correlation between the gross and microscopic changes is not precise, and the length of the transitional zone cannot be reliably predicted from the gross appearance. Furthermore, the proximal margin of the transitional zone is variable and difficult to define because the transition to normal gut is gradual. In some cases, a severe paucity of ganglion cells (hypoganglionosis), a dramatic excess of submucosal ganglion cells (hyperganglionosis), and/or displaced ganglion cells are easily recognizable features of the transition zone. Mild-to-moderate hypoganglionosis or hyperganglionosis may be very difficult to recognize and often requires quantitative studies that are impractical in routine practice.[17] Displaced ganglion cells can be found in the lamina propria, within the muscle fascicles of the muscularis propria, or in the subserosa.[36, 39-43] Subserosal ganglion cells are normal in the vermiform appendix, so it should not be evaluated for this feature. Many of the histologic changes evident in the transitional zone of some patients have been termed *neuronal intestinal dysplasia* (NID). Neuronal intestinal dysplasia has also been observed in the intestinal tracts of individuals with symptoms like those of HSCR, but no aganglionic segment. Isolated NID is a controversial subject, and the reader is referred to a previous paper in this series for an excellent discussion of this topic.[44]

The physiologic significance of the transitional zone is controversial. Empirical evidence suggests that persistence of symptoms may result if at least portions of the transitional zone are not surgically resected with the aganglionic gut.[40, 41] Unfortunately, accurate quantitation of ganglion cells cannot be practically achieved by gross or microscopic criteria at the time of resection, beyond the presence or absence of ganglion cells. Therefore, inadequate resection of the transitional zone is often only recognized when symptoms recur and a second operative procedure is performed.

Proximal to the transitional zone, the gut contains normal numbers of ganglion cells but may have evidence of the secondary effects of distal aganglionosis.[45] The latter include dilatation, hypertrophy, and enterocolitis. The term *congenital megacolon* is sometimes used in reference to HSCR in recognition of these secondary consequences. Dilatation and hypertrophy result from fecal impaction and prolonged peristaltic activity against the increased resistance afforded by the aganglionic segment. These changes can be so profound that the abdomen becomes markedly distended and peristaltic contractions are visible externally. The muscular layers of the intestinal wall are grossly and microscopically thickened. Chronic inflammation is often present in megacolon, and patients occasionally suffer from repeated episodes of acute enterocolitis. Rarely, overt ulcers exist. These features are not specific for HSCR but can be seen with other forms of chronic intestinal pseudo-obstruction.

LONG-SEGMENT VS. SHORT-SEGMENT HIRSCHSPRUNG DISEASE

Hirschsprung disease is subclassified according to the relative length of the aganglionic region (see Table 1). In the vast majority (75% to 85% of patients in most series), aganglionosis is restricted to the rectum and distal end of the sigmoid colon (short-segment disease). The remaining cases are referred to as long-segment disease. However, some recent classification schemes reserve the latter term for situations in which ganglion cells are not present proximal to the splenic flexure, in which case long-segment disease accounts for fewer than 10% of all cases.[50, 51]

TABLE 1.
Proximal Extent of Aganglionosis in Patients With Hirschsprung Disease

Proximal Margin of Aganglionic Segment	Fraction of Patients in Respective Series, %				
	Wyllie[46] (n = 152)	Foster[47] (n = 63)	Garver[48] (n = 134)	Bodian[49] (n = 207)	Badner[50] (n = 416)*
Small intestine	2	10	7	4	6
Ascending or transverse colon	1	5	3	4	4
Descending colon	14	9	13	10	11
Rectosigmoid	81	76	77	82	79

*Some of these patients have previously been reported by Garver et al.[48] and Bodian and Carter.[49]

ULTRASHORT-SEGMENT DISEASE

Ultrashort-segment HSCR is a controversial entity, in large part because it has been defined differently by various investigators.[52] Initially, ultrashort-segment HSCR was reserved to describe patients with clinical and radiologic symptoms similar to those of HSCR, but with ganglion cells in their rectal biopsy samples.[53] Others have claimed that such patients have fewer than normal numbers of ganglion cells in the terminal portion of the rectum (reviewed by Neilson and Yazbeck).[52] However, the paucity of ganglion cells in biopsy specimens from the terminal 2 to 3 cm has questionable significance since this area is aganglionic or hypoganglionic in normal individuals.[18, 54] Since it is probable that aganglionosis is a feature of the normal terminal rectum, use of the term "ultrashort HSCR" promotes confusion.

In reality, patients who fulfill the original criteria for ultrashort HSCR (Table 2) probably have a heterogeneous set of disorders more appropriately referred to as anal achalasia or internal sphincter achalasia. Conceivably the same clinical findings can be due to psychogenic, myogenic, or neurogenic causes. Recent data suggest that reduced nicotinamide-adenine dinucleotide phosphate (NADPH)- diaphorase activity (nitric oxide synthase), a marker for enteric nonadrenergic, noncholinergic nerve fibers, may be absent in the internal sphincter of some patients with anal achalasia.[8]

ZONAL AGANGLIONOSIS AND SKIP AREAS

Two rare patterns of congenital aganglionosis in which the aganglionic segment is contiguous and extends to the anorectal junction contrast with classic HSCR (Fig 2).[55] The first pattern consists of "skip areas" in a patient with total colonic aganglionosis. Skip areas are segments that contain ganglion cells flanked proximally and distally by aganglionic gut. Eleven cases have been reported to date.[43] In all instances, aganglionosis extended to the anorectal junction and the appendix was aganglionic, but a highly variable length of intervening colon contained ganglion cells.

It is important that pathologists be aware of this entity to avoid the inappropriate practice of intraoperative examination of the appendix in

---

TABLE 2.

Criteria for the Diagnosis of Ultrashort-Segment Hirschsprung Disease*

Chronic constipation from birth or childhood

Abdominal distension of fecal soiling and the presence of stool in the rectal ampulla

Presence of ganglion cells on suction rectal biopsy 3 cm from the anal verge

Barium enema without a funnel-shaped "transitional zone" typical of Hirschsprung disease

Manometry showing failed anorectal reflex

Clinical improvement after anal myomectomy

*Adapted from Neilson IR, Yazbeck S: *J Pediatr Surg* 25:1135–1138, 1990.

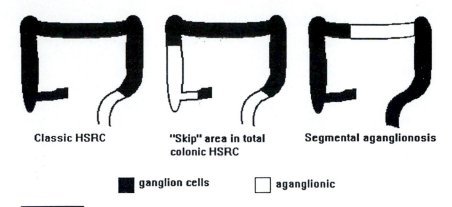

FIGURE 2.

Three patterns of aganglionosis observed in humans. "Classic" Hirschsprung disease *(HSCR)* accounts for the ovewhelming majority of cases of aganglionosis in humans. This pattern is characterized by the absence of ganglion cells from the terminal portion of the rectum plus a variable length of contiguous gut. In severe cases, the entire gut may be aganglionic. "Skip" areas are ganglionated segments that separate two zones of aganglionic gut. As in classic HSCR, the distal end of the rectum is always involved, and typically, the entire colon is aganglionic except for the skip area. "Segmental" aganglionosis describes a localized lesion flanked by gut that contains ganglion cells. In such cases, the distal portion of the rectum contains ganglion cells. Segmental aganglionosis is thought to represent an acquired lesion.

an effort to diagnose total colonic aganglionosis. Even in patients with long-segment HSCR and aganglionosis of the appendix, relatively large segments of colon may contain ganglion cells. In at least one patient, the ganglionic skip area has been spared from surgical resection and functionally anastomosed to the small intestine.[56]

The existence of skip areas is difficult to understand given the concept that HSCR is due to incomplete colonization by vagal neural crest cells, and unidirectional spread of these cells is cranial to caudal. However, a notable exception to the intramural progression of vagal neural crest cells occurs at the ileocecal junction, where these cells appear to migrate extramurally along the mesenteric border of the proximal portion of the large intestine before colonizing the latter segment. This phenomenon of extramural spread has been invoked as one explanation for rare cases of skip areas in patients with otherwise total colonic aganglionosis.[43] According to this hypothesis, vagal neural crest cells, which bypass the ileocecal region via the mesentery, re-enter the midcolon but fail to colonize both the proximal and distal portions of the large intestine.

Zonal or segmental aganglionosis refers to situations in which ganglion cells are present in the terminal portion of the colon but missing in a segment of gut more proximally.[32, 57] Zonal aganglionosis is thought to be an acquired lesion (disruption) in which ganglion cells are lost because of ischemic, viral, or other types of injury.[58, 59] In some cases, supportive evidence for such insults can be found (i.e., a history of necrotizing enterocolitis, viral inclusions).[60−62] An alternative hypothesis is that segmental aganglionosis results from failure of the vagal and sacral neural crest cells to converge and neuronal differentiation of both cell populations in the cranial and caudal portions of the gut, respectively. This seems unlikely since, as noted earlier, survival and/or differentiation of the sacral neural crest cells is thought to be dependent on convergence of the two populations. However, it is conceivable that these events could occur independently as part of a malformation process.

DIAGNOSIS OF HIRSCHSPRUNG DISEASE IN RECTAL BIOPSY TISSUE

Two diagnostic methods are widely used for HSCR, full-thickness rectal biopsies and suction biopsies of the rectal mucosa and submucosa. In either case, it is critical that the biopsy be taken at least 2 cm above the anorectal mucocutaneous junction because ganglion cells are frequently absent or sparse distal to this point.[18] Full-thickness biopsy specimens are harvested with the patient under general anesthesia but are generally easier to interpret since they contain portions of the myenteric plexus. Ganglion cells in this region between the inner circular and outer longitudinal layers of the muscularis propria are so numerous that they are easily found in normal specimens. In contrast, nerve cell bodies are conspicuously absent from this region in the aganglionic gut from patients with HSCR despite the persistence of prominent nerve processes. For intraoperative frozen sections, examination of a well-oriented 8- to 10-mm-long segment of intestinal musculature is generally adequate to exclude ganglion cells.

Suction biopsy specimens are smaller and can be obtained without general anesthesia. The principle limitations with such biopsies are the scattered distribution and relative paucity of submucosal ganglion cells coupled with the small amount of submucosa sampled in most cases. Although the presence of even a single ganglion cell in such biopsy samples excludes the diagnosis of HSCR, failure to identify such cells in suction biopsy specimens is insufficient to establish the diagnosis. A number of histochemical and immunohistochemical techniques have been advocated to facilitate the identification of ganglion cells in suction biopsy specimens or otherwise increase the diagnostic value of this procedure. Currently, the most valuable approach involves histochemical staining for AChE activity. This procedure is relatively simple but requires frozen sections.[63] Acetylcholinesterase activity is present in nerve fibers that normally exist in the submucosa and muscularis mucosa. In specimens from aganglionic gut, the fibers in the muscularis mucosa are numerous and large. In addition, AChE-positive nerve fibers are often present in the lamina propria in affected gut.

Since the changes evident in AChE staining are more quantitative than qualitative, interpretation of such preparations requires experience and quality histologic preparations. Under such conditions, the positive predictive value and false-negative rates with this method (as reported in the literature) are good. Some of the practical considerations inherent in AChE staining and interpretation are discussed elsewhere.[63, 64]

GENETICS OF HIRSCHSPRUNG DISEASE

Long-segment disease, defined as aganglionosis that extends either proximal to the splenic flexure or sigmoid colon, is epidemiogically and perhaps genetically distinct from short-segment disease. The incidence of short-segment HSCR in males is approximately four times that of females, in contrast with long-segment disease in which the male:female ratio is less than 2:1.[50, 65] In addition, the risk to siblings increases dramatically with long-segment disease but is 5% or less for siblings of patients with short-segment disease. On the basis of statistical analyses of long- and short-segment disease within first-degree relatives, Badner et al. proposed that long-segment disease is an autosomal dominant disorder with incomplete penetrance.[50] They concluded that short-segment disease, defined as aganglionosis of the rectum and/or sigmoid colon, could be either multifactorial or due to an autosomal recessive allele with very low penetrance.

Hirschsprung disease is usually an isolated birth defect. However, it has been reported in association with many other congenital conditions[65, 66] (Table 3). Some of these individual reports may represent the chance association of two independent events. However, frequently recognized associations probably indicate a single underlying etiology. The association of HSCR with trisomy 21 is particularly well established. In the most recent series, trisomy 21 occurred in 10% to 15% of all patients with HSCR.[4, 8, 65, 90–93] Conversely, 1% to 4% of individuals with trisomy 21 have HSCR.[121] The vast majority of patients with trisomy 21 have short-segment disease with a male-to-female ratio of 10:1.[50] Similar statistical associations between HSCR and atrial septal defects and urinary tract defects have been established independent of trisomy 21.[50, 122]

Among the group of disorders that have been reported in association with HSCR are many malformations of other tissues derived from the neural crest ("neurocristopathies"). Waardenburg syndrome type II/piebald trait, DiGeorge syndrome, neuroblastoma, neurofibromatosis type I, and multiple endocrine neoplasia (MEN) types 2A and 2B show varying phenotypic abnormalities in neural crest derivatives and have been associ-

TABLE 3.

Reported Conditions Associated With Hirschsprung Disease

Associated Disorder	Reference
DiGeorge syndrome	67
Facial clefts/mental retardation	68–71
Smith-Lemli-Opitz syndrome, type II	66, 72–77
Waardenburg syndrome, type II/piebald trait	78–89
Trisomy 21	4, 8, 65, 90–97
Multiple endocrine neoplasia, types 2A or 2B	98–102
Neurofibromatosis, type I	103
Ondine's curse (failure of automatic respiration during sleep)	104–117
Neuroblastoma/pheochromocytoma	103, 118–120
Congenital heart malformations	65
Urinary tract malformations	65
Dandy-Walker malformation	65

ated with HSCR. Since enteric ganglia are derived from the neural crest, the concept of HSCR as one component of a generalized "neurocristopathy" has appeal.

MUTATIONS IN THE RECEPTOR TYROSINE KINASE, *RET*, AND HIRSCHSPRUNG DISEASE

Perhaps the most exciting recent discovery regarding the pathogenesis of HSCR is that mutations in both the *ret* gene in mice and the homologous *RET* gene in humans are associated with aganglionosis coli. *RET* is a proto-oncogene that is widely expressed in many parts of the embryo, including the CNS, neural crest cells, and metanephric kidneys. The *RET* gene was initially discovered as part of DNA rearrangements that were associated with neoplastic transformation *in vitro* and *in vivo*.[123-127] In humans, several types of mutations of the *RET* gene have been linked with familial and sporadic HSCR.[128] *RET* is located on chromosome 10, and mutations in *RET* that cause HSCR behave as autosomal dominant traits with variable incomplete penetrance.[129, 130] Within individual families, the same *RET* mutation can be associated with variable phenotypes, including long-segment disease, short-segment disease, or no clinical manifestations. The factors that influence this variable penetrance are not known at present. Mutations in *RET* that are associated with HSCR include deletions of the gene and point mutations that eliminate the tyrosine kinase activity of the molecule. Therefore it appears that at least some forms of human HSCR are associated with haploid insufficiency for the *RET* gene. Most reported cases of HSCR associated with *RET* mutations have been familial long-segment disease. The prevalence of *RET* mutations among all patients with HSCR, particularly the common sporadic short-segment type, has not yet been established.

The protein encoded by the *RET* gene is a receptor tyrosine kinase. This protein spans the plasma membrane and serves as a receptor for one or more ligands that are unknown at present. The receptor protein is expressed on the surfaces of enteric neural crest cells and is presumably activated by interaction with ligand(s) present in the embryonic gut.[131] At this time, the ligand for *RET* is unknown. As with other receptor tyrosine kinases, receptor-ligand interaction should promote *RET* protein tyrosine kinase activity within neural crest cells and stimulate a cascade of intracellular phosphorylation events that may influence the replication, migration, survival, or differentiation of these cells (Fig 3).

Other hereditary disorders have also been associated with mutations in the *RET* proto-oncogene. These include familial medullary thyroid carcinoma (FMTC) and MEN 2A and 2B. In these families, mutations in the *RET* gene also act in a autosomal dominant fashion and appear to promote neoplasms in a variety of neural crest derivatives. However, a relatively small set of defined missense mutations of specific amino acids are found in these neoplastic syndromes, in contrast with the deletions, truncations, and other heterogeneous mutations observed in patients with familial HSCR. Although HSCR probably results from the loss of functional inactivity of one *RET* allele, it is likely that neoplastic transformation in FMTC and MEN, types 2A and 2B, results from mutations that cause ac-

NORMAL

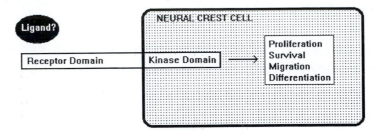

MEN2A/MEN2B DUE TO PRESUMPTIVE ACTIVATING MUTATIONS OF THE RET RECEPTOR TYROSINE KINASE

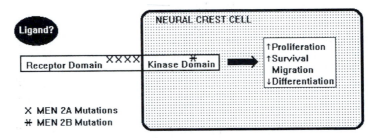

HIRSCHSPRUNG DISEASE DUE TO PRESUMPTIVE INACTIVATING MUTATIONS OF THE RET RECEPTOR TYROSINE KINASE

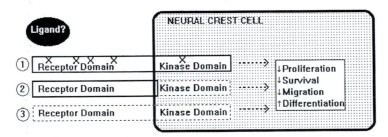

FIGURE 3.

Putative role of the RET receptor tyrosine kinase in enteric neurodevelopment and associated neurocristopathies. RET is a transmembrane protein with an extracellular receptor domain and a cytoplasmic kinase domain. The protein is expressed in enteric neural crest cells and presumably interacts with an unidentified extracellular ligand/growth factor via its receptor domain. Ligand-RET interaction is thought to activate the molecule's kinase activity and initiate a cascade of intracellular phosphorylation reactions that influence the proliferation, survival, migration, and/or differentiation of neural crest cells. Mis-sense mutations that cause amino acid substitutions in a restricted subset of sites in RET have been associated with multiple endocrine neoplasia types 2A (MEN 2A) and 2B (MEN 2B). These mutations presumably superactivate RET kinase activity and increase the risk for neoplastic transformation. Mis-sense mutations and mutations that delete all or part of the RET gene have been associated with some cases of HSCR. Hirschsprung disease–related mutations are believed to inactivate the activity of one of the RET alleles and thereby hinder colonization of the gut by enteric neural crest cells.

tivation of the *RET* tyrosine kinase and chronic "stimulation" of affected cells (Fig 3). Hence, gastrointestinal ganglioneuromas develop in patients with MEN, type 2B, presumably because of *RET*-mediated mitogenic stimulation of enteric neural crest cells.

An appropriate level of *RET* activity seems to be critical to normal colonization of the gut by neural crest cells. Although most cases of HSCR that are associated with *RET* mutations probably result from reduced *RET* activity, it is interesting that a small number of patients with MEN 2A have been reported with HSCR. Thus too much *RET* activity may also impair normal enteric neurodevelopment and promote HSCR. This concept may explain why both hypoganglionosis and hyperganglionosis have been reported in the transitional zones of patients with HSCR. It remains to be determined whether those with hyperganglionosis have specific types of *RET* mutations or whether *RET* mutations are associated with neuronal intestinal dysplasia.

Creation and analysis of mice that lack the *ret* gene have confirmed the suggestion that deficient *ret* activity results in aganglionosis coli.[132] In *ret-null* mice, mice in which both *ret* alleles have been disrupted, death occurs shortly after birth and they have no ganglion cells in their entire gastrointestinal systems. In addition, they have variable types of renal dysgenesis. Unlike many humans with familial HSCR and *RET* mutations, mice heterozygous for the disrupted allele have no phenotypic abnormalities. However, the effect of the murine mutation has not been examined against many genetic backgrounds.

CELL INTERACTIONS AND THE PATHOGENESIS OF HIRSCHSPRUNG DISEASE

It is clear from murine models and human studies that mutations in the *RET* gene only account for a fraction of HSCR cases. The molecular basis for HSCR is likely to be heterogeneous and complex. It is clear that mutations at more than one genetic locus can result in HSCR.[50, 133, 134] This is most evident in murine models for HSCR, where alleles at four loci on different chromosomes have been shown to produce aganglionosis coli. These include an autosomal dominant mutation, *dominant megacolon (Dom)*, and the autosomal recessive mutations *lethal spotted (ls)*, *piebald lethal (s')*, and *ret-null*. The molecular basis for aganglionosis in each of these mice is now known, with the exception of *Dom* (see later). In both humans and some murine models, the genetics are complicated by incomplete penetrance of the HSCR phenotype, depending on the genetic background.[130, 133, 135, 136]

The aforementioned murine models have been valuable systems with which to study the pathogenesis of aganglionosis coli. Like humans with Waardenburg syndrome or piebald trait, the phenotypes of all three of the spontaneous murine mutants include variable degrees of "spotting" and an absence of melanocytes from portions of the coat. The association of spotting and aganglionosis has also been observed in other species, further strengthening the concept that at least some forms of HSCR represent a more general neurocristopathy.[78, 137–139] Among the spontaneous mutants, *ls* and *s'* have been studied most extensively.[24, 29] The results of these studies have led to insights into the pathogenesis of aganglionosis coli that have implications for the human condition. In the case of *ls* and *s'* embryos which are destined to have the murine equivalent of short-segment disease, retarded neural crest cell colonization is evident throughout the entire length of the large intestine, not just in the segment destined to be aganglionic.[29]

The results from a series of experiments suggested that the primary defect in *ls/ls* embryos is not intrinsic to the individual neural crest cells, but rather exists in the microenvironment provided by surrounding cells.[35, 143, 144] Until recently, the molecular nature of the *ls* and *s'* mutations was unknown. However, experimental mutagenesis of the endothelin receptor B *(etr-B)* gene has led to the unexpected realization that the *s'* allele is a deletion of *etr-B* and the *ls* allele is a missense mutation in a gene that encodes a ligand for the receptor, endothelin-3 *(et-3)*.[140, 141] Endothelins are a family of closely related peptides synthesized by a variety of cells including enteric neurons. Until recently, endothelins and their receptors were studied primarily by vascular biologists interested in their vasoactive properties. In the gut, it appears that both *et-3* and the receptor are expressed by neurons and presumably their precursors and probably regulate autocrine or paracrine communication between neuronal precursors. Coincident with the murine studies,[133] Chakravarti and colleagues found evidence that some familial forms of HSCR are linked to a locus on chromosome 13 in a region syntenic with the murine *s'* locus.[142] Subsequently they have demonstrated that mutations in human *ETR-B* are associated with HSCR. Thus mutations of at least two discrete loci, *RET* and *ETR-B*, appear to cause some cases of HSCR, and in each instance the genes affected encode proteins involved in intercellular signaling.

The downstream effects of abnormal intercellular signals in the developing ENS remain to be worked out. However, one event in the pathogenesis of aganglionosis may be abnormal synthesis and/or accumulation of extracellular matrix components, such as laminin, that inhibit the proliferation or migration of enteric neural crest cells. Excess amounts of laminin and other extracellular matrix abnormalities have been demonstrated in mutant murine embryos and aganglionic intestines from mice and humans.[33-38]

The combined evidence to date suggests that most if not all cases of congenital aganglionosis coli are malformations caused by a failure of vagal neural crest cells to colonize distal portions of the intestinal tract. Intercellular signals mediated by receptor tyrosine kinases (e.g., *RET*), receptors coupled to G proteins (e.g., *ETR-B*), cell matrix components (e.g., laminin), or other factors appear to be important for normal neural crest cell migration, proliferation, survival, and differentiation. Abnormalities in these signaling processes, whether genetic or environmentally imposed, are likely to underlie the pathogenesis of HSCR. As our understanding of the dynamic interactions between neural crest cells and their microenvironments increases, it is likely that rapid, accurate, and possibly noninvasive diagnostic tests for HSCR will be developed to complement or replace the traditional approaches currently available. In addition, it will be possible to prenatally identify individuals at risk for HSCR and counsel families as to their risks for offspring with this condition.

REFERENCES

1. Cass D: Hirschsprung disease: An historical review. *Prog Pediatr Surg* 20:199–214, 1986.
2. Ehrenpreis T: *Hirschsprung's disease.* St Louis, Mosby, 1970, p 57.
3. Taguchi T, Tanaka K, Ikeda K, et al: Double zonal aganglionosis with a skipped oligoganglionic ascending colon. *Z Kinderchir* 38:312–315, 1983.
4. Klein MD, Coran AG, Wesley JR, et al: Hirschsprung disease in the newborn. *J Pediatr Surg* 19:370–374, 1984.
5. Kleinhaus S, Boley SJ, Sheran M, et al: Hirschsprung's disease: A survey of the members of the surgical section of the American Academy of Pediatrics. *J Pediatr Surg* 14:588–597, 1979.
6. Martin LW, Torres AM: Hirschsprung's disease. *Surg Clin North Am* 65:1171–1180, 1985.
7. Thomas DFM, Malone M, Fernie DS, et al: Association between Clostridium difficile and enterocolitis in Hirschsprung's disease. *Lancet* 1:78–79, 1982.
8. Quinn FMJ, Surana R, Puri P: The influence of trisomy 21 on outcome in children with Hirschsprung's disease. *J Pediatr Surg* 29:781–783, 1994.
9. Christensen J: Gross and microscopic anatomy of the large intestine, in Phillips SF, Pemberton JH, Shorter RG (eds): *The Large Intestine: Physiology, Pathophysiology, and Disease.* New York, Raven Press, 1991, pp 13–35.
10. Costa M, Furness JB, Llewellyn-Smith IJ: Histochemistry of the enteric nervous system, in Johnson LR (ed): *Physiology of the Gastrointestinal Tract,* ed 2. New York, Raven Press, 1987, pp 1–39.
11. Gershon MD, Rothman TP: Enteric glia. *Glia* 4:195–204, 1991.
12. Furness JB, Llewellyn-Smith IJ, Bornstein JC, et al: Chemical neuroanatomy and the analysis of neuronal circuitry in the enteric nervous system, in Bjorklund A, Hokfelt T, Owman C (eds): *Handbook of Chemical Neuroanatomy.* Amsterdam, Elsevier, 1988, pp 161–218.
13. Furness JB, Costa M: Types of nerves in the enteric nervous system. *Neuroscience* 5:1–20, 1980.
14. Wells TR, Landing BH, Ariel I, et al: Normal anatomy of the myenteric plexus of infants and children. *Perspect Pediatr Pathol* 11:152–174, 1987.
15. Smith VV: Intestinal neuronal density in childhood: A baseline for the objective assessment of hypo- and hyperganglionosis. *Pediatr Pathol* 12:225–237, 1993.
16. Irwin DA: The anatomy of Auerbach's plexus. *Am J Anat* 49:141–166, 1931.
17. Krishnamurthy S, Heng Y, Schuffler MD: Chronic intestinal pseudo-obstruction in infants and children caused by diverse abnormalities of the myenteric plexus. *Gastroenterology* 104:1398–1408, 1993.
18. Aldridge RT, Cambell PE: Ganglion cell distribution in the normal rectum and anal canal: A basis for the diagnosis of Hirschsprung's disease by anorectal biopsy. *J Pediatr Surg* 3:475–489, 1968.
19. Simpser E, Kahn E, Kenigsberg K, et al: Neuronal intestinal dysplasia: Quantitative diagnostic criteria and clinical management. *J Pediatr Gastroenterol Nutr* 12:61–64, 1991.
20. Thuneberg L: Interstitial cells of Cajal, in Schultz SG, Wood JD, Rauner BB (eds): *Handbook of Physiology, part I, The Gastrointestinal System.* Bethesda, Md, American Physiological Society, 1989.
21. Faussone-Pellegrini MS: Histogenesis, structure and relationships of interstitial cells of Cajal (ICC): From morphology to function. *Eur J Morphol* 30:137–148, 1992.
22. Faussone-Pellegrini MS, Cortesini C: The muscle coat of the lower esophageal sphincter in patients with achalasia and hypertensive sphincter. An electron microscopic study. *J Submicrosc Cytol* 17:673–685, 1985.

23. Le Douarin N: *The Neural Crest.* Cambridge, Mass, Cambridge University Press, 1982.

24. Gershon MD, Chalazonitis A, Rothman TP: From neural crest to bowel: Development of the enteric nervous system. *J Neurobiol* 24:199–214, 1993.

25. Kapur RP: Contemporary approaches toward understanding the pathogenesis of Hirschsprung disease. *Pediatr Pathol* 13:83–100, 1993.

26. Peters–van der Sanden M: *The Hindbrain Neural Crest and the Development of the Enteric Nervous System* (thesis). Erasmus Universiteit Rotterdam, The Netherlands, 1994.

27. Baetge G, Pintar JE, Gershon MD: Transiently catecholaminergic (TC) cells in the bowel of fetal rats and mice: Precursors of non-catecholaminergic enteric neurons. *Dev Biol* 141:353–380, 1990.

28. Troy CM, Brown K, Greene LA, et al: Ontogeny of the neuronal intermediate filament protein, peripherin, in the mouse embryo. *Neuroscience* 36:217–237, 1990.

29. Kapur RP, Yost C, Palmiter RD: A transgenic model for studying development of the enteric nervous system in normal and aganglionic mice. *Development* 116:167–175, 1992.

30. Yntema CL, Hammond WS: The origin of intrinsic ganglia of trunk viscera from vagal neural crest in the chick embryo. *J Comp Neurol* 101:515–542, 1954.

31. Yntema CL, Hammond WS: Experiments on the origin and development of the sacral autonomic nerves in the chick embryo. *J Exp Zool* 129:375–414, 1955.

32. Weinberg AG: Hirschsprung's disease—a pathologist's view. *Perspect Pediatr Pathol* 2:207–239, 1975.

33. Tennyson VM, Pham TD, Rothman TP, et al: Abnormalities of smooth muscle, basal laminae, and merves in the aganglionic segments of the bowel of lethal spotted mutant mice. *Anat Rec* 215:267–281, 1986.

34. Vaos GC, Lister J: Anatomic evidence for coexistence of cholinergic and adrenergic neurons in the developing human intestine: New aspects in the pathogenesis of developmental neuronal abnormalities. *J Pediatr Surg* 23:237–242, 1988.

35. Jacobs-Cohen RJ, Payette RF, Gershon MD, et al: Inability of neural crest cells to colonize the presumptive aganglionic bowel of ls/ls mutant mice: Requirement for a permissive microenvironment. *J Comp Neurol* 255:425–438, 1987.

36. Payette RF, Tennyson VM, Pomeranz HD, et al: Accumulation of components of basal laminae: Association with the failure of neural crest cells to colonize the presumptive aganglionic bowel of ls/ls mutant mice. *Indian J Gastroenterol* 7:53–54, 1988.

37. Tennyson VM, Payette RF, Rothman TP, et al: Distribution of hyaluronic acid and chondroitin sulfate proteoglycans in the presumptive aganglionic terminal bowel of ls/ls fetal mice: An ultrastructural analysis. *J Comp Neurol* 291: 345–362, 1990.

38. Parikh DH, Tam PKH, Lloyd DA, et al: Quantitative and qualitative analysis of the extracellular matrix protein, laminin, in Hirschsprung's disease. *J Pediatr Surg* 27:991–996, 1992.

39. Puri P, Lake BD, Nixon HH, et al: Neuronal colonic dysplasia: An unusual association of Hirschsprung's disease. *J Pediatr Surg* 12:681–685, 1977.

40. Briner J, Oswald HW, Hirsig J: Neuronal intestinal dysplasia—clinical and histochemical findings and its association with Hirschsprung's disease. *Z Kinderchir* 41:282–286, 1986.

41. Fadda B, Pistor G, Meier-Ruge W, et al: Symptoms, diagnosis and therapy

of neuronal intestinal dysplasia masked by Hirschsprung's disease. *J Pediatr Surg Int* 2:76–80, 1987.

42. Tennyson VM, Gershon MD, Sherman DL, et al: Structural abnormalities associated with congenital megacolon in transgenic mice that overexpress the Hoxa-4 gene. *Dev Dyn* 198:28–53, 1993.

43. Kapur RP: Hypothesis: Pathogenesis of skip areas in long-segment Hirschsprung disease. *Pediatr Pathol* 15:23–37, 1995.

44. Schofield DE, Yunis EJ: What is intestinal neuronal dysplasia? *Arch Ophthalmol* 110:233–235, 1992.

45. Madsen CM: *Hirschsprung's Disease.* Springfield, Ill, Charles C Thomas, 1964, pp 25–31.

46. Wyllie GG: Treatment of Hirschsprung's disease by Swenson's operation. *Lancet* 1:850–855, 1957.

47. Foster P, Cowan G, Wrenn ELJ: Twenty-five years' experience with Hirschsprung's disease. *J Pediatr Surg* 25:531–534, 1990.

48. Garver KL, Law JC, Garver B: Hirschsprung disease: A genetic study. *Clin Genet* 28:503–508, 1985.

49. Bodian M, Carter CO: A family study of Hirschsprung's disease. *Ann Hum Genet* 26:261–277, 1963.

50. Badner JA, Sieber WK, Garver KL, et al: A genetic study of Hirschprung disease. *Am J Hum Genet* 46:568–580, 1990.

51. Lyonnet S, Bolino A, Pelet A, et al: A gene for Hirschsprung disease maps to the proximal long arm of chromosome 10. *Nat Genet* 4:346–350, 1993.

52. Neilson IR, Yazbeck S: Ultrashort Hirschsprung's disease: Myth or reality. *J Pediatr Surg* 25:1135–1138, 1990.

53. Davidson M, Bauer CH: Studies of distal colonic motility in children. IV: Achalasia of the distal rectal segment despite presence of ganglia in the myenteric plexuses of this area. *Pediatrics* 21:746–761, 1958.

54. Weinberg AG: The anorectal myenteric plexus: Its relation to hypoganglionosis of the colon. *Am J Clin Pathol* 54:637–642, 1970.

55. Yunis E, Sieber WK, Akers DR: Does zonal aganglionosis really exist? Report of a rare variety of Hirschsprung's disease and review of the literature. *Pediatr Pathol* 1:33–49, 1983.

56. Martin LW, Buchino JJ, LeCoultre C, et al: Hirschsprung's disease with skip area (segmental aganglionosis). *J Pediatr Surg* 14:686–687, 1979.

57. Holschneider AM (ed): *Hirschsprung's Disease.* Stuttgart, Hippokrates-Verlag, 1982, pp 143–147.

58. Sprinz A, Cohen A, Heaton L: Hirschsprung's disease with skip area. *Ann Surg* 146:143–147, 1961.

59. Touloukian RJ, Duncan R: Acquired aganglionic megacolon in a premature infant: Report of a case. *Pediatrics* 56:459–462, 1975.

60. Dimmick JE, Bove KE: Cytomegalovirus infection of the bowel in infancy: Pathogenic and diagnostic significance. *Pediatr Pathol* 2:95–102, 1984.

61. Hershlag A, Ariel I, Lernau OI, et al: Cytomegalic inclusion virus and Hirschsprung's disease. *Z Kinderchir* 39:253–254, 1984.

62. Tam PKH, Quint WGV, Van Velzen D: Hirschsprung's disease: A viral etiology? *Pediatr Pathol* 12:807–810, 1992.

63. Lake BD, Malone MT, Risdon RA: The use of acetylcholinesterase (AChE) in the diagnosis of Hirschsprung's disease and intestinal neuronal dysplasia. *Pediatr Pathol* 9:351–354, 1989.

64. Lake BD, Puri P, Nixon HH, et al: Hirschsprung's disease. *Arch Pathol Lab Med* 102:244–247, 1978.

65. Ryan ET, Ecker JL, Christakis NA, et al: Hirschsprung's disease: Associated abnormalities and demography. *J Pediatr Surg* 27:76–81, 1992.

66. Cass D: Aganglionosis: Associated anomalies. *J Paediatr Child Health* 26:351–354, 1990.

67. Muller W, Peter HH, Wilken M, et al: The DiGeorge syndrome I. Clinical evaluation and course of partial and complete forms of the syndrome. *Eur J Pediatr* 147:496–502, 1988.

68. Kumasaka K, Clarren SK: Familial patterns of central nervous system dysfunction, growth deficiency, facial clefts and congenital megacolon: A specific disorder? *Am J Med Genet* 31:465–466, 1988.

69. Bruroni D, Joffe R, Farah LMS, et al: Syndrome identification case report 92: Hirschsprung megacolon, cleft lip and palate, mental retardation, and minor congenital malformations. *J Clin Dysmorphol* 1:20–22, 1983.

70. Goldberg RB, Shprintzen RJ: Hirschsprung megacolon and cleft palate in two sibs. *J Craniofac Genet Dev Biol* 1:185–189, 1981.

71. Yomo A, Taira T, Kondo I: Goldberg-Shprintzen syndrome: Hirschsprung disease, hypotonia, and ptosis in two sibs. *Am J Med Genet* 41:188–191, 1991.

72. Curry CJR, Carey JC, Hollan JS: Smith-Lemli-Opitz syndrome–type II: Multiple congenital anomalies with male pseudohermaphroditism and frequent early lethality. *Am J Med Genet* 26:45–57, 1987.

73. Lowry RB, Miller JR, MacLean JR: Micrognathia, polydactyly, and cleft palate. *J Pediatr* 72:859–861, 1968.

74. Kim EH, Boutwell WC: Smith-Lemli-Opitz syndrome and Hirschsprung disease. *J Pediatr* 106:861, 1985.

75. Lipson A, Hayes A: Smith-Lemli-Opitz syndrome and Hirschsprung disease. *J Pediatr* 105:177, 1984.

76. Patterson K, Toomey KE, Chandra RS: Hirschsprung disease in a 46, XY phenotypic girl with Smith-Lemli-Opitz syndrome. *J Pediatr* 103:425–427, 1983.

77. Le Merrer M, Briard ML, Girard S, et al: Lethal acrodysgenital dwarfism: A severe lethal condition resembling Smith-Lemli-Opitz syndrome. *J Med Genet* 25:88–95, 1988.

78. Omenn GS, McKusick VA: The association of Waardenburg syndrome and Hirschsprung megacolon. *Am J Med Genet* 3:217–223, 1979.

79. Goldberg MF: Waardenburg's syndrome with fundus and other anomalies. *Arch Ophthalmol* 76:797–810, 1966.

80. Reed WB, Stone VM, Boder E, et al: Hereditary syndromes with auditory and dermatological manifestations. *Arch Dermatol* 95:456–461, 1967.

81. McKusick VA: Congenital deafness and Hirschsprung's disease. *N Engl J Med* 288:691, 1973.

82. Bard LA: Heterogeneity in Waardenburg's syndrome. *Arch Ophthalmol* 96:1193–1198, 1978.

83. Branski D: Hirschsprung's disease and Waardenburg's syndrome. *Pediatrics* 63:803–805, 1979.

84. Mahakrishnan A, Srinivasan MS: Piebaldism with Hirschsprung's disease. *Arch Dermatol* 116:1102, 1980.

85. Kelley RI, Zackai EH: Congenital deafness, Hirschsprung's and Waardenburg syndrome (abstract). *Am J Hum Genet* 33:65, 1981.

86. Shah KN, Dalal SJ, Desai MP, et al: White forelock, pigmentary disorder of the irides, and long segment Hirschsprung's disease: Possible variant of Waardenburg syndrome. *J Pediatr* 99:432–435, 1981.

87. Currie ABM, Haddad M, Honeyman M, et al: Associated developmental abnormalities of the anterior end of the neural crest: Hirschsprung's disease– Waardenburg's syndrome. *J Pediatr Surg* 21:248–250, 1986.

88. Meire F, Standaert L, De Laey JJ, et al: Waardenburg syndrome, Hirschsprung megacolon, and Marcus Gunn ptosis. *Br J Surg* 74:668–670, 1987.
89. Kaplan P, de Chaderévian JP: Piebaldism–Waardenburg syndrome: Histopathologic evidence for a neural crest syndrome. *Am J Med Genet* 31:465–466, 1988.
90. Ikeda K, Goto S: Diagnosis of Hirschsprung's disease in Japan. An analysis of 1628 patients. *Ann Surg* 199:400–405, 1984.
91. Harrison MW, Deitz DM, Campbell JR, et al: Diagnosis and management of Hirschsprung's disease: A 25-year perspective. *Am J Surg* 152:49–56, 1986.
92. Polley TZ, Coran AG: Hirschsprung's disease in the newborn. *Pediatr Surg Int* 1:80–83, 1986.
93. Caniano DA, Teitelbaum DH, Qualman S: Management of Hirschsprung's disease in children with trisomy 21. *Am J Surg* 159:402–404, 1990.
94. Carter C: A life table for mongols with the cause of death. *J Mental Def Res* 2:64–74, 1958.
95. Rowe R, Uchida I: Cardiac malformation in mongolism. *Am J Med* 31:726–735, 1961.
96. Fabia J, Drolette M: Malformations and leukemia in children with Down's syndrome. *Pediatrics* 45:60–70, 1970.
97. Knox G, Ten Bensel R: Gastrointestinal malformations in Down's syndrome. *Minn Med* 55:542–544, 1972.
98. Le Marec B, et al: Cancer de la thyroide a stroma amyloide, syndrome de Sipple, megacolon congenital avec hyperplasia des plexus: Une seule et meme affection autosomique dominante a penetrance complete. *J Genet Hum* 28:169–174, 1980.
99. Verdy M, Weber AM, Roy CC, et al: Hirschsprung's disease in a family with multiple endocrine neoplasia type 2. *J Pediatr Gastroenterol Nutr* 1:603–607, 1982.
100. Khan AH, Desjardins JG, Youssef S, et al: Gastrointestinal manifestations of Sipple syndrome in children. *J Pediatr Surg* 22:764–766, 1987.
101. Michna BA, McWilliams NB, Krummel TM, et al: Multifocal ganglioneuroblastoma coexistent with total colonic aganglionosis. *J Med Genet* 25:204–205, 1988.
102. Mahaffey SM, Martin LW, McAdams AJ, et al: Multiple endocrine neoplasia type II B with symptoms suggesting Hirschsprung's disease: A case report. *J Pediatr Surg* 25:101–103, 1990.
103. Shockett E, Telok HA: Aganglionic megacolon, pheochromocytoma, megalureter, and neurofibroma: Co-occurrence of several neural abnormalities. *Am J Dis Child* 94:185–191, 1957.
104. El-Halaby E, Coran AG: Hirschsprung's disease associated with Ondine's curse: Report of three cases and review of the literature. *J Pediatr Surg* 29:530–535, 1994.
105. Haddad GG, Mazza NM, Defendini R, et al: Congenital failure of automatic control of ventilation, gastrointestinal motility, and heart rate. *Medicine (Baltimore)* 57:517–526, 1978.
106. Bower RJ, Adkins JC: Ondine's curse and neurocristopathy. *Clin Pediatr (Phila)* 19:665–668, 1980.
107. Stern M, Hellwege HH, Gravinghoff L, et al: Total aganglionosis of the colon (Hirschsprung's disease) and congenital failure of autonomic control of ventilation (Ondine's curse). *Acta Pediatr Scand* 70:121–124, 1981.
108. Guilleminault C, McQuitty J, Ariagno RL, et al: Congenital central alveolar hypoventilation syndrome in six infants. *Pediatrics* 70:684–694, 1982.
109. O'Dell K, Staren E, Bassuk A: Total colonic aganglionosis (Zuelzer-Wilson

syndrome) and congenital failure of automatic control of ventilation (Ondine's curse). *Langenbecks Arch Chir* 372:747–750, 1987.

110. Poceta JS, Strandjord TS, Badura RJJ, et al: Ondine's curse and neurocristopathy. *Pediatr Neurol* 3:370–372, 1987.

111. Roshkow JE, Haller JO, Berdon WE, et al: Hirschsprung's disease, Ondine's curse, and neuroblastoma—manifestations of neurocristopathy. *Radiol Diagn Berl* 29:681–688, 1988.

112. Wesse-Mayer DE, Brouillette RT, Naidich TP, et al: Magnetic resonance imaging and computerized tomography in central hypoventilation. *Am Rev Respir Dis* 173:393–398, 1988.

113. Hamilton J, Bodurtha JN: Congenital central hypoventilation syndrome and Hirschsprung's disease in half sibs. *J Med Genet* 26:272–274, 1989.

114. Minutillo C, Pemberton PJ, Goldblatt J: Hirschsprung's disease and Ondine's curse: Further evidence for a distinct syndrome. *Clin Genet* 36:200–203, 1989.

115. Gaisie G: Hirschsprung's disease, Ondine's curse, and neuroblastoma—manifestations of neurocristopathy. *Pediatr Radiol* 20:136, 1989.

116. Fodstad H, Ljunggren B, Shawis R: Ondine's curse with Hirschsprung's disease. *Br J Neurosurg* 4:87–93, 1990.

117. Mukhopadhyay S, Wilkinson PW: Cerebral arteriovenous malformation. Ondine's curse and Hirschsprung's disease. *Dev Med Child Neurol* 32:1087–1089, 1990.

118. Duffy TJ, Erickson EE, Jordan GL, et al: Megacolon and bilateral pheochromocytoma. *Am J Gastroenterol* 38:555–563, 1962.

119. Chatten J, Voorhess ML: Familial neuroblastoma. *N Engl J Med* 277:1230–1236, 1967.

120. Gaisie G, Kook SO, Young LW: Coexistent neuroblastoma and Hirschsprung's disease—another manifestation of neurocristopathy. *Pediatr Radiol* 8:161–163, 1979.

121. Levy J: Gastrointestinal concerns, in Pueschel SM, Pueschel JK (eds): *Biomedical Concerns in Persons With Down Syndrome.* Baltimore, Paul H Brookes, 1992, pp 119–125.

122. Spouge D, Baird PA: Hirschsprung disease in a large birth cohort. *Teratology* 32:171–177, 1985.

123. Takahashi M, Ritz J, Cooper GM: Activation of a novel human transforming gene, *ret,* by DNA rearrangement. *Cell* 42:581–588, 1985.

124. Takahashi M, Cooper GM: *Ret* transforming gene encodes a fusion protein homologous to tyrosine kinases. *Mol Cell Biol* 7:1378–1385, 1987.

125. Bongarzone I, Pierotti MA, Monzini N, et al: High frequency of activation of tyrosine kinase oncogenes in human papillary thyroid carcinoma. *Oncogene* 4:1457–1462, 1989.

126. Grieco M, Santoro M, Berlingieri MT, et al: PTC is a novel rearranged form of the *ret* proto-oncogene and is frequently detected in vivo in human thyroid papillary carcinomas. *Cell* 60:557–563, 1990.

127. Kunieda T, Matsui M, Nomura N, et al: Characterization of an activated human *ret* gene with a novel 5' sequence fused by DNA rearrangement. *Gene* 107:323–328, 1991.

128. van Heyningen V: One gene—four syndromes. *Nature* 367:319–320, 1994.

129. Hofstra RM, Landsvater RM, Ceccherini I, et al: A mutation in the RET proto-oncogene associated with multiple endocrine neoplasia type 2B and sporadic medullary thyroid carcinoma. *Nature* 367:375–376, 1994.

130. Romeo G, Ronchetto P, Luo Y, et al: Point mutations affecting the tyrosine kinase domain of the RET proto-oncogene in Hirschsprung's disease. *Nature* 367:377–378, 1994.

131. Pachnis V, Mankoo B, Costantini F: Expression of the c-ret proto-oncogene during mouse embryogenesis. *Development* 119:1005–1017, 1993.

132. Schuchardt A, D'Agati V, Larsson BL, et al: Defects in the kidney and enteric nervous system of mice lacking the tyrosine kinase receptor Ret. *Nature* 367:380–383, 1994.

133. Puffenberger EG, Kauffman ER, Bolk S, et al: Identity-by-descent and association mapping of a recessive gene for Hirschsprung disease on human chromosome 13q22. *Hum Mol Genet* 3:1217–1225, 1994.

134. Dow E, Cross S, Wolgemuth DJ, et al: Second locus for Hirschsprung disease/Waardenburg syndrome in a large Mennonite kindred. *Am J Med Genet* 53:75–80, 1994.

135. Edery P, Lyonnet S, Mulligan LM, et al: Mutations of the RET proto-oncogene in Hirschsprung's disease. *Nature* 367:378–380, 1994.

136. Lane PW, Liu HM: Association of megacolon with a new dominant spotting gene (Dom) in the mouse. *J Hered* 75:435–439, 1984.

137. Bolande RP: Animal model of human disease: Aganglionic megacolon in piebald and spotted mutant mouse strains. *Am J Pathol* 79:189–192, 1975.

138. McCabe L, Griffin LD, Kinzer A, et al: Overo lethal white foal syndrome: Equine model of aganglionic megacolon (Hirschsprung disease). *Am J Med Genet* 36:336–340, 1990.

139. Cass D: Aganglionosis in rodents. *J Pediatr Surg* 27:351–356, 1992.

140. Hosoda K, Hammer RE, Richardson JA, et al: Targeted and natural (piebald lethal) mutations of endothelin-B receptor gene produce aganglionic megacolon associated with white-spotted coat color in mice. *Cell* 79:1267–1276, 1994.

141. Greenstein-Baynash A, Hosoda K, Giaid A, et al: Interaction of endothelin-3 with endothelin-B receptor is essential for development of neural crest-derived melanocytes and enteric neurons. *Cell* 79:1277–1285, 1994.

142. Puffenberger EG, Hosoda K, Washington SS, et al: A missense mutation of the endothelin-B receptor gene in multigenic Hirschsprung disease. *Cell* 79:1257–1266, 1994.

143. Kapur RP, Yost C, Palmiter RD: Aggregation chimeras demonstrate that the primary defect responsible for aganglionic megacolon in lethal spotted mice is not neuroblast autonomous. *Development* 117:993–999, 1993.

144. Rothman TP, Goldowitz D, Gershon MD: Inhibition of migration of neural crest–derived cells by the abnormal mesenchyme of the presumptive aganglionic bowel of ls/ls mice: Analysis with aggregation and interspecies chimeras. *Dev Biol* 159:559–573, 1993.

Small Round Cell Tumors of Childhood: Importance of Cytogenetics in Prognosis and Diagnosis*

David M. Parham, M.D.
Department of Pathology and Laboratory Medicine, St. Jude Children's Research Hospital, Department of Pathology, University of Tennessee, Memphis, College of Medicine, Memphis, Tennessee

C hildhood neoplasms represent a diverse group of tumors that are unique in their tendency to recapitulate embryonic morphogenetic events and to contain characteristic chromosomal aberrations, generally balanced translocations, that are unique to each histologic group.[1] These features contrast with adult tumors, which generally display gradual morphologic diversion from a well-differentiated phenotype to a progressively more dysplastic lesion with accompanying progressive biological and genetic aberrations associated with malignant transformation.[2] In spite of this basic histogenetic distinction, childhood cancers nevertheless display a tendency, similar to that of adult malignancy, for loss of genetic controls of growth and invasiveness associated with karyotypic disturbances of prognostic significance. In addition, detection of characteristic cytogenetic aberrations by standard methods, the polymerase chain reaction (PCR), or in situ hybridization assists in the definition of diagnostic groups and subgroups with well-characterized clinical behavior.

Small cell neoplasms of childhood constitute a group of morphologically similar and clinically aggressive tumors that are notable for the frequent difficulty posed in their proper recognition.[3] These diagnostic dilemmas stem from their primitive nature, which is analogous to the pluripotent blastema of early embryonal tissues. Recognition of these lesions as discrete morphologic entities was initially enhanced by the use of electron microscopy, followed by immunohistochemical staining. More recently, cytogenetic studies have further enabled pathologists to separate entities with morphologic similarity but different responses to adjuvant therapy, thereby leading to sharp dissimilarity in treatment protocols. In this fashion, among the diagnostically heterogeneous group of small cell

*Supported by National Cancer Institute Center Support Grant P30 CA217657 and American Lebanese Syrian Associated Charities.

neoplasms, cytogenetics can be used to help define prognostic and therapeutic tumor categories that are also inherent to well-established histologic categories.

WILMS' TUMOR (NEPHROBLASTOMA)

Wilms' tumor is in many respects a quintessential childhood neoplasm, for it is composed of a mixture of embryonic and differentiated tissues that may exhibit wide histologic diversification, has characteristic aberrations associated with parental inheritance and multiorgan dysgenesis, is composed of good- and bad-prognosis groups that may be separated morphologically or cytogenetically, and displays a remarkable sensitivity to modern-day chemotherapy with gratifyingly high survival rates.[4, 5] Many of these advances in treatment and tumor biology result from the formation of large collaborative groups among numerous pediatric hospitals in the United States, Great Britain, and the European continent. Such groups as the National Wilms' Tumor Study (NWTS), the Manchester Tumor Registry, and the Société Internationale d'Oncologie Pédiatrique (SIOP) have devised strategies for the systematic study of tumor histology and cell biology as they relate to large numbers of similarly treated neoplasms. As a result, pathologists and biologists have been able to test features of potential prognostic significance in a short length of time when compared with single-institution retrospective analyses. Also, provision has been made for tissue banking via overnight shipment to a central collecting point, so studies on large amounts of fresh tumor tissue have been possible even with material from institutions that normally lack provision for detailed biological analysis. Thus a large body of knowledge currently exists for the relationship between Wilms' tumor biology and prognosis, and similar arrangements are in place for other childhood tumors.

KARYOTYPIC ANOMALIES OF WILMS' TUMOR

WT1

Work on the basic genetic dysfunction of Wilms' tumor was facilitated by the recognition of a group of associated phenotypic anomalies. One such lesion is aniridia, or absence of the iris, in which Wilms' tumor occurs in about one third of cases.[6] It became apparent that a large number of these patients also display genitourinary anomalies such as cryptorchidism or hypospadias, as well as mental retardation. Thus these four phenotypic features—Wilms' tumor, aniridia, genitourinary malformations, and mental retardation—form a quartet of childhood anomalies that appeared to result from the dysfunction of closely linked genetic loci.[7] Chromosomal analyses of peripheral lymphocytes of this group of patients demonstrated deletion of a portion of the short arm of chromosome 11 (or 11p), and a similar finding became apparent in studies of cultured Wilms' tumor cells taken from patients lacking this constitutional anomaly.[8] The number of cases found to be affected by this genetic alteration can be increased by more sensitive techniques that demonstrate deletion of a smaller portion of the DNA sequence.

One such technique, Southern blotting, can be used to detect the absence of gene segments by a lack of the heterozygous pattern seen as a consequence of the restriction enzyme–detected polymorphism (or "DNA fingerprint") that is apparent in a normal genome. This polymorphism results from the slight differences in DNA sequences inherited from maternal vs. paternal genes (Fig 1). This phenomenon, known as "loss of heterozygosity," became apparent in a large number of Wilms' tumor cells on probing DNA sequences of genes located in a narrow region of 11p.[9] Further definition of this deleted locus by sophisticated genetic methods led to the isolation of the first Wilms' tumor gene, or WT1.[10, 11] This gene is characterized as a "tumor suppressor" gene, or one whose proper function prevents the expression of a tendency for neoplasms to develop.[12] Loss of critical portions of the DNA sequence from WT1 and other tumor suppressor genes results in the formation of protein moieties that do not bind correctly to ligands related to cell division, thus adversely affecting the negative-feedback loops that normally prevent uncontrolled cell proliferation.[13, 14] In the case of WT1, the affected protein functions as a "transcription factor,"[15] a molecule that binds to a specific DNA sequence and leads to the formation of critical RNA sequences. These RNA molecules are transported to the cell cytoplasm and translated into proteins that as a general rule are associated with either cell division or differentiation. The protein produced by WT1, or WT1 (note that genes are italicized and proteins are not), is a unique transcription factor in that its expression is primarily restricted to the prenatal kidney,[16, 17] particularly

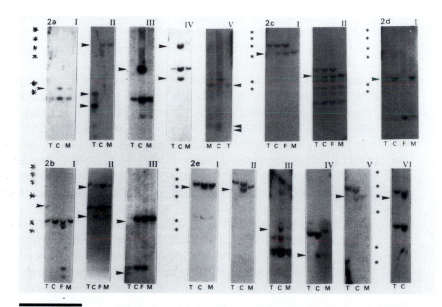

FIGURE 1.

Series of Southern blots illustrating loss of heterozygosity in a series of five Wilms' tumors (cases 2a to 2e). These blots represent the migration patterns of several genes (I to VI) located on 11p following digestion with a DNase, electrophoresis, and hybridization with gene-specific probes. The *arrowheads* mark the sites of allelic loss or alteration in the tumor lanes (T = tumor; C = constitutional tissues; M = mother; F = father). (From Mannens M, Slater RM, Heyting C, et al: *Hum Genet* 81:41–48, 1988. Used by permission.)

the glomerulus, although it is also found in smaller amounts in the developing mesothelium and genitourinary tract, particularly sex cord tissues.[18] Because of these associations, it is logical that another genetic syndrome, the Denys-Drash syndrome, which is composed of gonadal dysgenesis, glomerulosclerosis, and a tendency to the development of Wilms' tumor and granulosa cell tumor, is also caused by a dysfunctional WT1.[19]

Histologic investigation of the expression of WT1 by using mRNA in situ hybridization or immunohistochemistry paradoxically reveals increased amounts of WT1 production in the blastemal portions of Wilms' tumors rather than decreased amounts.[17, 20, 21] However, in tumors showing a predominance of stromal differentiation, there are decreased intracellular levels of WT1, thus indicating that this variety of Wilms' tumor is the type associated with WT1 deletions.[17] Intralobar nephrogenic rests, persistent foci of incompletely developed fetal-type tissue,[22] also demonstrate similar WT1 deletions[23] and are typically seen adjacent to stromal-predominant lesions (Fig 2). This association of a genetic event with a precursor lesion that later becomes neoplastic is consonant with the Knudson-Strong "two-hit" hypothesis of tumorigenesis,[24] which postulates that two separate mutations are required to effect the development of a neoplasm.

WT2

More recently, another putative Wilms' tumor gene, WT2, has been found on a different segment of 11p, specifically 11p15; WT1 is located on 11p13.[25-27] WT2 appears to be operative in the Beckwith-Weidemann syndrome, another childhood malformation complex that is associated with the development of Wilms' tumors as well as several other small cell neoplasms, particularly rhabdomyosarcoma and hepatoblastoma.[28] Children affected with the Beckwith-Weidemann syndrome are characteristically large with sizable heads, viscera, tongues, and abdomens. The overgrowth of the abdomen during prenatal development may be clinically manifested as an omphalocele. One peculiar feature of this syndrome is the overgrowth of individual cells, or cytomegaly, of the adrenal cortex. Besides the generalized somatic overgrowth connected with Beckwith-Weidemann syndrome, some patients with Wilms' tumor may exhibit hemihypertrophy,[6] which may be localized and manifested as overgrowth of a single extremity or truncal region.

WT2 appears to be associated with the production of insulin-like growth factor type II (IGF-II), a protein structurally and physiologically similar to insulin and capable of initiating either cell division or locomotion.[29] In Wilms' tumor, both IGF-II and one of its ligands, the IGF-I receptor, are expressed at high levels, so an autocrine mechanism of hormonally induced growth appears to be operative.[30] Alterations in serum levels of IGF-II binding proteins or peculiar chromatographic forms of IGFs may also be observed.[31] Observations on the parental source of the WT2 gene and the IGF2 gene indicate that they are normally imprinted, or functioning only if paternally inherited.[32] In this non-Mendelian form of inheritance, only paternal (or in some cases maternal) alleles function to produce RNA, so normally only half of the expected levels of the re-

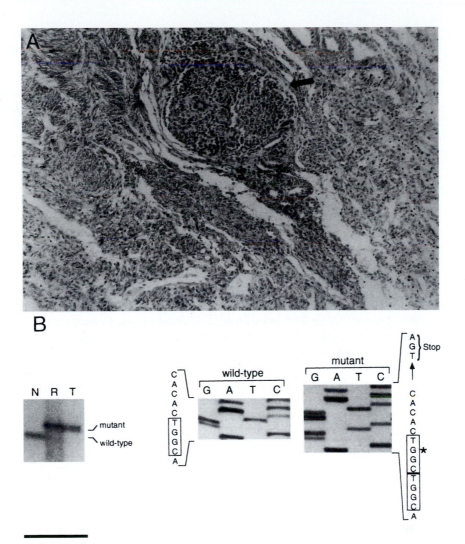

FIGURE 2.

A, intralobar nephrogenic rest *(arrow)* (Hematoxylin-eosin, ×80). **B,** mutation of *WT1* in a nephrogenic rest. On the *left* side of the figure, a mutated *WT1* is seen in polymerase chain reaction–amplified fragments from the rest (R) and adjacent tumor *(T)* as compared with normal kidney *(K)*. On the right side of the figure, nucleotide sequence analysis is illustrated. The mutant *WT1*, found in the rest and the tumor, contains a different nucleotide sequence from the wild-type *WT1* found in normal kidney. The mutation, caused by the duplication of four nucleotides (TGGC, or thymidine, guanine, guanine, cytosine), causes a premature stop codon (TGA) to arise and results in a severely shortened (or truncated), ineffectual WT1 protein. (From Park S, Bernard A, Bove KE, et al: *Nat Genet* 5:363–367, 1993. Used by permission.)

sultant protein are actually produced.[33] In some neoplasms such as Wilms' tumor, there is preferential "relaxation," or loss, of this imprinting mechanism, through loss of heterozygosity so that both alleles function as paternal alleles, with presumably twice the normal amount of a particular protein being produced.[34, 35] If the protein is a proto-oncogene or growth factor such as IGF-II, one then might hypothesize that unbridled cell proliferation could result from the double dose of DNA function.

Other Wilms' Tumor Genes

Current research indicates that a third Wilms' tumor gene is located on 16q. This gene appears to be associated with tumor progression and may thus be a prognostic factor.[36, 37] In one study, loss of heterozygosity for chromosome 16q was associated with a marked increase in tumor relapse and mortality.[38] Even more Wilms' tumor genes have been hypothesized inasmuch as families with heritable tumors but no alterations in currently described genes exist.[36, 37, 39] Wilms' tumor genes may serve as a paradigm for understanding the complexities of small cell tumor cytogenetics, and their recognition as a constitutional disorder is important in genetic counseling.

PLOIDY DETERMINATION IN WILMS' TUMOR

Studies of the incidence and prognostic import of aneuploidy in Wilms' tumor have been accomplished by using both flow cytometry and image analysis on fresh and paraffin-embedded tissues. Perhaps as a result, reported findings and conclusions display a moderate degree of variance. In a retrospective analysis performed at St. Jude Children's Research Hospital (SJCRH) on 48 tumors, there was a significant relationship between ploidy and both histology and clinical outcome.[40] In this study, DNA indices (DIs) of over 1.5 (or 1.5 times the normal diploid level) were strongly associated with subsequent relapse and anaplastic histology. Other studies have not demonstrated identical findings, although associations with either anaplasia[41–44] or suboptimal clinical outcome[41, 45–48] have been noted. When one examines these latter articles, one notes that either the exact DI was not recorded or that tumors having values of less than 1.5 and more than 1.0, being technically aneuploid, were included with this group when statistical testing was performed.[44, 46] Thus it is apparent that low levels of aneuploidy are not uncommon in Wilms' tumor, even in predictably good behavers such as the cystic, partially differentiated type,[44] but this factor in itself is not indicative of a poor prognosis. On the other hand, in studies besides that performed at SJCRH,[44, 49] tumors having markedly high DI values were typically clinically aggressive, anaplastic lesions.

Another factor complicating assessment of ploidy in Wilms' tumors is the not uncommon presence of intratumoral heterogeneity.[50] This feature could be responsible for some of the divergence in reported results. Nevertheless, when present, intratumor heterogeneity is associated with unfavorable histology and a poor clinical outcome.

One reason for the association between marked aneuploidy and histology is apparent when one considers a typical karyotype from an anaplastic Wilms' tumor. As seen in Figure 3, there is striking duplication of multiple chromosomes with accumulation of greatly increased amounts of DNA. In a similar vein, the criteria for a diagnosis of Wilms' tumor include hyperchromasia, marked nuclear enlargement, and atypical, multipolar mitoses. All of these phenomena might result from an abnormally

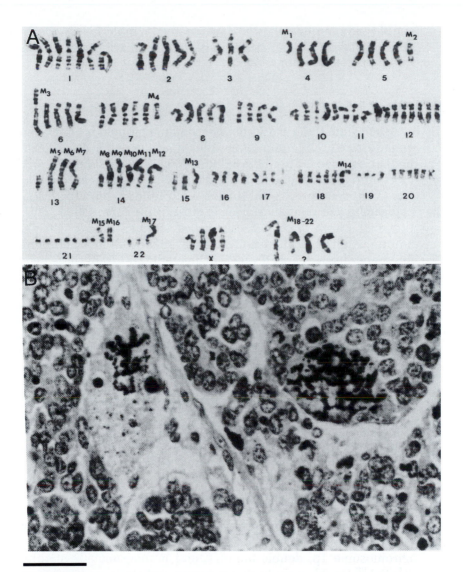

FIGURE 3.

A, karyotype of anaplastic Wilms' tumor containing numerous duplications and markers. **B,** Photomicrograph of anaplastic Wilms' tumor containing large, multipolar, atypical mitoses. (**A** from Douglass EC, Look AT, Webber B, et al: *J Clin Oncol* 4:975–981, 1986. **B** from Webber BL, Parham DM, Drake LG, et al: *Pathol Annu* 27:191–232, 1992. Both used by permission.)

large amount of basophilic DNA by routine histology, complemented by marked duplication as demonstrated by cytogenetic analysis. Anaplasia has a strong independent value as a predictor of clinical outcome, as demonstrated in a large number of patients in several NTWS studies,[51] possibly as a result of an increase in the production of growth factors and proto-oncogenes because of genetic duplication. However, the changes in growth control in these neoplasms are probably more complex because there appear to be cell-type–related alterations of growth factor and tumor suppressor gene expression that are not currently explicable by simple gene amplification.[52, 53] Alternatively, mutations in the tumor suppressor gene p53[54] may be responsible for the aggressive clinical behavior of anaplastic Wilms' tumor.

NEUROBLASTOMA

Neuroblastoma, the most common nonhematopoietic, non–central nervous system (CNS) tumor of childhood, accounts for 8% of pediatric malignancies. It arises from the autonomic nervous system and produces tumors of the adrenal glands, neck, mediastinum, retroperitoneum, and pelvis. Of all round cell solid tumors of childhood, the prognostic value of cytogenetics in neuroblastomas is most firmly established. This observation stems from three well-established factors, the frequent presence of amplification of the N-*myc* proto-oncogene, deletions of chromosome 1p, and hyperdiploidy (or DI values of greater than 1.0) in these neoplasms.[55]

N-*myc* AMPLIFICATION

N-*myc* encodes a protein that functions as a transcription factor that binds to specific DNA sequences (so-called homeobox genes) to promote neuronal proliferation and differentiation.[56] Its uncontrolled expression leads to neoplastic transformation of the cell, and indeed this class of genes was recognized early in recent genetic studies as one of a set of oncogenes (or tumor-promoting genes) responsible for a number of human cancers.[57] One member of this class, C-*myc*, has been shown to be altered in Burkitt's lymphoma by its juxtaposition with the immunoglobulin promoter gene in the 5(8;14) translocation.[58] Another, L-*myc*, is associated with small cell carcinoma of the lung. Isolation of the N-*myc* gene proceeded from the discovery that some neuroblastomas grew exceedingly well in cell cultures and could easily be propagated to form cell lines, which are immortalized lineages of tumor cells that do not die out in vitro if adequate media conditions are maintained.[59] Cytogenetic studies of these cells revealed three common observations: deletion of portions of chromosome 1p, double minutes, and homogeneously staining regions (HSRs).[60] Double-minute chromosomes and HSRs are similar cytogenetic phenomena that are both caused by over-replication of DNA sequences, small reduplicated fragments being formed in the former structures and long repeating segments with pale tinctorial qualities being produced in the latter (Fig 4).

After the N-*myc* gene was isolated from neuroblastoma cells and probes produced, hybridization studies were carried out via Southern blotting.[61] In this technique, portions of DNA fragmented by sequence-specific restriction enzymes migrate in a soft gel under the stimulus of an electrophoretic current, are blotted onto a more stable plastic medium, and are targeted by hybridization to complementary segments of probe gene sequences (in this case N-*myc*). The DNA probes are covalently attached to signal molecules, such as biotin or various radioisotopes, that are capable of producing a visible pattern. Depending on the intensity of the signal, comparison to specimens and standards in other lanes, and the assumption that equal amounts were loaded in each lane, a rough es-

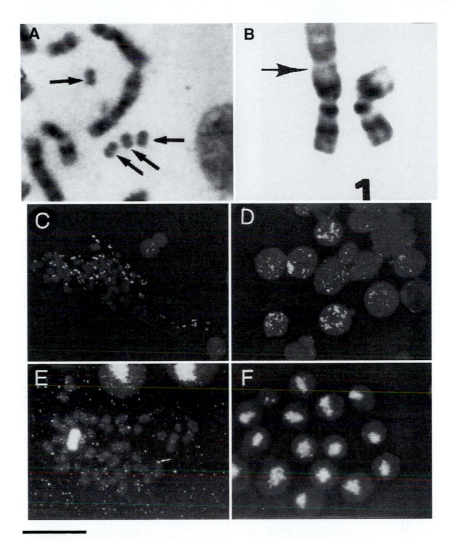

FIGURE 4.
A, double-minute chromosomes *(arrows).* **B,** homogeneously staining region *(arrow).* **C–F,** fluorescence in situ hybridization studies of N-*myc* amplification in mitotic **(C, E)** and interphase **(D, F)** nuclei. Signals from double minutes are seen in **C** and **D,** and homogeneously staining regions fluoresce in **E** and **F.** (**A** and **B** courtesy of Marc Valentine. **C–F** from Shapiro DN, Valentine MB, Rowe ST, et al: *Am J Pathol* 142:1339–1346, 1993. Used by permission.)

timate of the amount of DNA per cell can be obtained. With this method it was quickly apparent that N-*myc* was amplified, i.e., that multiple copies were present per cell, in those neuroblastomas capable of being easily propagated (Fig 5). When this observation was compared with the outcome of affected patients in standardized treatment protocols, it was found to be an indicator of a distinctly poor prognosis independent of surgical stage, presumably because an abnormally large dose of this growth inducer was being produced in affected cells.[55] The abnormally high levels of N-*myc* also appear to disrupt the responsiveness of neuroblastoma cells to extracellular signals that may normally arrest growth and induce differentiation.[62]

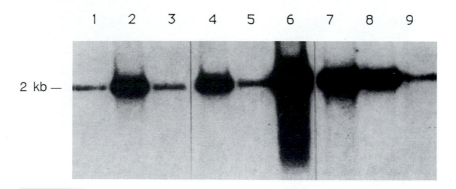

FIGURE 5.
Southern blot study of N-*myc* amplification. Neuroblastoma samples in lanes 2, 4, 6, 7, and 8 show markedly increased amounts of signal, representing gene amplification, as compared with the other samples, which show normal levels of N-*myc*. (From Brodeur GM, Fong C: *Cancer Genet Cytogenet* 41:153–174, 1989. Used by permission.)

More recently, the fluorescence in situ hybridization (FISH) technique has been used for N-*myc* quantitation.[63] With this method, the actual cells are visualized by fluorescence microscopy, and the presence of the target gene is detected by permeabilization of the cell membranes, diffusion of signal molecule–tagged DNA probes into the cell, and development of a visible signal via hybridization of the probe sequence with the target gene. Whole cells must be used to ensure that the entire genome of each cell is tested, but this can be accomplished via tumor imprints, cytologic preparations, or the isolation of whole nuclei from 50-μm-thick sections of tumor. In neuroblastomas with N-*myc* amplification, the signal is visualized in the double-minute chromosomes or the heterogeneously staining regions, thus furnishing a link between these two separate cytogenetic observations (Fig 5). The FISH technique does not require attention to standardized loading of lanes or precise quantitation and is more sensitive than the Southern blot technique. As with Southern blotting, detection of N-*myc* amplification via FISH has great clinical significance and is a portent of a poor outcome.

PLOIDY IN NEUROBLASTOMA

Neuroblastoma offers a distinct contrast with the usual bleak scenario painted by the discovery of hyperdiploidy in most adult tumors because its presence is associated with a good prognosis in this neoplasm independent of stage.[55, 64, 65] This association of hyperdiploidy with improved survival is not unique to neuroblastoma among childhood neoplasms, however, and has been observed with acute lymphoblastic leukemia. medulloblastoma, and rhabdomyosarcoma.[66, 67] Diploidy in neuroblastoma tends to be associated with other poor prognostic indicators such as N-*myc* amplification and unfavorable histology via newer subclassifications.[65]

1P DELETIONS

Loss of genetic material on chromosome 1p has been found to be the most common cytogenetic abnormality in neuroblastoma. This deletion is particularly common at the distal portion of the short arm of chromosome 1, from 1p36.1 to 1p36.3, and may be detected by loss-of-heterozygosity studies more commonly than by routine cytogenetics. It does not appear to have independent prognostic value, but probably involves alteration or loss of a tumor suppressor gene that is relatively specific for neuroblastoma.[55] One candidate gene for this phenomenon, *PITSLRE*, has been recently characterized.[68] It is located on chromosome 1p36.3 and appears to transcribe a protein kinase, $p58^{cdc2L1}$, that normally functions as a signal for apoptosis, so deletions could lead to a selective growth advantage.[69]

RHABDOMYOSARCOMA

Rhabdomyosarcoma is a neoplasm resulting from the malignant transformation of primitive mesenchyme. Although it often arises in and usually duplicates the histologic features of skeletal muscle, it does not necessarily result from malignant transformation of these tissues, for pediatric rhabdomyosarcoma often arises in regions such as the prostate, uterus, and biliary tract, areas that are normally devoid of striated musculature. Newer histologic classifications have been devised,[70] but they are primarily modifications of the basic scheme of Horn and Enterline, which separates rhabdomyosarcoma into embryonal, alveolar, botryoid, and pleomorphic subtypes. Although these subtypes constitute a group of tumors that all show morphologic evidence of myogenesis, they possess distinct histologic, clinical, and biological characteristics, although hybrid versions occasionally occur.

KARYOTYPIC ANOMALIES

11p Deletions

Like Wilms' tumor, embryonal rhabdomyosarcoma is genetically characterized by the presence of deletions of 11p, more easily detectable by demonstration of loss of heterozygosity than by standard karyotyping.[71] Occasional cell lines with bizarre karyotypic findings such as duplication of multiple chromosomes have also been established,[72] but these are only isolated findings when compared with the common observation of 11p deletions. Again, similar to Wilms' tumor, overexpression of IGF-II is common in these neoplasms, and a parental imprinting relaxation mechanism and autocrine stimulation of growth may be involved.[73] Readers will recall that the Beckwith-Weidemann syndrome is associated with an increased incidence of rhabdomyosarcoma as well as Wilms' tumor. Along these lines, it is fascinating to note that the genitourinary tract, the site unique to the action of WT1, is the most common site for the development of embryonal and botryoid variants of rhabdomyosarcoma and that myogenesis is a common event in Wilms' tumor, particularly those with alterations of *WT1*.

Analysis of the rhabdomyosarcoma gene proposed for the 11p locus has revealed that a second locus on the long arm of chromosome 11 may also be operative. These observations have resulted from studies in which normal portions of chromosome 11 were inserted into embryonal rhabdomyosarcoma cell lines.[74]

t(2;13)

Alveolar rhabdomyosarcomas possess a unique translocation between chromosomes 2 and 13, t(2;13)(q35;q14)[75] (Fig 6). This genetic aberration juxtaposes the *PAX3* gene on chromosome 2q13 and the *FRKR* (or *ALV*) gene on chromosome 13q14.[76] The *PAX3* gene is a "segmentation" gene, that is, it plays a key role during gastrulation, that period of early embryogenesis when basic body domains are determined.[77] Segmentation genes are also disrupted in other pediatric malignancies.[56, 78] *PAX3* is also abnormal in patients with Waardenburg's syndrome, an autosomal dominant genetic disorder with deafness and pigmentary anomalies,[79] but they do not suffer from a susceptibility to alveolar rhabdomyosarcoma. Rather it is the union of the *PAX3* protein, a DNA transcription factor, with the product of the *FRKR* gene that yields the oncogenetic properties of this karyotypic disruption. *PAX3* is noted to be transformative when overexpressed in vivo or in vitro, so it is the unrestrained action of the protein that appears critical in the production of rhabdomyosarcoma.[80] Another translocation affecting chromosome 13q14, t(1;13)(p36;q14), also produces alveolar rhabdomyosarcoma by fusing the *PAX7* gene with the *FKHR* gene.[81]

At present, the clinical significance of t(2;13) lies in its utility in iden-

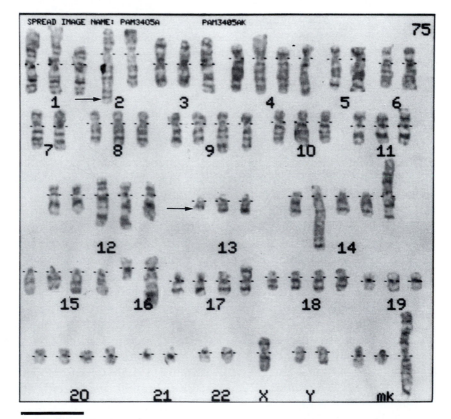

FIGURE 6.

Karyotype of alveolar rhabdomyosarcoma containing t(2;13). Note the lengthening of one chromosome 2q and the shortening of one chromosome 13q relative to their normal counterparts *(arrows)*. Chromosomal duplication is also present. (From Parham DM: *Semin Diagn Pathol* 11:39–46, 1994. Used by permission.)

tification of rhabdomyosarcomas of the alveolar type, which may be difficult to diagnose and show an aggressive behavior with poor outcome. Although most alveolar tumors have a "typical" histology with well-defined fibrous septa from which cells hang in a picket-row arrangement, some tumors have a "solid" pattern in which the production of stroma is inconspicuous (Fig 7).[82] Nevertheless, these lesions have the primitive, round cell cytology of typical alveolar tumors, display a similar aggressive behavior, and possess an identical t(2;13) karyotypic anomaly.[83] In addition, this genetic distinction has the potential utility of discriminating tumors with "mixed" histology, i.e., possessing both alveolar and embryonal features, from lower-grade embryonal tumors with stroma production. Routine cytogenetic analysis has the disadvantages of requiring special equipment, qualified technologists, and optimal tumor cell growth and has a slow turnaround time. However, newer techniques such as FISH and the reverse transcriptase PCR (RT-PCR) offer rapid turnaround time and easy accessibility.[84] The RT-PCR technique, which is based on the enzymatic amplification of hybridization sequencing that spans the site of the translocation break point, has the potential to detect the signal in a very few tumor cells. However, because of its extreme sensitivity, this method has a great potential for specimen contamination and thus requires meticulous attention to technique. As noted earlier, FISH does not have this drawback but requires whole cells, as are available from imprints, cytologic preparations, or thick (50-μm) sections.

Ploidy in Rhabdomyosarcoma

As with Wilms' tumor, the prognostic value of ploidy determination in rhabdomyosarcomas has received mixed reports in the literature. In studies

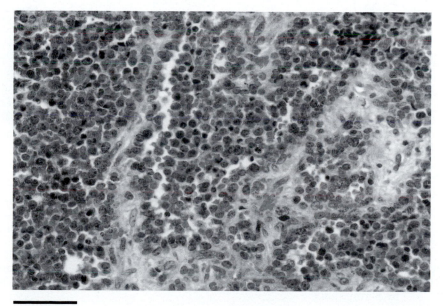

FIGURE 7.

Photomicrograph of alveolar rhabdomyosarcoma illustrating the typical picket-row appearance of tumor cells suspended from fibrous septa. The recently recognized "solid variant" of this tumor shows similar cytologic features but contains cells arrayed in solid sheets (hematoxylin-eosin, ×400). (From Shapiro DN, Parham DM, Douglass EC, et al: *J Clin Oncol* 9:159–166, 1991. Used by permission.)

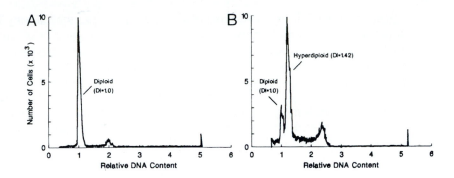

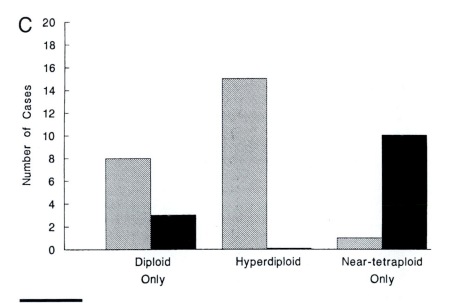

FIGURE 8.

A and **B,** illustrative ploidy studies performed by flow cytometry on two cases of unresectable embryonal rhabdomyosarcoma. Case **A** is diploid (DNA index *[DI]* = 1.0) and case **B** shows a hyperdiploid (DI > 1.0) peak. **C,** bar graph showing the relationship between histology and ploidy in rhabdomyosarcoma. Alveolar tumors *(dark-shaded bars)* were near tetraploid (DI ≈ 2.0) or diploid, whereas embryonal tumors were with one exception either hyperdiploid or diploid. (From Shapiro DN, Parham DM, Douglass EC, et al: *J Clin Oncol* 9:159–166, 1991. Used by permission.)

performed initially on material from SJCRH[85] and later from the Intergroup Rhabdomyosarcoma Study (IRS),[86] there was a fairly dramatic difference in the outcome of group III embryonal rhabdomyosarcoma patients with hyperdiploid tumors vs. those with diploid tumors. In this clinical grouping, which comprises patients with gross residual disease following initial surgical therapy but no evidence of metastasis, hyperdiploid embryonal tumors showed a significantly better outcome. In addition, hyperdiploidy was essentially confined to rhabdomyosarcomas with embryonal histology, near-tetraploidy (DI values of or near 2.0) was a feature of alveolar tumors, and diploidy was seen in both tumor types (Fig 8). These observations have been confirmed by some investigators,[87–90] but other studies that include tumors of diverse stages have reported results that indicate no prognostic value for ploidy determination.[91, 92]

EWING SARCOMA/PERIPHERAL PRIMITIVE NEUROECTODERMAL TUMORS

Ewing sarcoma is perhaps the most undifferentiated and monomorphous of all pediatric round cell sarcomas and has historically been the most difficult to diagnose, particularly when it occurs in extraosseous locations. In spite of this most basic of appearances, we now recognize Ewing sarcoma as a member of a family of embryonic neoplasms that have a capacity for differentiation into primitive neural tumors as well as epithelial, glial, and even mesenchymal tissues. Thus these lesions show a capacity for development analogous to that normally displayed by the primitive neural crest cells from which they may be derived. Discussion of the relationship between Ewing sarcoma of bone or soft tissue and primitive neuroectodermal tumors (PNETs) is beyond the scope of this chapter (see Dehner[93]), but suffice it to note that regardless of morphology, they share a characteristic cytogenetic anomaly, t(11;22)(q24;q12).[94] This translocation joins the genetic sequences of the *Fli-1* gene on 11q24 and the *EWS* gene on 22q12.[95, 96] The *Fli-1* gene was identified because of its homology with published sequences of a similarly named mouse oncogene that is induced by the Friend erythroleukemia virus. Like *PAX3*, *Fli-1* is capable of producing cell transformation and malignancy when it is inappropriately expressed in vitro or in vivo. This cell-transforming property is enhanced by fusion of the gene with *EWS*.[95]

In t(11;22), *Fli-1*, which encodes a DNA-binding transcription factor, is joined to *EWS*, which encodes an RNA-binding protein. A variety of fusion points produce the resultant oncogenic molecule, which contains functioning subunits at both ends.[97] This "combinatorial fusion" has implications for laboratory detection because hybridization sequences must span a sufficient width of the midportion of the combined gene in order to display maximum sensitivity. A similar molecule is obtained by t(21;22), which is present in a minority of Ewing sarcomas instead of t(11;22) and which joins *EWS* with another transcription factor, ERG.[98, 99] Isolated cases of mesenchymal chondrosarcoma and small cell osteosarcoma, bone tumors that are also at least partially composed of small undifferentiated cells, have been reported to contain t(11;22)(q24;q12).[100, 101] In fact, morphologically unrelated tumors such as myxoid chondrosarcoma, clear cell sarcoma, and others have been found to contain break points that may produce fusion genes pairing *EWS* with a transcription factor partner,[102–106] so this gene appears to be of prime importance in the genesis of a number of sarcomas.

Besides t(11;22) and t(21;22), other nonrandom, recurring translocations appear in both Ewing sarcoma and its differentiated cousin PNET.

These include the derivative chromosome der(16)t(1;13)(q21;q17) and trisomy 8.[107, 108] The clinical significance of these genetic anomalies and the exact identification of the involved DNA sequences are unknown at present.

As with the other translocations noted earlier, identification of t(11;22) and t(21;22) in primitive round cell tumors offers the opportunity of another avenue for diagnostic confirmation and possibly for future therapy. Both RT-PCR (Fig 9) and FISH (Fig 10) have been exploited as techniques for rapid and sensitive identification of these tumors,[109, 110] and when combined with t(2;13) in a "multiplex" test,[84] there is further diagnostic application. Currently in our own laboratory, fresh tissue is preferable for RT-PCR and FISH testing (see Figure 10), which unfortunately limits the applicability of these methods for archival studies. This drawback is primarily a result of the extensive molecular cross-linking that occurs during the fixation process, and to further complicate matters, the use of different fixatives has varying methodologic implications. In this regard, B5 and Bouin's fixatives appear more deleterious to DNA-based procedures than do routinely used formaldehyde solutions.[111]

As for prognosis, there are no currently available cytogenetic markers that appear to affect the clinical behavior of Ewing sarcoma/PNET. Mutations in *p53* have been identified in several cases,[112] and several proto-oncogenes are expressed at high levels.[113] A number of investigators have performed ploidy analyses, but these studies, including our own unpublished observations, generally reveal that the overwhelming majority of these tumors are diploid and that tetraploidy occurs infrequently.[114]

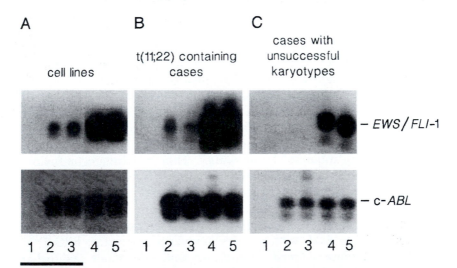

FIGURE 9.

Polymerase chain reaction studies on *Fli-1/EWS* fusion RNA transcripts in a series of Ewing sarcoma/primitive neuroectodermal tumors. Lane 1 in each study is a negative control, and the bottom lanes test for a ubiquitously expressed gene, *c-abl*, as a positive control. The panels show the results of testing a series of Ewing sarcoma cell lines **(A)**, tumors demonstrated to contain t(11;22) by routine cytogenetics **(B)**, and tumors in which attempts at karyotyping were unsuccessful **(C)**. All tumors are positive except for cases C2 and C3. (From Downing JR, Head DR, Parham DM, et al: *Am J Pathol* 5:1294–1300, 1993. Used by permission.)

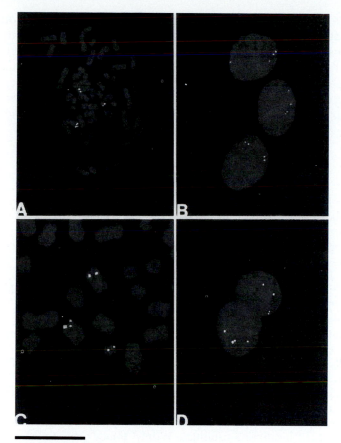

FIGURE 10.

Fluorescence in situ hybridization study of chromosomes (**A** and **C**) and inter-phase nuclei (**B** and **D**) in Ewing sarcoma primitive neuroectodermal tumor cell lines. Testing was performed by using two separate cosmids (large strands of DNA) binding to genes located on either side of the translocation break point on chromosome 11. **A** and **C** illustrate translocation of two signals to chromosome 22, so three chromosomes instead of the expected two are labeled. In the inter-phase nuclei there is separation of two signals in the translocated genes instead of the juxtaposition of signals that should occur normally (as in the lowest cell **B**). Because one chromosome is normal and the other is translocated, the signals appear as two adjacent points and two separate points within the tumor cell nu-clei (as in **D**). (From Giovannini M: *J Clin Invest* 90:1911–1918, 1992. Used by permission.)

However, some have recently demonstrated aneuploidy with apparent prognostic implications in Ewing sarcoma/PNET.[115] The clinical signifi-cance of identification of t(11;22) and other markers unique to Ewing sar-coma/PNET lies in their assistance in defining a group of neoplasms with a distinct behavior and responsiveness to chemotherapeutic and radio-therapeutic agents.

SUMMARY

In summary, our current knowledge of the expected behavior of child-hood round cell tumors has been greatly enhanced by recent findings in cytogenetics. To a large degree, these advances have increased our ability to separate these tumors into well-defined diagnostic groups and have confirmed categorical divisions initially devised via morphologic studies. In certain tumors, prognostic indicators such as ploidy have also been well characterized. Finally, the identification and study of discrete genetic events associated with particular tumor categories offer hope for future therapy aimed at total elimination of disease while avoiding excessive treatment morbidity.

REFERENCES

1. Donner LR: Cytogenetics and molecular biology of small round-cell tumors and related neoplasms. Current status. *Cancer Genet Cytogenet* 54:1–10, 1991.
2. Weinberg RA: Oncogenes and tumor suppressor genes. *CA Cancer J Clin* 44:160–170, 1994.
3. Triche TJ, Askin FB, Kissane J: Neuroblastoma, Ewing's sarcoma, and the differential diagnosis of small-, round-, blue-cell tumors, in Finegold M (ed): *Major Problems in Pathology*, vol 18, *Pathology of Neoplasia in Children and Adolescents*. Philadelphia, WB Saunders, 1986, pp 145–195.
4. National Wilms' Tumor Study Committee: Wilms' tumor: Status report, 1990. *J Clin Oncol* 9:877–887, 1991.
5. Donaldson SS: Lessons from our children. *Int J Radiat Oncol Biol Phys* 26:739–749, 1993.
6. Bolande RP: Neoplasia of early life and its relationships to teratogenesis. *Perspect Pediatr Pathol* 3:145–183, 1976.
7. Rose EA, Glaser T, Jones C, et al: Complete physical map of the WAGR region of 11p13 localizes a candidate Wilms' tumor gene. *Cell* 60:495–508, 1990.
8. Wang-Wuu S, Soukup S, Bove K, et al: Chromosome analysis of 31 Wilms' tumors. *Cancer Res* 50:2786–2793, 1990.
9. Mannens M, Devilee P, Bliek J, et al: Loss of heterozygosity in Wilms' tumors, studied for six putative tumor suppressor regions, is limited to chromosome 11. *Cancer Res* 50:3279–3283, 1990.
10. Ton CCT, Huff V, Call KM, et al: Smallest region of overlap in Wilms tumor deletions uniquely implicates an 11p13 zinc finger gene as the disease locus. *Genomics* 10:293–297, 1991.
11. Call KM, Glaser T, Ito CY, et al: Isolation and characterization of a zinc finger polypeptide gene at the human chromosome 11 Wilms' tumor locus. *Cell* 60:509–520, 1990.
12. Haber DA, Buckler AJ. WT1: A novel tumor suppressor gene inactivated in Wilms' tumor. *New Biol* 4:97–106, 1992.
13. Rauscher FJ III, Morris JF, Tournay OE, et al: Binding of the Wilms' tumor locus zinc finger protein to the EGR-1 consensus sequence. *Science* 250:1259–1262, 1990.
14. Madden SL, Cook DM, Morris JF, et al: Transcriptional repression mediated by the WT1 Wilms tumor gene product. *Science* 253:1550–1553, 1991.
15. Rauscher FJ III: The WT1 Wilms tumor gene product: A developmentally regulated transcription factor in the kidney that functions as a tumor suppressor. *FASEB J* 7:896–903, 1993.
16. Pritchard-Jones K, Fleming S, Davidson D, et al: The candidate Wilms' tumour gene is involved in genitourinary development. *Nature* 346:194–197, 1990.

17. Miwa H, Tomlinson GE, Timmons CF, et al: RNA expression of the WT1 gene in Wilms' tumors in relation to histology. *J Natl Cancer Inst* 84:181–187, 1992.

18. Pelletier J, Bruening W, Li FP, et al: *WT1* mutations contribute to abnormal genital system development and hereditary Wilms' tumour. *Nature* 353:431–434, 1991.

19. Pelletier J, Bruening W, Kashtan CE, et al: Germline mutations in the Wilms' tumor suppressor gene are associated with abnormal urogenital development in Denys-Drash syndrome. *Cell* 67:437–447, 1991.

20. Mundlos S, Pelletier J, Darveau A, et al: Nuclear localization of the protein encoded by the Wilms' tumor gene *WT1* in embryonic and adult tissues. *Development* 119:1329–1341, 1993.

21. Pritchard-Jones K, Fleming S: Cell types expressing the Wilms' tumour gene (WT1) in Wilms' tumours: Implications for tumour histogenesis. *Oncogene* 6:2211–2220, 1991.

22. Beckwith JB, Kiviat NB, Bonadio JF: Nephrogenic rests, nephroblastomatosis, and the pathogenesis of Wilms' tumor. *Pediatr Pathol* 10:1–36, 1990.

23. Park S, Bernard A, Bove KE, et al: Inactivation of *WT1* in nephrogenic rests, genetic precursors to Wilms' tumour. *Nat Genet* 5:363–367, 1993.

24. Knudson AG Jr, Strong LC: Mutation and cancer: A model for Wilms' tumor of the kidney. *J Natl Cancer Inst* 48:313–324, 1972.

25. Wadey RB, Pal N, Buckle B, et al: Loss of heterozygosity in Wilms' tumour involves two distinct regions of chromosome 11. *Oncogene* 5:901–908, 1990.

26. Dowdy SF, Fasching CL, Araujo D, et al: Suppression of tumorigenicity in Wilms tumor by the p15.5-p14 region of chromosome 11. *Science* 254:293–295, 1991.

27. Reeve AE, Sih SA, Raizis AM, et al: Loss of allelic heterozygosity at a second locus on chromosome 11 in sporadic Wilms' tumor cells. *Mol Cell Biol* 9:1799–1803, 1989.

28. Sotelo-Avila C, Gooch WM: Neoplasms associated with the Beckwith-Wiedemann syndrome. *Perspect Pediatr Pathol* 3:255–272, 1976.

29. Garvin AJ, Gansler T, Gerald W, et al: Insulin-like growth factor production by childhood solid tumors. *Perspect Pediatr Pathol* 15:106–116, 1992.

30. Gansler T, Furlanetto R, Gramling TS, et al: Antibody to type I insulinlike growth factor receptor inhibits growth of Wilms' tumor in culture and in athymic mice. *Am J Pathol* 135:961–966, 1989.

31. Zumkeller W, Schwander J, Mitchell CD, et al: Insulin-like growth factor (IGF)-I, -II and IGF binding protein-2 (IGFBP-2) in the plasma of children with Wilms' tumour. *Eur J Cancer* 29A:1973–1977, 1993.

32. Henry I, Puech A, Riesewijk A, et al: Somatic mosaicism for partial paternal isodisomy in Beckwith-Wiedemann syndrome: A post-fertilization event. *Eur J Hum Genet* 1:19–29, 1993.

33. Sapienza C: Genome imprinting and cancer genetics. *Semin Cancer Biol* 3:151–158, 1992.

34. Junien C: Beckwith-Wiedemann syndrome, tumourigenesis and imprinting. *Curr Opin Genet Dev* 2:431–438, 1992.

35. Brown KW, Gardner A, Williams JC, et al: Paternal origin of 11p15 duplications in the Beckwith-Wiedemann syndrome. A new case and review of the literature. *Cancer Genet Cytogenet* 58:66–70, 1992.

36. Huff V, Saunders GF: Wilms tumor genes. *Biochim Biophys Acta Rev Cancer* 1155:295–306, 1993.

37. Coppes MJ, Williams BRG: The molecular genetics of Wilms tumor. *Cancer Invest* 12:57–65, 1994.

38. Grundy PE, Telzerow PE, Breslow N, et al: Loss of heterozygosity for chromosomes 16q and 1p in Wilms' tumors predicts an adverse outcome. *Cancer Res* 54:2331–2333, 1994.
39. Schwartz CE, Haber DA, Stanton VP, et al: Familial predisposition to Wilms tumor does not segregate with the WT1 gene. *Genomics* 10:927–930, 1991.
40. Douglass EC, Look AT, Webber B, et al: Hyperdiploidy and chromosomal rearrangements define the anaplastic variant of Wilms' tumor. *J Clin Oncol* 4:975–981, 1986.
41. Misra M, Rohatgi M, Mathur M, et al: Flow cytometric analysis of DNA ploidy in 62 patients with Wilms' tumor. *Pediatr Surg Int* 7:51–54, 1992.
42. Layfield LJ, Ritchie AW, Ehrlich R: The relationship of deoxyribonucleic acid content to conventional prognostic factors in Wilms tumor. *J Urol* 142:1040–1043, 1989.
43. Kumar S, Marsden HB, Cowan RA, et al: Prognostic relevance of DNA content in childhood renal tumours. *Br J Cancer* 59:291–295, 1989.
44. Schmidt D, Wiedemann B, Keil W, et al: Flow cytometric analysis of nephroblastomas and related neoplasms. *Cancer* 58:2494–2500, 1986.
45. Oppedal BR, Glomstein A, Zetterberg A: Feulgen DNA values in Wilms' tumour in relation to prognosis. *Pathol Res Pract* 183:756–760, 1988.
46. Gururangan S, Dorman A, Ball R, et al: DNA quantitation of Wilms' tumour (nephroblastoma) using flow cytometry and image analysis. *J Clin Pathol* 45:498–501, 1992.
47. Chen F, Li ZC, Ge RQ, et al: The measurement of DNA content in Wilms' tumor and its clinical significance. *J Pediatr Surg* 29:548–550, 1994.
48. Barrantes JC, Muir KR, Toyn CE, et al: Thirty-year population-based review of childhood renal tumours with an assessment of prognostic features including tumour DNA characteristics. *Med Pediatr Oncol* 21:24–30, 1993.
49. Rainwater LM, Hosaka Y, Farrow GM, et al: Wilms tumors: Relationship of nuclear deoxyribonucleic acid ploidy to patient survival. *J Urol* 138:974–977, 1987.
50. Yildiz I, Jaffe N, Aksoy F, et al: Regional DNA content heterogeneity in Wilms' tumor: Incidence and potential clinical relevance. *Anticancer Res* 14:1365–1370, 1994.
51. Zuppan CW, Beckwith JB, Luckey DW: Anaplasia in unilateral Wilms' tumor: A report from the National Wilms' Tumor Study Pathology Center. *Hum Pathol* 19:1199–1209, 1988.
52. Hazen-Martin DJ, Re GG, Garvin AJ, et al: Distinctive properties of an anaplastic Wilms' tumor and its associated epithelial cell line. *Am J Pathol* 144:1023–1034, 1994.
53. Waber PG, Chen J, Nisen PD: Infrequency of *ras*, p53, WT1, or RB gene alterations in Wilms tumors. *Cancer* 72:3732–3738, 1993.
54. Bardeesy N, Falkoff D, Petruzzi M-J, et al: Anaplastic Wilms' tumour, a subtype displaying poor prognosis, harbours p53 gene mutations. *Nat Genet* 7:91–97, 1994.
55. Brodeur GM, Azar C, Brother M, et al: Neuroblastoma: Effect of genetic factors on prognosis and treatment. *Cancer* 70(suppl):1685–1694, 1992.
56. Beardsley T: Smart genes. *Sci Am* 265:86–95, 1991.
57. Lebovitz RM: Oncogenes as mediators of cell growth and differentiation (editorial). *Lab Invest* 55:249–251, 1986.
58. Van Krieken JHJM, Kluin PM: The association of c-*myc* rearrangements with specific types of human non-Hodgkin's lymphomas. *Leuk Lymphoma* 7:371–376, 1992.
59. Pahlman S, Mamaeva S, Meyerson G, et al: Human neuroblastoma cells in culture: A model for neuronal cell differentiation and function. *Acta Physiol Scand Suppl* 592:25–37, 1990.

60. Reynolds CP, Biedler JL, Spengler BA, et al: Characterization of human neuroblastoma cell lines established before and after therapy. *J Natl Cancer Inst* 76:375–387, 1986.

61. Oppedal BR, Oien O, Jahnsen T, et al: N-*myc* amplification in neuroblastomas: Histopathological, DNA ploidy, and clinical variables. *J Clin Pathol* 42:1148–1152, 1989.

62. Bernards R: N-*myc* disrupts protein kinase C–mediated signal transduction in neuroblastoma. *EMBO J* 10:1119–1125, 1991.

63. Shapiro DN, Valentine MB, Rowe ST, et al: Detection of N-*myc* gene amplification by fluorescence in situ hybridization. *Am J Pathol* 142:1339–1346, 1993.

64. Look AT, Hayes FA, Shuster JJ, et al: Clinical relevance of tumor cell ploidy and N-*myc* gene amplification in childhood neuroblastoma: A Pediatric Oncology Group study. *J Clin Oncol* 9:581–591, 1991.

65. Joshi VV, Cantor AB, Brodeur GM, et al: Correlation between morphologic and other prognostic markers of neuroblastoma: A study of histologic grade, DNA index, N-*myc* gene copy number, and lactic dehydrogenase in patients in the Pediatric Oncology Group. *Cancer* 71:3173–3181, 1993.

66. Shapiro DN, Parham DM, Douglass EC, et al: Relationship of tumor-cell ploidy to histologic subtype and treatment outcome in children and adolescents with unresectable rhabdomyosarcoma. *J Clin Oncol* 9:159–166, 1991.

67. Gansler T: Applications of DNA cytometry in pediatric pathology. *Perspect Pediatr Pathol* 15:83–105, 1992.

68. Lahti JM, Valentine M, Xiang J, et al: Alterations in the PITSLRE protein kinase gene complex on chromosome 1p36 in childhood neuroblastoma. *Nat Genet* 7:370–375, 1994.

69. Lahti JM, Xiang J, Heath LS, et al: PITSLRE protein kinase activity is associated with apoptosis. *Mol Cell Biol* 15:1–11, 1995.

70. Asmar L, Gehan EA, Newton WA, et al: Agreement among and within groups of pathologists in the classification of rhabdomyosarcoma and related childhood sarcomas: Report of an international study of four pathology classifications. *Cancer* 74:2579–2588, 1994.

71. Scrable H, Witte D, Shimada H, et al: Molecular differential pathology in rhabdomyosarcoma. *Genes Chromosome Cancer* 1:23–35, 1989.

72. Calabrese G, Guanciali Franchi P, Stuppia L, et al: Translocation (8;11)(q12-13;q21) in embryonal rhabdomyosarcoma. *Cancer Genet Cytogenet* 58:210–211, 1992.

73. Zhan S, Shapiro DN, Helman LJ: Activation of an imprinted allele of the insulin-like growth factor II gene implicated in rhabdomyosarcoma. *J Clin Invest* 94:445–448, 1994.

74. Loh WE Jr, Scrable HJ, Livanos E, et al: Human chromosome 11 contains two different growth suppressor genes for embryonal rhabdomyosarcoma. *Proc Natl Acad Sci U S A* 89:1755–1759, 1992.

75. Whang-Peng J, Knutsen T, Theil K, et al: Cytogenetic studies in subgroups of rhabdomyosarcoma. *Genes Chromosom Cancer* 5:299–310, 1992.

76. Shapiro DN, Sublett JE, Li B, et al: Fusion of *PAX3* to a member of the forkhead family of transcription factors in human alveolar rhabdomyosarcoma. *Cancer Res* 53:5108–5112, 1993.

77. Hill RE, Hanson IM: Molecular genetics of the Pax gene family. *Curr Opin Cell Biol* 4:967–972, 1992.

78. Lawrence HJ, Largman C: Review: Homeobox genes in normal hematopoiesis and leukemia. *Blood* 80:2445–2453, 1992.

79. Tassabehji M, Read AP, Newton VE, et al: Waardenburg's syndrome patients

have mutations in the human homologue of the Pax-3 paired box gene (see comments). *Nature* 355:635–636, 1992.

80. Maulbecker CC, Gruss P: The oncogenic potential of Pax genes. *EMBO J* 12:2361–2367, 1993.

81. Davis RJ, D'Cruz CM, Lovell MA, et al: Fusion of *PAX7* to *FKHR* by the variant t(1;13)(p36;q14) translocation in alveolar rhabdomyosarcoma. *Cancer Res* 54:2869–2872, 1994.

82. Tsokos M, Webber B, Parham D, et al: Rhabdomyosarcoma: A new classification scheme related to prognosis. *Arch Pathol Lab Med* 116:847–855, 1992.

83. Parham DM, Shapiro DN, Downing JR, et al: Solid alveolar rhabdomyosarcomas with the t(2;13): Report of two cases with diagnostic implications. *Am J Surg Pathol* 18:474–478, 1994.

84. Downing JR, Head D, Parham DM, et al: A multiplex RT-PCR assay for the diagnosis of alveolar rhabdomyosarcoma and Ewing's sarcoma (abstract). *Mod Pathol* 7:146, 1994.

85. Shapiro DN, Parham DM, Douglass EC, et al: Relationship of tumor-cell ploidy to histologic subtype and treatment outcome in children and adolescents with unresectable rhabdomyosarcoma. *J Clin Oncol* 9:159–166, 1991.

86. Pappo AS, Crist WM, Kuttesch J, et al: Tumor-cell DNA content predicts outcome in children and adolescents with clinical group III embryonal rhabdomyosarcoma. The Intergroup Rhabdomyosarcoma Study Committee of the Children's Cancer Group and the Pediatric Oncology Group. *J Clin Oncol* 11:1901–1905, 1993.

87. Boyle ET Jr, Reiman HM, Kramer SA, et al: Embryonal rhabdomyosarcoma of bladder and prostate: Nuclear DNA patterns studied by flow cytometry. *J Urol* 140:1119–1121, 1988.

88. Wijnaendts LC, van der Linden JC, van Diest P, et al: Prognostic importance of DNA flow cytometric variables in rhabdomyosarcomas. *J Clin Pathol* 46:948–952, 1993.

89. Jung WH, Jung SH, Yoo CJ, et al: Flow cytometric analysis of DNA ploidy in childhood rhabdomyosarcoma. *Yonsei Med J* 35:34–42, 1994.

90. Niggli FK, Powell JE, Parkes SE, et al: DNA ploidy and proliferative activity (S-phase) in childhood soft-tissue sarcomas: Their value as prognostic indicators. *Br J Cancer* 69:1106–1110, 1994.

91. Kowal-Vern A, Gonzalez-Crussi F, Turner J, et al: Flow and image cytometric DNA analysis in rhabdomyosarcoma. *Cancer Res* 50:6023–6027, 1990.

92. Dias P, Kumar P, Marsden HB, et al: Prognostic relevance of DNA ploidy in rhabdomyosarcomas and other sarcomas of childhood. *Anticancer Res* 12:1173–1178, 1992.

93. Dehner LP: Primitive neuroectodermal tumor and Ewing's sarcoma. *Am J Surg Pathol* 17:1–13, 1993.

94. Delattre O, Zucman J, Melot T, et al: The Ewing family of tumors—A subgroup of small-round-cell tumors defined by specific chimeric transcripts. *N Engl J Med* 331:294–299, 1994.

95. May WA, Lessnick SL, Braun BS, et al: The Ewing's sarcoma *EWS/FLI-1* fusion gene encodes a more potent transcriptional activator and is a more powerful transforming gene than *FLI-1*. *Mol Cell Biol* 13:7393–7398, 1993.

96. Stephenson CF, Bridge JA, Sandberg AA: Cytogenetic and pathologic aspects of Ewing's sarcoma and neuroectodermal tumors. *Hum Pathol* 23:1270–1277, 1992.

97. Zucman J, Melot T, Desmaze C, et al: Combinatorial generation of variable fusion proteins in the Ewing family of tumours. *EMBO J* 12:4481–4487, 1993.

98. Sorensen PHB, Lessnick SL, Lopez-Terrada D, et al: A second Ewing's sarcoma translocation, t(21;22), fuses the EWS gene to another ETS-family transcription factor, ERG. *Nat Genet* 6:146–151, 1994.

99. Giovannini M, Biegel JA, Serra M, et al: EWS-erg and EWS-Fli1 fusion transcripts in Ewing's sarcoma and primitive neuroectodermal tumors with variant translocations. *J Clin Invest* 94:489–496, 1994.

100. Sainati L, Scapinello A, Montaldi A, et al: A mesenchymal chondrosarcoma of a child with the reciprocal translocation (11;22)(q24;q12). *Cancer Genet Cytogenet* 71:144–147, 1993.

101. Noguera R, Navarro S, Triche TJ: Translocation (11;22) in small cell osteosarcoma. *Cancer Genet Cytogenet* 45:121–124, 1990.

102. Reeves BR, Fletcher CDM, Gusterson BA: Translocation t(12;22)(q13;q13) is a nonrandom rearrangement in clear cell sarcoma. *Cancer Genet Cytogenet* 64:101–103, 1992.

103. Rey JA, Bello MJ, Kusak ME, et al: Involvement of 22q12 in a neurofibrosarcoma in neurofibromatosis type 1. *Cancer Genet Cytogenet* 66:28–32, 1993.

104. Mandahl N: Genetic changes in bone and soft tissue tumors (abstract). Presented at the Fifth International Workshop on Chromosomes in Solid Tumors, Tucson, Ariz, January 1993.

105. Cordoba JC, Parham DM, Meyer WH, et al: A new cytogenetic finding in an epithelioid sarcoma, t(8;22)(q22;q11). *Cancer Genet Cytogenet* 72:151–154, 1994.

106. Ladanyi M, Gerald W: Fusion of the EWS and WT1 genes in the desmoplastic small round cell tumor. *Cancer Res* 54:2837–2840, 1994.

107. Mugneret F, Lizard S, Aurias A, et al: Chromosomes in Ewing's sarcoma. II. Nonrandom additional changes, trisomy 8 and der(16)t(1;16). *Cancer Genet Cytogenet* 32:239–245, 1988.

108. Douglass EC, Rowe ST, Valentine M, et al: A second nonrandom translocation, der(16)t(1;16)(q21;q13), in Ewing sarcoma and peripheral neuroectodermal tumor. *Cytogenet Cell Genet* 53:87–90, 1990.

109. Giovannini M, Selleri L, Biegel JA, et al: Interphase cytogenetics for the detection of the t(11;22)(q24;q12) in small round cell tumors. *J Clin Invest* 90:1911–1918, 1992.

110. Downing JR, Head DR, Parham DM, et al: Detection of the (11;22)(q24;q12) translocation of Ewing's sarcoma and peripheral neuroectodermal tumor by reverse transcriptase polymerase chain reaction. *Am J Pathol* 143:1–7, 1993.

111. Rogers BB: Application of the polymerase chain reaction to archival material. *Perspect Pediatr Pathol* 16:99–119, 1992.

112. Komuro H, Hayashi Y, Kawamura M, et al: Mutations of the p53 gene are involved in Ewing's sarcomas but not in neuroblastomas. *Cancer Res* 53:5284–5288, 1993.

113. Tsokos M: Peripheral primitive neuroectodermal tumors: Diagnosis, classification, and prognosis. *Perspect Pediatr Pathol* 16:27–98, 1992.

114. Kowal-Vern A, Walloch J, Chou P, et al: Flow and image cytometric DNA analysis in Ewing's sarcoma. *Mod Pathol* 5:56–60, 1992.

115. Dierick AM, Langlois M, Van Oostveldt P, et al: The prognostic significance of the DNA content in Ewing's sarcoma: A retrospective cytophotometric and flow cytometric study. *Histopathology* 23:333–339, 1993.

Granulomas of the Liver*

Kamal G. Ishak, M.D., Ph.D.
Department of Hepatic and Gastrointestinal Pathology, Armed Forces Institute of Pathology, Washington, D.C.

The liver is involved in many diseases that are histologically manifested, wholly or in part, by a granulomatous response. Some are intrinsic hepatic diseases, for example, primary biliary cirrhosis (PBC), whereas others are systemic diseases in which the liver is but one of many affected organs. Most of the granulomatous diseases involve the liver diffusely, but a few are surface or superficial reactions, usually related to previous surgery, for example, granulomas associated with suture material, starch, or talc. In the diffuse granulomatous diseases with a known etiology the inciting agent may reach the liver via the arterial circulation (e.g., most of the infectious diseases), portal venous system (e.g., eggs of *Schistosoma mansoni* or *japonicum*), bile ducts (e.g., eggs of *Fasciola hepatica*, *Ascaris lumbricoides*, or *Clonorchis sinensis*), or lymphatics (e.g., mineral oil or lymphangiographic contrast material). In some instances the granulomatous response is to extruded cell components such as lipid (lipogranuloma) or extravasated bile (bile granuloma).

Up to 10% of liver biopsy specimens in general hospitals may reveal granulomas. As pointed out by Fauci and Wolff,[1] anywhere from 13% to 36% of granulomas in the liver have no known etiology. These figures, however, should not deter the pathologist and clinician from making every effort to arrive at a diagnosis in each patient.

Granulomatous diseases involving the liver may not be accompanied by symptoms or signs. When the patient is symptomatic, there may be fever, abdominal pain, weight loss, hepatomegaly, splenomegaly, and lymphadenopathy. Symptoms and signs related to other organ systems such as the lung or central nervous system may completely dominate the clinical picture. Biochemical evidence of hepatic involvement is also often nonspecific. Hyperglobulinemia is a common finding. Hypoalbuminemia may occur in some granulomatous diseases, e.g., visceral leishmaniasis. Elevations in serum bilirubin are found in about half of the patients with tuberculosis, but fewer than a tenth of the patients are jaundiced. Other diseases that may be associated with hyperbilirubinemia and jaundice include primary biliary cirrhosis, primary sclerosing cholangitis, the chronic cholestatic syndrome of sarcoidosis, and some instances of drug-induced liver injury, for example, injury related to phe-

---

*The opinions or assertions contained herein are the private views of the author and are not to be construed as official or as representing the views of the Departments of the Army and Defense.

Advances in Pathology and Laboratory Medicine, vol. 8
© 1995, Mosby–Year Book, Inc.

nylbutazone. The serum alkaline phosphatase activity may be elevated, with the highest values in patients with chronic cholestatic syndromes, for example, primary biliary cirrhosis. Serum aminotransferase values will vary with the basic disease; for example, they are likely to be normal or slightly increased in sarcoidosis but moderately increased in some drug-induced injuries. Elevation of the activity of serum angiotensin converting enzyme may be helpful in supporting a diagnosis of sarcoidosis, but the activity of this enzyme may be increased in a number of other diseases, for example, primary biliary cirrhosis, leprosy, and histoplasmosis.[2] A positive antimitochondrial antibody test (>1:40) helps to confirm the diagnosis of primary biliary cirrhosis.

Hematologic findings in the granulomatous diseases are likely to show too much variation for generalization. Peripheral eosinophilia is frequent in many of the parasitic diseases, for example, visceral larva migrans, but can also occur in drug-induced granulomatous diseases. Additionally, Guckian and Perry[3] found eosinophilia in 50% of patients with sarcoidosis and in 31% of patients with granulomas of unknown cause. Pancytopenia may occur as a result of splenomegaly secondary to hepatosplenic schistosomiasis and other conditions.

Investigation of patients with hepatic granulomas should include a careful history that stresses possible exposure to infectious diseases (including previous residence or travel to tropical or subtropical countries), types of sexual activity, a detailed drug history (including the use of nonprescription or recreational drugs), an occupational history, possible domestic exposure to granuloma-inciting agents, and information on previous abdominal surgery. When appropriate, investigation of the patient should include cultures of blood for bacteria, mycobacteria, fungi, and viruses; skin tests; serologic tests for infectious diseases; and molecular diagnostic techniques such as the polymerase chain reaction (PCR).[4-8]

Other than biochemical tests, imaging studies in selected cases may include chest radiography, ultrasonography, computed tomography of the liver and biliary tree, and endoscopic retrograde cholangiopancreatography (ERCP). Biopsy of the liver, usually percutaneous, is firmly established in the workup of granulomatous diseases of the liver and other organs and is helpful in subsequent documentation of the clinical course and response to therapy.

In addition to sections stained with hematoxylin-eosin (HE), the pathologist's armamentarium includes a multitude of special stains, polarizing and phase-contrast microscopy, ultraviolet microscopy, scanning electron microscopy, energy-dispersive x-ray analysis, and transmission electron microscopy. Immunopathologic techniques, particularly in the diagnosis of infectious diseases, have had limited application, but their use is likely to increase in the future.

For purposes of this review, a *granuloma* is defined as a focal aggregate of epithelioid cells derived from the mononuclear phagocyte system. It should be emphasized at the outset that the term "granulomatous hepatitis" is meaningless and should not be used.[9, 10] Epithelioid cells are distinguished from macrophages by their abundant homogeneous cytoplasm free of ingested particulate matter, their ill-defined cell membrane, and their often peripherally located, curved nuclei.[10] The nuclei are vesicular and contain small but distinct nucleoli. The definition of a granuloma does not include the focal aggregates of hypertrophied Kupffer cells commonly seen in acute viral (e.g., acute viral hepatitis and infectious mononucleosis) or bacterial infectious diseases (e.g., typhoid fever); these are more appropriately referred as *granulomatoid* foci. The term "microgranuloma" has been used for such foci.[9] Other granulomatoid lesions that may be mentioned include aggregates of foam cells (xanthomatous or pseudoxanthomatous cells) that are characteristic of chronic cholestasis, for example, primary biliary cirrhosis. Focal, organized clusters of markedly hypertrophied macrophages that have not been transformed to epithelioid cells are referred to in this review as *macrophagic granulomas*. Typical examples include *Mycobacterium avium-intracellulare* (MAI) infection (in which the macrophagic granulomas are packed with acid-fast bacilli) and chronic granulomatous disease of childhood (in which the macrophages are full of lipofuscin).

Epithelioid cells evolve from stimulated, activated macrophage cells. The activators and immunomodulators of macrophage cells and their signal products are beyond the scope of this presentation; they have been reviewed recently by Decker.[11] Experimentally, granulomas have been shown to be mediated by cytokines. Depending on the inciting agent (e.g. purified protein derivative [PPD] vs. schistosomal antigen in one study), granulomas can be induced by different cytokines, a finding that may have therapeutic implications.[12] Epithelioid cells, in contrast to macrophages, are poorly phagocytic but are highly secretory.[13, 14] In sarcoidosis, for example, the sarcoid granuloma secretes angiotensin converting enzyme, lysozyme, glucuronidase, collagenase, elastase, and calcitriol.[15] At the ultrastructural level, epithelioid cells are interdigitated; the secretory activity is paralleled by a marked proliferation of rough endoplasmic reticulum and no or few phagocytic vacuoles. By scanning electron microscopy, the pseudopodia and ruffles of the typical macrophage are lost, and the surface of the epithelioid cell becomes smooth. Other cells that may be found between and around epithelioid cells include lymphocytes, plasma cells, eosinophils and fibroblasts. Multinucleated giant cells, which are found in many granulomas, are formed by the fusion of epithelioid cells.[16, 17] Clustering and cell-to-cell adhesion of the epithelioid cells are enhanced by various cytokines, of which interferon-γ appears to be the most potent.[17] Interferon-γ exerts its effect in part by changes in the expression of intercellular adhesion molecule 1.[17]

Granulomas may have necrotic centers, and several types of necrosis are recognized—fibrinoid, fibrillogranular (caseation), purulent, and eosinophilic.[10] Granulomas may contain within them the inciting agents. These include microorganisms, parasitic eggs, larvae or even adult parasites, or foreign materials (such as silk sutures), all of which may be associated with the *Splendore-Hoeppli phenomenon*.[18-21] This phenomenon is histopathologically characterized by radiating, eosinophilic deposits around the causative agent and is due to precipitation of an antigen-antibody complex.

In this review, *foreign body granulomas* (also termed "mature granulomas" by Adams[22]) are included in the spectrum of the granulomatous inflammatory response. It is worth noting at this juncture that some diseases may be characterized by both epithelioid and foreign body granulomas, the best example being schistosomiasis. According to Adams,[22]

TABLE 1.
Etiology of Granulomas in Reported Series

Series	Location	Idiopathic	Sarcoidosis	Tuberculosis	Schistosomiasis	Brucellosis	Primary Biliary Cirrhosis	Drug Induced	Neoplasm
Guckian and Perry,[3] 1966	Galveston, Tex	20.0*	12.0	53.0	—	—	—	—	5.0
Neville et al.,[25] 1975	London	10.0	54.0	2.0	—	—	19.0	—	1.4
Klatskin,[26] 1977	New Haven, Conn	6.5	38.0	12.4	—	—	10.4	—	4.4
McMaster and Hennigar,[27] 1981	Charleston, SC	12.0	31.0	8.4	—	—	—	29.0	3.0
Cunningham et al.,[28] 1982	Glasgow, Scotland	31.2	10.4	—	—	6.5	—	—	7.8
Diaz Curiel et al.,[29] 1983	Madrid, Spain	10.1	—	34.8	—	7.3	—	—	17.4 (Hodgkin's)
Satti et al.,[30] 1990†	Dammam, Saudi Arabia	—	—	22.2	54.2	6.7	—	3.38	—
Ferrell,[9] 1990‡	San Francisco	20.0	20.0	2.5	—	—	22.8	—	8.5
Sartin and Walker,[31] 1991	Rochester, Minn	50.0	21.6	3.4	—	—	—	5.9	—
McCluggage and Sloan,[32] 1994	Belfast, N. Ireland	11.0	18.4	—	—	55.2	1.2	—	—

*Values are percentages.
†Granulomas with no etiology not included.
‡Only epithelioid granulomas included.

TABLE 2.
Causes of Hepatic Granulomas

Causes	Examples
Infectious diseases	
Viral infections	Infectious mononucleosis, cytomegalovirus infection
Rickettsial infections	Q fever, boutonneuse fever
Clamydial infections	Psittacosis
Bacterial infections	Brucellosis, listeriosis, yersiniosis
Mycobacterial infections	Tuberculosis, leprosy
Spirochetal infections	Syphilis
Mycotic infections	Histoplasmosis, coccidioidomycosis
Protozoal infections	Visceral leishmaniasis, toxoplasmosis
Helminthic infections	Visceral larva migrans, schistosomiasis
Sarcoidosis	
Chronic cholestatic disorders	Primary biliary cirrhosis
Gastrointestinal diseases	Chronic ulcerative colitis, regional ileitis
Vascular/connective tissue diseases	Polymyalgia arteritica, giant cell arteritis
Drug-induced injury	Quinidine, hydralazine, phenylbutazone, phenytoin
Metal-induced injury	Berylliosis, copper toxicity, hyperalbuminemia
Foreign particulate material	Talc, starch, silica
Extruded cell components	Lipogranuloma, bile granuloma
Inherited metabolic diseases	Chronic granulomatous disease
Neoplasms	Hodgkin's disease, primary liver tumors
Miscellaneous	Familial granulomatous hepatitis, granulomatous hepatitis with prolonged fever

granulomas develop in three stages: (1) the formation of a monocytic infiltrate; (2) the aggregation, maturation, and organization of these cells into a mature granuloma; and (3) the further evolution of this granuloma into an epithelioid one. The progression to and persistence of an epithelioid granuloma require the continued presence of the inciting agent or the development of delayed hypersensitivity. For further information on the pathogenetic and immunologic aspects of granulomas, the reader is referred to other reviews.[22–25]

Of the many diseases that are histologically expressed by granuloma formation, a considerable number can affect the liver. Even a cursory review of the world literature on hepatic granulomas discloses striking etiologic differences in series from various countries and even from the same country (reflecting in part the interest of the clinicians performing the biopsies).[3, 9, 26–32] A few examples are listed in Table 1. For this reason, the present review is intentionally comprehensive so that it may have general relevance in various geographic settings.

The causes of hepatic granulomas, with examples, are listed in Table 2, which also serves as an outline for the succeeding review.

VIRAL INFECTIONS

INFECTIOUS MONONUCLEOSIS.—Histopathologic changes in the hepatitis of infectious mononucleosis have been described by a number of authors.[33–38] Typical changes include moderate anisocytosis and anisonucleosis of liver cells, increased mitotic activity in hepatocytes and Kupffer cells, apoptosis, multiple small focal necroses, and mild or no cholestasis. Kupffer cells and portal macrophages are markedly hypertrophied and focally hyperplastic (granulomatoid foci) but generally contain little or no lipofuscin pigment. True noncaseating granulomas are seen in about 15% of cases (Fig 1).[38] Sinusoids are hypercellular, and lymphocytes may be arranged in an "Indian-file" pattern. Portal areas are moderately to heavily infiltrated with lymphocytes, as well as some eosinophils and neutrophils. Bile duct cells may reveal occasional mitoses. Nenert et al.[39] reported fibrin ring granulomas in the liver of a 38-year-old man with Epstein-Barr virus infection. Multiple epithelioid granulomas were noted by Rothwell[40] in the bone marrow of a young woman with infectious mononucleosis.

The hepatitis of infectious mononucleosis generally resolves without sequelae. Rare instances of fatal fulminant liver failure have been reported.[37, 41–43]

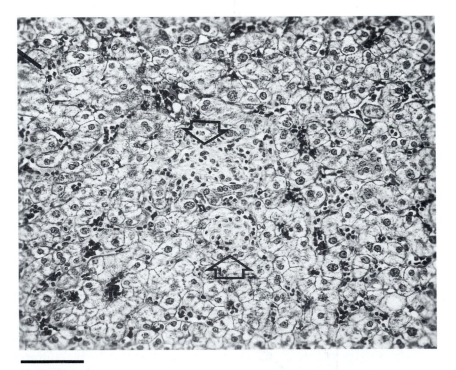

FIGURE 1.

Infectious mononucleosis hepatitis with two small epithelioid granulomas (arrows) and sinusoidal lymphocytosis (hematoxylin-eosin [HE], ×250).

Cytomegalovirus Infection.—One of the clinical expressions of cytomegalovirus (CMV) infection in immunocompetent adults is an acute febrile illness with lymphocytosis and many atypical lymphocytes that has been termed CMV mononucleosis because of its resemblance to infectious mononucleosis.[44, 45] Histologically, CMV mononucleosis resembles infectious mononucleosis, although the granulomatous component appears to be more prominent.[44–48] The granulomas are epithelioid and noncaseating, and giant cells have been reported in only one instance.[44] Fibrin ring granulomas have been observed in a case of CMV hepatitis[49] and in CMV infection of the bone marrow in another case.[50] Intranuclear inclusions have not been identified in hepatic biopsy material from the reported cases. It is worth noting at this junction that neonatal CMV infection and CMV infections in immunocompromised patients are not associated with granuloma formation. Instead, these infections reveal the characteristic cytomegaly of liver and duct cells, nuclear and cytoplasmic inclusions, and a focal neutrophilic inflammatory response.

Hepatitis A Virus Infection.—Fibrin ring granulomas have been described in two cases of acute hepatitis A.[51, 52] It must be emphasized at this juncture that this pattern of injury is most unusual for hepatitis A; the typical histopathology is one of acute hepatocellular injury with spotty necrosis and apoptosis.[53] Severe injury is characterized by zone 1 necrosis.[53]

Hepatitis C Virus Infection.—Epithelioid granulomas were found in 10% of 52 cases of hepatitis C virus–related cirrhosis by Emile et al.[54] There was no detectable cause for the granulomas other than the virus infection.

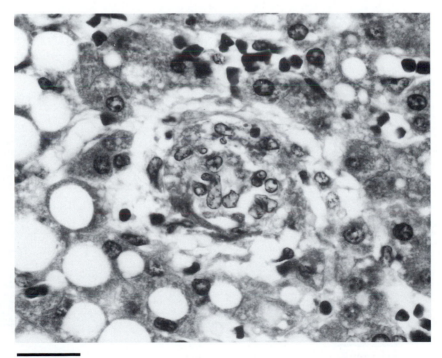

FIGURE 2.
AIDS: small, nondescript parenchymal granuloma (HE, ×720).

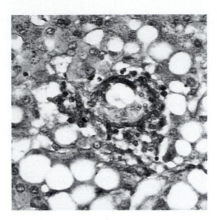

FIGURE 3.
AIDS: fibrin ring and central vacuole in a small granuloma (periodic acid–Schiff [PAS] after diastase digestion ×300).

ACQUIRED IMMUNODEFICIENCY SYNDROME.—The liver is involved by granulomas in many patients with acquired immunodeficiency syndrome (AIDS). The most frequent causes of granulomas are disseminated infections, with MAI heading the list; these infections are discussed throughout this review. Other than infections, granulomas in the liver of patients with AIDS may be drug induced or have no known etiology. Rarely, fibrin ring granulomas unrelated to Q fever have been reported in the liver[55]; one example is illustrated in Figures 2 to 4.

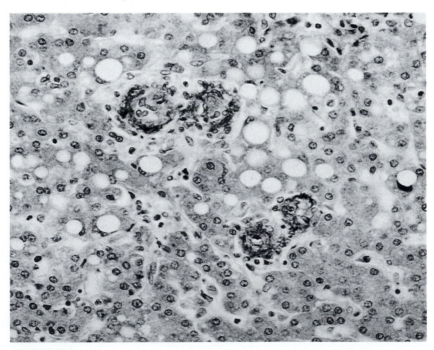

FIGURE 4.
AIDS: fibrin rings in several granulomas identified immunohistochemically with the use of antifibrin antibodies (×300).

RICKETTSIAL DISEASES

Q FEVER.—Granulomas or granulomatoid lesions have been described in most cases with hepatic involvement. They are usually located within the acini but can be found in portal areas. A highly distinctive feature of the granulomas of *acute* Q fever, both in the bone marrow and liver, is a central empty space surrounded by histiocytes or epithelioid cells with a ring of fibrin, hence the term "fibrin ring" granulomas (Figs 5 to 7).[56-63] That space is believed to be an entrapped fat vacuole. The liver is also involved in *chronic* Q fever, as was the case in all 16 patients reported by Turck et al.[64] The changes were nonspecific, but several livers contained granulomas (not referred to as fibrin ring in type).

Fibrin ring granulomas are most frequently observed in the liver and bone marrow in acute Q fever. They are not pathognomonic; other causes of fibrin ring granulomas are listed in Table 3. The largest series of diseases associated with hepatic fibrin ring granulomas was reported in 1991 by Marazuela et al.,[62] who also reviewed the literature. They are mentioned in the appropriate sections throughout this review.

It should be emphasized that a fibrin ring granuloma is by no means the only lesion seen in acute Q fever hepatitis. Some granulomas may have no central vacuole, others may contain only irregular strands of fibrin, and still others may be entirely epithelioid, with or without giant cells.[56, 58, 60, 62] Additionally, a variety of other lesions are present, including focal necrosis, microabscesses, apoptotic bodies, hypertrophy and hyperplasia of Kupffer cells, and variable steatosis (Fig 8). In two studies with follow-up biopsies the fibrin ring granulomas evolved into

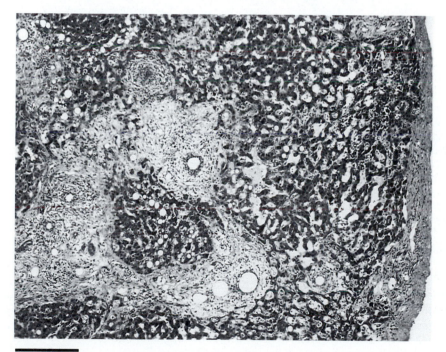

FIGURE 5.
Q fever hepatitis. Several granulomas contain vacuoles (HE, ×60).

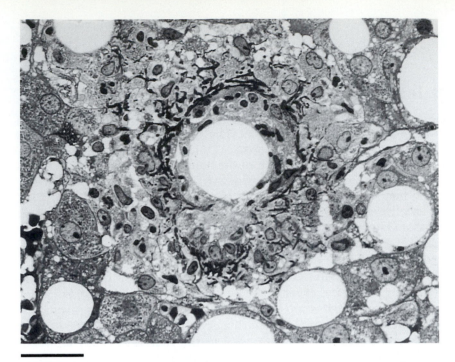

FIGURE 6.

Q fever hepatitis. Strands of fibrin *(black)* form an incomplete ring, together with epitheliod cells, around an empty space (toluidine blue stain of an Epon-embedded section 1 μm thick, ×720).

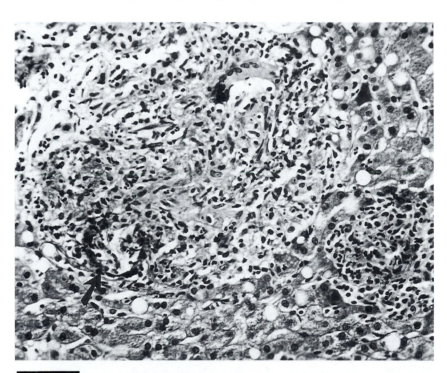

FIGURE 7.

Q fever hepatitis: epithelioid granuloma with an eccentrically located fibrin ring *(arrow)*. Note the multinucleated giant cell at the opposite end of the granuloma (HE, ×250).

TABLE 3.
Diseases Associated With Hepatic Fibrin
Ring Granulomas

Acquired immunodeficiency syndrome
Allopurinol drug injury
Boutonneuse fever
Cytomegalovirus hepatitis
Giant cell arteritis
Hepatitis A
Hodgkin's disease
Infectious mononucleosis
Lupus erythematosus
Q fever
Staphylococcal sepsis
Toxoplasmosis
Visceral leishmaniasis

"atypical" granulomas that did not contain fibrin.[58, 60] The causative organism, *Coxiella burnetti,* was not been identified by either light or electron microscopic examination.[60]

BOUTONNEUSE FEVER.—Also known as Mediterranean exanthematous fever, this disease is caused by *Rickettsia conorii* and transmitted by the bite of

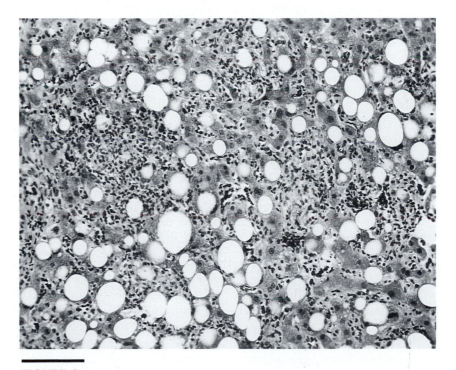

FIGURE 8.
Q fever hepatitis with numerous foci of necrosis (HE, ×160).

Rhipicephalus sanguineus (a dog tick). Histologically, there is hypertrophy of Kupffer cells, focal necrosis, and small granulomas. Fibrin ring granulomas have also been reported in the liver in this disease.[62, 65]

CHLAMYDIAL INFECTIONS

PSITTACOSIS.—Hepatic histologic changes include focal necrosis, hyperplasia of Kupffer cells with erythrophagocytosis and leukophagocytosis, and variable infiltration of portal areas by mononuclear cells.[66-68] Noncaseating granulomas have been described in liver biopsy sections from several patients.[69, 70]

LYMPHOPATHIA VENEREUM.—Granulomas are mentioned in two patients with this disease in a series of 38 cases of hepatic granulomas reported by Wagoner et al.[71]

BACTERIAL INFECTIONS

MELIOIDOSIS.—This disease is caused by *Pseudomonas pseudomallei* and prevails in Southeast Asia and northern Australia. Clinical manifestations range from subclinical infections to overwhelming septicemia.[72] All but a few cases among residents of the United States have been associated with foreign travel.[73] It is estimated that 225,000 U.S. citizens of the total of 2.5 million who served in Vietnam may have acquired subclinical melioidosis.[72] In acute septicemic melioidosis the liver contains multiple small abscesses; bacilli can easily be recognized with special stains. They are gram-negative with bipolar staining. The lesions in chronic melioidosis are a combination of necrosis and granulomatous inflammation.[74, 75] The central area of the larger lesions usually consists of a purulent exudate surrounded by a granulomatous reaction with macrophage or epithelioid cells, giant cells, proliferating fibroblasts, and collagen deposition (Fig 9). Bacteria are difficult to identify in the chronic lesions.

YERSINIOSIS.—*Yersinia enterocolitica* infections lead to enterocolitis or to fever and pain in the right upper quadrant secondary to terminal ileitis or mesenteric adenitis. Extraintestinal manifestations include arthritis, erythema nodosum, and hepatic involvement. Half of the patients with septicemia have jaundice. Hepatic abscesses occur in some of these patients.[76] A granulomatous hepatitis has been reported in both acute[77] and chronic[78] infections (Fig 10). Patients with iron-overload states are predisposed to infection with *Y. enterocolitica*.[79]

BRUCELLOSIS.—Granulomas in the liver are a frequent finding in infections with *Brucella abortus* and *Brucella melitensis* in both the acute and chronic forms of the disease.[80-85] More granulomas apparently occur in chronic infections (100%) than in acute infections (60%).[82] There is general agreement that the granulomas are noncaseating and resemble those seen in sarcoidosis. In addition to the granulomas, various nonspecific changes have been observed in brucellosis, including focal necrosis, Kupffer cell hypertrophy, and portal area inflammation. Brucellosis may also rarely lead to hepatic abscess formation.[86, 87]

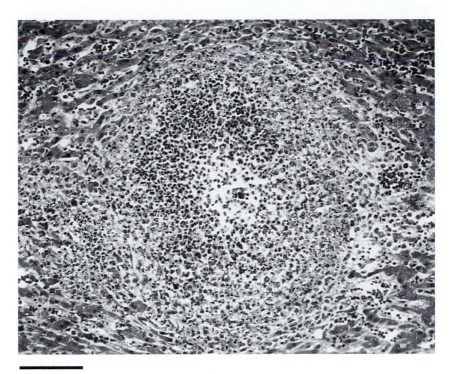

FIGURE 9.
Subacute melioidosis. An abscess has an organized granulomatoid periphery (HE, ×160).

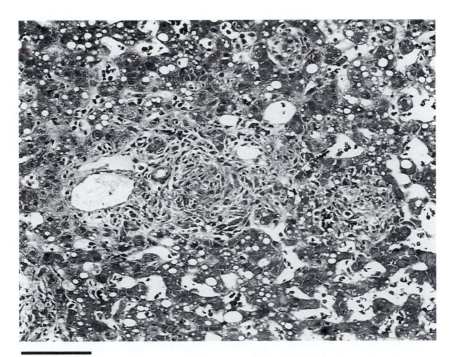

FIGURE 10.
Yersiniosis with several small epithelioid granulomas (HE, ×200).

TYPHOID FEVER.—The liver is almost always involved in typhoid fever, but overt liver disease is uncommon.[88–97] In one series, hepatic dysfunction occurred in 55%, but jaundice was noted in only 8% of the cases.[95] In the series of Morganstern and Hayes,[96] liver test abnormalities were found in 100% of the patients. Histologic lesions include marked Kupffer cell hypertrophy and hyperplasia, the latter forming so-called typhoid nodules, which may undergo necrosis[89, 93, 97] (Fig 11). Granulomas have been observed rarely.[91, 92] Other lesions include focal necrosis, rare sinusoidal acidophilic bodies, and very mild patchy portal inflammation. *Salmonella typhi* is a rare cause of hepatic abscess.[98]

LISTERIOSIS.—Hepatic involvement in this disease is characterized by focal necrosis and microabscess or abscess formation. In neonatal listeriosis, some of the lesions may appear granulomatoid or even granulomatous; the granulomas are either macrophagic or epithelioid and contain lymphocytes, but giant cells are not seen (Fig 12).[99] The causative organism, *Listeria monocytogenes*, can be identified in the liver and other organs as a gram-positive pleomorphic rod (Fig 13). An acute listerial hepatitis has been reported in several adult patients, one of whom was a liver transplant recipient.[100, 101] Hepatic abscess is also a recognized complication of listeriosis.[102–104] Several reviews of listeriosis are recommended for further reading.[105–107]

TULAREMIA.—Hepatic involvement occurs in the majority of cases.[108–111] Grossly, the lesions are grayish yellow and average 1 to 2 mm in diameter. Microscopically, acute lesions consist of small focal necroses infil-

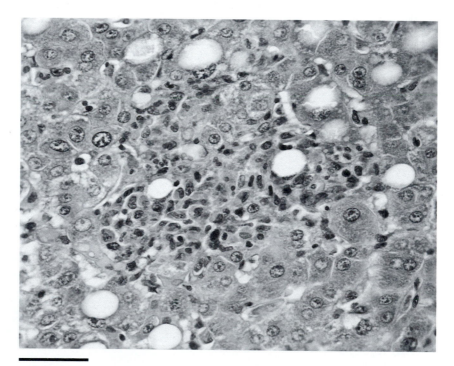

FIGURE 11.

Typhoid fever. A typhoid nodule consists of an organized cluster of histiocytes (HE, ×250).

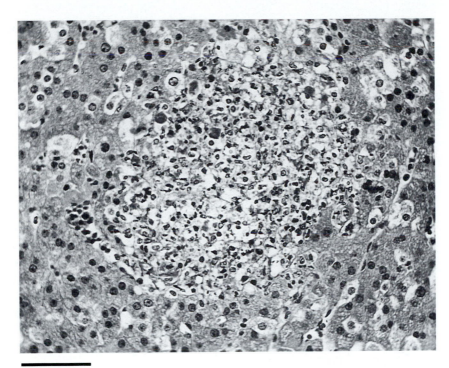

FIGURE 12.
Neonatal listeriosis: microabscess with a vague granulomatoid appearance (HE, ×245).

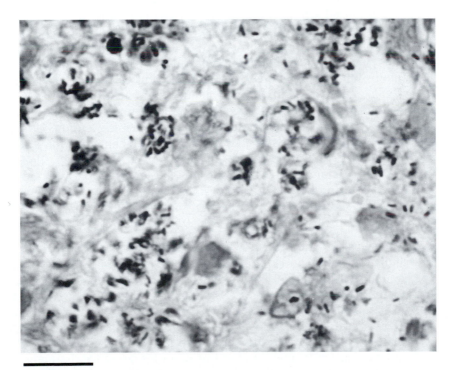

FIGURE 13.
Neonatal listeriosis: numerous pleomorphic gram-positive rods in the focus of necrosis (Brown and Brenn, ×1,500).

trated by neutrophils. In subacute cases, centrally suppurative lesions are surrounded by a layer of epithelioid cells and fibroblasts in a radial arrangement and a peripheral zone of lymphocytes, among which are scattered a few giant cells.[110] A cholestatic hepatitis with focal coagulative necrosis was reported by Ortego et al.[112]

BOTRYOMYCOSIS.—This chronic suppurative inflammation of the skin, or less often the viscera, is also referred to as "bacterial pseudomycosis." It is characterized by a purulent center containing structures resembling actinomycotic granules, as well as a peripheral granulomatous response.[113, 114] Although the causative agent is usually a staphylococcus, other bacteria such as streptococci, Escherichia coli, Proteus vulgaris, and Pseudomonas species have been incriminated.

In HE-stained sections, the granules in the abscess cavities are indistinguishable from those of actinomycosis and may display peripheral clubbing (Splendore-Hoeppli phenomenon).[21] Special stains can serve to distinguish the botryomycotic from actinomycotic granules, in particular, tissue Gram stains that reveal cocci or gram-negative bacilli, respectively. The central abscess cavities are usually walled off by granulation tissue that may also have a granulomatous component with ill-defined collections of epithelioid cells and giant cells of the foreign body or even Langhans' type.

ACTINOMYCOSIS.—Infection in man is usually caused by Actinomyces israelii.[115-120] The liver is involved in almost 20% of cases of abdominal actinomycosis. The infectious agent reaches the liver from the intestine via the portal vein. The resultant abscess is usually single, but multiple abscesses may develop. Microscopically, the abscess has a fibrous wall with proliferating fibroblasts and capillaries, foamy macrophages, lymphocytes, plasma cells, and neutrophils (Fig 14). A granulomatous response with foreign body or Langhans' giant cells may be seen peripherally. The abscess is filled with pus in which actinomycotic granules can be identified (see Fig 14). The granules are round to oval and basophilic, except for an eosinophilic clubbed periphery (Splendore-Hoeppli phenomenon) (Fig 15). Each granule, which represents a colony of A. israelii, is composed of an intertwined mass of gram-positive filaments (Fig 16). The filaments are also intensely stained with periodic acid–Schiff (PAS) and Gomori methenamine stain (GMS). Detailed descriptions of the granules and their staining reactions are provided by Brown[119] and Hotchi and Schwartz.[120]

NOCARDIOSIS.—The liver may be involved in nocardiosis, but other organs such as the brain and kidneys are more frequently affected when extrapulmonary dissemination occurs.[121] The majority of infections affect immunocompromised hosts.[121-124] Organisms lodging in the liver lead to the formation of abscesses that may become walled off; a granulomatous response is less frequent. Nocardia asteroides has delicate branched filaments that are gram-positive and acid-fast. The property of acid-fastness and the lack of formation of sulfur granules serve to distinguish the visceral lesions of nocardiosis from those of actinomycosis.[125]

It is appropriate to point out at this juncture that bacterial infections

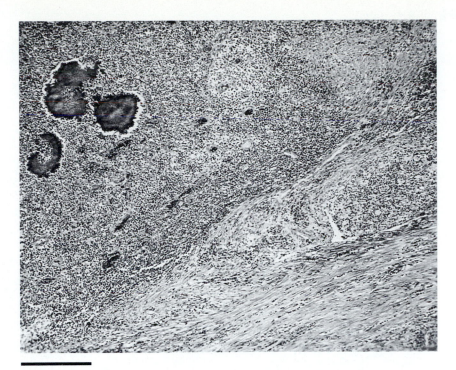

FIGURE 14.
Actinomycosis with a segment of the actinomycotic abscess containing typical granules *(top left)* suspended in pus. Note the fibrous wall with xanthomatous cells. Some foreign body giant cells (not shown) were also present (HE, ×60).

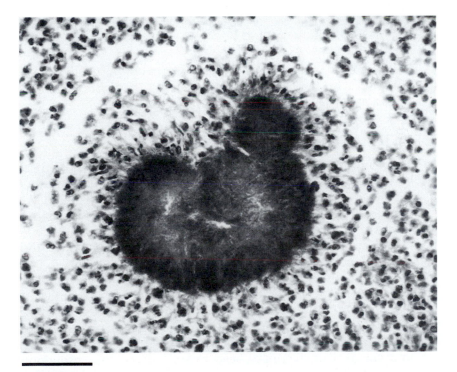

FIGURE 15.
Actinomycosis. A granule with a felt-like structure and a clubbed periphery is surrounded by pus cells (HE, ×400).

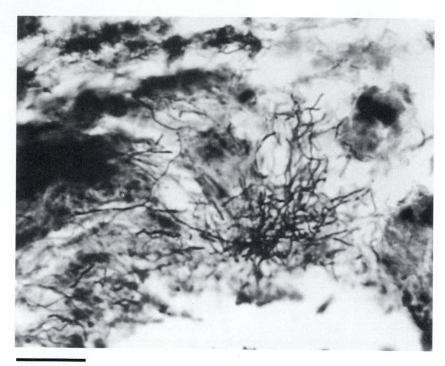

FIGURE 16.

Actinomycosis. The granule consists of intertwined gram-positive filaments (Brown and Brenn, ×1,100).

have not been incriminated in the induction of fibrin ring granulomas in the liver, with the exception of one case of *Staphylococcus epidermidis* sepsis.[126]

MYCOBACTERIAL DISEASES

TUBERCULOSIS.—Worldwide there are an estimated 7.5 million cases of tuberculosis, with 2.5 million yearly deaths.[127] The highest prevalence and estimated annual risk of tuberculosis are in sub-Saharan Africa and Southeast Asia.[127] The increase in the number of tuberculosis cases, particularly in Africa, is being caused by AIDS. If worldwide control of tuberculosis does not improve, 90 million new cases and 30 million deaths are to be expected in the decade 1990 through 1999.[127]

Hepatic tuberculosis caused by *Mycobacterium tuberculosis* has been classified into five types: primary acute pulmonary tuberculosis with liver involvement, miliary tuberculosis, "primary" tuberculosis, tuberculoma (conglomerate granuloma), and chronic pulmonary tuberculosis with liver involvement.[128] Grossly, conglomerate tuberculomas (larger than 2 to 3 cm in diameter) have been called "tuberculous pseudotumors" or "macronodular tuberculosis."[129–135] Rupture of tuberculomas into the bile ducts can lead to tuberculous cholangitis, also referred to as "tubular tuberculosis" of the liver in the past.[136] However, extensive involvement of the intrahepatic bile ducts has also been reported in a case of miliary tuberculosis.[137] Imaging studies of that case revealed saccular dilatation of the bile ducts with areas of stenosis and narrowed intrahepatic bile ducts. Tuberculosis of the common hepatic duct has also been reported.[138] Tuberculous involvement of hepatic hilar or peripancreatic lymph nodes can lead to obstructive jaundice.[139-142] It should be remembered that miliary tuberculosis can also be manifested by jaundice and hepatic failure.[143-147]

There has been marked variation in the reported incidence of hepatic granulomas in tuberculosis. Although a number of factors are undoubtedly responsible, the most important one is probably the type of involvement. Thus, Klatskin[38] found that whereas the incidence of granulomas is close to 100% in acute miliary tuberculosis and in "primary" miliary tuberculosis, it is near 50% in other forms of the disease. In a recent series of 109 cases of miliary tuberculosis from South Africa, granulomas were found in 100% of hepatic biopsy specimens.[148]

Granulomas in hepatic tuberculosis resemble those occurring in other organs. They are composed of epithelioid cells, variable numbers of Langhans' giant cells, and an outer rim of lymphocytes and histiocytes (Figs 17 and 18). Healing is associated with fibrosis and sometimes calcification. Fibrillogranular necrosis (caseation) is less often seen in biopsy (29%) than in autopsy (78%) material, probably because of better sampling and greater severity of the disease in the latter (Fig 19).[3] For the same reason, acid-fast bacilli are more frequently found in autopsy (31%) than in biopsy (13%) material (Fig 20).[3] Polymerase chain reaction has been found useful in detecting mycobacterial DNA in paraffin-embedded

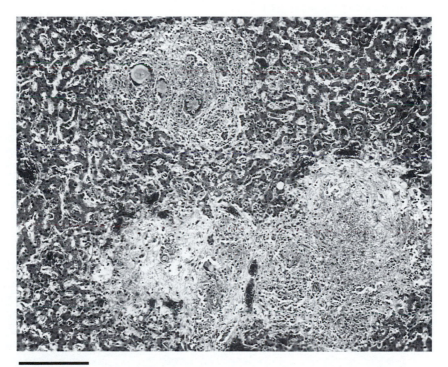

FIGURE 17.
Miliary tuberculosis with three granulomas, one of which *(top)* contains Langhans' giant cells (HE, ×100).

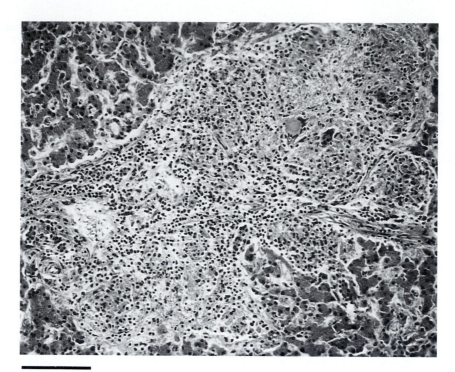

FIGURE 18.
Miliary tuberculosis with confluent granulomas surrounded by a mononuclear inflammatory response (HE, ×160).

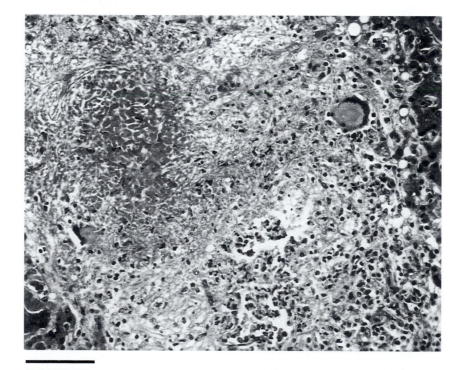

FIGURE 19.
Miliary tuberculosis with fibrillogranular (caseation) necrosis in the center of a tuberculoma. Note the Langhans' giant cell (HE, ×250).

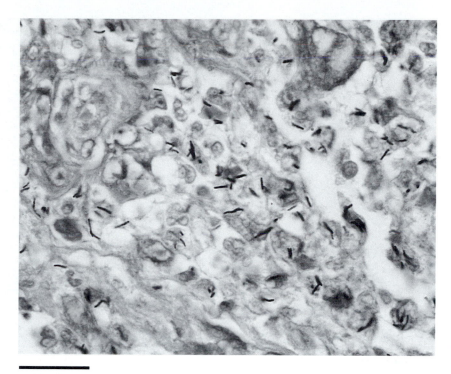

FIGURE 20.

Miliary tuberculosis with tubercle bacilli in the necrotic center of a tuberculoma (Kinyoun stain, ×1,500).

tissues from patients with tuberculosis (with acid-fast–negative histology).[149] In addition to granulomas (with or without necrosis), the morphologic expression of hepatic tuberculosis includes tuberculomas (formed by the confluence of multiple granulomas with a central cavity filled with necrotic material) and, rarely, tuberculous cholangitis, which is characterized by granulomatous inflammation and destruction of the intrahepatic bile ducts (Fig 21). Nonspecific changes such as focal necrosis, apoptotic bodies, and focal hypertrophy and hyperplasia of Kupffer cells are also frequent findings in extrapulmonary tuberculosis.[150, 151]

ATYPICAL MYCOBACTERIOSES.—The bacillus most frequently reported in cases with hepatic involvement has been MAI, which is particularly frequent in disseminated infections in patients with AIDS. Studies of the cumulative incidence of disseminated MAI infection have indicated that it occurs in 15% to 24% of patients with AIDS.[152] The frequency of hepatic involvement in two series was 46% and 57%.[153, 154] Histopathologic features have been described in many reports.[153–157] Hundreds of bacilli are present in granulomatoid aggregates of hypertrophied Kupffer cells and portal macrophages (macrophagic granulomas); they excite very little if any inflammatory response (Fig 22). The inability of patients with AIDS to respond effectively to MAI infection may be related to the recent finding that coinfection of monocytoid cells with human immunodeficiency virus (HIV) and MAI in vitro results in reciprocal enhancement of multiplication.[158] The cells containing the MAI organisms are granular and basophilic in HE-stained sections. They are GMS-positive and PAS-positive,

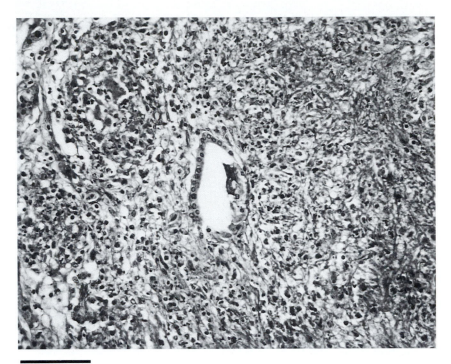

FIGURE 21.
Miliary tuberculosis. An interlobular bile duct in the center of a granuloma is undergoing necrosis (HE, ×250).

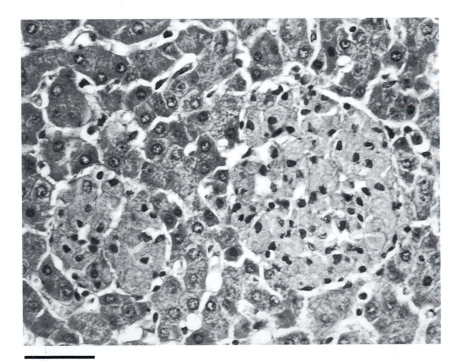

FIGURE 22.
Mycobacterium avium-intracellulare infection. Two granulomas are composed of clusters of hypertrophied macrophages. Note the absence of inflammatory response or necrosis (HE, ×400).

in addition to being acid-fast (Fig 23).[159] Patients with MAI infection who are not immunocompromised have noncaseating epithelioid granulomas resembling those seen in tuberculosis; only two thirds of the granulomas in these patients contain acid-fast bacilli.[155]

A pseudosarcomatous "histoid" variant of MAI infection with nodule formation has been reported in the liver of children with AIDS.[160]

Disseminated infections with atypical mycobacteria other than MAI have been reported in immunocompromised patients. Those in which specific mention of hepatic involvement has been noted include infections by *Mycobacterium kansasii*,[161, 162] *Mycobacterium xenopi*,[163] *Mycobacterium scrofulaceum*,[164] *Mycobacterium genavense*,[165, 166] and Battey bacillus.[167] For further information on the atypical mycobacterioses and associated diseases the reader is referred to several reviews.[166–170]

INFECTIONS WITH BACILLUS CALMETTE-GUÉRIN.—Disseminated lesions have been reported to follow either bacillus Calmette-Guérin (BCG) vaccination (including vaccinated AIDS patients) or immunotherapy[171–194] or occur rarely after intravesical instillation.[195, 196] Lesions complicating vaccination occur at a rate of 0.72 per million vaccinated. Most of the severe disseminated cases have been fatal, and many have occurred in patients with altered immune states such as severe combined immunodeficiency, chronic granulomatous disease, or AIDS.

Epithelioid granulomas are found in the liver in the majority of disseminated BCG infections, whether resulting from vaccination or cancer-immunotherapy (Fig 24). Acid-fast bacilli have been identified in some

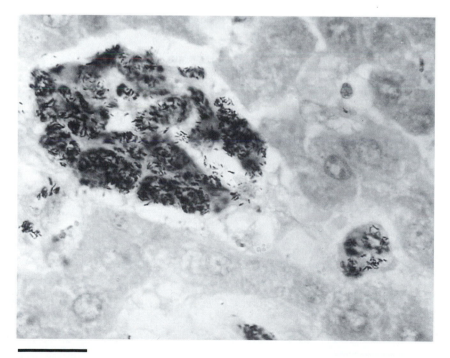

FIGURE 23.

Mycobacterium avium-intracellulare infection. Hundreds of acid-fast bacilli are present in the macrophagic granulomas (Kinyoun stain, ×1,000).

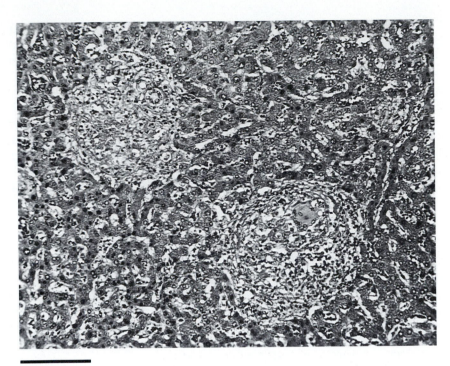

FIGURE 24.
Bacillus Calmette-Guérin (BCG) infection with two epithelioid granulomas (HE, ×120).

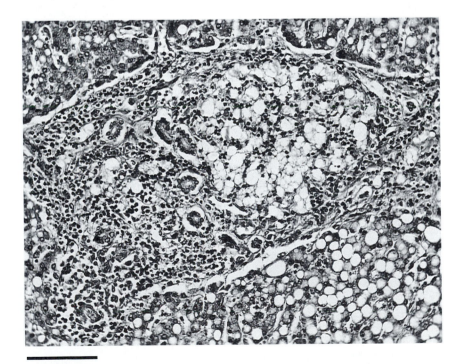

FIGURE 25.
Lepromatous leprosy. This well-defined granuloma in a portal area is composed of vacuolated cells (HE, ×195).

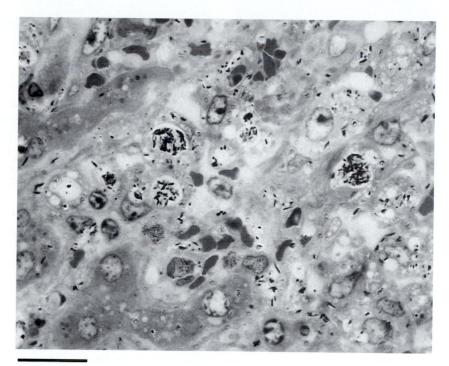

FIGURE 26.

Lepromatous leprosy. Small, acid-fast lepra bacilli are present in hypertrophied Kupffer cells (Kinyoun stain, ×1,000).

cases but not in others. Cultures, when reported, have been either negative or positive.

LEPROSY.—Estimates of involvement of the liver in biopsy material vary from 60% to 90% in lepromatous leprosy to about 20% in tuberculoid leprosy. Lesions in the liver in the two principal types resemble those in other sites.[197–201] In *lepromatous leprosy* there are multiple, varying-sized clusters of hypertrophied Kupffer cells or portal macrophages with a foamy cytoplasm; they contain numerous acid-fast lepra bacilli *(Mycobacterium leprae)* (Fig 25). Single Kupffer cells loaded with the bacilli are also frequently seen (Fig 26). The histiocytic nodules are located within the acini as well as in portal areas.

The hepatic lesions in tuberculoid leprosy consist of epithelioid cells, with or without Langhans' giant cells, and a variable cuff of lymphocytes. Bacilli are absent or found infrequently. Lepra bacilli were demonstrated immunohistochemically in 50% of skin biopsy samples that were acid-fast–negative in a series of 56 patients with early leprosy,[202] but the method has not been applied to liver biopsy tissue. Other sensitive techniques such as in situ hybridization and PCR have been used to identify lepra bacilli in skin specimens.[203]

SPIROCHETAL DISEASES

SYPHILIS.—Hepatic involvement occurs in all stages of syphilis. Congenital syphilis leads to a diffuse hepatitis without the formation of granulomas.[204] Healing results in diffuse intra-acinar fibrosis; microgummas may be present in this stage of the disease. Giant cell hepatitis has been reported after treatment.[205]

The incidence of involvement of the liver in early acquired syphilis is unknown. Granulomas resembling those of tuberculosis or sarcoidosis were found in hepatic biopsy specimens from four patients with secondary and one patient with tertiary syphilis by Wagoner et al.[71] Two other cases were mentioned by Frank and Raffensperger,[206] who also referred to earlier published examples. Histologic changes in subsequently reported cases have included portal inflammation, usually with a predominance of neutrophils, and focal necrosis.[207-216] Infiltration of portal connective tissue near bile ducts by neutrophils ("pericholangitis") was observed in some cases,[208, 209, 211] whereas an actual cholangitis with bile duct damage was noted in one case.[212] Vasculitis was described in the cases of Feher et al.[210] and the patient reported by Romeu et al.[212] These investigators and others identified spirochetes in liver biopsy specimens.

The gumma is the hallmark of late syphilis.[217-219] Gummas are more frequently multiple than single and can measure up to 6 cm in diameter. They have a center of coagulative necrosis and, as healing progresses, a fibrous wall of varying thickness that is infiltrated by many inflammatory cells (plasma cells, lymphocytes, histiocytes) and scattered granulomas; syphilitic vascular lesions are frequently observed in the wall of active gummas. Spirochetes are either absent or identified with difficulty. Calcification may be present and, when marked, may simulate a hydatid cyst.[219] Healing of the gummas leads to hepar lobatum, whereas healing of gummas in the porta hepatis can cause portal hypertension.[219] Reviews of syphilitic involvement of the liver by Davies[219] and Veeravahu[220] are recommended for further reading.

LYME DISEASE.—Hepatic granulomas have been reported in experimental infections of mice with severe combined immunodeficiency inoculated with *Borrelia burgdorferi*.[221] A liver biopsy specimen from a patient with recurrent Lyme disease revealed necroinflammatory changes but no granulomas.[222]

MYCOTIC INFECTIONS

CANDIDIASIS.—Involvement of the liver in systemic candidiasis in reported series has varied from less than 10% to over 75%.[223-228] This variability may be related to the underlying condition, as was clearly shown in the study of Myerowitz et al.[226] in which the liver was involved in 75% of patients with acute leukemia as compared with 17% of patients with other diseases (e.g., after abdominal surgery). In addition to involvement of the liver there have been reports of candidiasis of the extrahepatic bile ducts (including the gallbladder), often with obstructive jaundice.[229-231]

Candida in the liver may excite little or no reaction, particularly in a granulocytopenic patient. The lesions appear as radially arranged waves of pseudohyphae associated with hemorrhagic necrosis of the advancing edge and little or no inflammation. In some patients the fungus may lead to the formation of microabscesses, with or without a palisaded granulomatous periphery.[227, 228] Granulomas are generally considered to occur infrequently.[122, 225]

Candida in tissue sections is best demonstrated with the GMS, Gridley, and PAS stains, although the organisms can be seen in HE-stained sections. The blastospores are 3 to 5 μm in diameter and often show budding or the formation of pseudohyphae.

CRYPTOCOCCOSIS.—This infectious disease is caused by *Cryptococcus neoformans*. The majority of infected persons have no immunologic defect or underlying disease. Predisposing factors include lymphoreticular malignancies, collagen vascular diseases, diabetes mellitus, therapy with corticosteroid or cytotoxic drugs, and AIDS.[232–239] The incidence of this infection in AIDS is 7%, with half of the patients having disseminated disease.[238, 239] The capsular polysaccharide of the organism is believed to enhance HIV infection.[240] The primary portal of entry of *C. neoformans* is usually the lung, where the disease may localize, or there may be widespread dissemination, especially to the central nervous system. "Primary" hepatic cryptococcosis, possibly resulting from infection via the oral route, has been reported.[241] Other cases of cryptococcal "hepatitis" with hepatic failure or features mimicking primary sclerosing cholangitis have been reported.[242–244] The tissue response to invasion by cryptococci is either gelatinous or granulomatous.[234, 245] There may be microabscess formation, or the fungal spores may be phagocytosed by Kupffer cells and portal macrophages. The gelatinous foci consist of cystic areas packed with fungal spores; the spores are initially located in macrophages but later become extracellular (Fig. 27). The foci in the liver are generally smaller than the size of an acinus, but large confluent areas of necrosis have been observed. The cryptococci are colorless or faintly stained by HE; they are spherical to oval and measure 4 to 7 μm in diameter. Budding may be seen. A clear halo surrounding the organisms corresponds to a thick mucinous capsule that is stained positively by PAS, mucicarmine, Alcian blue, or colloidal iron (Fig. 28). Granulomas induced by cryptococci contain only a few organisms.

ASPERGILLOSIS.—Clinical evidence of hepatic involvement in disseminated aspergillosis is rare.[246, 247] In the series of Young et al.,[246] 12 of 78 patients had tender hepatomegaly, and 3 were jaundiced or had marked liver test abnormalities. Lesions in the liver were found in 25% to 35% of autopsy cases. Invasion of the liver is associated with the formation of miliary abscesses 0.5 to 1.0 cm in diameter; microscopically, the abscesses are filled with the fungus. Granuloma formation is exceptionally rare. Some patients may have widespread hepatocellular damage from abscess formation and infarction as a result of vascular invasion. Invasion of the hepatic veins may lead to the Budd-Chiari syndrome.[248] The hyphae of *Aspergillus* are 3 to 4 μm in diameter and reveal dichotomous branching and septae.

MUCORMYCOSIS.—This disease is caused by fungi belonging to genera within the taxonomic order Mucorales, usually *Rhizopus, Absidia, Mortierella,* and *Mucor.* Ketoacidotic diabetes are susceptible to pulmonary or disseminated infections.[249] The liver is infrequently involved in dis-

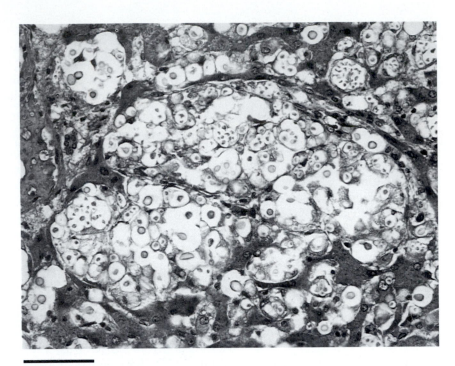

FIGURE 27.
Cryptococcosis: gelatinous focus in the liver of an AIDS patient with disseminated infection. Fungal spores surrounded by lytic spaces have excited no inflammatory response (HE, ×300).

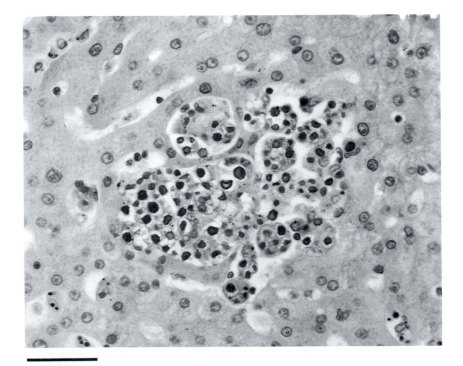

FIGURE 28.
Cryptococcosis. The capsule of the fungal spores is carminophilic (mucicarmine, ×400).

seminated mucormycosis.[249, 250] In one literature survey of 57 cases, only 5 disclosed hepatic lesions.[249] The fungi usually involve vessels in the liver and may lead to necrosis or infarction.[251] Granulomas have not been reported in the liver, although they are occasionally seen in chronic infections in other sites.[122] The fungal hyphae are broad (10 to 15 μm in diameter), appear distorted or twisted, and exhibit infrequent septation and haphazard branching.

HISTOPLASMOSIS.—In most countries this disease is caused by *Histoplasma capsulatum*, but African histoplasmosis is due to infection by *Histoplasma duboisii*.

The majority of human infections in normal hosts are asymptomatic.[252] The lung is primarily affected, but severe infection may lead to advanced lesions of the hilar lymph nodes and mediastinum.[252] Residua of the primary infection in endemic areas are discrete splenic and hepatic calcifications.[253] Disseminated histoplasmosis is rare and mainly affects patients who are immunocompromised,[254–256] including patients with AIDS.[257] Many of the disseminated cases are endogenous reinfections. Liver involvement is common in disseminated histoplasmosis. Histopathologic aspects of histoplasmosis are covered in the publications of Binford[258] and Schwartz.[259] *Histoplasma capsulatum* in tissue sections is round to ovoid with little variation in size (1 to 5 μm) and shows occasional budding. Atypical forms, including occasional hyphal elements, may occur. A halo often surrounds each organism, but there is no true capsule. While the organism can be seen in HE-stained sections (generally as a blue dot with a faintly stained oval envelope around it), special stains, particularly the GMS stain, should be performed in every case. Ultrastructural features of the fungus have been described by Dumont and Piché.[260]

In an immunologically virginal organism the tissue response to *H. capsulatum* is predominantly histiocytic. The histiocytes engulfing the organisms may remain interspersed within normal tissue elements or may excite a granulomatous reaction. When an immune response develops, there is fibrillogranular necrosis (caseation) and confluence of lesions. The three main types of active tissue response include (1) a large number of organisms in greatly hypertrophied Kupffer cells and portal macrophages with no associated inflammatory response; (2) scattered varying-sized epithelioid granulomas, with or without giant cells or necrosis (Figs 29 to 31); and (3) inconspicuous foci of necrosis (sometimes with a granulomatoid appearance) containing Kupffer cells with phagocytosed organisms. Occasional sinusoidal acidophilic bodies and variable degrees of portal inflammation are seen, particularly in the third type of hepatic involvement.[91] As noted earlier, the healed lesions of the primary infection may be noted on the surface of the liver and spleen at laparotomy or autopsy.[253] They consist of a globular or wedge-shaped mass of dense, hyalinized collagen with varying degrees of calcification; a few chronic inflammatory cells or isolated multinucleated giant cells may be seen at the periphery (Fig 32). Organisms are often demonstrable with the GMS stain, although they may be faintly stained (Fig 33).

In African histoplasmosis the tissue response is dominated by giant cells containing numerous fungi.[261, 262] The organisms are larger than those of *H. capsulatum* and have a diameter ranging from 8 to 15 μm.

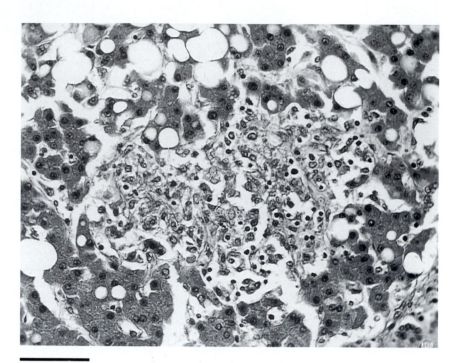

FIGURE 29.
Histoplasmosis with a granuloma composed of epithelioid cells (HE, ×245).

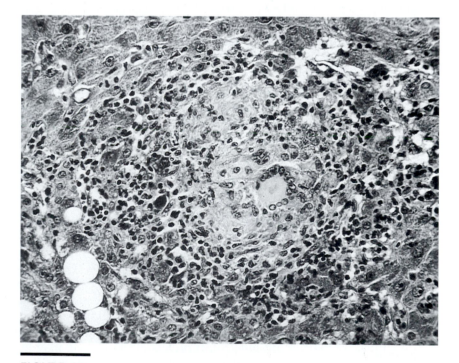

FIGURE 30.
Histoplasmosis with a granuloma containing a Langhans' giant cell surrounded
by epithelioid cells and a ring of mononuclear inflammatory cells (HE, ×300).

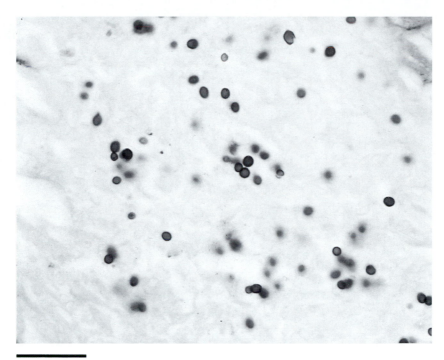

FIGURE 31.
Histoplasmosis. Fungal spores are small and round to ovoid. Note the occasional budding (Gomori methenamine silver, ×1,000).

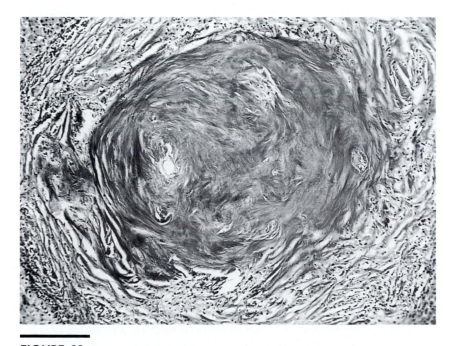

FIGURE 32.
Histoplasmosis. Granulomatous lesions have been replaced by a fibrous scar (HE, ×75).

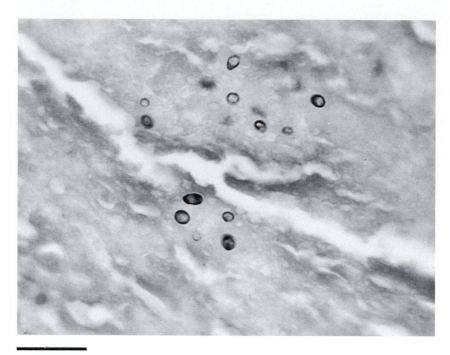

FIGURE 33.
Histoplasmosis: same case illustrated in Figure 32 but showing scattered *Histoplasma capsulatum* spores (Gomori methenamine silver, ×1,500).

NORTH AMERICAN BLASTOMYCOSIS.—The tissue response to *Blastomyces dermatitidis* is a combination of suppuration and an epithelioid cell granulomatous reaction with giant cells (Fig 34).[263, 264] Involvement of the liver and spleen occurs in only a few of the widely disseminated cases. The incidence of blastomycosis appears to be increased in patients with AIDS.[265] The organisms in the granulomas measure 8 to 15 μm in diameter and have a sharply defined, "doubly contoured" wall and several nuclei per cell (Fig 35). Budding may be identified in tissue sections.

PARACOCCIDIOIDOMYCOSIS.—This disease, also known as South American blastomycosis, is called by *Paracoccidioides brasiliensis*. Hepatic involvement occurs in about 57% of cases; in the majority the tissue response is granulomatous.[266] The fungal spores in the lesions in paracoccidioidomycosis vary from 5 to 60 μm in diameter and reproduce by single or multiple budding.

COCCIDIOIDOMYCOSIS.—This disease is caused by *Coccidioides immitis*. Infection occurs by inhalation of airborne arthrospores. Primary pulmonary infection is followed by dissemination in fewer than 10% of cases. Dissemination with frequent hepatic involvement has been reported in neonates,[267] children,[268] and the immunocompromised,[269] including patients with AIDS.[270, 271] Liver involvement in one series of disseminated coccidioidomycosis was 60%,[272] with diagnosis by liver biopsy in a number of cases.[273, 274] The lesions in the liver are granulomatous and contain histiocytes, epithelioid cells, giant cells of the Langhans' or foreign body type, and a variable number of mononuclear cells; fibrillogranular

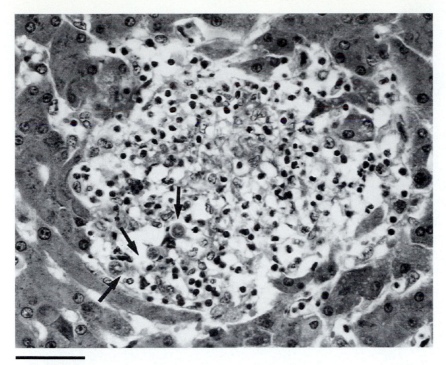

FIGURE 34.
North American blastomycosis with a granuloma composed of an admixture of epithelioid and inflammatory cells. Fungal spores are present (*arrows*) but not easily seen in this HE-stained section (×400).

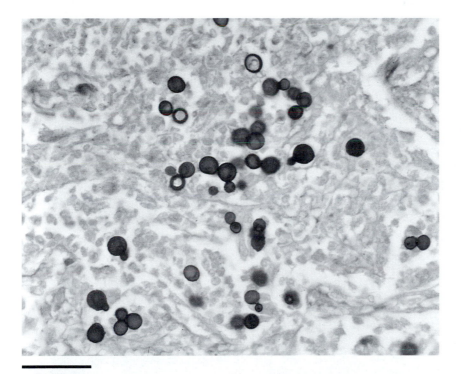

FIGURE 35.
North American blastomycosis: same case illustrated in Figure 34 but showing numerous fungal spores. Note the thick walls of the spores and budding (Gomori methenamine silver, ×400).

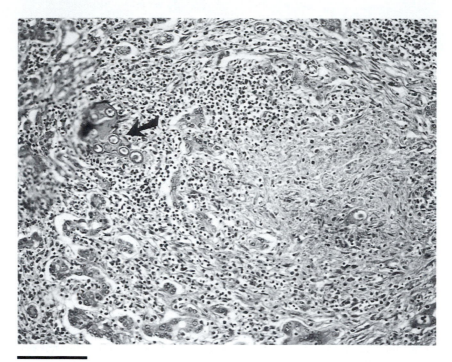

FIGURE 36.
Coccidioidomycosis: granuloma with central necrosis *(lower right)*. Note the giant cell with several fungal spores *(arrow)* (HE, ×160).

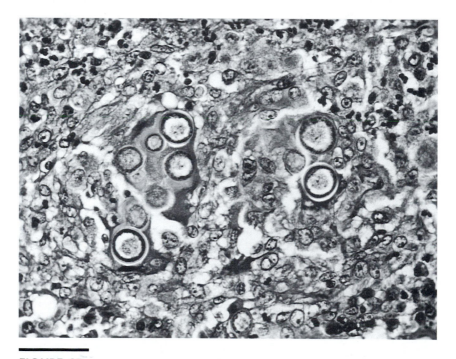

FIGURE 37.
Coccidioidomycosis. Fungal spores with a thick wall are present in a granuloma (PAS, ×485).

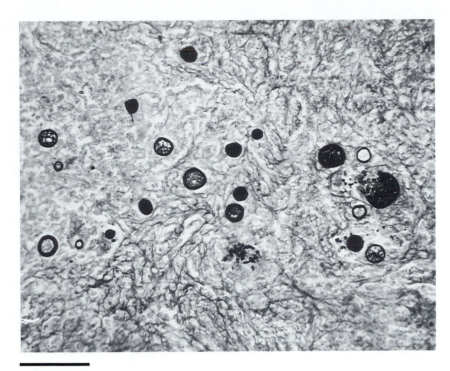

FIGURE 38.

Coccidioidomycosis. Sporangia and small sporangiospores are well demonstrated by the Gomori methenamine silver stain (×400).

necrosis may be present (Fig 36). The fungus can often be identified within the giant cells or the granulomas or, rarely, in Kupffer cells (Figs 36 to 38). Mature sporangia (30 to 60 μm in diameter) form by cleavage of spherules; they have a thick, double-contoured wall, and the surface may reveal the Splendore-Hoeppli phenomenon. Each sporangium contains numerous sporangiospores (endospores) with a diameter of 1 to 5 μm; these are released when the sporangium ruptures.

PROTOZOAL INFECTIONS

VISCERAL LEISHMANIASIS.—Visceral leishmaniasis (kala-azar) is a disseminated infection caused by *Leishmania donovani*. The disease is endemic in India and other countries in Asia, the Middle East and Mediterranean littoral, Africa, and South America. Seven cases of visceral leishmaniasis were reported among the approximately 500,000 military personnel from the United States who participated in Operation Desert Storm, 1990 to 1991.[275, 276] These soldiers did not have the classic signs and symptoms of visceral leishmaniasis. *Leishmania tropica*, which usually causes only cutaneous disease, was isolated from 6 patients.[276] Cases of visceral leishmaniasis have been reported in immunocompromised patients, including renal transplant recipients[277, 278] and patients with AIDS.[279–283] Hepatic involvement (hepatomegaly, abnormal liver tests) in this disease is frequent.[284] A chronic or relapsing course has been described in 42.5% of the patients with AIDS.[281] The reported incidence of jaundice has varied from 1.2% to 15%.[285, 286] Portal hypertension is rare.[287]

In all cases Kupffer cells and portal macrophages are markedly hypertrophied and full of parasitized Leishman-Donovan bodies or leishmanias (Fig 39).[284] Each organism measures 4 to 5 μm in diameter and has a dark blue nucleus (1 to 2 μm in diameter) and a dot-like or rod-shaped kinetoplast.[288] The organisms are well demonstrated in sections stained with Wilder's reticulum or Giemsa stains (Fig 40).[288] Granulomas in the liver have been reported by several investigators.[287, 289, 290] In one study they were found in the liver of patients who survived longer than 2 months after infection; they showed a central area of necrosis and mild fibrosis surrounded by plasma cells, lymphocytes, and macrophages.[289] Kupffer cells contained parasites only at the margins of the granulomas.[289] Epithelioid or giant cells were noted by one group of investigators.[290] Fibrin ring granulomas were reported by Moreno et al.[291] and Marazuela et al.[62] The ultrastructural appearance of the organisms has been described by Tanikawa and Hojiro[292] and by Daneshbod.[289] Fibrosis of terminal hepatic venules and pericellular fibrosis were reported in the series of El Hag et al.[293] A more diffuse fibrosis has also been observed in some cases.[284]

TOXOPLASMOSIS.—Toxoplasmosis in adults may occasionally involve the liver, with manifestations resembling those of infectious mononucleosis or viral hepatitis.[294, 295] Acute toxoplasmic hepatitis with extensive coagulative necrosis developed in one patient with AIDS.[296] Noncaseating granulomas have been described in two cases of acquired toxoplasmo-

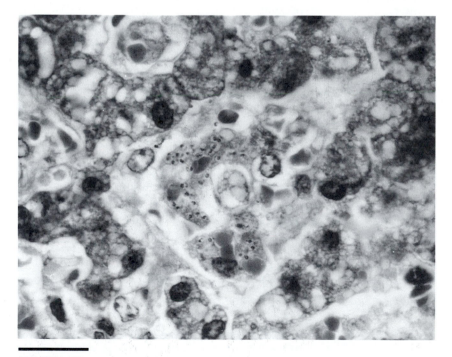

FIGURE 39.
Visceral leishmaniasis. A cluster of markedly hypertrophied Kupffer cells contain dot-like leishmaniae (HE, ×1,000).

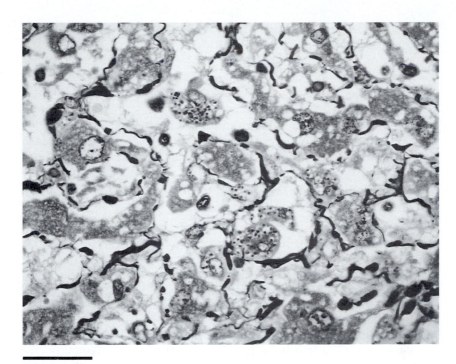

FIGURE 40.
Visceral leishmaniasis: same case illustrated in Figure 39. The hypertrophied Kupffer cells in sinusoids contain silvered dot-like leishmaniae (Wilders' reticulum stain, ×750).

sis.[297, 298] Neonatal toxoplasmosis is a generalized infection with encephalitis, pneumonia, and myocarditis. Liver involvement is characterized by areas of necrosis, giant cells, and extramedullary hematopoiesis.[299] Usually, no organisms are found in sections stained with HE or with Giemsa or Bodian stains, but they have been identified by immunohistopathologic methods[300, 301] or by PCR,[302] mostly in extrahepatic sites.

A useful model for studying disseminated toxoplasmosis in AIDS was recently reported in the nude rat infected with *Toxoplasma gondii*.[303] Macrophagic or epithelioid granulomas developed in the livers of some of the rats.

HELMINTHIC INFECTIONS

STRONGYLOIDIASIS.—Disseminated strongyloidiasis has been reported in immunocompromised patients, including those with AIDS.[304-310] In such patients the filariform larvae of *Strongyloides stercoralis* can circulate throughout the body and invade multiple organs and tissues, including the liver. The proximal segment of the small intestine and the lungs bear the heaviest parasite burden.[311] In the liver, larvae can be found in sinusoids and portal area vessels. Dead larvae may excite a focal inflammatory, or granulomatous response, with many eosinophils.[305-307, 310]

VISCERAL LARVA MIGRANS.—This syndrome, first reported by Beaver et al.,[311] is caused by the erratic visceral migration of helminth larvae for which humans are incidental hosts. Most of the cases are caused by the larvae of *Toxocara canis* and less often *Toxocara cati*. The hog ascaris

(*Ascaris suum*), *Capillaria hepatica,* and the raccoon ascarid (*Baylisas-caris procyonis*) may occasionally be the etiologic agent.[312, 313] The majority of cases occur in children between 18 months and 4 years of age. Infection results from ingestion of soil contaminated by infective eggs. Most of the patients are young children, and fever, hepatomegaly, respiratory symptoms, ocular and central nervous system disturbances, hypergammaglobulinemia, and eosinophila may be present.[311, 314–318] Diagnosis is established by enzyme-linked immunosorbent assay (ELISA) for serum antibodies to excretory-secretory antigens of toxocaral larvae.[319, 320]

Grossly, the lesions of visceral larva migrans consist of grayish white or tan nodules that vary in size from 0.1 to 1 cm or more in diameter. Microscopically, the initial exudative response to the larvae is primarily an outpouring of eosinophils, the abscess-like areas being haphazardly distributed. Larvae are rarely found except by serial sectioning. As the lesions get older, the periphery becomes granulomatous, with palisaded epithelioid cells and multinucleated giant cells forming a ring around the often confluent abscesses (Figs 41 and 42). The contents of the central abscesses then consist of structureless material (including keratin-like debris that may represent the molted skin of dead larvae), rare larvae (Fig 43), granules of eosinophils, and Charcot-Leyden crystals. The crystals are colorless or lightly eosinophilic and have a hexagonal or dipyramidal shape (Fig 44). Both the crystals and the granules of eosinophils are stained a bright red color by Luna's Biebrich scarlet stain (Fig 44). The crystals are also well visualized by scanning electron microscopy (Fig 45). In addition to eosinophils, other inflammatory cells (lymphocytes, plasma

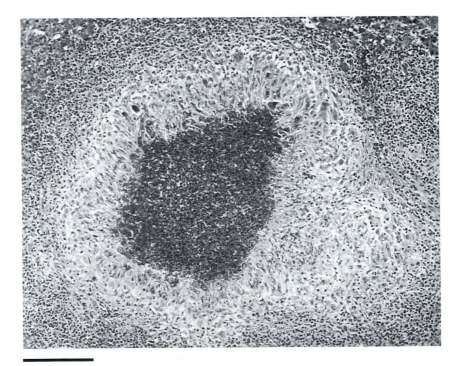

FIGURE 41.
Visceral larva migrans. A darkly stained central area of necrosis is surrounded by a granulomatous mantle (HE, ×100).

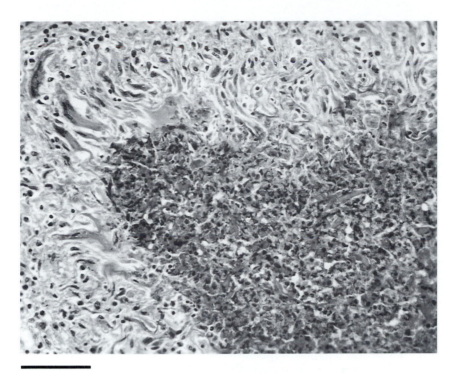

FIGURE 42.
Visceral larva migrans: same case illustrated in Figure 41. A segment of the lesion discloses a palisaded granulomatous periphery and an amorphous necrotic center (HE, ×160).

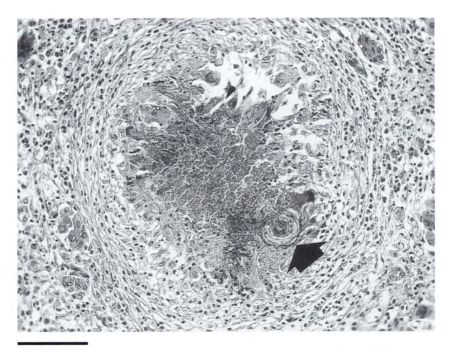

FIGURE 43.
Visceral larva migrans. A degenerating larva within a granuloma (*arrow*) was found in this case by serial sectioning (HE, ×165).

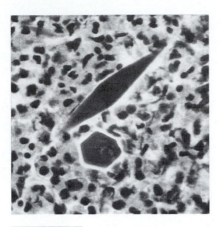

FIGURE 44.

Visceral larva migrans. Charcot-Leyden crystals have hexagonal or dipyramidal shapes (Biebrich scarlet stain, ×575).

cells) are noted in the granulomatous areas. Veins entrapped in the lesions often show a phlebitis with eosinophilic infiltration, and there may be an eosinophilic cholangitis. There is progressive proliferation of fibroblasts and collagen deposition as the lesions become older, eventually all that remain are focal scars (Fig 46).

CAPILLARIASIS.—Lesions in the liver are usually a reaction to the eggs of *C. hepatica,* but adult worms may also be found.[321–325] Lesions in the liver of mammals (mostly rodents) resemble those in humans.[326] They may contain recognizable parasites or their disintegrated remnants with an

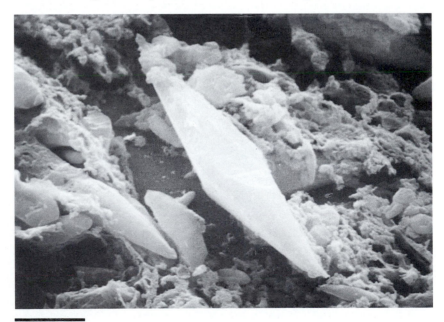

FIGURE 45.

Visceral larva migrans. The dipyramidal shape of a Charcot-Leyden crystal is well demonstrated in this scanning electron micrograph (×2,500).

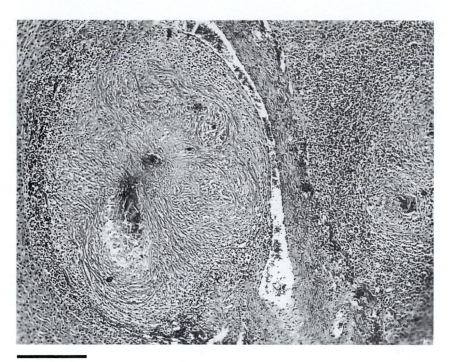

FIGURE 46.

Visceral larva migrans. This healing granuloma *(left)* is composed of fibrous tissue except for a small, darkly stained necrotic center. An active granuloma surrounded by many eosinophils is noted to the right (HE, ×70).

outpouring of eosinophils. Granulomas contain eggs resembling those of *Trichuris trichiura*, they measure 48 to 66 by 28 to 36 μm, are barrel-shaped, and have a double shell, and the outer shell is distinctly striated. Healing of granulomas can lead to extensive scarring. Intestinal capillariasis caused by *Capillaria philippinensis* can occasionally lead to migration of adult parasites into the liver, but a granulomatous response has not been observed.[327]

ASCARIASIS.—More than a quarter of the world's population is infected with *A. lumbricoides*.[328] Ascariasis is usually a benign disease, but migration of the adult worms into the biliary tract can lead to serious complications. Biliary ascariasis has been reported most frequently from China, South Africa, and India (see the review of Kamath[329]). Adult worms may migrate from the intestine into the ampulla of Vater and thence into the pancreatic ducts or the extrahepatic and intrahepatic bile ducts. There may be an associated bacterial cholangitis with severe suppuration and the formation of cholangitic abscesses, as well as a chronic cholangitis; other complications include acute pancreatitis, acute cholecystitis, pylephlebitis, and intrahepatic lithiasis[329–333] (Fig 47). Death of parasites trapped in the liver can lead to the release of many eggs, which then excite a granulomatous response. Fertilized ascaris eggs (45 to 75 by 35 to 50 μm) are round to ovoid and mamillated and may contain a dividing embryo. The shell is not birefringent or acid-fast but acquires a deep blue color in sections stained with Masson's trichrome stain (Fig

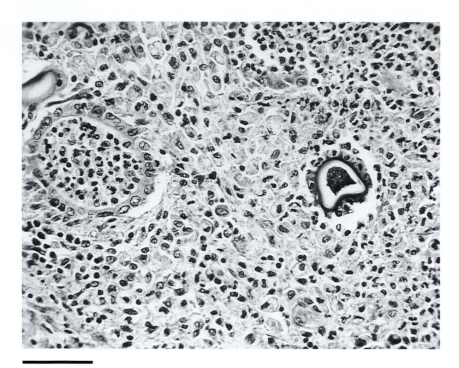

FIGURE 47.

Ascariasis with acute suppurative cholangitis *(left)*. One egg *(right)* is surrounded by xanthomatous cells and neutrophils (HE, ×300).

48). Unfertilized eggs are longer than the fertilized ones and have an irregular shape and a thin shell.

Chronic changes in the bile ducts in ascariasis resemble those of recurrent pyogenic cholangitis (Oriental cholangiohepatitis).[332, 334] In addition to intraductal stones there may be metaplastic and proliferative lesions such as pyloric and intestinal metaplasia, hyperplasia, adenomatous proliferation, and intraductal papillomas.[332, 334] Extensive fibroplasia can lead to portal-to-portal bridging fibrosis and even a secondary biliary cirrhosis.[334]

SCHISTOSOMIASIS.—Schistosomes are trematode blood flukes that infect over 200 million persons worldwide.[335] Five species infect humans, but two, *S. mansoni* and *S. japonicum*, are responsible for most cases of hepatosplenic schistosomiasis. The clinical, radiographic, and pathogenetic aspects and treatment of hepatosplenic schistosomiasis have been periodically reviewed[335–343] and will not be dwelled on because of the limitations of space.

Numerous contributions to the pathologic aspects of schistosomiasis, based on observations of human cases and experimentally infected animals, have been published over the past several decades. A number of reviews have summarized these contributions and are recommended for further reading.[344–350] Tissue injury in schistosomiasis is caused predominantly by eggs deposited in various organs. The eggs of *S. mansoni* (about 60 to 170 μm) have a large lateral spine, whereas those of *Schistosoma haematobium* (approximately the same size) have a pointed ter-

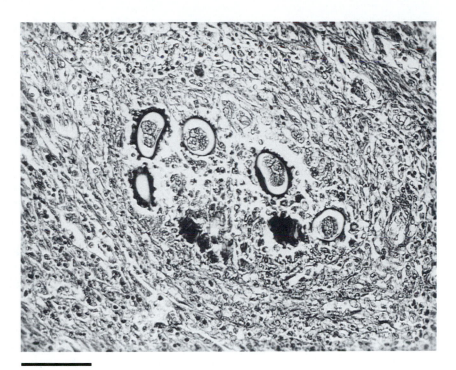

FIGURE 48.

Ascariasis. *Ascaris lumbricoides* eggs, neutrophils, and darkly stained, amorphous bile are present in a bile duct that has lost its epithelium. Note the periductal fibrosis and chronic inflammation. The ascaris eggs have a thick, knobby shell, and several contain dividing embryos (Masson, ×210).

minal spine. Eggs of S. *japonicum* (70 to 100 by 50 to 70 μm) have a small spine and an indistinct knob-like protuberance on the opposite end. Eggs that reach the liver lodge in the small intrahepatic portal vessels. The resultant granulomatous lesions and eventual development of chronic liver disease depend on the intensity of infection, the host immune response, and the schistosome species. Chronic hepatitis and cirrhosis caused by either hepatitis B virus or hepatitis C virus have been reported in a significant number of patients with schistosomiasis.[351–353] A possible synergistic role of schistosomiasis and hepatitis B infection in the induction of hepatocellular carcinoma in Japan has been postulated.[354]

The evolution of the host response to schistosome eggs in experimental animals has been divided into five stages[355]: (1) a nonreactive or weakly reactive stage when the egg is immature, at which time it gradually attracts mononuclear cells, neutrophils, and eosinophils; (2) an exudative stage when the egg matures and is surrounded by a microabscess, with many neutrophils and some eosinophils; (3) an exudative-productive stage when histiocytes and epithelioid cells surround the egg and microabscess and are in turn encircled by fibroblasts; (4) a productive stage in which the granuloma surrounding the egg consists of three zones—an inner zone of epithelioid cells, histiocytes, and occasional giant cells; a middle zone of fibroblasts; and an outer zone of lymphocytes, histiocytes, plasma cells, and sometimes eosinophils—and the miracidium may be alive or dead during this stage; and (5) an involutional stage in which the egg is reduced in size and the shell is surrounded by some collagen fibers; the egg is usually disintegrated and may be calcified.

Most of the experimentally produced stages just described can be seen in human biopsy or autopsy material (Figs 49 to 51). The eggs of S. *mansoni* and S. *japonicum* are acid-fast, a property useful in identifying small chitinous remnants that may be missed in sections stained with HE (Fig 52). Calcification of often intact eggs is characteristic of S. *japonicum* infections (Figs 53 to 56).

Descriptions of vascular lesions in hepatic schistosomiasis in humans have included obstruction by granulomas, sclerotic narrowing, and thrombophlebitis.[356] Experimental studies have subsequently confirmed and extended these studies.[357, 358] Obliteration of many of the intrahepatic portal vein branches leads to the formation of new vessels ("angiomatoids") in portal areas, a compensatory phenomenon[359–361] (Fig 57).

Intrahepatic bile duct lesions were found in 55.3% of cases of hepatosplenic schistosomiasis mansoni by Vianna et al.[362] They included epithelial hyperplasia and various patterns of mucopolysaccharide production.

The portal and septal fibrosis in advanced schistosomiasis is characterized by a complex matrix with marked hyperplasia of connective tissue, several collagen isotypes (I, III, procollagen III, IV, and V), actin, desmin, fibronectin, and laminin in a richly vascularized connective tissue.[363] Capillarization of sinusoids has been described in chronic schistosomiasis mansoni.[364] A highly characteristic type of fibrosis resembling pipestems ("pipestem cirrhosis") was described many years ago by Sym-

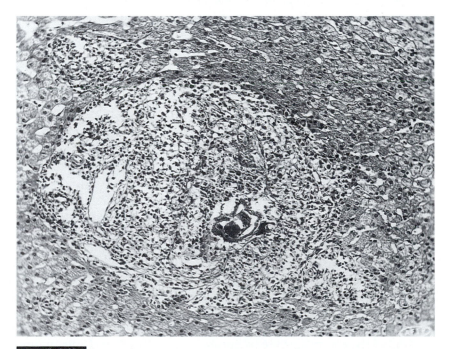

FIGURE 49.

Schistosomiasis mansoni. A cross section of crumpled egg is present in a young, loosely structured granuloma (HE, ×145).

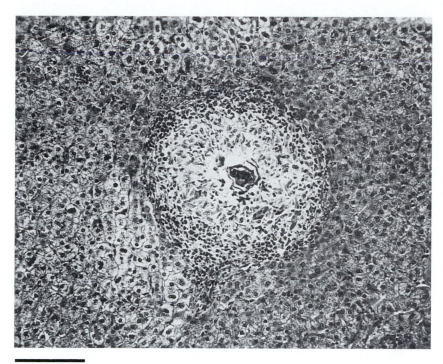

FIGURE 50.

Schistosomiasis mansoni. Epithelioid cells and a ring of eosinophils surround an egg (HE, ×160).

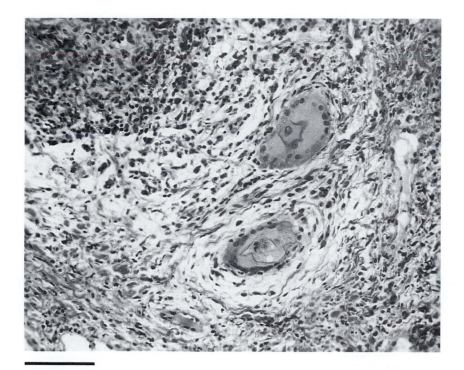

FIGURE 51.

Schistosomiasis mansoni. Residual Langhans' giant cells contain chitinous remnants of schistosome eggs (HE, ×250).

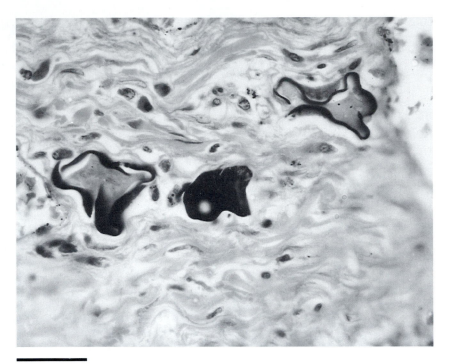

FIGURE 52.
Schistosomiasis mansoni. Chitinous remnants of eggs *(black)* embedded in fibrous tissue are acid-fast (Kinyoun stain, ×630).

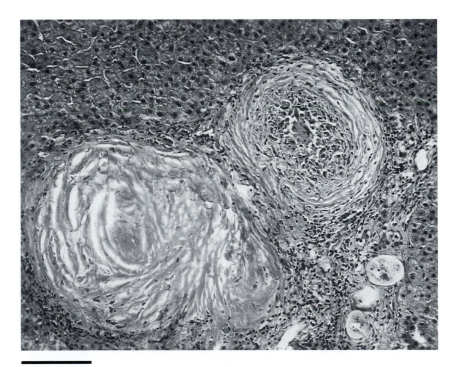

FIGURE 53.
Schistosomiasis japonica. One granuloma *(top right)* is surrounded by a fibrous capsule, whereas the other *(lower left)* is completely replaced by a fibrous scar. Note the eggs in *lower right* corner (HE, ×160).

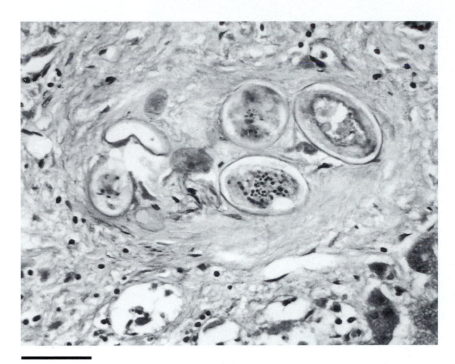

FIGURE 54.

Schistosomiasis japonica. Calcified eggs, some intact and others distorted, are embedded in dense fibrous tissue (HE, ×400).

mers[365] (Fig 58). On the basis of experimental studies in mice, Warren[366] determined that it resulted from the formation of fibrotic bands derived from residual collagen originating about granulomas. Of interest is the recent report of a unique case of hepar lobatum in a patient with advanced schistosomiasis.[367]

Schistosomal pigment accumulation in the reticuloendothelial cells of the liver is a frequent finding in hepatosplenic schistosomiasis, both human and experimental.[368, 369] The pigment is a breakdown product of the hemoglobin of red cells ingested and then regurgitated by adult schistosome worms; it can be seen in the gastrointestinal tract of sections of the worms. In the liver it can be identified in Kupffer cells, portal macrophages, and phagocytic cells entrapped in the granulomas (Fig 59). It is finely granular, dark brown, and birefringent. Ultrastructurally, the pigment is composed of dense ovoid and doughnut-shaped structures that are intensely osmiophilic.[368] Although it resembles malarial pigment histopathologically, it differs from that pigment both chemically and ultrastructurally.[370]

FASCIOLIASIS.—This disease is caused by the liver fluke *F. hepatica*. It is endemic in South America, Puerto Rico, Africa, China, and Australia. Patients with fascioliasis diagnosed in this country have usually acquired the infection by travel to an endemic area.[371] Humans, who are accidental hosts, acquire the infection by ingesting metacercariae on water plants. These penetrate the intestinal wall, migrate into the peritoneal cavity, and penetrate Glisson's capsule to enter the liver. After gaining access to the

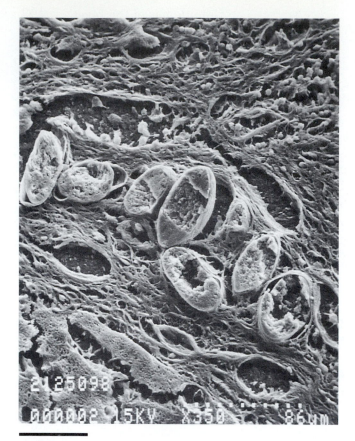

FIGURE 55.

Schistosomiasis japonica. A scanning electron micrograph of the same case illustrated in Figure 54 discloses sections of completely calcified eggs entrapped in a meshwork of collagen fibrils (×350).

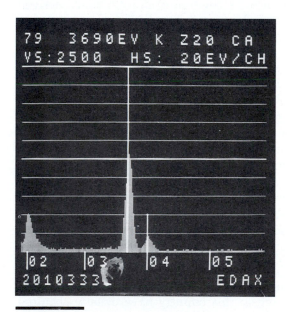

FIGURE 56.

Schistosomiasis japonica. Energy-dispersive x-ray microanalysis of the eggs depicted in Figure 55 shows them to be composed of calcium *(two right peaks)* and phosphorus *(left peak)*.

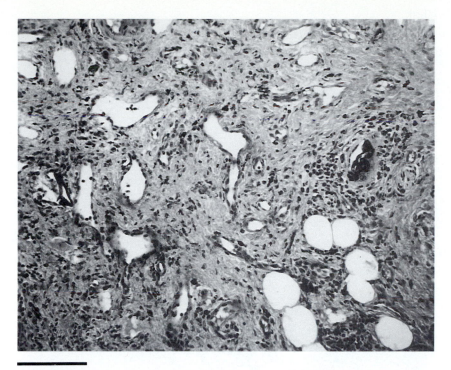

FIGURE 57.
Schistosomiasis mansoni. A fibrosed portal area contains numerous newly formed vessels ("angiomatoids"). Note the darkly stained crumpled egg *(right)* (PAS, ×160).

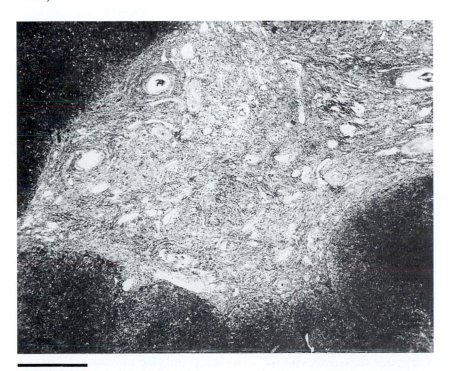

FIGURE 58.
Schistosomiasis mansoni. A markedly expanded portal area with many newly formed vessels and residual inflammation is the histologic equivalent of a "pipestem" (Masson, ×40).

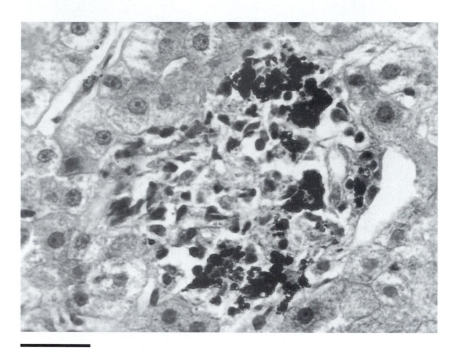

FIGURE 59.

Schistosomiasis mansoni. Macrophages laden with schistosomal pigment *(black)* have formed a granulomatoid lesion (HE, ×700).

bile ducts, they mature into adult worms in 3 to 4 months. Clinically, patients have fever, upper abdominal pain, hepatomegaly, and eosinophilia. Blockage of the common bile duct can lead to obstructive jaundice. The diagnosis is established by finding eggs in the stool or duodenal aspirates by ELISA or imaging studies.[371, 372] The egg of *F. hepatica* measures 130 to 140 by 50 to 90 μm and has a thin shell and an operculum at one end.

In the acute invasive stage the metacercariae burrow into the liver, which leads to necrotic, hemorrhagic tunnels with ragged edges and leukocytic infiltration.[373, 374] These fill in by granulation tissue and are later transformed into linear scars. The chronic phase is characterized grossly by multiple nodules.[373–375] Adult worms are found in the intrahepatic or extrahepatic bile ducts, the cystic duct, or the gallbladder. The ducts are dilated and have thickened walls, and there may be an associated choledocholithiasis or cholelithiasis.[373, 374] Histopathologically, the ducts reveal acute and/or chronic inflammation, epithelial hyperplasia, and mucous gland metaplasia. Eggs released by death of the worms can excite a granulomatous response.[374, 375] Calcification of the wall of the ducts and a secondary biliary cirrhosis may occur.

OPISTHORCHIASIS AND CLONORCHIASIS.—The adult flukes *(Opisthorchis viverrini, Opisthorchis felineus,* and *C. sinensis)* inhabit the entire biliary system and may also migrate into the pancreatic ducts. In both diseases the bile ducts are dilated and often thick walled as a result of epithelial hyperplasia, mucous gland hyperplasia, and acute and/or chronic cholangitis (Fig 60). Clonorchiasis may be associated with intrahepatic or extra-

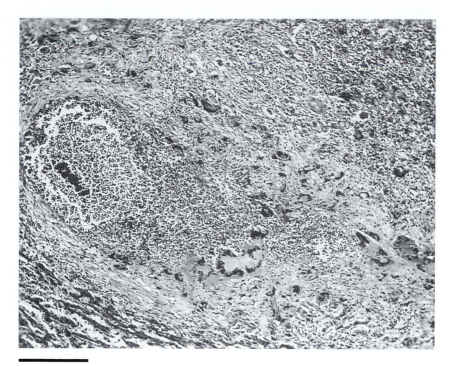

FIGURE 60.

Clonorchiasis. A cholangitic abscess *(left)* has caused the release of eggs of *Clonorchis sinensis*, which have excited a foreign body reaction (HE, ×70).

hepatic lithiasis. A granulomatous reaction to the eggs may occur (Fig 61).[376, 377] These parasitic infections are considered to predispose to intrahepatic cholangiocarcinoma.[378–381]

PARAGONIMIASIS.—Most of the infections are caused by *Paragonimus westermani,* but other species have been implicated. The eggs (or less often the adult parasites) are associated with abscess formation followed by encystation.[382, 383] The fully developed cyst contains necrotic debris with numerous eggs located at the periphery or embedded in the fibrous wall; some of the eggs may be associated with a foreign body, giant cell reaction.[382, 383] The eggs (80 to 120 by 45 to 65 µm) are ovoid and thick shelled, have a flattened operculum at one end, and are birefringent.

ECHINOCOCCOSIS.—The cyst of *Echinococcus granulosus* is generally not associated with granulomas, although some cysts may contain a foreign body or Langhans' giant cells in the fibrous (adventitial) wall. These are usually a reaction to disintegration of the inner germinal layer.

The alveolar echinococcal cyst caused by *Echinococcus multilocularis* is composed of multiple small cysts lined by a laminated membrane and surrounded by a variable amount of chronically inflamed fibrous tissue. Scoleces are found in fewer than 10% of the cysts.[384] Many multinucleated giant cells, frequently engulfing pieces of the germinal layer, are noted in the fibrous tissue. *Echinococcus vogeli* leads to multilocular cysts that histopathologically resemble those of alveolar echinococcosis.[385]

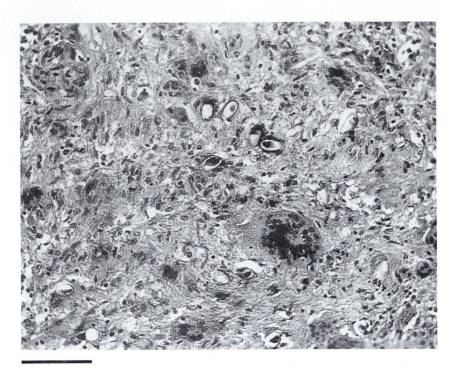

FIGURE 61.

Clonorchiasis. A higher magnification of the case illustrated in Figure 60 shows eggs of *C. sinensis* and an associated foreign body, giant cell reaction (HE, ×70).

PENTASTOMIASIS.—Synonyms for this infection, caused by members of the class Pentastomida, including tongue worm infection, linguatuliasis, and porocephaliasis.[386, 387] There are two orders of pentastomids: Porocephalida and Cephalobaenida. Two families of Porocephalida are of medical importance to humans—Porocephalidae and Linguatulidae. Ninety-nine percent of infections in humans are accounted for by two species, *Armillifer armillatus* and *Linguatula serrata*. Pentastomiasis has been reported from many countries in Africa, Asia, Europe, and the Americas. The autopsy incidence of infection may be quite high in some populations, for example, Malaysian aborigines, where 45% of adults autopsied are infected.[388]

Humans usually become infected by ingesting embryonated eggs discharged into water by infected reptiles or by eating snakes, thus becoming an aberrant intermediate host; for details of the life cycle, the reader is referred to other sources.[386, 387] Infections are generally asymptomatic, and evidence for pentastomiasis is usually found incidentally by roentgenographic studies or at surgery or autopsy. Larvae liberated from the eggs can migrate widely and encyst in many organs, including the liver. The encysted larvae are surrounded by a thick, fibrous wall with eventual disintegration, inflammation, fibrosis, and/or calcification. Often, all that remains of the parasite are fragments of the cuticle, which may be engulfed by foreign body giant cells. Although the term "healed granulomas" has been used in connection with the lesions in the liver,[389] an epithelioid granulomatous response is not generally seen.

MISCELLANEOUS PARASITIC INFECTIONS.—A number of other parasitic infections such as ectopically located *Enterobius vermicularis*,[390–394] *Giardia lamblia*,[395, 396] and *Alaria americana*[397] can elicit a granulomatous response in the liver. In the case of *G. lamblia* infections, abnormal liver tests and nonspecific necroinflammatory changes were described in hepatic biopsy material from 20 patients by Sotto et al.[397] Liver tests and histologic changes reverted to normal in 12 of the 20 patients after eradication of the infection.

SARCOIDOSIS

The reported incidence of hepatic granulomas in sarcoidosis varies from 50% to 100%.[3, 206] Analysis of autopsy material shows that the liver is third only to the lungs and lymph nodes in frequency of involvement, despite which clinical and/or laboratory evidence of liver disease is found in only 39% of patients.[398] Hepatomegaly occurs in 28% of cases.[206] Fever is not usually a prominent feature of sarcoidosis, but it may be more common among patients with hepatic involvement.[399] Jaundice is rare. The chronic cholestatic syndrome of sarcoidosis shares a number of features with primary biliary cirrhosis: pruritus, jaundice, hepatomegaly, and striking elevations of the serum levels of alkaline phosphatase and cholesterol.[400] Unlike primary biliary cirrhosis, however, no mitochondrial antibodies are found in the serum. Furthermore, the patients have indisputable clinical evidence of sarcoidosis antedating the onset of cholestasis.[400]

In addition to the "pure" form of chronic cholestasis of sarcoidosis,[400–405] it has become evident that sarcoidosis can coexist with primary biliary cirrhosis,[406–410] and less often with primary sclerosing cholangitis.[411, 412] It should be remembered that cholestasis in sarcoidosis, may also be secondary to extrahepatic biliary obstruction caused by strictures of the bile ducts[413, 414] or enlarged lymph nodes in the porta hepatis.[10] The chronic cholestatic syndrome of sarcoidosis may be accompanied by portal hypertension.[408, 415] On the other hand, portal hypertension may complicate sarcoidosis in the absence of chronic cholestasis.[408, 415–419] In the cases associated with chronic cholestasis, the portal hypertension is usually a manifestation of biliary fibrosis or cirrhosis. In other cases it is presinusoidal and probably secondary to compromise of portal area vessels by the granulomas.[408]

Laboratory abnormalities in hepatic sarcoidosis include hyperglobulinemia and moderate increases in serum alkaline phosphatase activity. In the chronic cholestatic syndrome, serum bilirubin levels are elevated (usually below 5 mg/dL), whereas alkaline phosphatase values are elevated from 2-fold to over 30-fold. Transaminase values are only mildly abnormal. Serum angiotensin converting enzyme levels are elevated in sarcoidosis[420–422] and other conditions (with or without associated granulomas). Serial assays of this enzyme are useful in assessing the response to therapy and warning of impending relapse. Serum collagenase activity (also significantly elevated in sarcoidosis) is considered a less sensitive index of sarcoidosis activity than that of angiotensin converting enzyme.[423] Immunologic aspects of sarcoidosis have recently been reviewed by several investigators[424-426] and will not be further commented on here.

Sarcoid granulomas in the liver are generally scattered widely, but most tend to be portal or periportal. The smallest and presumably earliest lesions are best appreciated within acini and consist of a few loosely arranged epithelioid cells (Fig 62). Older lesions are globular or ovoid and sharply defined (Figs 62 and 63). In cases with severe hepatic involvement there may be a confluence of the granulomas (Fig 64). The epithelioid cells tend to be radially oriented, and there may be one or more multinucleated giant cells. Angiotensin converting enzyme has been demonstrated in these cells by immunohistochemical methods.[427] A variable but usually minimal inflammatory cell response consisting of lymphocytes, plasma cells, and eosinophils is present. The epithelioid cells in the granulomas are supported by a delicate network of reticulin fibers.[428] Fibrillogranular necrosis (caseation) is usually absent, but some granulomas may have central fibrinoid necrosis.

Several types of inclusions may be found in sarcoid granulomas; none are pathognomonic.[429-431] Asteroid bodies (5 to 20 μm in overall diameter) resembling a sea anemone are found in multinucleated giant cells; they often lie in globular vesicles (Figs 65 and 66). Asteroid bodies appear to be composed of noncollagenous filamentous[432, 433] and myelinoid membranes.[433] Microtubular material derived from the cytoskeleton was found in one ultrastructural study[432] but not in another.[433] The asteroid bodies in sarcoid granulomas can be immunostained with antibodies to ubiquitin (see Fig 66), as has been demonstrated in silicone-induced

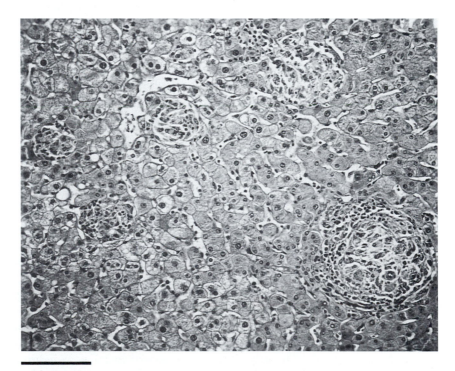

FIGURE 62.

Sarcoidosis. Several epithelioid granulomas of varied size are scattered in the parenchyma. The largest *(bottom right)* is in a portal area (HE, ×160).

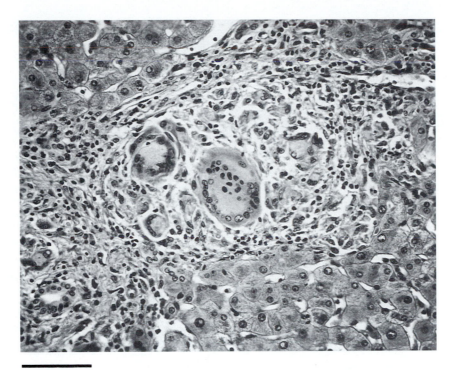

FIGURE 63.

Sarcoidosis. Periportal epithelioid granulomas contain several multinucleated, Langhans' giant cells (HE, ×250).

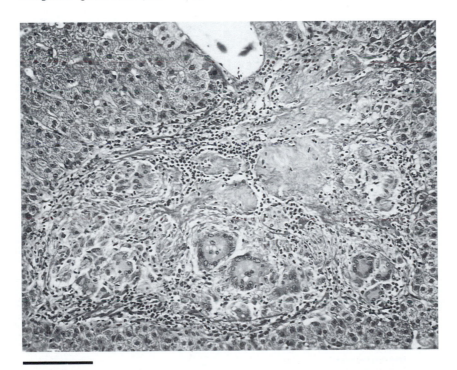

FIGURE 64.

Sarcoidosis with confluent epithelioid granulomas. The *uppermost* is undergoing fibrosis (HE, ×250).

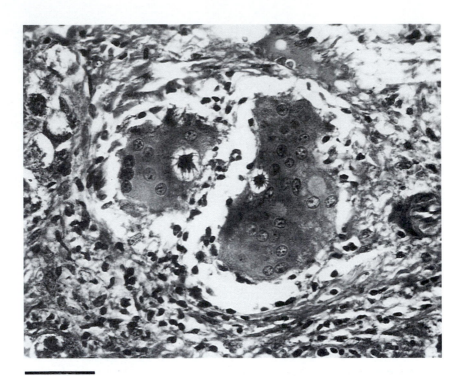

FIGURE 65.
Sarcoidosis. Each of two giant cells contains one darkly stained asteroid body suspended in a vacuole (Masson, ×400).

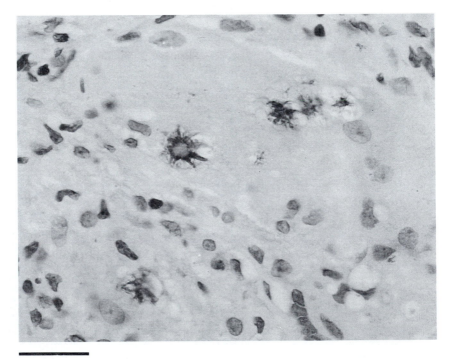

FIGURE 66.
Sarcoidosis. Asteroid bodies are decorated by antiubiquitin antibodies (×600).

granulomas.[434] Schaumann ("conchoidal") bodies are large (25 to 200 μm), round to roughly oval in configuration, and concentrically laminated (Fig 67). They are composed of calcium phosphate or carbonate and iron.[433] Crystals of calcium oxalate have also been identified in giant cells; they are birefringent (Fig 68).[435, 436] Schaumann bodies are infrequently found in the giant cells of sarcoid granulomas in the liver. Centrospheres, the third type of inclusion seen in sarcoid granulomas, are small homogeneous vesicles that are single or multiple and may displace the nucleus to the cell margin.[429]

Sarcoid granulomas heal by fibrosis (Figs 64, 69, and 70). Early resolution is characterized by an accumulation of fibroblasts that tend to arrange themselves concentrically around the granulomas. There is progressive formation of collagen, which may become very hyalinized (paramyloid), the end stage being a focal scar that eventually disappears. The giant cells containing asteroids or Schaumann bodies tend to be the last vestiges of the granulomatous response in the fibrous tissue (see Fig 70).

It should be emphasized that involvement of the liver in sarcoidosis is not confined to infiltration by noncaseating granulomas. In a series of 100 patients with hepatic sarcoidosis, "cholestatic" features were found in 58%.[437] The changes included duct lesions that resembled those of primary biliary cirrhosis (Fig 71) or primary sclerosing cholangitis, ductopenia, and chronic cholestasis (Figs 72 and 73). Necroinflammatory changes in the form of random small foci of necrosis, sinusoidal acidophilic bodies, and mild to moderate portal inflammation were also found. As al-

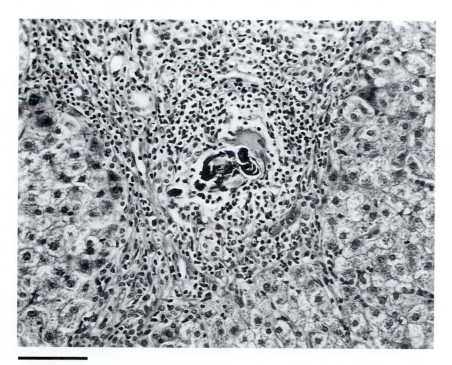

FIGURE 67.
Sarcoidosis with a conchoidal Schaumann body in the center of a sarcoid granuloma (HE, ×160).

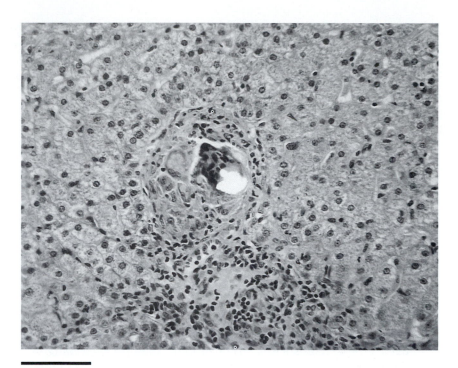

FIGURE 68.
Sarcoidosis. The calcium oxalate in a giant cell (within a sarcoid granuloma) is birefringent. Note the focus of necrosis beneath the granuloma (HE, ×250).

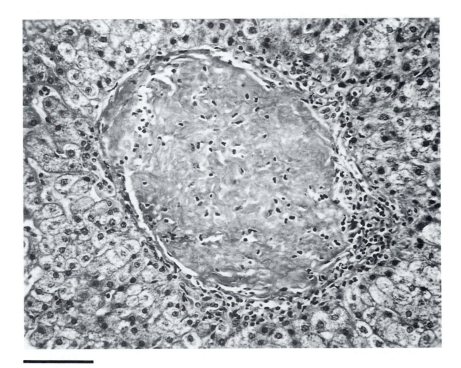

FIGURE 69.
Sarcoidosis. A round scar is all that remains of a sarcoid granuloma (HE, ×160).

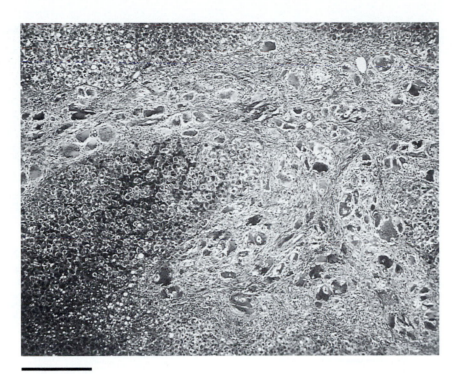

FIGURE 70.
Sarcoidosis. Extensive fibrosis has followed the healing of multiple, confluent sarcoid granulomas. The fibrous tissue contains residual multinucleated giant cells but no epithelioid granulomas (Masson, ×60).

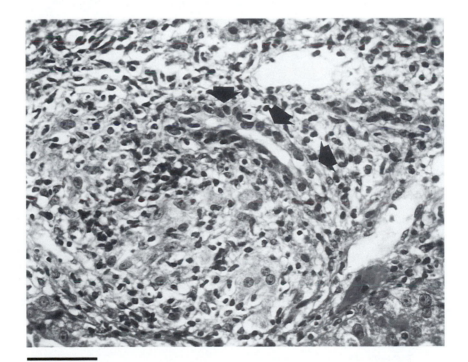

FIGURE 71.
Sarcoidosis. A bile duct (arrow) is being infiltrated and destroyed by a sarcoid granuloma (HE, ×400).

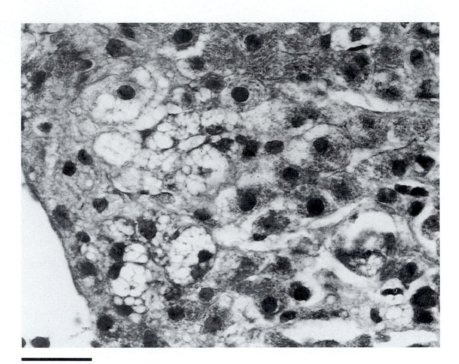

FIGURE 72.
Sarcoidosis: granulomatoid aggregate of pseudoxanthomatous cells *(left)* in a case of chronic cholestatic syndrome of that disease (×720).

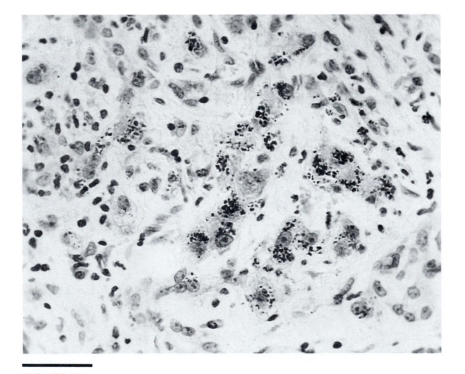

FIGURE 73.
Sarcoidosis with marked copper accumulation *(black granules)* in the periportal liver cells in chronic cholestatic syndrome of that disease (rhodanine, ×400).

ready noted, there may be severe fibrosis and actual cirrhosis with portal hypertension in sarcoidosis. Cirrhosis was noted in 6% of the cases reported by Devaney et al.[437] Nodular regenerative hyperplasia was found in 9% of cases in the same series.[437] Finally, note should be made of the rare complication of the Budd-Chiari syndrome in sarcoidosis.[438, 439]

A mycobacterial etiology for sarcoidosis has been suggested for many years (see the discussion by Popper et al.[149]). The detection of mycobacterial DNA and RNA in sarcoid lesions by several groups of investigators lends support to that association.[149, 440, 441] It is of interest in this context that a case of disseminated sarcoidosis was reported in a patient 2 years after successful therapy for isolated hepatic tuberculosis.[442]

CHRONIC CHOLESTATIC DISORDERS

PRIMARY BILIARY CIRRHOSIS.—Epithelioid granulomas have been reported with varying frequency in this disease (Figs 74 to 76). The percentage of cases with granulomas in three series was 18.3,[443] 23.0,[444] and 36.4.[445] When present, the granulomas are helpful in differentiating primary biliary cirrhosis from chronic hepatitis. However, the histopathologic diagnosis of primary biliary cirrhosis depends largely on the presence of other lesions such as degeneration and destruction of bile ducts (chronic nonsuppurative destructive cholangitis), chronic cholestasis (location of cholestasis in periportal areas, pseudoxanthomatous transformation, copper accumulation, and sometimes Mallory bodies), portal inflammation, and periportal fibrosis eventually leading to a micronodular cirrhosis.

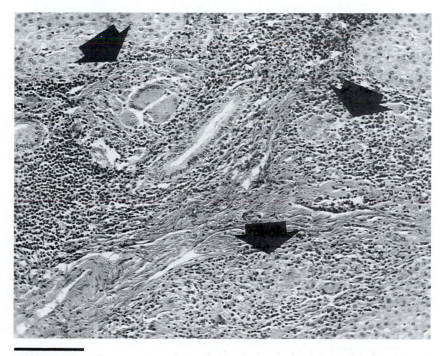

FIGURE 74.
Primary biliary cirrhosis. Several small epithelioid granulomas are incorporated into an expanded portal area (HE, ×145).

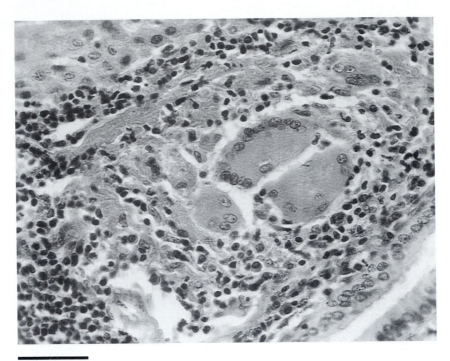

FIGURE 75.
Primary biliary cirrhosis: higher magnification of one of granulomas depicted in Figure 72 (HE, ×395).

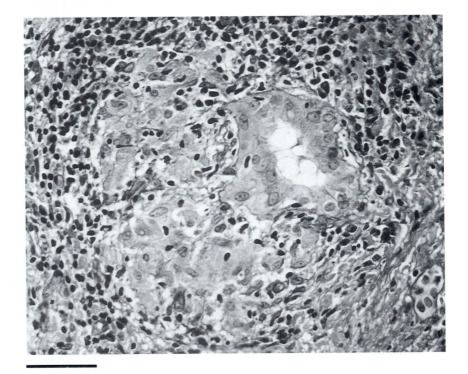

FIGURE 76.
Primary biliary cirrhosis. An epithelioid granuloma is closely apposed to a degenerating bile duct (HE, ×400).

PRIMARY SCLEROSING CHOLANGITIS.—In my experience, granulomas are exceptionally rare in this disease. They were found in 10% of a series of 29 patients,[446] but none were described in a larger series of 43 patients.[447]

GASTROINTESTINAL DISEASES

CHRONIC ULCERATIVE COLITIS.—The incidence of granulomas in chronic ulcerative colitis is thought to be about 1%.[448]

CROHN'S DISEASE.—Noncaseating granulomas have been reported in a number of studies.[449-452] Their incidence has varied from 2.5% to about 23%.

EOSINOPHILIC GASTROENTERITIS.—Granulomas are rarely reported in the liver in this disorder. In one case the granulomas contained many eosinophils in addition to epithelioid and giant cells, a feature probably reflecting the marked (62%) peripheral eosinophila.[453]

WHIPPLE'S DISEASE.—Hepatic granulomas have been reported in several cases of this disease (Fig 77).[454-458] A more frequent change, which was found in two thirds of the cases in one series, is hypertrophy of Kupffer cells and portal macrophages, which are packed with a granular, PAS-positive material (Fig 78).[459] The bacilli can also be demonstrated by the Warthin-Starry stain (Fig 79). They were identified in Kupffer cells by electron microscopy in one case.[458] The causative organism has been detected by a PCR technique and named *Tropheryma whippelii*.[460]

JEJUNOILEAL BYPASS.—Hepatic granulomas have been reported following jejunoileal bypass surgery for morbid obesity.[461-465] The incidence in three series was 4%,[461] 7%[463] and 24%.[462] Other organs may be involved si-

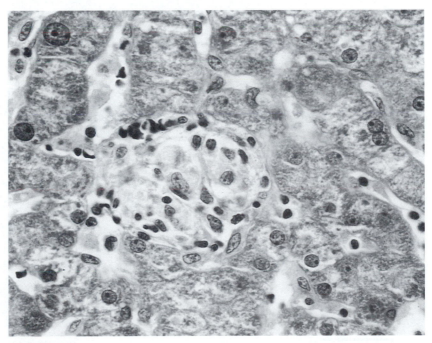

FIGURE 77.
Whipple's disease with a tiny epithelioid granuloma (HE, ×630).

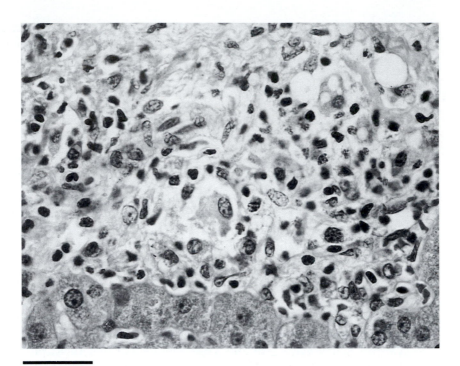

FIGURE 78.

Whipple's disease: same case illustrated in Figure 77. A portal area reveals an ill-defined, granulomatoid inflammatory response with hypertrophied macrophages, lymphocytes, and plasma cells (HE, ×630).

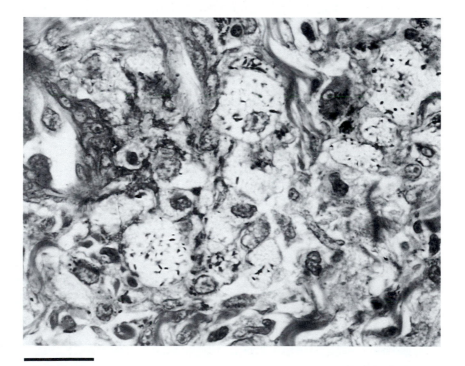

FIGURE 79.

Whipple's disease: same case illustrated in Figures 77 and 78. Numerous short bacilli are present in the hypertrophied portal macrophages (Warthin-Starry, ×1,000).

multaneously, for example, the kidney, bone marrow, lymph nodes, and lung. The four patients of Bruce and Wise[461] were determined to have tuberculosis, as were the two cases of intrathoracic tuberculosis reported by Pickleman et al.[466] The etiology of the hepatic granulomas in the remaining cases has not been elucidated and is largely of academic interest since the procedure has now been abandoned.

VASCULAR/CONNECTIVE TISSUE DISEASES

Granulomas may involve vessels in the liver, particularly those in portal areas, in a number of diseases such as sarcoidosis, tuberculosis, drug reactions, mycotic infections, and some parasitic diseases (for example, schistosomiasis). The liver may also be involved in several vasculitides, as discussed in the following sections:

DISSEMINATED VISCERAL GIANT CELL ARTERITIS.—Several examples of this entity,[467–471] one with fibrin ring granulomas,[470] have been reported.

ALLERGIC GRANULOMATOSIS.—Hepatic vascular lesions and extravascular granulomas were noted in the first report of this disease and in subsequent case reports.[471–473] Veno-occlusive liver disease developed in one patient with allergic granulomatosis.[474]

POLYMYALGIA ARTERITICA.—This term has been proposed to include the closely related disease temporal arteritis and polymyalgia rheumatica with arteritis. Hepatic granulomas have been described in occasional patients with polymyalgia rheumatica, with or without temporal arteritis.[475–477] Cases of giant cell arteritis involving hepatic arteries in portal areas, as well as the temporal arteries, have been reported rarely. Affected vessels in portal areas revealed transmural inflammation with giant cells and destruction of elastic lamina.

WEGENER'S GRANULOMATOSIS.—Epithelioid hepatic granulomas have been described in two patients with this disease.[3, 478] In one patient some of the granulomas revealed central necrosis.[420]

SYSTEMIC LUPUS ERYTHEMATOSUS.—Hepatic involvement in this disease is variable and often nonspecific but may be severe, for example, steatosis, arteritis, chronic hepatitis, or cirrhosis.[479–481] A few examples of nodular regenerative hyperplasia were reported by Matsumoto et al.[480] Granulomas have been found in a number of cases.[481–484] One example of fibrin ring granulomas was reported by Murphy et al.[485]

RHEUMATOID ARTHRITIS.—The majority of patients with rheumatoid arthritis have nonspecific histopathologic changes, even though they often have hepatosplenomegaly and evidence of hepatocellular dysfunction.[486, 487] Rheumatoid nodules, identical to those in subcutaneous tissue near joints, were reported in one patient.[488] Of interest is the report of similar granulomas in a patient with extrahepatic biliary atresia.[489]

DRUG-INDUCED GRANULOMAS

Many drugs have been implicated in the causation of hepatic granulomas[27, 490, 491] (Table 4). Some granulomatous reactions have been isolated

---

TABLE 4.

Drugs Causing Hepatic Granulomas

Allopurinol	Oral contraceptives
Aspirin	Oxacillin
Carbamazepine	Oxyphenbutazone
Carbutamide	Papaverine
Cephalexin	Penicillin
Chlorpromazine	Phenazone
Chlorpropamide	(antipyrine)
Diazepam	Phenprocoumon
Diltiazem	Phenylbutazone
Disopyramide	Phenytoin
Gold salts	Procainamide
Glibenclamide	Procarbazine
Halothane	Quinidine
Hydralazine	Quinine
Isoniazid	Ranitidine
Methyldopa	Sulfonamides*
Metolazone	Tocainide
Mineral oil	Tolbutamide
Nitrofurantoin	Trichlormethiazide
Nomifensine	

---

*Sulphanilamide, sulfadiazine, salicylazosulfa-
pyridine (sulfasalazine) sulfadoxine + py-
rimethamine, sulphamethoxazole-trimethoprim,
succinylsulphathiazole.

---

examples, whereas others have been reported repeatedly with certain drugs. Drug-induced granulomatous reactions are not as rare as previously thought; in one series from the United States, such reactions were diagnosed in 6% of liver biopsy samples studied over a period of 10 years.[27] In the same study, drugs accounted for 29% of all cases of granulomatous hepatitis, being almost equal in frequency to sarcoidosis.[27] The major causes of drug-induced granulomatous reactions include mineral oil lipogranulomas and granulomas induced by BCG (already discussed), the sulfonamides, sulphonylurea compounds, quinidine, phenylbutazone (Figs 80 and 81), phenytoin, allopurinol, and carbamazepine.[490, 491]

Drug-induced hepatic granulomas are distributed in portal areas and throughout the hepatic acinus and are of variable size. When tissues from other organs are studied, it is found that granulomas are often simultaneously present in multiple extrahepatic sites. The granulomas in the liver have no specific features that distinguish them from those of sarcoidosis or sarcoid-like processes except for tissue eosinophila, when present (see Fig 80). In the experience of the author, the tissue eosinophilia is frequently accompanied by peripheral blood eosinophilia. Moreover, eosinophils are present in sinusoids and other vessels, in addition to those in the granulomas. Histologic features not seen in drug-induced

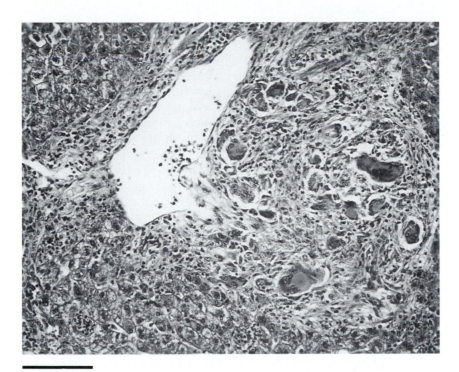

FIGURE 80.
Phenylbutazone injury. An epithelioid granuloma with several multinucleated giant cells is located in a portal area. Note the encroachment of the granuloma on a portal vein branch (HE, ×160).

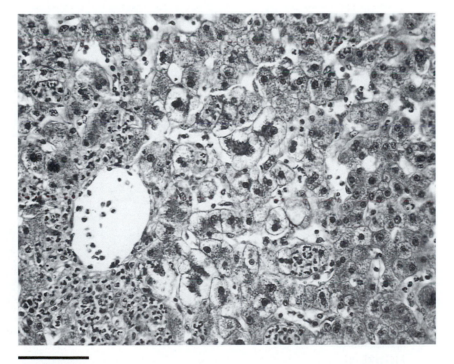

FIGURE 81.
Phenylbutazone injury: same case illustrated in Figure 80. There is ballooning degeneration of liver cells in zone 3 (HE, ×160).

hepatic granulomas include central necrosis and various inclusions in giant cells such as Schaumann or asteroid bodies. Differentiation of parasitic granulomas from drug-induced ones (which are also accompanied by marked tissue eosinophilia) requires clinicopathologic correlation and identification of parasitic eggs, pigment, of larvae in the former.

Many drug-induced granulomatous reactions are accompanied by minimal and inconstant intra-acinar changes. On the other hand, significant hepatocellular and/or cholestatic injury may accompany the granulomatous response, as has been reported with phenylbutazone and phenytoin (see Fig 81). The hepatocellular injury may include ballooning degeneration (usually in acinar zone 3) or haphazardly distributed sinusoidal acidophilic bodies. Cholestasis, both cytoplasmic and canalicular, is located predominantly in zone 3. Other associated lesions such as a cholangitis (e.g., in cases related to allopurinol, chlorpromazine, methyldopa, or chlorpropamide) or a vasculitis (e.g., in cases caused by penicillin, the sulfonamides, glibenclamide, allopurinol, and phenytoin) may also be helpful in the differential diagnosis.[490] Fibrin ring granulomas attributed to allopurinol in one patient[492] have been subsequently found to not be a common lesion in six other patients with granulomatous liver injury induced by this drug.[493] Healing of drug-induced granulomatous reactions is not known to be associated with any sequelae.

Mineral oil used for the relief of constipation is listed as one of the causes of drug-induced hepatic granulomas (see Table 4). However, the origin of mineral oil in the liver, spleen, and abdominal lymph nodes is likely to include nonmedicinal sources such as the extensive use of min-

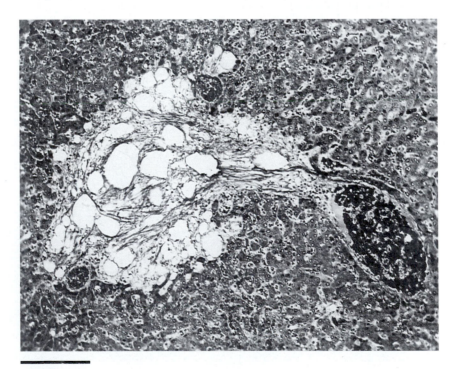

FIGURE 82.
Mineral oil lipogranuloma adjacent to a terminal hepatic venule (Masson, ×140).

eral oil in food processing in the United States.[494, 495] Mineral oil lipogranulomas are a frequent finding in hepatic biopsy or autopsy material in North America.[496–499] The mineral oil accumulates mainly in portal macrophages or perivenular Kupffer cells, which are markedly hypertrophied and vacuolated and are often clustered to form granulomatoid foci (Fig 82). The lipogranulomas can lead to occlusion of terminal hepatic venules[498] or to appreciable inflammation and scarring in portal areas.[500]

METAL-INDUCED INJURY

BERYLLIUM.—Chronic beryllium disease (berylliosis) is an occupational disease that resembles sarcoidosis, the most severe manifestations being related to involvement of the lungs.[501, 502] Hepatic biopsy specimens from some patients have revealed noncaseating epithelioid granulomas.[502–504] Tissue assays for beryllium were positive in two of the three cases analyzed by Stoeckle et al.[502] Experimental work suggests that the histologic changes induced by beryllium compounds are immunologic reactions of the delayed or tuberculin type.[505] A murine model of granulomatous lung disease induced by beryllium has proved useful in understanding the genetic and immunologic factors that determine the response to that metal.[506]

COPPER.—A variety of hepatic lesions have developed in vineyard sprayers exposed to copper sulfate (mostly by inhalation) for 3 to 45 years (mean of 10 years).[507, 508] All of the 30 reported cases had swelling of Kupffer cells, 7 had granulomas, 8 had fibrosis, 3 had cirrhosis, and 1 had an angiosarcoma. Portal hypertension developed in 2 patients. Two of the livers with severe fibrosis revealed areas of nodular regeneration. Copper accumulation was demonstrated by special stains in Kupffer cells, portal macrophages, and granulomas and in focal areas of fibrosis.

BARIUM.—Barium enemas may be rarely complicated by intravasation of the contrast material into the portal venous system and thence into the liver. The two reported patients with that complication had chronic ulcerative colitis, which may have allowed access of the contrast material to veins through the damaged mucosa.[509, 510] In one patient the intravasation resulted in a liver abscess.[509] In the second patient, intrahepatic branches of the portal vein were filled with barium suspension and revealed thrombosis with organization.[510] That case was accessioned and reviewed at this institute. A foreign body, giant cell reaction to the barium suspension was seen in some of the veins. The barium suspension was finely granular, grayish green and refractile, and faintly birefringent. The birefringence is due to talc in the suspension rather than the barium itself.[511] Barium in tissue sections can be positively identified by energy-dispersive x-ray analysis.

ALUMINUM.—Granulomas containing aluminum have been detected in the liver of two patients with hyperaluminemia from long-term hemodialysis.[512] Macrophages in the granulomas contained a brown pigment. The presence of aluminum in the granulomas was confirmed by x-ray microanalysis. A case of pulmonary granulomatosis associated with inhalation of aluminum was reported by Chen et al.[513]

GOLD.—Gold therapy in rheumatoid arthritis results in the accumulation of gold particles in portal lipophages and lipogranulomas, as well as in hypertrophied Kupffer cells.[514] The gold is granular and black in HE-stained sections. The gold particles are birefringent. In my experience the birefringence is golden, but two groups of investigators describe the birefringence (in extrahepatic tissues) as orange-red.[515, 516] Additionally, an unreported feature is the presence of a black (isotropic) cross in each polarized particle; because of the small size of the particles this feature is best appreciated when the oil immersion objective is used. The gold particles are readily recognized by scanning electron microscopy with the backscatter technique, and the element gold can be identified by x-ray microanalysis.

TITANIUM.—Titanium admixed with talc has been reported in the lungs, liver, and spleen of two intravenous abusers of drugs[517] and in an autopsied liver (as well as the lungs) of one patient occupationally exposed to titanium dioxide.[518] In drug addicts the titanium may be admixed with talc.[517] The titanium granules are black and display pink birefringence.[517, 518] In the lungs they are found in perivascular granulomas, but in the liver and spleen they are present in macrophages in portal areas and the red pulp, respectively. The metal is also stored in the liver, bile ducts, and endothelial cells. X-ray microanalysis identifies the element titanium in the black particles and silicon and magnesium in the talc particles.

OTHER FOREIGN PARTICULATE MATERIALS

In addition to the particulate metals mentioned in the previous section, the materials in the following sections have been recognized.

STARCH.—The surface of the liver may be acutely involved in starch peritonitis; more frequently, old fibrous surface adhesions may be found to contain starch particles in surgical biopsy or autopsy material (Figs 83 and 84). The initial response to starch is isolation of the particles by fibrin.[519] This is followed by a granulomatous reaction that eventually leads to disintegration of the particles and their transport to regional lymphatics.[519] That this is not always the case is attested to by the presence of starch particles that have presumably escaped destruction by the inflammatory response within old adhesions. The granulomatous response to starch is usually of the phagocytic foreign body type, but tuberculoid granulomas, with or without caseation, may develop.[520]

Starch particles are not easily visualized in sections stained with HE. They are best identified by their "Maltese cross" birefringence (see Fig 84). Starch can be stained with Lugol's iodine solution and the PAS reagent.[520] The particles have a roughly spherical configuration with a central depression when viewed by the scanning electron microscope.[520]

Hydroxethyl starch (HES) has been used as a colloidal plasma substitute. Ascites developed in several patients who were maintained on di-

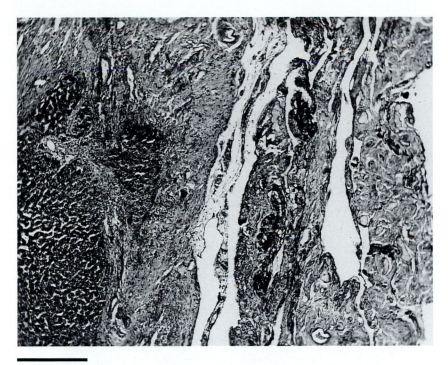

FIGURE 83.
Adhesions on the surface of the liver from previous surgery (Masson, ×50).

alysis and had received repeated infusions of HES, presumably because of massive storage of that material in sinusoidal lining cells.[521, 522] Affected cells are enlarged and have a foamy appearance; they may be clustered together, but true granulomas are not formed. The ultrastructural appearance of the stored material was reported by Pfeifer et al.[521]

CELLULOSE.—Cellulose fibers (from swabs, drapes, etc.) may contaminate the peritoneum during surgery and lead to a granulomatous peritonitis.[523-525] The lint fibers in the resultant granulomas are PAS-positive and birefringent and have a trilaminar structure. It is worth noting at this juncture that cellulose fibers from crushed tablets injected intravenously by drug addicts may disseminate widely and have been identified in portal macrophages and Kupffer cells.[526]

   Oxidized regenerated cellulose (Oxycel), a topical hemostatic agent widely used to control surgical bleeding at many different sites, may lead to tissue reactions,[527] including reactions in the liver.[528] In several cases involving the pelvic peritoneum, phagocytic cells contained basophilic cytoplasmic inclusions that were isotropic and stained positively with mucicarmine, Alcian blue, and the PAS reagent.[527]

TALC.—In addition to starch and cellulose, talc may be found in adhesions on the surface of the liver, usually from previous abdominal surgery (see Figs 83 and 84). Contamination of surgical gloves by talc has been demonstrated by two groups of investigators.[529, 530] The major source of talc in the liver, however, is the filler material that is admixed with drugs injected intravenously by drug addicts.

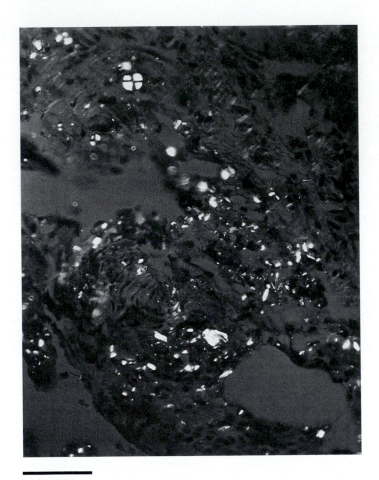

FIGURE 84.
Same case illustrated in Figure 83. Adhesions viewed in polarized light reveal numerous birefringent talc particles and a Maltese cross of starch particle *(top)* (HE, ×300).

Talc in the liver of drug addicts is generally located in hypertrophied portal macrophages or Kupffer cells. The former may cluster to form granulomatoid foci; foreign body giant cells are an exceptionally rare response to talc in the liver. As already noted, the talc may be admixed with titanium[517] or other adulterants.[531-534]

Talc crystals in the reticuloendothelial cells of the liver or in lipogranulomas are colorless, refractile, and birefringent (Fig 85). They are needle shaped but may aggregate to form craggy masses. Scanning electron microscopy reveals irregular plates that often show characteristic "flaking" (Fig 86). Ultrastructurally, the talc crystals are electron dense and elongated, with sharp edges and apparent lamination.[535] The magnesium and silicon in talc can be definitively identified by x-ray microanalysis (Fig 87).[536, 537]

In addition to the accumulation of talc and other particulate material and their consequences in cells of the mononuclear-phagocyte system throughout the body, intravenous abusers of drugs also suffer from a variety of infections transmitted by contaminated needles and syringes. Examples include disseminated histoplasmosis,[538] miliary tuberculosis,[539] CMV infection,[540] HIV infection, and the hepatitis viruses B, delta, and C.

SUTURE MATERIAL.—Suture material (usually catgut) left in the liver from previous surgery excites a foreign body, giant cell reaction (Fig 88) that ultimately leads to a focal scar. Catgut is birefringent, and its fibers in cross section are doughnut shaped (see Fig 88).

POLYVINYLPYRROLIDONE.—Polyvinylpyrrolidone (PVP) is a water-soluble, hydrophilic, high-molecular-weight product of the polymerization of vinylpyrrolidone. It was formerly used as a plasma expander[541–543] and continues to be used as a retarding agent for drugs injected subcutaneously.[544] A substantial amount of the compound is stored in cells of the reticuloendothelial system for many years, but long-term sequelae have not been reported. In the liver, PVP accumulates in markedly hypertrophied Kupffer cells and portal macrophages; the former may be converted into multinucleated giant cells, but granuloma formation does not occur (Fig 89). The affected cells have a granular, basophilic cytoplasm. The PVP stains positively with Lugol's iodine solution (mahogany brown), Congo red, and Sirius red (Fig 90). Unlike amyloid deposits, Congo red–stained PVP does not disclose apple-green birefringence. Ultrastructurally, Kupffer cells contain vacuoles surrounded by a membrane; granular or thread-like material may be present in the vacuoles.[544]

SILICONE.—Degeneration (variance) of the silicone rubber poppet of Starr-Edwards heart valve replacement prostheses is well known. Material from

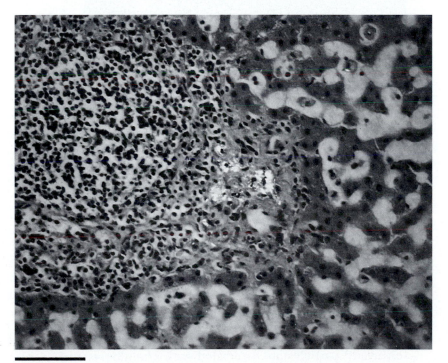

FIGURE 85.

Talc particles in portal macrophages are birefringent *(center)*. Note the lymphoid aggregate characteristic of chronic hepatitis C (HE, partially polarized, ×250).

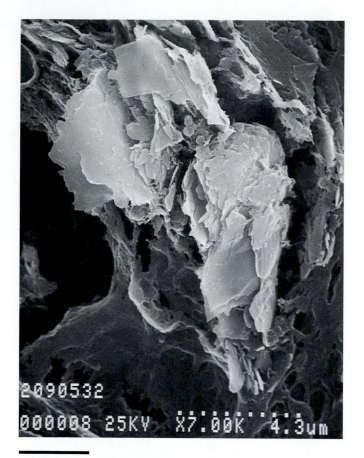

FIGURE 86.

Talc particles are composed of irregular plates (scanning electron micrograph, ×7,000).

the damaged poppet may disseminate widely and has been found in reticuloendothelial cells of the liver and spleen, as well as in other organs and tissues.[545, 546] Liver biopsy has been suggested as perhaps the best technique available for diagnosing ball variance.[545, 546] In the liver the silicone rubber excites a marked granulomatous reaction. Kupffer cells and portal macrophages are replaced by multinucleated, foreign body–type giant cells containing irregular colorless fragments of silicone rubber (Fig 91). It is of interest in this regard that Kupffer cells maintained in culture are capable of cell division and giant cell formation.[547] The silicone rubber is refractile and faintly birefringent and is brightly illuminated by phase-contrast microscopy (Fig 92). It has a sculpted appearance when viewed by scanning electron microscopy (Fig 93). Silicon can be detected in the particles by x-ray microanalysis.

Silicone has also been identified in the liver and spleen of patients undergoing maintenance hemodialysis.[548–554] The refractile (but not birefringent) particles are associated with granulomas and, in some cases, chronic portal inflammation, fibrosis, and focal necrosis. The source of the material is believed to be the tubing used in hemodialysis equipment. Silicone spallation from silicone tubing has been demonstrated *in vitro* at flow rates similar to those during hemodialysis.[555] Hepatic accumula-

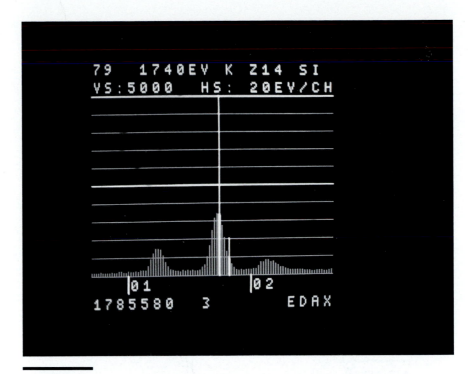

FIGURE 87.
Talc particles are readily identified by x-ray microanalysis. Note the peaks for the elements silicon *(center)* and magnesium *(left)*.

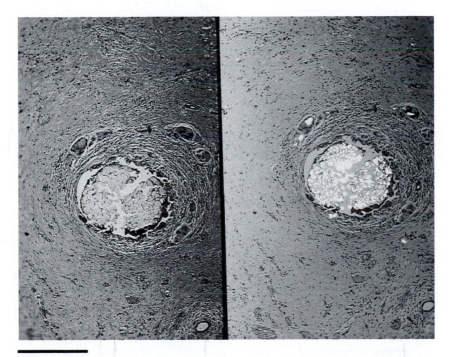

FIGURE 88.
Suture granuloma. Catgut, which is surrounded by fibrous tissue and foreign body giant cells *(left)*, is birefringent *(right)*. Note the portal area in the *lower right-hand corner* (HE, ×50).

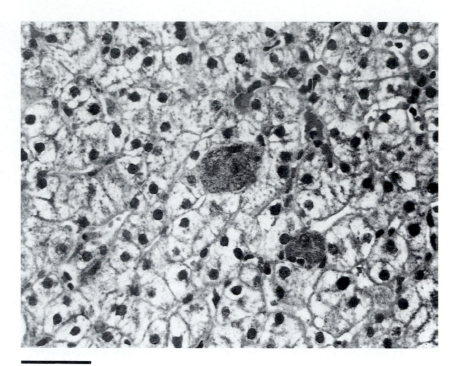

FIGURE 89.
Polyvinylpyrrolidone. Markedly hypertrophied Kupffer cells contain a darkly stained granular material (basophilic in an HE-stained section, ×400).

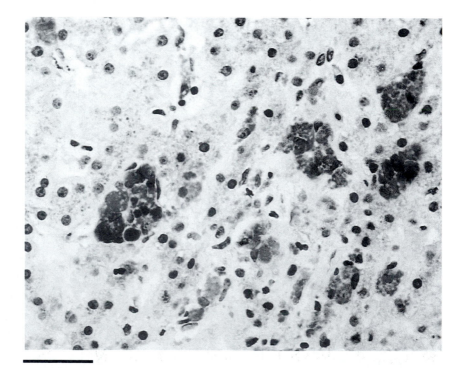

FIGURE 90.
Polyvinylpyrrolidone in hypertrophied Kupffer cells is stained with Congo red (×450).

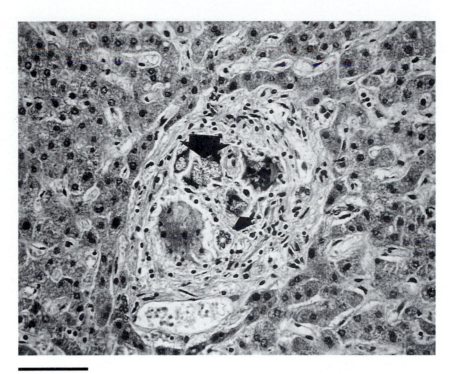

FIGURE 91.
Silicone foreign body giant cells in a portal area contain colorless, slightly refractile material (HE, ×250).

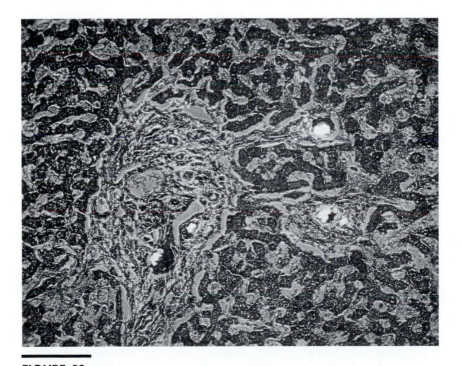

FIGURE 92.
Silicone in portal macrophages and Kupffer cells (right) is brightly illuminated by phase-contrast microscopy (HE, ×160).

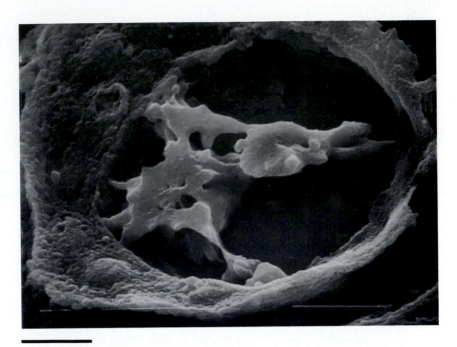

FIGURE 93.
Silicone appears suspended in a vacuole in a giant cell and has a "sculpted" structure (scanning electron micrograph, ×2,500).

tion of silicone in four patients, with granuloma formation in three of those patients, was reported following silicone injections for breast augmentation; the presence of the silicone was confirmed by atomic emission spectrography.[556]

THOROTRAST.—This material, which was formerly used for radiographic opacification, may accumulate in the reticuloendothelial cells of the liver (as well as in the spleen, bone marrow, and lymph nodes) or may be entrapped extracellularly in dense periportal or subcapsular fibrous tissue. The Thorotrast particles are colorless, but in sections stained with HE, they usually have a pink-brown color. They are coarsely granular, refractile, and brilliantly illuminated by phase-contrast microscopy (Fig 94). Rarely, Thorotrast aggregates in the liver may excite a granulomatous response. They are readily detected by scanning electron microscopy (Fig 95), and the element thorium can be positively identified by energy-dispersive x-ray analysis (Fig 96).[557, 558] The late effects of Thorotrast are well known and include the development of cholangiocarcinoma, angiosarcoma, and hepatocellular carcinoma.

ANTHRACOSILICOSIS.—The majority of reported cases have been a consequence of occupational exposure (e.g., miners, sandblasters, quarry workers)[559–566] and, rarely, of inhalational abuse of commercial cleansing[567] or talcum[568] powders. In most of the reported cases the silica and anthracotic pigment were identified in portal macrophages as well as in aggregates of Kupffer cells (Figs 97 and 98). Hemosiderin may also accumulate in the cells containing the silica and anthracotic pigment. The granulomas in the liver are noncaseating and rarely contain giant cells.

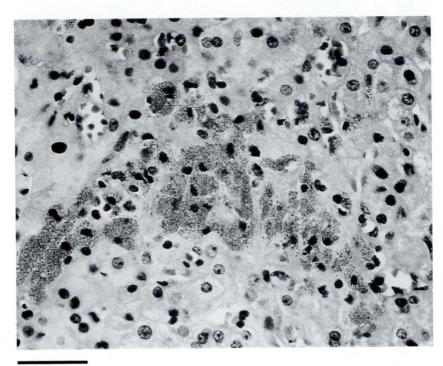

FIGURE 94.
Thorotrast particles phagocytosed by Kupffer cells that have formed a granulomatoid aggregate (HE, ×450).

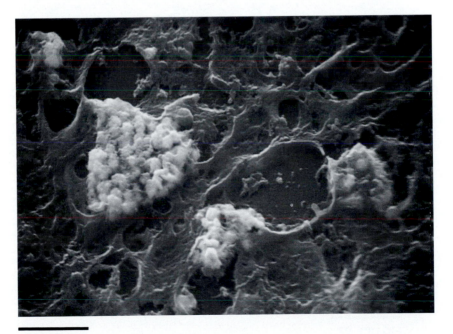

FIGURE 95.
Thorotrast particles in Kupffer cells have a uniform, roughly spherical shape (scanning electron micrograph, ×2,500).

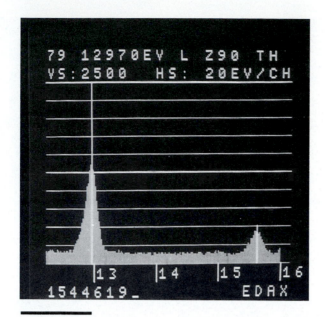

FIGURE 96.
Energy dispersive x-ray analysis of Thorotrast particles in the case illustrated in Figures 94 and 95 discloses two peaks of the element thorium.

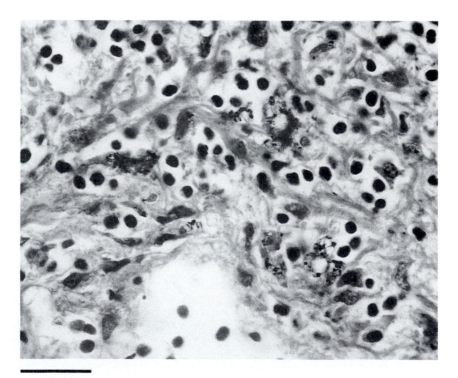

FIGURE 97.
Anthracosilicosis. Several markedly hypertrophied portal macrophages contain anthracotic pigment granules. A few silica particles were also identified by polarizing microscopy (not shown) (HE, ×400).

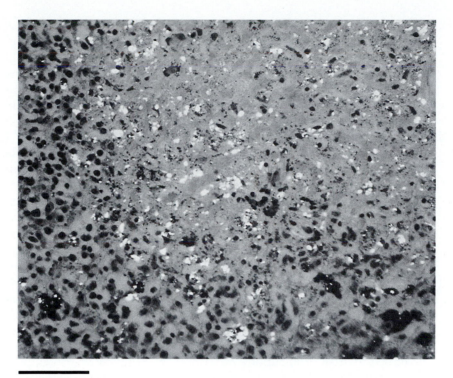

FIGURE 98.

Anthracosilicosis. A section of a pulmonary hilar lymph node of the same patient depicted in Figure 97 shows numerous birefringent silica particles as well as black anthracotic pigment (HE, partially polarized, ×300).

They undergo progressive fibrosis and are ultimately transformed into rounded, hyalinized scars. In addition to granulomas noted in the portal or periportal areas, a perivenular location has been emphasized by some investigators.[560, 563] The silica particles in reticuloendothelial cells and granulomas have generally been visualized by their birefringence in polarized light, but positive identification can be accomplished by x-ray microanalysis. For further information on extrapulmonary anthracosilicosis the reader is referred to the comprehensive review of Slavin et al.[566]

EXTRUDED CELL COMPONENTS

LIPOGRANULOMA.—Lipogranulomas consist of varying-sized aggregates of lymphocytes and lipid-laden macrophages (lipophages) surrounding one or more droplets of fat; a few eosinophils, neutrophils, and plasma cells may be present (see Fig. 82). There are no epitheliod cells, but multinucleated giant cells with a foamy cytoplasm may be present infrequently. In one series of liver biopsies with steatosis (mainly alcoholic), 43 (64%) revealed lipogranulomas.[569] They were found throughout the hepatic acinus and were classified into three types. Type 1 consists of a large extracellular vacuole surrounded by histiocytes and some lymphocytes and eosinophils; this corresponds to the "fat cyst" of Leevy et al.[570] Type 2 consists of a nodule composed of histiocytes, most of which are lipophages, together with lymphocytes and sometimes eosinophils and giant cells; serial sections reveal a centrally located extracellular lipid vacuole. Type 3 is a multinodular structure formed by the confluence of type 1 and type 2 lipogranulomas. Fibroblasts and collagen fibrils are found between the component nodules. Ultrastructural studies have shown that a fat droplet that is destined to become a lipogranuloma protrudes through one side of the plasma membrane of a hepatocyte, whereupon it becomes surrounded by histiocytes and lymphocytes.[571] Remnants of the cell membrane may be seen between the fat droplets and the histiocytes.[571] In fully developed lipogranulomas, the fat droplets are entirely extracellular.[571]

The aforementioned studies focused on parenchymal lipogranulomas and their pathogenesis. In another study of lipogranulomas located in portal areas it was suggested that these lesions originated from parenchymal fat transported to portal areas.[572] The portal lipogranulomas were also seen predominantly in liver biopsy samples from chronic alcoholics.

In my experience and that of others,[494–500] the majority of lipogranulomas seen in biopsy or autopsy material in North America are due to ingested mineral oil, as already noted in the section on drug-induced granulomas. They are not usually associated with hepatic steatosis, and in the reported autopsy series, the spleen and abdominal lymph nodes were also the seat of numerous lipogranulomas.[496–498] Mineral oil lipogranulomas are morphologically indistinguishable from those presumed to arise from rupture of fat cysts or from transport of lipid to portal areas. In the large series of cases from North America, the mineral oil composition of the lipogranulomas in the liver and other organs was conclusively established by chemical analysis.[494–499]

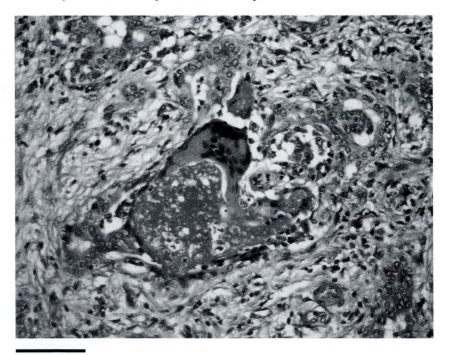

FIGURE 99.
Bile granuloma. Extravasated bile has excited a foreign body, giant cell response (HE, ×250).

BILE GRANULOMA.—Extravasated bile is often surrounded by a ring of foamy and bile-stained macrophages (pseudoxanthomatous) cells). In some instances there may be scattered foreign body giant cells that contain phagocytosed bile (Fig 99). Bile lakes and extravasates generally occur in prolonged extrahepatic biliary obstruction, e.g., extrahepatic biliary atresia. A granulomatous response to the extracellular bile, when present, is usually portal or periportal in location. It is worth noting at this juncture that granulomatoid clusters of xanthomatous and pseudoxanthomatous cells (formed by accumulation of the lipid component of bile in macrophages or epithelial cells, respectively) are frequently encountered in chronic cholestasis. These foamy, often bile-tinged cells are an important histologic hallmark of chronic cholestasis, regardless of etiology.

INHERITED METABOLIC DISEASES

CHRONIC GRANULOMATOUS DISEASE.—Characteristic findings in the liver in chronic granulomatous disease include the marked accumulation of lipofuscin in Kupffer cells and portal macrophages, epithelioid granulomas, and abscesses.[573-576] The portal macrophages are often clustered in granulomatoid foci. The granulomas may contain a few giant cells and many plasma cells. Special stains for microorganisms are generally negative. Abscesses in the liver are usually caused by staphylococci, Enterobacteriaceae, or *Serratia marcescens*. Other nonspecific changes in the liver include portal inflammation, periportal fibrosis, and steatosis; cirrhosis is rare.

NEOPLASMS

LANGERHANS' CELL HISTIOCYTOSIS.—This disorder of unknown etiology is characterized by abnormal proliferation of activated Langerhans' cells. Their Langerhans' cell lineage is confirmed by expression of S100 protein and CD1a antigen and by the presence of Birbeck granules in the cytoplasm by electron microscopic examination.[577] The majority of cases occur in early childhood. Multisystem involvement is rare, with the lungs, bone marrow, and liver most often affected. Hepatic involvement is manifested by features of sclerosing cholangitis or cirrhosis.[578-580] Langerhans' cells may infiltrate and progressively destroy bile ducts and also infiltrate the portal connective tissue. Focal granulomatoid aggregates of these cells may be present, typically in a periportal location (Figs 100 and 101). Ductopenia is accompanied by features of chronic cholestasis (pseudoxanthomatous change and copper accumulation), and there is increasing periportal fibrosis with eventual bridging and development of a biliary cirrhosis.

HODGKIN'S LYMPHOMA.—Epithelioid ("pseudosarcoid") granulomas in the liver have been described in this disease by many authors.[581-587] In one case the granulomas were "caseating."[587] It has been proposed that the presence of granulomas has favorable prognostic implications.[583] The etiology and pathogenesis of the granulomas in the liver, spleen, and lymph nodes in patients with Hodgkin's disease remain undetermined. In one

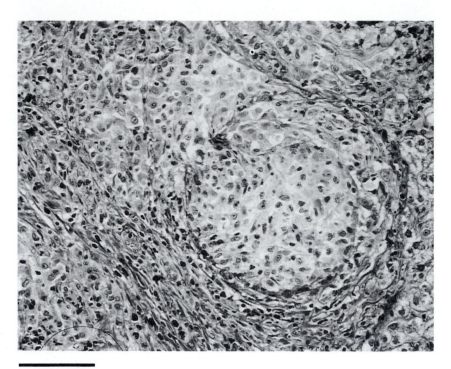

FIGURE 100.
Langerhans' cell histiocytosis with a focal granulomatoid aggregate of Langerhans' cells (HE, ×300).

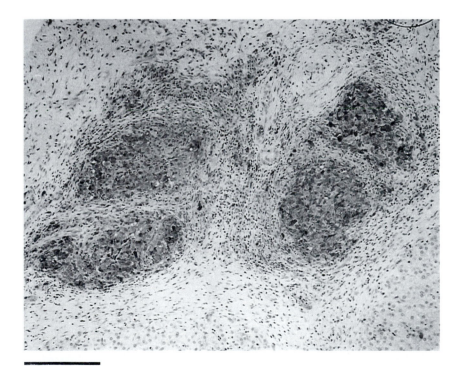

FIGURE 101.
Same case illustrated in Figure 100 with several aggregates of Langerhans' cells immunoreactive to anti-S100 protein (×150).

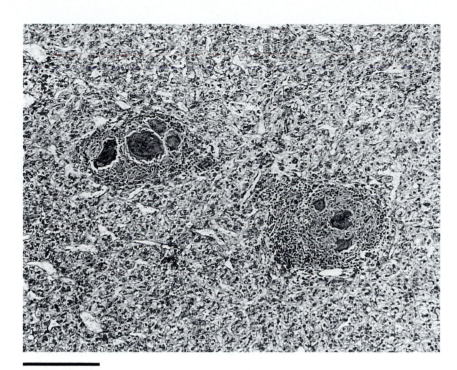

FIGURE 102.

Epithelioid granulomas in a hepatocellular adenoma (HE, ×100).

series of 332 cases of Hodgkin's disease studied by Delsol et al.,[588] fibrin ring granulomas were found in 4 cases (3 in the liver and 1 in the bone marrow).

NON-HODGKIN'S LYMPHOMA.—Epithelioid granulomas were reported by Saito et al.[589] in the liver of a patient with peripheral T-cell lymphoma and by Aderka et al.[586] in a patient with histiocytic lymphoma.

HYPERNEPHROMA.—Hepatic granulomas have been reported as a possible paraneoplastic manifestation in a patient with hypernephroma.[591]

PRIMARY HEPATIC TUMORS.—In cases on file at the Armed Forces Institute of Pathology, epithelioid granulomas have been observed in occasional primary tumors such as hepatocellular adenoma, focal nodular hyperplasia, hepatoblastoma, and hepatocellular carcinoma, both the usual and the fibrolamellar types (Fig 102). There are also scattered case reports in the literature.[592–595] The granulomas are typically confined to the tumor, and special stains for microorganisms have been consistently negative.

MISCELLANEOUS

FAMILIAL GRANULOMATOUS HEPATITIS.—A systemic illness was reported in two West Indian parents and their seven offspring who were studied for a 12-year period by Mahida et al.[596] In addition to the liver, granulomas were variably found in muscle, lymph nodes, and the pleura of some of the affected family members.

GRANULOMATOUS LIVER DISEASE OF THE INTRAHEPATIC VEINS.—This entity was reported in a 72-year-old man who had portal hypertension and refractory ascites.[597] Widespread epithelioid granulomas and phlebitis involving small hepatic and portal veins were found at necropsy.

GRANULOMATOUS HEPATITIS WITH PROLONGED FEVER.—This term has been used by Simon and Wolff[598] for patients with granulomatous hepatitis and prolonged fever that averaged 3.6 years from onset to referral to the authors. Extensive studies in the majority of these and other cases have failed to establish an etiology.[598–600] Most of the patients have responded well to corticosteroids. Histopathologic studies have not revealed differences between the granulomas in this condition and those of other diseases. The role of liver biopsy in the evaluation of fever of unknown origin was recently reviewed by Holz et al.[601]

PATHOLOGIC DIFFERENTIAL DIAGNOSIS

The final diagnosis in many cases of granulomatous liver disease depends on careful assessment of all clinical, laboratory, imaging, and histologic findings. On the other hand, histologic evaluation alone may be diagnostic or may suggest further investigations that ultimately lead to the correct diagnosis.

In studying hepatic (particularly needle) biopsy material the pathologist should examine every fragment on the slide. Serial sections are helpful in searching for etiologic agents, for example, eggs on their remnants in schistosomiasis or larvae in visceral larva migrans.

Gross examination of needle biopsy specimens is not likely to provide much useful information but should be recorded before fixation. Wedge biopsy and autopsy specimens may reveal changes that could be helpful, for example, the size and color of focal granulomatous lesions, confluence of the lesions, central necrosis or caseation, associated focal or diffuse fibrosis, "pipestem" fibrosis, cirrhosis, bile stasis, steatosis, etc.

Special stains are essential in studying granulomatous lesions of the liver, and their applications have been considered in the preceding sections. Those useful in identifying infectious agents are summarized in Table 5.

In reviewing sections of the liver containing granulomas the pathologist should seek answers to the following questions: (1) is the basic structure of the granulomas, in particular, the types of inflammatory cells, helpful in the differential diagnosis? (2) Do the granulomas contain some "object" in them that is of etiologic significance? (3) Do the granulomas contain microorganisms that are visible in HE-stained sections or in sections stained with special stains? (4) Do the granulomas contain particulate material that can only be seen (or is better visualized) by special microscopy such as polarizing or phase-contrast microscopy? (5) Can the particulate material in the granulomas be positively identified by energy-dispersive x-ray analysis or other special techniques? (6) Are there associated hepatic parenchymal changes that are helpful in the differential diagnosis?

BASIC STRUCTURE OF HEPATIC GRANULOMAS

1. Epithelioid granulomas in North America, Europe, and many other countries are most frequently related to sarcoidosis. They are, how-

TABLE 5.

Special Stains in Diagnosing Hepatic Granulomas

Stains	Application
Brown and Brenn or Brown/Hopps	Gram-positive and gram-negative bacteria, actinomycetes
Giemsa	Bacteria, *Toxoplasma*, leishmanias, rickettsiae
Periodic acid–Schiff	Fungi, *Mycobacterium avium-intracellulare*
Gridley fungus	Fungi
Gomori methenamine silver	Fungi, mycobacteria
Mucicarmine, Alcian blue, colloidal iron	Cryptococci
Kinyoun's stain	Mycobacteria, *Nocardia asteroides*, eggs of *Schistosoma mansoni* and *japonicum*, hooklets of *Echinococcus granulosus*
Warthin-Starry	Spirochetes
Machiavello	Rickettsiae
Wilder's reticulum stain	Leishmanias

ever, seen in a variety of infectious diseases (e.g., tuberculosis, tuberculoid leprosy, disseminated BCG infections, brucellosis, mycotic infections) as well as noninfectious disease (e.g., drug-induced liver injury). The differential diagnosis includes an assessment of the morphologic features and clinicopathologic correlation, as discussed in the preceding sections.

2. Granulomas containing many vacuolated macrophages may or may not be lipogranulomas. The term *lipogranuloma* has been used for the lesions resulting from the extrusion of neutral lipid from liver cells (which are usually intra-acinar in location) or for portal lipogranulomas that are thought to be due to migration of lipid from the parenchyma. Much more commonly, lipogranulomas are of mineral oil origin and are perivenular or portal in location. The lesions of lepromatous leprosy resemble lipogranulomas but are composed of vacuolated "lepra cells" that contain many lepra bacilli demonstrable by stains for acid-fast bacilli. Some particulate materials, e.g., talc or gold, may be entrapped in lipogranulomas; they are birefringent and can be positively identified by x-ray microanalysis.

3. Granulomas composed of aggregates of hypertrophied Kupffer cells or portal macrophages with a granular basophilic cytoplasm (macrophagic granulomas) are usually due to disseminated infection with MAI. The organisms are PAS-positive and acid-fast.

4. Lesions with suppurative centers and a granulomatous and sometimes palisaded periphery are likely to be related to infections caused by bacteria or higher bacteria; examples of diseases with these lesions include listeriosis, melioidosis, tularemia, and actinomycosis.

5. Palisading may also be seen in parasitic infections such as visceral larva migrans or capillariasis, the centers of the granulomatous lesions having eosinophilic necrotic centers. Rarely, palisaded granulomas have been noted in rheumatoid arthritis and extrahepatic biliary atresia.

6. Fibrin ring ("doughnut") granulomas are typical of Q fever but have been reported in other diseases (see Table 3). The classic fibrin ring granuloma has a central vacuole, a fibrin ring, histiocytes, and less often epithelioid cells and a few inflammatory cells.

7. Granulomas with many eosinophils are usually caused by drug-induced injury or helminthic infections. The latter may contain parasitic eggs or larvae, or there may be parasitic (schistosomal) pigment in reticuloendothelial cells. Some drug-induced granulomas may be accompanied by hepatocellular and/or cholestatic injury and infrequently by cholangitis or vasculitis.

8. The type of necrosis, when present, can be helpful in the differential diagnosis. Fibrillogranular (caseous) necrosis is typical of tuberculosis but can be seen in some mycotic granulomas, for example, in coccidioidomycosis or histoplasmosis. An amorphous, eosinophilic necrosis is typical of syphilitic gummas, which are also often associated with an endarteritis. A fibrillary type of necrosis may be occasionally seen in sarcoidosis. An eosinophilic granular necrosis is typical of granulomas associated with helminthic infections, for example, visceral larva migrans, capillariasis, and schistosomiasis. The eosinophilic center of such granulomas contains the extruded granules of degenerated eosinophils, Charcot-Leyden crystals, and in some cases, the parasite or parasitic eggs.

EXOGENOUS OR ENDOGENOUS STRUCTURES IDENTIFIED IN GRANULOMAS IN SECTIONS STAINED WITH HEMATOXYLIN-EOSIN.—These include some bacteria, fungi, protozoal organisms, parasitic larvae or eggs, extruded endogenous cell components (lipid, bile), or exogenous particulate material such as suture material, talc, starch, silica, anthracotic pigment (black), gold (black), titanium (black), barium (colorless), and Thorotrast (pinkish brown). Copper in visceral granulomas of vineyard sprayers exposed to copper sulfate is colorless but can be stained with rubeanic acid of rhodanine. Talc, silica, and the various metals are all readily identified by scanning electron microscopy coupled with x-ray microanalysis.

INFECTIOUS AGENTS IDENTIFIED BY SPECIAL STAINS.—These include rickettsiae, bacteria, mycobacteria, spirochetes, fungi, protozoa, and parasitic eggs (particularly the chitinous remnants of schistosome eggs (see Table 5).

SEQUELAE OF HEPATIC GRANULOMAS

Most of the sequelae listed in Table 6 have been discussed in the text and do not require further elaboration.

ACKNOWLEDGMENTS

The author is most grateful for the expert typing and editorial assistance of Ms. Fanny X. Revelo, secretary, Department of Hepatic and Gastroin-

TABLE 6.
Sequelae of Hepatic Granulomas and Underlying Diseases

Sequela	Example
Focal scarring ± calcification	Sarcoidosis, tuberculosis, histoplasmosis, schistosomiasis
Granulomatous pseudotumor	Sarcoidosis ("sarcoidoma"), tuberculosis
Irregular and deep scarring (hepar lobatum)	Tertiary syphilis, schistosomiasis
Diffuse fibrosis	Visceral leishmaniasis
Marked portal fibrosis ("pipestem type")	Schistosomiasis
Cirrhosis,* biliary	Primary biliary cirrhosis, sarcoidosis, ascariasis
Obliterative portal venopathy ± portal hypertension	Schistosomiasis, sarcoidosis
Nodular transformation	Primary biliary cirrhosis, schistosomiasis
Budd-Chiari syndrome†	Sarcoidosis, tertiary syphilis
Acute and chronic cholangitis ± intrahepatic lithiasis	Ascariasis, fascioliasis, clonorchiasis, opisthorchiasis
Destructive cholangitis, ductopenia, chronic cholestasis	Sarcoidosis, primary biliary cirrhosis
Rupture of tuberculoma into bile ducts with granulomatous cholangitis	Tuberculosis
Metaplasia, dysplasia, cancer in situ of the biliary epithelium	Clonorchiasis, opisthorchiasis, fascioliasis
Intrahepatic cholangiocarcinoma	Clonorchiasis, opisthorchiasis

*Cirrhosis may also be due to an associated disease, e.g., hepatitis B or C infection in patients with schistosomiasis.
†Vascular invasion by *Aspergillus* can lead to the Budd-Chiari syndrome, but the involvement is nongranulomatous.

testinal Pathology, and for the outstanding photographic support of Ms. Robin Anne V. Ferris, MFS, and Mr. BeeJay Jones, Medical Illustration Service, Armed Forces Institute of Pathology, Washington, DC.

REFERENCES

1. Fauci AS, Wolff SM: Granulomatous hepatitis. *Prog Liver Dis* 5:609–621, 1976.
2. Ryder KW, Jay SJ, Kiblawi SO, et al: Serum angiotensin converting enzyme activity in patients with histoplasmosis. *JAMA* 248:1888–1889, 1983.
3. Guckian JC, Perry JE: Granulomatous hepatitis: An analysis of 63 cases and review of the literature. *Ann Intern Med* 65:1081–1100, 1966.
4. Relman DA: The identification of uncultured microbial pathogens. *J Infect Dis* 168:1–8, 1993.
5. Naber SP: Molecular pathology–diagnosis of infectious disease. *N Engl J Med* 331:122–1215, 1994.

6. Hillyard DR: The molecular approach to microbial diagnosis. *Am J Clin Pathol* 101(suppl 1):518–521, 1994.

7. Versalovic J, Kapur V, Koeuth T, et al: DNA fingerprinting of pathogenic bacteria by fluorophore-enhanced repetitive sequence-base polymerase chain reaction. *Arch Pathol Lab Med* 119:23–29, 1995.

8. Montone KT, Litzky LA: Rapid method for detection of *Aspergillus* 55 ribosomal RNA using a genus-specific oligonucleotide probe. *Am J Clin Pathol* 103:48–51, 1995.

9. Ferrell LD: Hepatic granulomas: A morphologic approach to diagnosis. *Surg Pathol* 3:87–106, 1990.

10. Denk H, Scheuer PJ, Baptista A, et al: Guidelines for the diagnosis and interpretation of hepatic granulomas. *Histopathology* 25:209–218, 1994.

11. Decker K: The macrophages and their signal products, in Bianchi L, Gerok W, Maler K-P, et al: (eds): *Infectious Diseases of the Liver.* Dordrecht, Kluwer Academic, 1990, pp 49–71.

12. Chensue SW, Warmington K, Ruth J, et al: Cytokine responses during mycobacterial and schistosomal antigen–induced pulmonary granuloma formation. Production of Th1 and Th2 cytokines and relative contribution of tumor necrosis factor. *Am J Pathol* 145:1105–1113, 1991.

13. James EMV, Williams WJ: Fine structure and histochemistry of epithelioid cells in sarcoidosis. *Thorax* 29:115–120, 1974.

14. Murch AR, Grounds MD, Marshall CA, et al: Direct evidence that inflammatory multinucleate giant cells form by fusion. *J Pathol* 137:177–180, 1982.

15. James DJ, Scheuer PJ: Hepatic granulomas, in McIntyre N, Benhamou J-P, Bircher J, et al (eds): *Oxford Textbook of Clinical Hepatology,* vol 2. Oxford, Oxford University Press, 1991, pp 750–758.

16. van der Rhee HJ, van der Burgh–de Winter CPM, Daems WT: The differentiation of monocytes into macrophages, epithelioid cells and multinucleated giant cells in subcutaneous granulomas. *Cell Tissue Res* 197:355–361, 1979.

17. Fais D, Burgio VL, Silvestri M, et al: Multinucleated giant cells generation induced by interferon-γ. Changes in the expression of the intercellular adhesion molecule-1 during macrophages fusion and multinucleated giant cell formation. *Lab Invest* 71:737–744, 1994.

18. von Lichtenberg F, Smith JH, Cheever AW: The Hoeppli phenomenon in schistosomiasis: Comparative pathology and immunopathology. *Am J Trop Med Hyg* 15:886–895, 1966.

19. Williams AO: Pathology of phycomycosis due to *Entomophthora* and *Basidiobolus* species. *Arch Pathol* 87:13–20, 1973.

20. Liber AF, Choi H-S H: Splendore-Hoeppli phenomenon about silk sutures in tissue. *Arch Pathol* 95:217–220, 1973.

21. Johnson FB: Splendore-Hoeppli phenomenon, in Binford CH, Connor DH (eds): *Pathology of Tropical and Extraordinary Disease,* vol 2. Washington, DC, Armed Forces Institute of Pathology, 1976, pp 681–683.

22. Adams DO: The granulomatous inflammatory response. A review. *Am J Pathol* 84:164–191, 1976.

23. Epstein LW: Granuloma formation in man. *Pathobiology Annu* 7:1–30, 1977.

24. Adams DO: The biology of the granuloma, in Ioachim HL (ed): *Pathology of Granulomas.* New York, Raven Press, 1983, pp 1–20.

25. Neville E, Piyasena KHG, James DG: Granulomas of the liver. *Postgrad Med J* 15:361–365, 1975.

26. Klatskin G: Hepatic granulomata: Problems in interpretation. *Mt Sinai J Med* 44:798–812, 1977.

27. McMaster KR, Hennigar GR: Drug-induced granulomatous hepatitis. *Lab Invest* 44:61–73, 1982.

28. Cunningham D, Mills PR, Quigley EMM, et al: Hepatic granulomas: Experience over a 10-year period in the West of Scotland. *Q J Med* 51:162–170, 1982.

29. Diaz Curiel M, Guerrero F, De Miguel J, et al: Granulomatosis hepatica. Un estudio de 109 casos. *Rev Clin Esp* 170:265–269, 1983.

30. Satti MB, Al-Freihi H, Ibrahim EM, et al: Hepatic granulomas in Saudi Arabia: A clinicopathological study of 59 cases. *Am J Gastroenterol* 85:669–673, 1990.

31. Sartin JS, Walker RC: Granulomatous hepatitis: A retrospective review of 88 cases at the Mayo Clinic. *Mayo Clin Proc* 66:914–918, 1991.

32. McCluggage WG, Sloan JM: Hepatic granulomas in Northern Ireland: A thirteen year review. *Histopathology* 25:219–228, 1994.

33. Wadsworth RC, Keil PG: Biopsy of the liver in infectious mononucleosis. *Am J Pathol* 28:1003–1016, 1952.

34. Nelson RS, Darragh JH: Infectious mononucleosis hepatitis: A clinicopathologic study. *Am J Med* 21:26–33, 1956.

35. Kilpatrick SM: Structural and functional abnormalities of liver in infectious mononucleosis. *Ann Intern Med* 117:47–53, 1966.

36. Ishak KG: Granulomas of the liver, in Ioachim HL (ed): *Pathology of Granulomas.* New York, Raven Press, 1983, pp 307–369.

37. White NJ, Juel-Jensen BE: Infectious mononucleosis hepatitis. *Semin Liver Dis* 4:301–306, 1984.

38. Klatskin G: Hepatitis associated with systemic infections, in Schiff L (ed): *Diseases of the Liver,* ed 4. Philadelphia, JB Lippincott, 1975, pp 711–754.

39. Nenert M, Mavier P, Dubuc N, et al: Epstein-Barr virus infection and hepatic fibrin-ring granulomas. *Hum Pathol* 19:608–610, 1988.

40. Rothwell DJ: Bone marrow granulomas and infectious mononucleosis. *Arch Pathol* 100:508–509, 1975.

41. Harries JT, Ferguson AW: Fatal infectious mononucleosis with liver necrosis in two sisters. *Arch Dis Child* 43:480–485, 1968.

42. Chang MY, Campbell WG: Fatal infectious mononucleosis: Association with liver necrosis and herpes-like viral particles. *Arch Pathol* 99:185–191, 1975.

43. Tazawa Y, Nishinomiya F, Noguchi H, et al: A case of fatal infectious mononucleosis presenting with fulminant hepatic failure associated with an extensive CD8-positive lymphocyte infiltration in the liver. *Hum Pathol* 24:1135–1139, 1993.

44. Reller LB: Granulomatous hepatitis associated with acute cytomegalovirus infection. *Lancet* 1:20–22, 1973.

45. Bonkowsky HL, Lee RV, Klatskin G: Acute granulomatous hepatitis: Occurrence in cytomegalovirus mononucleosis. *JAMA* 233:1284–1288, 1975.

46. Clarke J, Craig RM, Saffro R, et al: Cytomegalovirus granulomatous hepatitis. *Am J Med* 66:264–269, 1979.

47. Snover DC, Horwitz CA: Liver disease in cytomegalovirus mononucleosis: A light microscopical and immunoperoxidase study of six cases. *Hepatology* 4:408–412, 1984.

48. Krech T, Wegmann T, Stanisic M: Granulomatose Zytomegalievirus-Hepatitis. *Schweiz Med Wochenschr* 114:469–475, 1984.

49. Lobdel DH: Ring granulomas in cytomegalovirus hepatitis. *Arch Pathol Lab Med* 111:881–882, 1987.

50. Young JF, Goulian M: Bone marrow fibrin ring granulomas and cytomegalovirus infection. *Am J Clin Pathol* 99:65–68, 1993.

51. Porz E, Garcia-Pagan JL, Bruguera M, et al: Hepatic fibrin-ring granulomas in a patient with hepatitis A. *Gastroenterology* 100:269–270, 1991.

52. Ruel M, Sevestre H, Biabaud H, et al: Fibrin ring granulomas in hepatitis A. *Dig Dis Sci* 17:1915–1917, 1992.

53. Ishak KG: Hepatitis A infection: Pathology, in Seeff LB, Lewis JH (eds): *Current Perspectives in hepatology. A Festschrift for Hyman J. Zimmerman, M.D.* New York, Plenum, 1989, pp 15–22.

54. Emile JF, Sebagh M, Feray C, et al: The presence of epithelioid granulomas in hepatitis C virus–related cirrhosis. *Hum Pathol* 10:1095–1097, 1993.

55. Reynolds TB, Campra JL, Peters RL: Hepatic granulomata, in Zakim D, Boyer TD (eds): *Hepatology. A Textbook of Liver Disease*, vol 2. Philadelphia, WB Saunders, 1990, pp 1098–1114.

56. Pellegrin M, Delsol G, Auvergnat JC, et al: Granulomatous hepatitis in Q fever. *Hum Pathol* 11:51–57, 1980.

57. Hofmann CE, Heaton JH: Q fever hepatitis: Clinical manifestations and pathological findings. *Gastroenterology* 83:474–479, 1982.

58. Qizilbash AH: The pathology of Q fever. *Arch Pathol Lab Med* 107:364–367, 1983.

59. Voigt J-J, Cassigneul J, Delsol G, et al: Hèpatite granulomateuse: A propos de 112 cas chez l'adulte. *Ann Pathol* 4:78–80, 1984.

60. Srigley JR, Geddie WR, Vellend H, et al: Q fever: The liver and bone marrow pathology. *Am J Surg Pathol* 9:752–758, 1985.

61. Travis LB, Travis WD, Li C-Y, et al: Q fever: A clinicopathologic study of five cases. *Arch Pathol Lab Med* 110:1017–1020, 1986.

62. Marazuela M, Moreno A, Yebra M, et al: Hepatic fibrin-ring granulomas: A clinicopathologic study of 23 patients. *Hum Pathol* 22:607–613, 1991.

63. Yale SH, DeGroen PC, Tooson JD, et al: Unusual aspects of acute Q fever–associated hepatitis. *Mayo Clin Proc* 69:769–773, 1994.

64. Turck WPG, Howitt G, Turnberg A, et al: Chronic Q fever. *Q J Med* 45:193–217, 1976.

65. Guardia J, Martinez-Vasquez, Moragas A, et al: The liver in boutonneuse fever. *Gut* 15:549–551, 1974.

66. Yow EM, Brennan JC, Preston K, et al: The pathology of psittacosis: Report of 2 cases with hepatitis. *Am J Med* 27:739–749, 1959.

67. Byron NP, Walls J, Mair HJ: Fulminant psittacosis. *Lancet* 1:353–356, 1979.

68. Macfarlane JT, Macrae AD: Psittacosis. *Br Med Bull* 39:163–167, 1983.

69. Cornog JL, Hanson W: Psittacosis as a cause of miliary infiltrates of the lung and hepatic granulomas. *Am Rev Respir Dis* 98:1033–1036, 1968.

70. Ragnaud JM, Dupon M, Echinard E, et al: Les manifestations hèpatiques de la psittacosis. *Gastroenterol Clin Biol* 10:234–237, 1986.

71. Wagoner GP, Anton AT, Gall EA, et al: Needle biopsy of the liver. VIII. Experience with hepatic granulomas. *Gastroenterology* 25:487–494, 1953.

72. Leelarasamee A, Bovarnkitti S: Melioidosis: Review and update. *Rev Infect Dis* 11:413–425, 1989.

73. Centers for Disease Control: Melioidosis—Pennsylvania. *MMWR* 25:419–420, 1977.

74. Piggott JA, Hochholzer L: Human melioidosis: A histopathologic study of acute and chronic melioidosis. *Arch Pathol* 90:101–111, 1970.

75. Piggott JA: Melioidosis, in Binford CH, Connor DH (eds): *Pathology of Tropical and Extraordinary Diseases*, vol 1. Washington, DC, Armed Forces Institute of Pathology, 1976, pp 169–174.

76. Colizza F, LePages, LaJoie J-F, et al: Multiple hepatic abscesses following Yersinia enterocolitica septicemia. *Can J Gastroenterol* 4:179–183, 1990.

77. Stjernberg U, Silseth C, Ritland S: Granulomatous hepatitis in *Yersinia enterocolitica* infection. *Hepatogastroenterology* 34:56–57, 1987.
78. Saebo A, Lassen J: Acute and chronic liver disease associated with Yersinia enterocolitica infection: A Norwegian 10-year follow-up study of 458 hospitalized patients. *J Intern Med* 231:531–535, 1992.
79. Cover TL, Aber RC: *Yersinia enterocolitica. N Engl J Med* 321:16–24, 1989.
80. Hunt AC, Bothwell PW: Histological findings in human brucellosis. *J Clin Pathol* 20:267–272, 1967.
81. Young EJ: Brucella melitensis hepatitis: The absence of granulomas. *Ann Intern Med* 91:414–415, 1979.
82. Molina JL, Cadaval RL, Guttierrez JMH, et al: Granulomatosis hepatica brucelòsica. *Rev Clin Esp* 152:465–468, 1979.
83. Masana L, Bernardo L, Bacardi R, et al: Brucella hepatitis. *Ann Intern Med* 92:709–710, 1980.
84. Cervantes F, Bruguera M, Carbonell J, et al: Liver disease in brucellosis. A clinical and pathological study of 40 cases. *Postgrad Med J* 58:346–350, 1982.
85. Williams RK, Crossley K: Acute and chronic hepatic involvement of brucellosis. *Gastroenterology* 83:455–458, 1982.
86. Naveau S, Poitrine A, Delfraissy JF, et al: Brucellosis hepatic abscesses and pregnancy (letter). *Gastroenterology* 84:1643, 1983.
87. Greiner VL, Franken FH, Schubert GE, et al: Solitare Leberabszesse bei chronischer Brucelloses. *Z Gastroenterol* 22:337–442, 1984.
88. Ramachandran S, Godfrey JJ, Perera MVF: Typhoid hepatitis. *JAMA* 230:236–240, 1974.
89. de Brito T, Vieira WT, Dias MD: Jaundice in typhoid hepatitis: A light and electron microscopy study based on liver biopsies. *Acta Hepatogastroenterol* 24:426–433, 1977.
90. Singh DS, Nair PNR, Krishnasamy S, et al: Jaundice in typhoid fever. *J Trop Med Hyg* 81:68–70, 1978.
91. El Kabbaj M, Bernard P, El Hachimi A, et al: Attiente hèpatique an cours de la fievre typhoide. *Gastroenterol Clin Biol* 3:651–656, 1979.
92. Zarate E, Sanchez L, Nava E, et al: Compromiso hepatico in Fiebre Tifoidea. *Rev Gastroenterol (Peru)* 4:88–91, 1984.
93. Dan M, Bar-Meir S, Jedevah M, et al: Typhoid hepatitis with immunoglobulin and complement deposits in bile canaliculi. *Arch Intern Med* 142:148–149, 1982.
94. Pais P: A hepatitis like picture in typhoid fever. *BMJ* 289:225–226, 1984.
95. Khosla SN, Singh R, Singh GP, et al: The spectrum of hepatic injury in enteric fever. *Am J Gastroenterol* 83:413–416, 1988.
96. Morgenstern R, Hayes PC: The liver in typhoid fever: Always affected, not just a complication. *Am J Gastroenterol* 86:1235–1239, 1991.
97. Chung WK, Yoo JY: Histologic study of typhoid fever, in Chung WK (ed): *Liver Diseases. An Atlas of Histopathology.* Amsterdam, Elsevier, 1993, pp 167–175.
98. Soni PN, Hoosen AA, Pillay DG: Hepatic abscess caused by *Salmonella typhi. Dig Dis Sci* 39:1694–1696, 1994.
99. Ishak KG: Listeriosis, in Binford CH, Connor DH (eds): *Pathology of Tropical and Extraordinary Diseases,* vol 1. Washington, DC, Armed Forces Institute of Pathology, 1976, pp 178–186.
100. Yu VL, Miller WP, Wing EJ, et al: Disseminated listeriosis presenting as acute hepatitis. Case reports and review of hepatic involvement in listeriosis. *Am J Med* 73:773–777, 1982.

101. Bourgeois N, Jacobs F, Tavares ML, et al: Listeria monocytogenes hepatitis in liver transplant recipient: A case report and review of the literature. *J Hepatol* 19:284–289, 1993.

102. Al-Dajani O, Khatib R: Cryptogenic liver abscess due to Listeria Monocytogenes. *J Infect Dis* 147:961–962, 1983.

103. Jenkins D, Richards J, Rees Y, et al: Multiple listerial liver abscesses. *Gut* 28:1661–1662, 1987.

104. Ribiere O, Coutarel P, Jarher V, et al: Abcès du foie á Listeria monocytogens chez un malade diabètique. *Presse Med* 19:1538–1540, 1990.

105. Lamont R, Postlewhaite R, McGowan A: Review. Listeria monocytogenes and its role in human infection. *J Infect* 17:7–28, 1988.

106. Gellin BG, Broome CV: Listeriosis. *JAMA* 281:1313–1320, 1988.

107. Armstrong D: Listeria monocytogenes, in Mandell GL, Bennett JE, Dolin R (eds): *Principles and Practice of Infectious Diseases*, ed 4. New York, Churchill Livingstone, 1995, pp 1880–1885.

108. Bernstein A: Tularemia: A report of three fatal cases with autopsies. *Arch Intern Med* 56:1117–1135, 1935.

109. Dienst FT: Tularemia: A perusal of three-hundred and thirty-nine cases. *J La State Med Soc* 115:114–127, 1963.

110. Francis E: A summary of present knowledge of tularaemia. *Medicine (Baltimore)* 8:411–532, 1928.

111. Pullen RL, Stuart BM: Tularemia: Analysis of 225 cases. *JAMA* 129:495–500, 1945.

112. Ortego TJ, Hutchins LF, Rice J, et al: Tularemic hepatitis presenting as objective jaundice. *Gastroenterology* 91:461–463, 1986.

113. Winslow DJ: Botryomycosis. *Am J Pathol* 35:153–167, 1959.

114. Greenblatt M, Heredia R, Rubenstein L, et al: Bacterial pseudomycosis ("botryomycosis"). *Am J Clin Pathol* 41:188–193, 1964.

115. Weed LA, Baggenstoss AH: Actinomycosis: A pathologic and bacteriologic study of twenty-one fatal cases. *Am J Clin Pathol* 7:201–219, 1949.

116. Putman HC Jr, Dockerty MB, Waugh JM: Abdominal actinomycosis. *Surgery* 28:781–800, 1950.

117. Meade RH: Primary hepatic actinomycosis. *Gastroenterology* 78:355–359, 1980.

118. Davies M, Keddie NC: Abdominal actinomycosis. *Br J Surg* 60:18–22, 1973.

119. Brown JR: Human actinomycosis: A study of 181 subjects. *Hum Pathol* 4:319–330, 1973.

120. Hotchi M, Schwarz J: Characterization of actinomycotic granules by architecture and staining methods. *Arch Pathol* 93:392–400, 1972.

121. Murray JF, Finegold SM, Froman S, et al: The changing spectrum of nocardiosis: A review and presentation of nine cases. *Am Rev Respir Dis* 83:315–330, 1961.

122. Emmons CW, Binford CH, Utz JP, et al: *Medical Mycology*, ed 3. Philadelphia, Lea & Febiger, 1977.

123. Cross RM, Binford CH: Is Nocardia asteroides an opportunist? *Lab Invest* 11:1103–1109, 1962.

124. Sen P, Louria DB: Higher bacterial and fungal infections, in Greico MH (ed): *Infections in the Abnormal Host*. New York, Yorke Medical Books, 1980, pp 325–359.

125. Robboy SJ, Vickery AL Jr: Tinctorial and morphologic properties distinguishing actinomycosis and nocardiosis. *N Engl J Med* 282:593–596, 1970.

126. Font J, Bruguera M, Perez-Villa F, et al: Hepatic fibrin ring granulomas caused by Staphylococcus epidermidis generalized infection. *Gastroenterology* 93:1449–1451, 1987.

127. Raviglione MC, Snider DE, Kochi A: Global epidemiology of tuberculosis: Morbidity and mortality of a worldwide epidemic. *JAMA* 273:220–226, 1995.

128. Alvarez SZ, Carpio R: Hepatobiliary tuberculosis. *Dig Dis Sci* 28:193–200, 1983.

129. Zipser RD, Rau JE, Ricketts RR, et al: Tuberculous pseudotumors of the liver. *Am J Med* 61:946–951, 1976.

130. Forward KR, Tong AY, Campbell RO, et al: Tuberculous pseudotumour of the liver developing during antituberculous chemotherapy. *Can Med Assoc J* 132:45–46, 1985.

131. Blangy S, Cornud F, Sibert A, et al: Hepatic tuberculosis presenting as tumoral disease on ultrasonography. *Gastrointest Radiol* 13:52–54, 1988.

132. Chan HS, Pang J: Isolated giant tuberculomata of the liver detected by computed tomography. *Gastrointest Radiol* 14:305–307, 1989.

133. Levine C: Primary macronodular hepatic tuberculosis: US and CT appearances. *Gastrointest Radiol* 15:307–309, 1990.

134. Kawamori Y, Matsui O, Ketagawa K, et al: Macronodular tuberculoma of the liver: CT and MR findings. *AJR Am J Roentgenol* 158:311–313, 1992.

135. Emre A, Akpinar E, Acarli K, et al: Primary solitary tuberculosis of the liver. *HPB Surg* 5:261–265, 1992.

136. Rosenkranz K, Howard LD: Tubular tuberculosis of the liver. *Arch Pathol* 22:743–754, 1936.

137. Abscal J, Martin F, Abreu L, et al: Atypical hepatic tuberculosis presenting as obstructive jaundice. *Am J Gastroenterol* 83:1183–1186, 1988.

138. Ratanarapee S, Pausawasdi A: Tuberculosis of the common bile duct. *HPB Surg* 3:205–208, 1991.

139. Murphy TF, Gray GF: Biliary tract obstruction due to tuberculous adenitis. *Am J Med* 68:452, 1980.

140. Lafay J-P, Fouet P: Adenopathie tuberculeuse compressive de la voie biliare principale: Guerison spontanee par fistulisation dans le choledoque. *Gastroenterol Clin Biol* 7:915–918, 1983.

141. Stanley JH, Yantis PL, Marsh WH: Periportal tuberculous adenitis: A rare cause of obstructive jaundice. *Gastrointest Radiol* 9:227–229, 1984.

142. Pombo F, Soler R, Arrojo L, et al: US and CT findings in biliary obstruction due to tuberculous adenitis in the periportal area: 2 cases. *Eur J Radiol* 9:71–163, 1990.

143. Essop AR, Posen JA, Hodkinson JH, et al: Tuberculous hepatitis: A clinical review of 96 cases. *Q J Med* 53:465–477, 1987.

144. Maharay B, Leary WP, Pudifin DJ: A prospective study of hepatic tuberculosis in 41 black patients. *Q J Med* 63:517–522, 1987.

145. Thomas MR, Goldin RD: Tuberculosis presenting as jaundice. *Br J Clin Pract* 44:161–163, 1990.

146. Asada Y, Hayashi T, Sumiyoshi A, et al: Miliary tuberculosis presenting as fever and jaundice with hepatic failure. *Hum Pathol* 22:92–94, 1991.

147. Mandak M, Kerbl U, Kleinert R, et al: Miliare Tuberkulose der Leber als Ursache eines septischen Schocks mit Multiorganversagen. *Wien Klin Wochenschr* 106:11–114, 1994.

148. Maartens G, Willcox PA, Benatar SR: Miliary tuberculosis: Rapid diagnosis, hematologic abnormalities, and outcome in 109 treated adults. *Am J Med* 89:291–296, 1990.

149. Popper HH, Winter E, Hofler G: DNA of *Mycobacterium* tuberculosis in formalin-fixed, paraffin embedded tissue in tuberculosis and sarcoidosis detected by polymerase chain reaction. *Am J Clin Pathol* 101:738–741, 1994.

150. Korn RJ, Kellow WF, Heller P, et al: hepatic involvement in extrapulmo-

nary tuberculosis: Histologic and functional characteristics. *Am J Med* 28:60–71, 1950.

151. Chung WK: *Liver Diseases. An Atlas of Histopathology.* Amsterdam, Elsevier, 1993.

152. Horsburgh CR: *Mycobacterium avium* complex infection in the acquired immunodeficiency syndrome. *N Engl J Med* 324:1332–1338, 1991.

153. Horsburgh CR, Mason UG, Farhi DC, et al: Disseminated infection with *Mycobacterium avium-intracellulare:* A report of 13 cases and a review of the literature. *Medicine (Baltimore)* 64:36–47, 1985.

154. Glasgow BJ, Anders K, Layfield LJ, et al: Clinical and pathologic findings in the acquired immune deficiency syndrome (AIDS). *Am J Clin Pathol* 83:582–588, 1985.

155. Farhi DC, Mason UG, Horsburgh CR: Pathologic findings in disseminated *Mycobacterium avium-intracellulare* infection; a report of 11 cases. *Am J Clin Pathol* 85:67–72, 1986.

156. Klatt EC, Jensen DF, Meyer PR: Pathology of *Mycobacterium avium-intracellulare* infection in acquired immunodeficiency syndrome. *Hum Pathol* 18:709–714, 1987.

157. Ludwig J, Ishak KG: *Proceedings of Slide Seminar "Diseases of the Liver."* Chicago, American Society of Clinical Pathologists, 1989.

158. Ghassemi M, Anderson BR, Reddy VM, et al: Human immunodeficiency virus and *Mycobacterium avis* complex coinfection of monocytoid cells results in reciprocal enhancement of multiplication. *J Infect Dis* 171:68–73, 1995.

159. Wear DJ, Hadfield TL, Connor DH, et al: Periodic acid–Schiff reaction stains *Mycobacterium tuberculosis, Mycobacterium leprae, Mycobacterium ulcerans, Mycobacterium chelonei (abscessus)* and *Mycobacterium kansasii. Arch Pathol Lab Med* 109:701–702, 1985.

160. Anderson VM, Kehn E, Greco MA: Pediatric AIDS pathology, in Weinstein RS (ed): *Advances in Pathology and Laboratory Medicine,* vol 6. St Louis, Mosby, 1993, pp 313–343.

161. Gruhl VR, Reese MH: Disseminated atypical mycobacterial disease presenting as "leukemia." *Am J Clin Pathol* 55:206–211, 1971.

162. Manes JL, Blair OM: Disseminated *Mycobacterium kansasii* complication of hairy cell leukemia. *JAMA* 236:1878–1879, 1976.

163. Weinberg JR, Dootson G, Gertner D, et al: Disseminated *Mycobacterium xenopi* infection. *Lancet* 1:1033–1034, 1985.

164. Patel KM: Granulomatous hepatitis due to *Mycobacterium scrofulaceum:* Report of a case. *Gastroenterology* 81:156–158, 1981.

165. Maschek H, Georgii A, Schmidt RE, et al: *Mycobacterium genavense:* Autopsy findings in three patients. *Am J Clin Pathol* 101:95–99, 1994.

166. Wolinsky E: Nontuberculous mycobacteria and associated diseases. *Am Rev Respir Dis* 119:107–159, 1979.

167. Voline F, Colton R, Lester W: Disseminated infection caused by Battey type mycobacteria. *Am J Clin Pathol* 43:39–46, 1965.

168. Gorse G, Fairshter RD, Friedly G, et al: Nontuberculosis mycobacterial disease: Experience in a Southern California hospital. *Arch Intern Med* 143:225–228, 1983.

169. Havur DV, Ellner JJ: Mycobacterium avium complex, in Mandell GL, Bennett JE, Dolin R (eds): *Principles and Practice of Infectious Diseases,* ed 4. New York, Churchill Livingstone, 1995, pp 2250–2264.

170. Horowitz EA, Sanders WE: Other mycobacterium species, in Mandell GL, Bennett JE, Dolin R (eds): *Principles and Practice of Infectious Diseases,* ed 4. New York, Churchill Livingstone, 1995, pp 2264–2273.

171. Gormsen H: On the occurrence of epithelioid cell granulomas in the organs of B.C.G-vaccinated human beings. *Acta Pathol Microbiol Scand Suppl* 11:117–118, 1955.
172. Bodurtha A, Kim YH, Laucius JF, et al: Hepatic granulomas and other hepatic lesions associated with B.C.G. immunotherapy for cancer. *Am J Clin Pathol* 61:747–752, 1964.
173. Carlgren LE, Hansson CG, Henricsson L, et al: Fatal B.C.G. infection in an infant with congenital, lymphopenic agammaglobulinemia. *Acta Paediatr Scand* 55:636–644, 1966.
174. Watanabe T, Tanaka K, Hajiwara Y: Generalized tuberculosis after B.C.G. vaccination: Report of an autopsy case. *Acta Pathol Jpn* 19:395–407, 1969.
175. Freundlich E, Suprun H: Tuberculoid granulomata in the liver after B.C.G. vaccination. *Isr J Med Sci* 5:108–113, 1969.
176. Esterly JR, Sturner WQ, Esterly NB, et al: Disseminated B.C.G. in twin boys with presumed chronic granulomatous disease of childhood. *Pediatrics* 48:141–144, 1971.
177. Hunt JS, Silverstein JJ, Sparks FC, et al: Granulomatous hepatitis: A complication of B.C.G. immunotherapy (letter). *Lancet* 2:13, 1973.
178. Hunt JS, Silverstein JJ, Sparks FC, et al: Granulomatous hepatitis: A complication of B.C.G. immunotherapy. *Lancet* 2:820–821, 1973.
179. Sparks FC, Silverstein MJ, Hunt JS, et al: Complications of B.C.G. immunotherapy in patients with cancer. *N Engl J Med* 289:827–830, 1973.
180. Grant RM, Mackie R, Cochran AJ, et al: Results of administering B.C.G. to patients with melanoma. *Lancet* 2:1096–1100, 1974.
181. Verronon P: Presumed disseminated B.C.G. in a boy with chronic granulomatous disease of childhood. *Acta Pediatr Scand* 63:627–630, 1974.
182. Aungst CW, Sokal JE, Jager BV: Complications of B.C.G. vaccination in neoplastic disease. *Ann Intern Med* 82:666–669, 1975.
183. Serrou B, Michel H, Dubois JB, et al: Granulomatous hepatitis caused by B.C.G. vaccination of a malignant melanoma. *Biomedicine* 23:236, 1975.
184. Passwell J, Katz D, Frank Y, et al: Fatal disseminated B.C.G. infection. *Am J Dis Child* 130:433–436, 1976.
185. Sharma MK, Foroozanfar N, Ala FA: Progressive B.C.G. infection in an immunodeficient child treated with transfer factor. *Clin Immunol Immunopathol* 10:369–380, 1978.
186. Lotte A, Waxz-Höckert O, Poisson N, et al: Complications induites par la. vaccination (BCG): Etude a rètrospective. *Bull Int Union Tuberc* 53:121–123, 1978.
187. Flippin T, Mukherji B, Dayal Y: Granulomatous hepatitis as a late complication of BCG immunotherapy. *Cancer* 46:1759–1762, 1980.
188. Catanzaro A, Melish ME, Minkoff DI: Disseminated B.C.G. infection. *J Pediatr* 99:268–271, 1981.
189. Kallenius G, Moller E, Ringden O, et al: The first infant to survive a generalized BCG infection. *Acta Pediatr Scand* 71:161–165, 1982.
190. Hadzitheofilou C, Obenchain DF, Porter DD, et al: Granulomas in melanoma patients treated with BCG immunotherapy. *Cancer* 49:55–60, 1982.
191. Molz G, Hartmann HP, Griesser HR: Genneralisierte BCG-Infektion bel einem 7 Wochen alten, plotzlich gestorbenen Saugling. *Pathologe* 7:216–221, 1986.
192. Winters RE: Disseminated Mycobacterium bovis infection from BCG vaccination of patient with acquired immunodeficiency syndrome. *MMWR* 34:227–228, 1986.
193. Ninane J, Grymonprez A, Burtonboy G, et al: Disseminated BCG in HIV infection. *Arch Dis Child* 63:1268–1269, 1988.

194. Besnard M: Bacillus Calmette-Guérin infection after vaccination of human immunodeficiency virus–infected children. *Pediatr Infect Dis J* 12:993–997, 1993.

195. Graziano DA, Jacobs D, Locano RG, et al: A case of granulomatous hepatitis after intravesical bacillus Calmette-Guérin administration. *J Urol* 146:118–119, 1991.

196. Proctor DD, Chopra S, Rubenstein SC, et al: Mycobacteremia and granulomatous hepatitis following initial intravesical bacillus Calmette-Guérin instillation for bladder carcinoma. *Am J Gastroenterol* 88:1112–1115, 1993.

197. Kramarsky B, Edmondson HA, Peters RL, et al: Lepromatous leprosy in reaction: A study of the liver and skin lesions. *Arch Pathol* 85:516–531, 1968.

198. Contreras F, Bernal FV: Lesiones hepaticas en al lepra lepromatosa. *Rev Clin Esp* 115:91–96, 1969.

199. Karat ABA, Job CK, Rao PSS: Liver in leprosy: Histological and biochemical findings. *BMJ* 1:307–310, 1971.

200. Sehgal VN, Tygai SP, Kumar S, et al: Microscopic pathology of the liver in leprosy patients. *Int J Dermatol* 11:168–172, 1972.

201. Chen TSN, Drutz DJ, Whelan GE: Hepatic granulomas in leprosy. *Arch Pathol Lab Med* 100:182–185, 1976.

202. de Almeida Barbosa A, Correia Silva T, Patel BN, et al: Demonstration of mycobacterial antigens in skin biopsies from suspected leprosy cases in the absence of bacilli. *Pathol Res Pract* 190:782–785, 1994.

203. Arrnoldi J, Schluter C, Duchrow M, et al: Species-specific assessment of Mycobacterium leprae in skin biopsies by in situ hybridization and polymerase chain reaction. *Lab Invest* 66:618–623, 1992.

204. Oppenheimer EH, Hardy JB: Congenital syphilis in the newborn infant: Clinical and pathological observations in recent cases. *Johns Hopkins Med J* 129:63–82, 1971.

205. Long WA, Ulshen MH, Lawson EE: Clinical manifestations of congenital syphilitic hepatitis: Implications for pathogenesis. *J Pediatr Gastroenterol Nutr* 3:551–555, 1984.

206. Frank BB, Raffensperger EC: Hepatic granulomata: Report of a case with jaundice improving on antituberculous therapy and review of the literature. *Arch Intern Med* 115:223–224, 1965.

207. Baker RD, Kaplan MM, Wolfe HJ, et al: Liver disease associated with early syphilis. *N Engl J Med* 284:1422–1423, 1971.

208. Lee RV, Thornton GF, Conn HO: Liver disease associated with secondary syphilis. *N Engl J Med* 284:1423–1425, 1971.

209. Sobel JH, Wolf EH: Liver involvement in early syphilis. *Arch Pathol* 93:565–568, 1971.

210. Feher J, Somogyi T, Timmer M, et al: Early syphilitic hepatitis. *Lancet* 2:896–899, 1975.

211. Brooks SEH, Hanchard B, Terry S, et al: Hepatic ultrastructure in secondary syphilis. *Arch Pathol Lab Med* 103:451–455, 1979.

212. Romeu J, Rybak B, Dave P, et al: Spirochetal vasculitis and bile ductular damage in early hepatic syphilis. *Am J Gastroenterol* 74:352–354, 1980.

213. Velasco M, Gonzales X: Enfermedad hepatica in el curso e sifilis secundaria. *Rev Med Chile* 108:330–331, 1980.

214. Tiliakos N, Shammaa JM, Nasrallah SM: Syphilitic hepatitis. *Am J Gastroenterol* 73:60–61, 1981.

215. Rampal P, Veyres B, Agrati D, et al: Les atteintes hepatiques de la syphilis. *Ann Gastroenterol Hepatol* 22:77–81, 1986.

216. Relvas S, Carreira F, Castro B: Liver involvement in secondary syphilis (letter). *Am J Gastroenterol* 87:1528, 1992.

217. Hahn RD: Syphilis of the liver. *Am J Syphil* 27:529–562, 1943.
218. Symmers D, Spain DM: Hepar lobatum: Clinical significance of the anatomic changes. *Arch Pathol* 42:64–67, 1946.
219. Davies PJ: Hepatic syphilis: An historical review. *J Gastroenterol Hepatol* 3:287–294, 1988.
220. Veeravahu M: Diagnosis of liver involvement in early syphilis: A critical review. *Arch Intern Med* 145:132–134, 1985.
221. Schaible UE, Gay S, Museteanu U, et al: Lyme borreliosis in the severe combined immunodeficiency (Scid) mouse manifests predominantly in the joints, heart, and liver. *Am J Pathol* 137:811–820, 1990.
222. Goellner KH, Agger WA, Gess JH, et al: hepatitis due to recurrent Lyme disease. *Ann Intern Med* 108:707–708, 1988.
223. Louria DB, Stiff D, Bennett B: Disseminated moniliasis in the adult. *Medicine (Baltimore)* 41:307–323, 1962.
224. Gaines JD, Remington JS: Disseminated candidiasis in the surgical patient. *Surgery* 72:730–736, 1972.
225. Parker JC, McCloskey JJ, Knauer KA: Pathobiologic features of human candidiasis: A common deep mycosis of the brain, heart and kidney in the altered host. *Am J Clin Pathol* 65:991–1000, 1976.
226. Myerowitz RL, Pazin GJ, Allen CM: Disseminated candidiasis: Changes in incidence, underlying disease, and pathology. *Am J Clin Pathol* 68:29–38, 1977.
227. Lewis JH, Patel HR, Zimmerman JH: The spectrum of hepatic candidiases. *Hepatology* 2:479–487, 1982.
228. Gordon SC, Watts JC, Veneri RJ, et al: Focal hepatic candidiasis with perihepatic adhesions: Laparoscopic and immunohistologic diagnosis. *Gastroenterology* 98:214–217, 1990.
229. Gupta NM, Chaudhary A, Talwar P: Candidal obstruction of the common bile duct. *Br J Surg* 72:13, 1985.
230. Irani M, Truong LD: Candidiasis of the extrahepatic biliary tract. *Arch Pathol Lab Med* 110:1087–1090, 1986.
231. Morris AB, Sands ML, Shiraki M, et al: Gallbladder and biliary tract candidiasis: Nine cases and review. *Rev Infect Dis* 12:483–489, 1990.
232. Zimmerman LE, Rappaport H: Occurrence of cryptococcosis in patients with malignant disease of reticuloendothelial system. *Am J Clin Pathol* 24:1050–1072, 1954.
233. Littman ML, Zimmerman LE: *Cryptococcosis.* New York, Grune & Stratton, 1956.
234. Littman ML, Walter JE: Cryptococcosis. Current status. *Am J Med* 45:922–932, 1968.
235. Lewis JL, Rabinovich S: The wide spectrum of cryptococcal infections. *Am J Med* 53:315–322, 1972.
236. Rinaldi MC: Cryptococcosis. *Lab Med* 13:11–19, 1982.
237. Diamond Rd: Cryptococcus neoformans, in Mandell GL, Bennett JE, Dolin R (eds): *Principles and Practice of Infectious Diseases,* ed 4. New York, Churchill Livingstone, 1995, pp 2331–2340.
238. Kovacs JA, Kovac AA, Polis M, et al: Cryptococcosis in the acquired immunodeficiency syndrome. *Ann Intern Med* 103:533–538, 1985.
239. Eng RH, Bishburg E, Smith SM, et al: Cryptococcal infections in patients with AIDS. *Am J Med* 81:19–23, 1986.
240. Pettoello-Mantovenia M, Casadevall A, Kollmann TR, et al: Enhancement of HIV-1 infection by the capsular polysaccharide of *Cryptococcus neoformans.* *Lancet* 339:21–23, 1992.
241. Das BC, Haynes I, Weaver RM, et al: Primary hepatic cryptococcosis. *BMJ* 287:464, 1983.

242. Sabesin SM, Fallon HJ, Andriole VT: Hepatic failure as a manifestation of cryptococcosis. *Arch Intern Med* 111:661–669, 1963.

243. Procknow JJ, Benfield JR, Rippon JW, et al: Cryptococcal hepatitis presenting as a surgical emergency. *JAMA* 191:269–274, 1965.

244. Lefton B, Farmer RG, Buchwald R, et al: Cryptococcal hepatitis mimicking primary sclerosing cholangitis. *Gastroenterology* 67:511–515, 1974.

245. Baker RD, Haugen RK: Tissue changes and tissue diagnosis in cryptococcosis: A study of 26 cases. *Am J Clin Pathol* 25:14–24, 1955.

246. Young RC, Bennett JE, Vogel CL, et al: Aspergillosis: The spectrum of the disease in 98 patients. *Medicine (Baltimore)* 49:147–173, 1970.

247. Khoo TK, Sugai K, Leong TK: Disseminated aspergillosis: Case report and review of the world literature. *Am J Clin Pathol* 45:697–703, 1966.

248. Young RC: The Budd-Chiari syndrome caused by Aspergillus: Two patients with vascular invasion of the hepatic veins. *Arch Intern Med* 124:754–757, 1969.

249. McBride RA, Corson JM, Dammin GJ: Mucormycosis: Two cases of disease with cultural identification of Rhizopus: Review of the literature. *Am J Med* 28:832–846, 1960.

250. Virmani R, Connor DH, McAllister HA: Cardiac mucormycosis: Report of five patients and review of 14 previously reported cases. *Am J Clin Pathol* 78:42–47, 1982.

251. Baker RD, Bassert DE, Remington E: Mucormycosis of the digestive tract. *Arch Pathol* 63:176–182, 1957.

252. Goodwin RA, Loyd JE, Des Prez RM: Histoplasmosis in normal hosts. *Medicine (Baltimore)* 60:231–266, 1981.

253. Okudaira M, Straub M, Schwartz J: The etiology of discrete splenic and hepatic calcifications in an endemic area of histoplasmosis. *Am J Pathol* 39:599–611, 1961.

254. Salfelder K, Brass K, Doehnert G, et al: Fatal disseminated histoplasmosis. *Virchows Arch* 350:303–335, 1970.

255. Smith JW, Utz JP: Progressive disseminated histoplasmosis: A prospective study of 26 patients. *Ann Intern Med* 76:557–665, 1972.

256. Davies SF, Khan M, Sarosi GA: Disseminated histoplasmosis in immunologically suppressed patients. *Am J Med* 64:94–100, 1978.

257. Wheat LJ, Connolly-Stringfield PA, Baker RL, et al: Disseminated histoplasmosis in the acquired immunodeficiency syndrome: Clinical findings, diagnosis and treatment, and review of the literature. *Medicine (Baltimore)* 69:361–374, 1990.

258. Binford CH: Histoplasmosis. Tissue reactions and morphologic variations of the fungus. *Am J Clin Pathol* 25:25–36, 1955.

259. Schwartz J: Histoplasmosis. *Pathol Annu* 3:335–336, 1968.

260. Dumont A, Piché C: Electron microscopic study of human histoplasmosis. *Arch Pathol* 87:168–178, 1969.

261. Cockshott WP, Lucas AO: *Histoplasmosis duboisii*. *Q J Med* 33:223–238, 1964.

262. Williams AO, Lawson EA, Lucas A: African histoplasmosis due to *Histoplasma duboisii*. *Arch Pathol* 92:306–318, 1971.

263. Weed LA: North American blastomycosis. *Am J Clin Pathol* 25:37–45, 1955.

264. Vanek J, Schwartz J, Hakim S: North American blastomycosis: A study of ten cases. *Am J Clin Pathol* 54:384–400, 1970.

265. Hardin CV: Blastomycosis and opportunistic infections in patients with acquired immunodeficiency syndrome. *Arch Pathol Lab Med* 115:1133–1136, 1991.

266. Teixeira F, Gayotto LC, De Brito T: Morphological patterns of the liver in South American blastomycosis. *Histopathology* 2:231–237, 1978.
267. Spark RP: Does transplacental spread of coccidioidomycosis occur? Report of a neonatal fatality and review of the literature. *Arch Pathol Lab Med* 105:347–350, 1981.
268. Kafka JA, Catanzaro A: Disseminated coccidioidomycosis in children. *J Pediatr* 98:355–361, 1981.
269. Deresinski SC, Stevens DA: Coccidioidomycosis in compromised hosts: Experience at Stanford University Hospital. *Medicine (Baltimore)* 54:377–395, 1974.
270. Fish DG, Ampel NM, Galgiani JN, et al: Coccidioidomycosis during human immunodeficiency virus infection: A review of 77 patients. *Medicine (Baltimore)* 69:384–391, 1990.
271. Ampel NM, Dols CL, Galgiani JN: Coccidioidomycosis during human immunodeficiency virus infection: Results of a prospective study in a coccidioidal endemic area. *Am J Med* 94:235–240, 1993.
272. Bayer AS, Yoshikawa TF, Galpin JE, et al: Unusual syndromes of coccidioidomycosis: Diagnostic and therapeutic consideration: A report of 10 cases and review of the English literature. *Medicine (Baltimore)* 55:131–152, 1976.
273. Howard PE, Smith JW: Diagnosis of disseminated coccidioidomycosis by liver biopsy. *Arch Intern Med* 143:1335–1338, 1983.
274. Dodd LG, Nelson SD: Disseminated coccidioidomycosis detected by percutaneous liver biopsy in a liver transplant recipient. *Am J Clin Pathol* 93:141–144, 1990.
275. Centers for Disease Control: Viscerotropic leishmaniasis in persons returning from operation Desert Storm 1990–1991. *MMWR* 41:131–134, 1992.
276. Magill AJ, Grögl M, Gasser RA, et al: Visceral infection caused by *Leishmania tropica* in veterans of operation Desert Storm. *N Engl J Med* 328:1383–1387, 1993.
277. Ma DD, Concannon AJ, Hayes J: Fatal leishmaniasis in renal-transplant patient. *Lancet* 2:311–312, 1979.
278. Broeckaert–van Orshoven A, Michielsen P, Vandepitte J: Fatal leishmaniasis in renal-transplant patient. *Lancet* 2:740–741, 1979.
279. Falk S, Helm EB, Hubner K, et al: Disseminated visceral leishmaniasis (kala azar) in acquired immunodeficiency syndrome (AIDS). *Pathol Res Pract* 183:252–255, 1988.
280. Sendino A, Javier Barbado F, Mostaza JM, et al: Visceral leishmaniasis with malabsorption syndrome in a patient with acquired immunodeficiency syndrome. *Am J Med* 89:673–675, 1990.
281. Montalban C, Calleja JL, Erica A, et al: Visceral leishmaniasis in patients infected with human immunodeficiency virus. *J Infect* 21:261–270, 1990.
282. Peters BS, Fish D, Golden R, et al: Visceral leishmaniasis in HIV infection and AIDS: Clinical features and response to therapy. *Q J Med* 77:1101–1111, 1990.
283. Baily GG, Nandy A: Visceral leishmaniasis: More prevalent and more problematic. *J Infect Dis* 29:241–247, 1994.
284. Bryceson ADM: The liver in leishmaniasis, in Bianchi L, Gerok W, Maier K-P, et al (eds): *Infectious Diseases of the Liver*. Dordrecht, Kluwer Academic, 1990, pp 215–223.
285. Thakur CP, Kumar M, Pathak PK: Kala-azar hits again. *J Trop Med Hyg* 84:271–276, 1981.
286. Aggarwal P, Wali JP, Chopra P: Liver in kala-azar. *Indian J Gastroenterol* 9:135–136, 1990.

287. Sen Gupta PC, Chankravarty NK, Ray HN, et al: The liver in kala-azar. *Ann Trop Med Parasitol* 50:252–259, 1956.

288. Winslow DJ: Kala-azar (visceral leishmaniasis), in Marcial-Rojas RA (ed): *Pathology of Protozoal and Helminthic Diseases.* Baltimore, Williams & Wilkins, 1971, pp 86–96.

289. Daneshbod K: Visceral leishmaniasis (kala-azar) in Iran: A pathologic and electron microscopic study. *Am J Clin Pathol* 57:156–166, 1972.

290. Pampiglione E, LaPlaca M, Schlick G: Studies on Mediterranean leishmaniasis. *Trans R Soc Trop Med Hyg* 68:349–359, 1974.

291. Moreno AM, Marazuela M, Yerba M, et al: Hepatic fibrin ring granulomas in visceral leishmaniasis. *Gastroenterology* 95:1123–1126, 1988.

292. Tanikawa K, Hojiro O: Electron microscopic observations of the liver in Kala-azar. *Kurume Med J* 2:148–154, 1965.

293. El Hag IA, Hashim FA, El Toum IA, et al: Liver morphology and function in visceral leishmaniasis. *J Clin Pathol* 47:547–551, 1994.

294. Remington JS, Jacobs L, Kaufman HE: Toxoplasmosis in the adult. *N Engl J Med* 262:180, 237–241, 1960.

295. Vischer TL, Bernheim C, Engelbrecht E: Two cases of hepatitis due to *Toxoplasma gondii*. *Lancet* 2:919–921, 1967.

296. Briton JP, Pelloux H, Le Marc'hadour F, et al: Acute toxoplasmic hepatitis in a patient with AIDS. *Clin Infect Dis* 15:183–184, 1992.

297. Weitberg AB, Alper JC, Diamond I, et al: Acute granulomatous hepatitis in the course of acquired toxoplasmosis. *N Engl J Med* 300:1093–1096, 1979.

298. Ortego TJ, Robey B, Morrison D, et al: Toxoplasmic chorioretinitis and hepatic granulomas. *Am J Gastroenterol* 85:1418–1420, 1990.

299. Frenkel JK: Toxoplasmosis, in Binford CH, Connor DH (eds): *Pathology of Tropical and Extraordinary Diseases,* vol 1. Washington, DC, Armed Forces Institute of Pathology, 1976, pp 284–300.

300. Andres TL, Dorman SA, Winn WC, et al: Immunohistochemical demonstration of *Toxoplasma gondii*. *Am J Clin Pathol* 75:431–434, 1981.

301. Conley FK, Jenkins KA, Remington JS: *Toxoplasma gondii* infection of the central nervous system: Use of the peroxidase-antiperoxidase method to demonstrate Toxoplasma in formalin-fixed, paraffin embedded tissue sections. *Hum Pathol* 12:690–698, 1981.

302. Tsai MM, O'Leary TJ: Identification of Toxoplasma gondii in formalin-fixed, paraffin-embedded tissue by polymerase chain reaction. *Mod Pathol* 6:185–188, 1993.

303. Foulet A, Zenner L, Darcy F, et al: Pathology of Toxoplasma gondii infection in the nude rat. *Pathol Res Pract* 190:775–781, 1994.

304. Purtilo DT, Meyers WN, Connor DH: Fatal strongyloidiasis in immunosuppressed patients. *Am J Med* 56:488–493, 1974.

305. Poltera AA, Katsimbura N: Granulomatous hepatitis due to *Strongyloides stercoralis*. *J Pathol* 113:241–246, 1974.

306. Meyers WM, Connor DH, Neafie RC: Strongyloidiasis, in Binford CH, Connor DH (eds): *Pathology of Tropical and Extraordinary Disease,* vol 2. Washington, DC, Armed Forces Institute of Pathology, 1976, pp 428–432.

307. Scowden EB, Schaffner W, Stone WJ: Overwhelming strongyloidiasis: An unappreciated opportunistic infection. *Medicine (Baltimore)* 57:527–544, 1978.

308. Milder JE, Walzer PD, Kilgore G, et al: Clinical features of *Strongyloides stercoralis* infection in an endemic area of the United States. *Gastroenterology* 80:1481–1488, 1981.

309. Davidson RA, Fletcher RA, Chapman LE: Risk factors for strongyloidiasis: A case-control study. *Arch Intern Med* 144:321–324, 1984.

310. Haque AK, Schnadig V, Rubin SA et al: Pathogenesis of human strongy-loidiasis: Autopsy and quantitative parasitological analysis. *Mod Pathol* 7:276–288, 1994.

311. Beaver PC, Snyder CH, Carrera GM, et al: Chronic eosinophilia due to viseral larva migrans. *Pediatrics* 9:7–19, 1952.

312. Phills JA, Harrold AJ, Whiteman GV, et al: Pulmonary infiltrates, asthma and eosinophilia due to *Ascaris suum* infestation in man. *N Engl J Med* 286:965–970, 1972.

313. Fox AS, Kazacos KR, Heydemann PT, et al: Fatal eosinophilic meningoen-cephalitis and visceral larva migrans caused by the raccoon ascarid *Bay-lisasaris procyonis. N Engl J Med* 312:1619–1623, 1985.

314. Huntly CC, Costas MC, Lyerly A: Visceral larva migrans syndrome: Clinical characteristics and immunologic studies in 51 patients. *Pediatrics* 36:523–536, 1965.

315. Woodruff AW: Toxocariasis. *BMJ* 2:663–669, 1970.

316. Zinham WH: Visceral larva migrans. *Am J Dis Child* 132:627–633, 1978.

317. Mok CH: Visceral larva migrans: A discussion based on review of the litera-ture. *Clin Pathol (Phila)* 7:565–573, 1988.

318. Bhatia V, Sarin SK: Hepatic visceral larva migrans: Evolution of the lesion, diagnosis, and role of high-dose albendazole therapy. *Am J Gastroenterol* 89:624–627, 1994.

319. De Savigny DH, Voller A, Woodruff AW: Toxocariasis: Serological diagno-sis by enzyme immunoassay. *J Clin Pathol* 32:284–288, 1979.

320. van Knapen F, van Leusden J, Polderman AM, et al: Visceral larva migrans: Examination by means of enzyme-linked immunosorbent assay of human sera for antibodies to excretory-secretory antigens of the second-stage lar-vae of *Toxocara canis. Z Parasitenkunde* 69:113–118, 1983.

321. Otto GF, Berthrong M, Appleby RE, et al: Eosinophilia and hepatomegaly due to *Capillaria hepatica* infection. *Bull Johns Hopkins Hosp* 94:319–336, 1954.

322. Arean VM: Capillariasis, in Marcial-Rojas RA (ed): *Pathology of Protozoal and Helminthic Diseases.* Baltimore, Williams & Wilkins, 1971, pp 666–676.

323. Neafie RL, Connor DH, Cross JH: Capillariasis (intestinal and hepatic), in Binford CH, Connor DH (eds): *Pathology of Tropical and Extraordinary Dis-eases,* vol 2. Washington, DC, Armed Forces Institute of Pathology, 1976, pp 402–408.

324. Attah EB, Nagaraja S, Obineche EN, et al: Hepatic capillariasis. *Am J Clin Pathol* 79:127–130, 1983.

325. Berger T, Degremont A, Gebbers JO, et al: Hepatic capillariasis in a 1-year-old child. *Eur J Pediatr* 149:333–336, 1990.

326. Solomon GB, Raybourne RB: Granulomatous lesions of helminth origin. *Comp Pathol Bull* 8:3–4, 1976.

327. Fresh JW, Cross JH, Reyes V, et al: Necropsy findings in intestinal capillari-asis. *Am J Trop Med* 21:169–173, 1972.

328. *WHO Tech Rep Ser* 666:57–59, 1981.

329. Kamath PS: Hepatobiliary and pancreatic ascariasis. *Indian J Gastroenterol* 10:137–139, 1991.

330. Piggott J, Hansbarger EA, Neafie RC: Human ascariasis. *Am J Clin Pathol* 53:223–234, 1970.

331. Arean VM, Crandall CA: Ascariasis, in Marcial-Rojas RA (ed): *Pathology of Protozoal and Helminthic Diseases.* Baltimore, Williams & Wilkins, 1971, pp 769–807.

332. Gayotto LC, Muszkat RML, Souza IV: Hepatobiliary alterations in massive

biliary ascariasis: Histopathological aspects of an autopsy case. *Rev Inst Med Trop Sao Paulo* 32:91–95, 1990.

333. Khuroo MS, Zargar SA, Mahajan R: Hepatobiliary and pancreatic ascariasis in India. *Lancet* 335:1503–1506, 1990.

334. Gayotto LC, DaSilva LC: Ascariasis, visceral larva migrans, capillariasis, strongyloidiasis, and pentastomiasis, in McIntyre N, Benhamou J-P, Bircher J, et al (eds): *Oxford Textbook of Clinical Hepatology*, vol 1. Oxford, Oxford University Press, 1991, pp 730–739.

335. Warren KS: The relevance of schistosomiasis. *N Engl J Med* 303:203–206, 1980.

336. Dunn MA, Kamel R: Hepatic schistosomiasis. *Hepatology* 1:653–661, 1981.

337. Warren KS: The kinetics of hepatosplenic schistosomiasis. *Semin Liver Dis* 4:293–306, 1984.

338. De Cock KM: Hepatosplenic schistosomiasis: A clinical review. *Gut* 27:734–745, 1986.

339. Warren KS: The liver in schistosomiasis, in Bianchi L, Gerok W, Maier K-P, et al (eds): *Infectious Diseases of the Liver*. Dordrecht, Kluwer Academic, 1990, pp 226–234.

340. Nompleggi DL, Farraye FA, Singer A, et al: Hepatic schistosomiasis: Report of two cases and literature review. *Am J Gastroenterol* 86:1658–1664, 1991.

341. Richter J, Zwingenberger K, Ali QM, et al: Hepatosplenic schistosomiasis: Comparison of sonographic findings with clinical symptoms. *Radiology* 184:711–716, 1992.

342. McKerrow JH, Sun E: Hepatic schistosomiasis. *Prog Liver Dis* 12:121–135, 1994.

343. Strickland GT: Gastrointestinal manifestations of schistosomiasis. *Gut* 35:1334–1337, 1994.

344. Andrade ZA: Hepatic schistosomiasis. *Prog Liver Dis* 2:228–241, 1965.

345. Winslow DJ: Histopathology of schistosomiasis, in Mostofi FK: *Bilharziasis*. New York, Springer-Verlag, 1967, pp 230–341.

346. Marcial-Rojas RA: Schistosomiasis mansoni, in Marcial-Rojas RA (ed): *Pathology of Protozoal and Helminthic Diseases With Clinical Correlation*. Baltimore, Williams & Wilkins, 1971, pp 373–413.

347. Miyake M: Schistosomiasis japonicum, in Marcial-Rojas RA (ed): *Pathology of Protozoal and Helminthic Diseases With Clinical Correlation*. Baltimore, Williams & Wilkins, 1971, pp 414–433.

348. McCully RM, Barron CN, Cheever AW: Schistosomiasis, in Binford CH, Connor DH (eds): *Pathology of Tropical and Extraordinary Diseases*, vol 2. Washington, DC, Armed Forces Institute of Pathology, 1976, pp 482–508.

349. Kage M, Nakashima T: The pathology of schistosomiasis, in Okuda K, Benhamou J-P (eds): *Portal Hypertension: Clinical and Physiologic Aspects*. Tokyo, Springer-Verlag, 1991.

350. Gutierrez Y: *Diagnostic Pathology of Parasitic Infections With Clinical Correlations*. Philadelphia, Lea & Febiger, 1990.

351. Lyra LG, Reboucas G, Andrade ZA: Hepatitis B surface antigen carrier state in hepatosplenic schistosomiasis. *Gastroenterology* 71:641–645, 1976.

352. Bassily S, Farid Z, Higashi GI, et al: Chronic hepatitis B antigenaemia in patients with hepatosplenic schistosomiasis. *J Trop Med Hyg* 82:248–251, 1979.

353. Koshy A, Al-Nakib B, Al-Mufti S, et al: Anti-HCV–positive cirrhosis associated with schistosomiasis. *Am J Gastroenterol* 88:1428–1431, 1993.

354. Kojiro M, Kakizoe S, Yano H, et al: Hepatocellular carcinoma and schistosomiasis japonica. *Acta Pathol Jpn* 36:525–532, 1986.

355. Hsü SYL, Hsü HF, Davis JR, et al: Comparative study on the lesions caused

by eggs of *Schistosoma japonicum* and *Schistosoma mansoni* in liver of albino mice and rhesus monkeys. *Ann Trop Med Parasitol* 66:89–97, 1992.

356. von Lichtenberg F: Lesions of the intrahepatic portal radicles in Manson's schistosomiasis. *Am J Pathol* 31:757–771, 1955.

357. Cheever AW: hepatic vascular lesions in mice infected with Schistosoma mansoni. *Arch Pathol* 72:648–657, 1961.

358. von Lichtenberg F, Sadum EH, Cheever AW, et al: Experimental infection with *Schistosoma japonicum* in chimpanzees. *Am J Trop Med Hyg* 20:850–893, 1971.

359. Aidaros SM, Soliman LAM: Portal vascular changes in human bilharzial cirrhosis. *J Pathol Bacteriol* 82:19–22, 1961.

360. Andrade ZA, Cheever AW: Alterations of the intrahepatic vasculature in hepatosplenic schistosomiasis mansoni. *Am J Trop Med Hyg* 20:425–432, 1971.

361. Alves CAP, Alves AR, Abreu WN, et al: Hepatic artery hypertrophy and sinusoidal hypertension in advanced schistosomiasis. *Gastroenterology* 72:126–128, 1977.

362. Vianna MR, Gayotto LC, Telma R, et al: Intrahepatic bile duct changes in human hepatosplenic schistosomiasis mansoni. *Liver* 9:100–109, 1989.

363. Andrade ZA, Peixoto LE, Guerret S, et al: Hepatic connective tissue changes in hepatosplenic schistosomiasis. *Hum Pathol* 23:566–573, 1992.

364. Grimaud J-A, Borojevic R: Chronic human schistosomiasis mansoni: Pathology of the Disse's space. *Lab Invest* 36:268–273, 1977.

365. Symmers WSTC: Note on a new form of liver cirrhosis due to the presence of ova of *Bilharzia haematobium*. *J Pathol* 9:237–239, 1994.

366. Warren KS: The pathogenesis of "clay-pipe stem cirrhosis" in mice with chronic schistosomiasis mansoni, with a note on the longevity of the schistosomes. *Am J Pathol* 49:477–489, 1966.

367. Tsui WMS, Chow LTC: Advanced schistosomiasis as a cause of hepar lobatum. *Histopathology* 23:495–497, 1993.

368. Stenger RJ, Warren KS, Johnson EA: An electron microscope study of the liver parenchyma and schistosome pigment in murine hepatosplenic schistosomiasis mansoni. *Am J Trop Med Hyg* 16:473–481, 1967.

369. Grimaud JA, Borojevic R, Santos HA: Schistosomal pigment in human and murine infections with *Schistosoma mansoni*. *Trans R Soc Trop Med Hyg* 70:73–77, 1976.

370. Moore G, Homewood CA, Gilles HM: A comparison of pigment from S. mansoni and P. berghei. *Ann Trop Med Parasitol* 69:373, 1975.

371. Price TA, Tuazon CU, Simon GL: Fascioliasis: Case reports and review. *Clin Infect Dis* 17:426–430, 1993.

372. de Miguel F, Carrasco J, Garcia N, et al: CT findings in human fascioliasis. *Gastrointest Radiol* 9:157–159, 1984.

373. Naquira-Vildose F, Marcial-Rojas RA: Fascioliasis, in Marcial-Rojas RA (ed): *Pathology of Protozoal and Helminthic Diseases With Clinical Correlation.* Baltimore, Williams & Wilkins, 1971, pp 477–489.

374. Accosta-Ferreira W, Vercelli-Reta J, Falconi LM: *Fasciola hepatica* human infection: Histopathological study of sixteen cases. *Virchows Arch* 383:319–327, 1979.

375. Jones WA, Kay JM, Mulligan HP, et al: Massive infection with Fasciola hepatica in man. *Am J Med* 63:836–842, 1977.

376. Viranuvatti V, Stitnimankarn T: Liver fluke infection and infestation in Southeast Asia. *Prog Liver Dis* 4:537–547, 1972.

377. Case Records of the Massachusetts General Hospital: Case 33-1990. *N Engl J Med* 323:467–475, 1990.

378. Schwartz DA: Helminths in the induction of cancer: *Opisthorchis viverrini*, *Clonorchis sinensis* and cholangiocarcinoma. *Trop Geogr Med* 32:95–100, 1980.
379. Sher L, Iwatsuki S, Lebeau G, et al: Hilar cholangiocarcinoma associated with clonorchiasis. *Dig Dis Sci* 34:1121–1123, 1989.
380. Srivatanakul P, Parkin M, Jiang Y-Z, et al: The role of infection by Opisthorchis viverrini, hepatitis B virus, and aflatoxin exposure in the etiology of liver cancer in Thailand: A correlation study. *Cancer* 68:2411–2417, 1991.
381. Haswell-Elkins MR, Satarug S, Elkins DB: *Opisthorchis viverrini* infestation in northeast Thailand and its relationship to cholangiocarcinoma. *J Gastroenterol hepatol* 7:538–548, 1992.
382. Meyers WM, Neafie RN: Paragonimiasis, in Binford CH, Connor DH (ed): *Pathology of Tropical and Extraordinary Diseases*, vol 2. Washington, DC, Armed Forces Institute of Pathology, 1976, pp 517–523.
383. Chung CH: Human paragonimiasis (pulmonary distomiasis, endemic hemoptysis), in Marcial-Rojas RA (ed): *Pathology of Protozoal and Helminthic Diseases*. Baltimore, Williams & Wilkins, 1971, pp 504–535.
384. Miguel JP, Bresson-Hadnic S, Vuitton D: Echinococcosis of the liver, in McIntyre N, Benhamou J-P, Bircher J, et al (eds): *Oxford Textbook of Clinical Hepatology*. Oxford, Oxford University Press, 1991, pp 721–730.
385. Menegelli UG, Martinelli ALC, Llorach Velludo MAS, et al: Polycystic hydatid disease: Clinical and morphological findings in nine Brazilian patients. *J Hepatol* 14:203–210, 1992.
386. Hopps HC, Keegan HC, Price DL, et al: Pentastomiasis, in Marcial-Rojas RA (ed): *Pathology of Protozoal and Helminthic Diseases With Clinical Correlation*. Baltimore, Williams & Wilkins, 1971, pp 970–989.
387. Meyers WM, Neafie RC, Connor DH: Diseases caused by pentastomids: Pentastomiasis, in Binford CH, Connor DH (eds): *Pathology of Tropical and Extraordinary Diseases*, vol 2. Washington, DC, Armed Forces Institute of Pathology, 1976, pp 546–550.
388. Prathap K, Lass KS, Bolton JM: Pentastomiasis: A common finding among Malaysian aborigines. *Am J Trop Med Hyg* 18:20–27, 1969.
389. Mendeloff J: Healed granulomas of the liver due to tongue worm infection. *Am J Clin Pathol* 43:433–437, 1965.
390. Symmers WS: Pathology of oxyuriasis with special reference to granuloma formation. *Arch Pathol* 50:475–516, 1950.
391. Slais J: A threadworm granuloma in the human liver. *Helminthologia* 4:479–483, 1963.
392. Little MD, Cuello CJ, D'Alessandro A: Granuloma of the liver due to *Enterobius vermicularis*: Report of a case. *Am J Trop Med Hyg* 22:567–569, 1973.
393. Daly JJ, Baker GF: Pinworm granulomas of the liver. *Am J Trop Med Hyg* 33:62–64, 1984.
394. Mondoci EN, Grepp DR: Hepatic granuloma resulting from *Enterobius vermicularis*. *Am J Clin Pathol* 91:97–100, 1989.
395. Roberts-Thomson IC, Anders RF, Bhathal PS: Granulomatous hepatitis and cholangitis associated with giardiasis. *Gastroenterology* 83:480–483, 1976.
396. Sotto A, Alvarez JL, Garcia B, et al: Lesiòn hepàtica aguda por *Giardia lamblia*. *Rev Esp Enferm Dig* 77:24–28, 1990.
397. Fernandes BJ, Cooper JD, Cullen JB, et al: Systemic infection with *Alaria americana* (Trematoda). *Can Med Assoc J* 115:111–114, 1976.
398. Branson JH, Park JH: Sarcoidosis—hepatic involvement. *Ann Intern Med* 40:111–154, 1954.
399. Israel HL, Goldstein RA: Hepatic granulomatosis and sarcoidosis. *Ann Intern Med* 79:669–678, 1973.

400. Rudzki C, Ishak KG, Zimmerman HJ: Chronic intrahepatic cholestasis of sarcoidosis. *Am J Med* 59:373–387, 1975.

401. Thomas E, Micci D: Chronic intrahepatic cholestasis with granulomas and biliary cirrhosis: Enigmatic disease and therapeutic dilemma. *JAMA* 238:337–338, 1977.

402. Pereira-Lima J, Schaffner F: Chronic cholestasis in hepatic sarcoidosis with clinical features resembling primary biliary cirrhosis: Report of two cases. *Am J Med* 83:144–148, 1987.

403. Bass NM, Burroughs AK, Scheuer PJ, et al: Chronic intrahepatic cholestasis due to sarcoidosis. *Gut* 23:417–421, 1982.

404. Chamuleau RAFM, Sprangers RIH, Alberts C, et al: Sarcoidosis and chronic intrahepatic cholestasis. *Neth J Med* 28:470–476, 1985.

405. Mayor JC, Cabrera J, Garcia J, et al: Chronic intrahepatic cholestasis and Sicca syndrome of sarcoidosis. *J Hepatol* 18:379–380, 1993.

406. Bories C, Certin M, Lavergne A, et al: Cirrhosis biliare primitive at sarcoidose. Association ou maladie unique? *Gastroenterol Clin Biol* 8:851–855, 1984.

407. Keeffe EB: Sarcoidosis and primary biliary cirrhosis: Literature review and illustrative case. *Am J Med* 83:977–980, 1987.

408. Valla D, Pessegueiro-Miranda H, Degott C, et al: Hepatic sarcoidosis with portal hypertension. A report of seven cases with a review of the literature. *Q J Med* 63:531–544, 1967.

409. Sherman S, Nieland NS, Van Thiel DH: Sarcoidosis and primary biliary cirrhosis: Coexistence in a single patient. *Dig Dis Sci* 33:368–374, 1988.

410. Xerri L, Nosny Y, Minko D, et al: Association de sarcoidose et de cirrhose biliare primitive: Etude clinique et anatomopathologique d'un cas suivi pendant 10 ans. *Gastroenterol Clin Biol* 13:513–516, 1989.

411. Ilan Y, Rappaport I, Feigin R, et al: Primary sclerosing cholangitis in sarcoidosis. *J Clin Gastroenterol* 16:326–328, 1993.

412. Murphy JR, Sjogren MH, Kikendall JW, et al: Small bile duct abnormalities in sarcoidosis. *J Clin Gastroenterol* 12:555–561, 1990.

413. Kusielewicz D, Duchatelle V, Valeyre D, et al: Ictere obstructif par sténose granulomatense des voies biliares extra-hepatiques an cours d'une sarcoidose. *Gastroenterol Clin Biol* 12:664–667, 1988.

414. Toda K, Souda S, Yoshikawa Y, et al: Narrowing of the distal common bile duct and the portal vein secondary to pancreatic sarcoidosis. *Am J Gastroenterol* 89:1259–1261, 1994.

415. Maddrey WC, Johns CJ, Boinott JK, et al: Sarcoidosis and chronic hepatic disease: A clinical and pathological study of 20 patients. *Medicine (Baltimore)* 49:375–395, 1970.

416. Vilinskas J, Joyeuse R, Serlin O: Hepatic sarcoidosis with portal hypertension. *Am J Surg* 120:393–396, 1970.

417. Le Verger J-C, Gosselin M, Launois B, et al: Sarcoidose et hypertension portale. *Gastroenterol Clin Biol* 1:661–669, 1977.

418. Leger L, Lemaigre G, Prémont M, et al: Hypertension portale an cours de la sarcoidose: trois observations dont une avec foie fibreux et hépatome malin à stroma osseux. *Presse Med* 9:1021–1024, 1980.

419. Tekeste H, Latour F, Levitt RE: Portal hypertension complicating sarcoid liver disease: Case report and review of the literature. *Am J Gastroenterol* 79:389–396, 1984.

420. Leiberman J: Elevation of serum angiotensin-converting enzyme (ACE) in sarcoidosis. *Am J Med* 59:365–372, 1975.

421. Studdy P, Bird R, James DG: Serum angiotensin-converting enzyme (SACE) in sarcoidosis and other granulomatous disorders. *Lancet* 2:1331–1334, 1978.

422. Lufkin EG, DeRemee RA, Rohrbach MS: The predictive value of serum angiotensin-converting enzyme activity in the differential diagnosis of hypercalcemia. *Mayo Clin Proc* 58:447–451, 1983.

423. Silverstein E, Lockerman E, Friedland J: Serum and lymph-node collagenase in sarcoidosis: Comparison with angiotensin-converting enzyme. *Am J Clin Pathol* 70:348–351, 1978.

424. James DG, Williams WJ: Immunology of sarcoidosis. *Am J Med* 72:5–8, 1982.

425. James DG, Williams WJ: *Sarcoidosis and Other Granulomatous Disorders.* Philadelphia, WB Saunders, 1985.

426. Kataria YP: Immunology of sarcoidosis, in Lieberman J (ed): *Sarcoidosis.* Orlando, Fla, Grune & Stratton, 1985, pp 39–63.

427. Pertschuk LP, Silverstein E, Friedland J: Immunohistologic diagnosis of sarcoidosis: Detection of angiotension-converting enzyme in sarcoid granulomas. *Am J Clin Pathol* 75:350–354, 1981.

428. Klatskin G, Yesner R: Hepatic manifestations of sarcoidosis and other granulomatous diseases. Study based on histologic examination of tissue obtained by needle biopsy of liver. *Yale J Biol Med* 23:207–248, 1950.

429. Uehlinger E: The sarcoid tissue reaction. The origin and significance of inclusion bodies. Differential diagnosis with particular delineation from tuberculosis, *Acta Med Scand* (suppl 425) 176:7–13, 1964.

430. Cunningham JA: Sarcoidosis. *Pathol Annu.* 31–46, 1967.

431. Rosen HD, Valetin JC, Pertschuk LP, et al: Sarcoidosis from the pathologist's vantage point. *Pathol Ann* 14:405–439, 1979.

432. Cain H, Kraus B: Asteroid bodies: Derivatives of the cytosphere. *Virchows Arch* 26:119–132, 1977.

433. Kirkpatrick CJ, Curry I, Bisset DL: Light and electron-microscopic studies on multinucleated giant cells in sarcoid granuloma: New aspects of asteroid and Schaumann bodies. *Ultrastruct Pathol* 12:581–597, 1988.

434. Okamoto K, Hirai S, Yoshida T, et al: Asteroid bodies in silicone-induced granulomas are ubiquinated. *Jpn J Pathol* 42:688–689, 1992.

435. Johnson FB, Pani K: Histochemical identification of calcium oxalate. *Arch Pathol* 74:347, 1962.

436. Reid JD, Andersen ME: Calcium oxalate in sarcoid granulomas with particular reference to the small ovoid body and a note on the finding of dolomite. *Am J Clin Pathol* 90:545–558, 1988.

437. Devaney K, Goodman ZD, Epstein MS, et al: Hepatic sarcoidosis. *Am J Surg Pathol* 17:1272–1280, 1993.

438. Natalino MB, Goyette RE, Owensby LC, et al: The Budd-Chiari syndrome in sarcoidosis. *JAMA* 239:2657–2658, 1978.

439. Russi EW, Bansky G, Pfalz M, et al: Budd-Chiari syndrome in sarcoidosis. *Am J Gastroenterol* 81:71–75, 1986.

440. Saboor SA, Johnson NM, McFadden J: Detection of mycobacterial DNA in sarcoidosis and tuberculosis with polymerase chain reaction. *Lancet* 339:1012–1015, 1992.

441. Mitchell IC, Turk JL, Mitchell DN: Detection of mycobacterial rRNA in sarcoidosis. *Lancet* 339:1015–1018, 1992.

442. Krulik M, Seroka J, Brissaud P, et al: Tuberculose hépatique pseudotumorale suivie d'une sarcoidose disséminée. *Semin Hop* 60:2803–2807, 1984.

443. Lee RG, Epstein O, Jauregui H, et al: Granulomas in primary biliary cirrhosis: A prognostic feature. *Gastroenterology* 81:983–986, 1981.

444. Hadziyannis S, Scheuer PJ, Feizi T, et al: Immunological and histological studies in primary biliary cirrhosis. *J Clin Pathol* 23:95–98, 1970.

445. Baggenstoss AH, Foulk WT, Butt HR, et al: The pathology of primary biliary cirrhosis with emphasis on histogenesis. *Am J Clin Pathol* 42:259–276, 1964.

446. Chapman RWG, Arborgh BAM, Rhodes JM, et al: Primary sclerosing cholangitis: A review of its clinical features, cholangiography, and hepatic histology. *Gut* 21:870–877, 1980.

447. Ludwig J, Barham SS, LaRusso NF, et al: Morphologic features of chronic hepatitis associated with primary sclerosing cholangitis and chronic ulcerative colitis. *Hepatology* 1:632–640, 1981.

448. Eade MN, Cooke WT, Brooke NB: Liver disease in ulcerative colitis. Analysis of operative liver biopsy in 138 consecutive patients having colectomy. *Ann Intern Med* 72:475–487, 1970.

449. Chapin LE, Scudamore HH, Baggenstoss AH, et al: Regional enteritis: Associated visceral changes. *Gastroenterology* 30:404–415, 1956.

450. Dordal E, Glogov S, Kirsner JB: Hepatic lesions in chronic inflammatory bowel disease. I. Clinical correlations with liver biopsy diagnoses in 103 patients. *Gastroenterology* 52:239–253, 1967.

451. Maurer LH, Hughes RW, Folley JL, et al: Granulomatous hepatitis associated with regional enteritis. *Gastroenterology* 53:301–305, 1967.

452. Eade MN, Coote WT, Brooke BN: Liver disease in Crohn's colitis: A study of 21 consecutive patients having colectomy. *Ann Intern Med* 74:518–528, 1971.

453. Everett GD, Mitros FA: Eosinophilic gastroenteritis with hepatic eosinophilic granulomas: Report of a case with 30-year follow-up. *Am J Gastroenterol* 74:519–521, 1980.

454. Apperly FL, Copley EL: Whipple's disease (lipophagia granulomatosis). *Gastroenterology* 1:461–470, 1943.

455. Cornet A, Barbier JP, Henry-Biabaud E, et al: Maladie de Whipple. Localizations granulomateuses hepatique decelees par ponction-biopsie due foie. (A propos de deux observations). *Ann Med Interne (Paris)* 127:139–146, 1976.

456. Brisseau JM, Rodat O, Buzelin F, et al: Localisations granulomateuses hépatiques au cours de la maladie de Whipple. *Semin Hop* 59:2889–2892, 1983.

457. Saint-Marc Girardin MF, Zafrani ES, Chaumette MT, et al: Hepatic granulomas in Whipple's disease. *Gastroenterology* 86:753–756, 1984.

458. Cho C, Linscheer WG, Hirschkorn MA, et al: Sarcoid like granulomas as an early manifestation of Whipple's disease. *Gastroenterology* 87:941–947, 1984.

459. Enzinger FM, Helwig EB: Whipple's disease: A review of the literature and report of fifteen patients. *Virchows Arch* 336:238–269, 1963.

460. Relman DA, Schmidt TM, MacDermott RP, et al: Identification of the uncultured bacillus of Whipple's disease. *N Engl J Med* 327:293–301, 1992.

461. Bruce RM, Wise L: Tuberculosis after jejunoileal bypass for obesity. *Ann Intern Med* 87:574–576, 1977.

462. Banner BF, Banner AS: Hepatic granulomas following ileal bypass for obesity. *Arch Pathol Lab Med* 102:655–657, 1978.

463. Halverson JD, Wise L, Wazna MF, et al: Jejunoileal bypass for morbid obesity. *Am J Med* 64:461–475, 1978.

464. Sweet RM, Smith CL, Berkseth RO, et al: Jejunoileal bypass surgery and granulomatous disease of the kidney and liver. *Arch Intern Med* 138:626–627, 1978.

465. Kalat ED, Martin DB: Granulomatous hepatitis associated with jejunoileal bypass surgery. *JAMA* 246:982, 1981.

466. Pickleman JR, Evans LS, Kane JM, et al: Tuberculosis after jejunoileal bypass for obesity. *JAMA* 234:744–745, 1975.

467. Litwack KD, Bohan A, Silverman L: Granulomatous liver disease and giant cell arteritis: Case report and literature review. *J Rheumatol* 4:307–312, 1977.

468. Lie JT: Disseminated visceral giant cell arteritis: Histopathologic description and differentiation from other granulomatous vasculitides. *Am J Clin Pathol* 69:299–305, 1978.

469. Pedro-Botet J, Lopez MJ, Barranco C, et al: Granulomatous hepatitis and giant cell arteritis. *Am J Gastroenterol* 89:1898–1899, 1994.

470. de Bayser L, Rodlot P, Ramassamy A, et al: Hepatic fibrin-ring granulomas in giant cell arteritis. *Gastroenterology* 108:272–273, 1993.

471. Churg J, Strauss L: Allergic granulomatosis, allergic angiitis, and periarteritis nodosa. *Am J Pathol* 27:277–301, 1951.

472. Sokolov RA, Rachmaninoff N, Kaine HD: Allergic granulomatosis. *Am J Med* 32:131–141, 1962.

473. Chumbley LC, Harrison EG, Deremee RA: Allergic granulomatosis and angiitis (Churg-Strauss syndrome): Report and analysis of 30 cases. *Mayo Clin Proc* 52:477–522, 1977.

474. Ito N, Kimura A, Nishikawa M, et al: Veno-occlusive disease of the liver in a patient with allergic granulomatous angiitis. *Am J Gastroenterol* 83:316–319, 1988.

475. Long R, James O: Polymyalgia rheumatica and liver disease. *Lancet* 1:77–79, 1994.

476. Kosolcharoen P, Magnin GE: Liver dysfunction and polymyalgia rheumatica: A case report. *J Rheumatol* 3:50–53, 1976.

477. Ogilvie AL, James PD, Toghil PJ: Hepatic artery involvement in polymyalgia arteritica. *J Clin Pathol* 34:769–772, 1981.

478. Chomet B, Pilz CG, Vosti K, et al: Case of Wegener's granulomatosis. *Arch Pathol* 66:100–107, 1958.

479. Kofman S, Hohnson CG, Zimmerman HJ: Apparent hepatic dysfunction in lupus erythematosus. *Arch Intern Med* 95:669–676, 1955.

480. Matsumoto T, Yoshimine T, Shimouchi K, et al: The liver in systemic lupus erythematosus: Pathologic analysis of 52 cases and review of Japanese autopsy registry data. *Hum Pathol* 23:1151–1158, 1992.

481. Leggett BA: The liver in systemic lupus erythematosus. *J Gastroenterol Hepatol* 8:84–88, 1993.

482. Harvey AMC, Shulman LE, Ttumulty PA, et al: Systemic lupus erythematosus: Review of the literature and clinical analysis of 138 cases. *Medicine (Baltimore)* 33:291–437, 1954.

483. Aronson AR, Montgomery MM: Chronic liver disease with a "lupus erythematosus–like syndrome." *Ann Intern Med* 104:544–552, 1959.

484. Runyon BA, La Brecque DR, Anuras S: The spectrum of liver disease in systemic lupus erythematosus: Report of 33 histologically-proved cases and review of the literature. *Am J Med* 69:187, 1980.

485. Murphy E, Griffiths MR, Hunter JA, et al: Fibrin-ring granulomas: A nonspecific reaction to liver injury? *Histopathology* 19:91–93, 1991.

486. Movitt ER, Davis AR: Liver biopsy in rheumatoid arthritis. *Am J Med Sci* 226:521–524, 1953.

487. Mills PR, MacSween RNM, Dick WC, et al: Liver disease in rheumatoid arthritis. *Scot Med J* 25:618–622, 1980.

488. Smits JG, Kooijman CD: Rheumatoid nodules in the liver. *Histopathology* 10:1211–1215, 1986.

489. Calder CJ, Hubscher SG: Extrahepatic biliary atresia with palisading granulomas. *Histopathology* 23:585–587, 1993.

490. Ishak KG, Zimmerman HJ: Drug-induced and toxic granulomatous hepatitis. *Baillieres Clin Gastroenterol* 2:463–480, 1988.

491. Farrell GC: *Drug-Induced Liver Disease.* Edinburgh, Churchill-Livingstone, 1994.

492. Vanderstigel M, Zafrani ES, Legonc JL, et al: Allopurinol hypersensitivity syndrome as cause of hepatic doughnut-ring granulomas. *Gastroenterology* 90:188–190, 1986.

493. Stricker BHC, Bloch APR, Babany G, et al: Fibrin ring granulomas and allopurinol. *Gastroenterology* 96:119–1203, 1989.

494. Boitnott JK, Margolis S: Mineral oil in human tissues. II. Oil droplets in lymph nodes of the porta hepatis. *Bull Johns Hopkins Hosp* 118:414–422, 1966.

495. Boitnott JK, Margolis D: Saturated hydrocarbons in human tissues. III. Oil droplets in the liver and spleen. *Johns Hopkins Med J* 127:65–67, 1970.

496. Dincsoy HP, Weesner RE, MacGee J: Lipogranulomas in non-fatty human livers: A mineral oil induced environmental disease. *Am J Clin Pathol* 78:35–41, 1982.

497. Cruickshank B, Thomas MJ: Mineral oil (follicular) lipidosis. II. Histologic studies of spleen, liver, lymph nodes, and bone marrow. *Hum Pathol* 15:731–737, 1984.

498. Keen ME, Engsbrand DA, Habez G-R: Hepatic lipogranulomatosis simulating veno-occlusive disease of the liver. *Arch Pathol Lab Med* 109:70–72, 1985.

499. Wanless IR, Geddie WR: Mineral oil lipogranulomata in liver and spleen. *Arch Pathol Lab Med* 109:283–286, 1977.

500. Blewitt RW, Bradbury K, Greenall MJ, et al: Hepatic damage with mineral oil deposits. *Gut* 18:476–479, 1977.

501. Scadding JG: *Sarcoidosis.* London, Eyre & Spottiswoode, 1967.

502. Stoeckle JD, Hardy HL, Weber AL: Chronic beryllium disease: Long-term follow-up of sixty cases and selective review of the literature. *Am J Med* 46:545–561, 1969.

503. Dutra FR: The pneumonitis and granulomatosis peculiar to beryllium workers. *Am J Pathol* 24:1137–1165, 1948.

504. Metzner F, Leiben J: Respiratory disease associated with beryllium refining and alloy fabrication. *J Occup Med* 3:341, 1961.

505. Chiappino G, Cirla A, Vigliani EC: Delayed-type hypersensitivity reactions to beryllium compounds. *Arch Pathol* 87:131–140, 1969.

506. Huang H, Meyer KC, Kubai L, et al: An immune model of beryllium-induced pulmonary granulomata in mice. *Lab Invest* 67:138–146, 1992.

507. Pimentel JC, Menezes AP: Liver granulomas containing copper in vineyard sprayer's lung: A new etiology of hepatic granulomatosis. *Am Rev Respir Dis* 111:189–195, 1975.

508. Pimentel JC, Menezes AP: Liver disease in vineyard sprayers. *Gastroenterology* 71:275–283, 1977.

509. Isaacs I, Nissen R, Epstein BS: Liver abscess resulting from barium enema in a case of chronic ulcerative colitis. *N Y State J Med* 50:332–334, 1950.

510. Salvo AF, Capron CW, Leigh KE, et al: Barium intravasation into portal venous system during barium enema examination. *JAMA* 235:749–751, 1976.

511. Marek J, Jurek K: Comparative light microscopical and x-ray microanalysis study of barium granuloma. *Pathol Res Pract* 171:293–302, 1981.

512. Kurumaya H, Kono N, Nakanuma Y, et al: Hepatic granulomata in long-term

hemodialysis patients with hyperaluminumemia. *Arch Pathol Lab Med* 113:1132–1134, 1989.

513. Chen W-J, Monnat RJ, Chen M, et al: Aluminum induced pulmonary granulomatosis. *Hum Pathol* 9:705–711, 1978.

514. Landas SK, Mitros FA, Furst DE, et al: Lipogranulomas and gold in the liver in rheumatoid arthritis. *Am J Surg Pathol* 16:171–174, 1992.

515. Al-Talib RK, Wright DH, Theaker JM: Orange-red birefringence of gold particles in paraffin wax embedded sections: An aid to the diagnosis of chrysiasis. *Histopathology* 24:176–178, 1994.

516. Keen CE, Brady K, Levison DA: Orange-red birefringence of gold particles. *Histopathology* 24:298, 1994.

517. Coelho Filho JC, Moreira RA, Crocker PR, et al: Identification of titanium pigment in drug addicts' tissues. *Histopathology* 19:190–192, 1991.

518. Moran CA, Mullick KG, Ishak KG, et al: Identification of titanium in human tissues: Probable role in pathologic processes. *Hum Pathol* 22:450–454, 1991.

519. Sternlieb JJ, McIlrath DC, van Heerden JA, et al: Starch peritonitis and its prevention. *Arch Surg* 112:458–461, 1977.

520. Nissim F, Ashkenazy M, Borenstein R, et al: Tuberculoid cornstarch granulomas with caseous necrosis: A diagnostic challenge. *Arch Pathol Lab Med* 105:86–88, 1981.

521. Pfeifer U, Kult J, Förster H: Ascites als Komplikation hepatischer Speicherung von Hosdroxyetheylstärke (HES) bei Langzeitdialyse. *Klin Wochenschr* 62:862–866, 1984.

522. Dienes HP, Gerharz C-D, Wagner R, et al: Accumulation of hydroxyethyl starch (HES) in the liver of patients with renal failure and portal hypertension. *J Hepatol* 3:223–227, 1986.

523. Saxen L, Myllärniemi H: Foreign material and post operative adhesions. *N Engl J Med* 279:200–202, 1968.

524. Janoff K, Wayne R, Hunt Work B, et al: Foreign body reactions to cellulose lint fibers. *Am J Surg* 147:598–600, 1984.

525. Brittan RF, Studley JGN, Parkin JV, et al: Cellulose granulomatous peritonitis. *Br J Surg* 71:452–453, 1984.

526. Tomashefski JF, Hirsch CS, Jolly PN: Microcrystalline cellulose pulmonary embolism and granulomatosis. *Arch Pathol Lab Med* 105:89–93, 1981.

527. Kershisnik MM, Ro JY, Cannon GH, et al: Histiocytic reaction in pelvic peritoneum associated with oxidized regenerated cellulose. *Am J Clin Pathol* 103:27–31, 1994.

528. Bradley M, Singh G: An oxidized cellulose granuloma: Another hepatic pseudotumor? *Clin Radiol* 44:206–207, 1991.

529. Henderson WJ, Melville-Jones C, Griffithes K, et al: Talc contamination of surgical gloves. *Lancet* 1:1419, 1975.

530. Tolbert TW, Brown JL: Surface powders on surgical gloves. *Arch Surg* 115:729–732, 1980.

531. Ishak BW, Ishak KG: Foreign-body reaction in the liver of a drug addict. *Forensic Sci* 14:515–520, 1969.

532. Hahn HH, Schweid AI, Beaty HN: Complications of injecting dissolved methylphenidate tablets. *Arch Intern Med* 123:656–659, 1969.

533. Groth DH, Mackay GR, Crable JV, et al: Intravenous injection of talc in narcotics addict. *Arch Pathol* 94:171–178, 1972.

534. Min K-W, Gyorkey F, Cain D: Talc granulomata in liver disease in narcotic addicts. *Arch Pathol* 98:331–335, 1974.

535. Buschmann RJ, Mir J: Electron microscopic identity of talc in the liver of a narcotic addict. *Hum Pathol* 10:736–739, 1979.

536. Terzakis JA, Eisenmenger WJ, Reidy JJ: X-ray microanalysis of crystalline material in the liver of a narcotics user. *Am J Clin Pathol* 82:236–239, 1984.

537. Allaire J, Goodman ZG, Ishak KG, et al: Talc in liver tissue of intravenous drug abusers with chronic hepatitis: A comparative study. *Am J Clin Pathol* 92:583–588, 1989.

538. Racela LS, Papasian CJ, Watanabe I, et al: Systemic talc granulomatosis associated with disseminated histoplasmosis in a drug abuser. *Arch Pathol Lab Med* 112:557–560, 1988.

539. Mariani-Constantini R, Jannotta FS, Johnson FB: Systemic visceral talc granulomatosis associated with miliary tuberculosis in a drug addict. *Am J Clin Pathol* 78:785–789, 1982.

540. Lewis JH, Sundeen JT, Simon GL, et al: Disseminated talc granulomatosis: An unusual finding in a patient with acquired immunodeficiency syndrome and fatal cytomegalovirus infection. *Arch Pathol Lab Med* 109:147–150, 1985.

541. Gall EA, Altemeier WA, Schiff L, et al: Liver lesions following intravenous administration of polyvinylpyrrolidone (PVP). *Am J Clin Pathol* 23:1187–1189, 1953.

542. Cabanne F, Michiels R, Dusserre P, et al: La maladie polyvinylique. *Ann Anat Pathol* 14:419–440, 1969.

543. Kuo T-T, Hsueh S: Mucicarminophilic histiocytosis: Polyvinylpyrrolidone (PVP) storage disease simulating signet-ring cell carcinoma. *Am J Surg Pathol* 8:419–428, 1984.

544. Reske-Nielsen E, Bojsen-Moller M, Vetner M, et al: Polyvinylpyrrolidone storage disease: Light microscopical, ultrastructural and chemical verification. *Acta Pathol Microbiol Scand* 84:397–405, 1976.

545. Hameed K, Ashfag S, Waugh DOW: Ball valve fracture and extrusion in Starr-Edwards aortic valve prosthesis with dissemination of ball material. *Arch Pathol* 86:520–524, 1968.

546. Ridolfi RL, Hutchins GM: Detection of ball variance in prosthetic heart valves by liver biopsy. *Johns Hopkins Med J* 134:131–140, 1974.

547. Pulford K, Souhami RL: Cell division and giant cell formation in Kupffer cell cultures. *Clin Exp Immunol* 42:67–76, 1980.

548. Bommer J, Ritz E, Waldherr R, et al: Silicone cell inclusions causing multi-organ body reaction in dialyzed patients. *Lancet* 1:1314, 1981.

549. Leong AS-Y, Disney APS, Gove DW: Silicone particles and hemodialysis. *Lancet* 2:210, 1981.

550. Leong AS-Y, Disney APS, Gove DW: Refractile particles in liver of hemodialysis patients. *Lancet* 1:889–890, 1981.

551. Parfrey PS, O'Driscoll JB, Paradinas FJ: Refractile material in the liver of hemodialysis patients. *Lancet* 2:1101–1102, 1981.

552. Leong AS-Y, Disney APS, Gove SW: Spallation and migration of silicone from blood-pump tubing in patients on hemodialysis. *N Engl J Med* 306:135–140, 1982.

553. Leong AS-Y: Silicone—a possible iatrogenic cause of hepatic dysfunction in hemodialysis patients. *Pathology* 15:193–195, 1983.

554. Hunt J, Farthing MJG, Baker LRI, et al: Silicone in the liver: Possible late effects. *Gut* 30:239–242, 1989.

555. Leong AS-Y, Gove DW: Pathological finding in silicone spallation in vitro studies. *Pathology* 15:189–192, 1983.

556. Ellenbogen R, Ellenbogen R, Rubin L: Injectable fluid silicone therapy: Human morbidity and mortality. *JAMA* 234:308–309, 1975.

557. Terzakis JA, Sommers SC, Snyder RW, et al: X-ray microanalysis of hepatic thorium deposits. *Arch Pathol* 98:241–242, 1974.

558. Bowen JH, Woodward BH, Mossler JA, et al: Energy dispersive x-ray detection of thorium dioxide. *Arch Pathol Lab Med* 104:459–461, 1980.

559. Cisno F, Azzalini M, Camagna MT: Considerazioni su 16 casi de silicosi del fegato e della milza. *Med Lav* 62:378–385, 1971.

560. Pacheco GO, Nuno AS: Silicosis hepatica: Analisis de 21 casos. *Rev Esp Enferm Dig* 46:107–130, 1975.

561. Langlois S de P, Sterrett GF, Henderson DW: Hepatosplenic silicosis. *Aust Radiol* 21:143–149, 1977.

562. Pimentel JC, Menezes AP: Pulmonary and hepatic granulomatous disorders due to the inhalation of cement and mica ducts. *Thorax* 33:219–227, 1978.

563. Dirschmid K, Kicsler J: Die Morphologie der Leber bei der Anthrakosilikose. *Leber Magen Darm* 10:115–118, 1980.

564. Lefevre ME, Green FHY, Joel DD, et al: The frequency of black pigment in livers and spleens of coal workers: Correlation with pulmonary pathology and occupational information. *Hum Pathol* 13:1121–1126, 1982.

565. Eide J, Gylseth B, Skaug V: Silicotic lesions of the bone marrow: Histopathology and microanalysis. *Histopathology* 8:693–703, 1984.

566. Slavin RE, Swedo JL, Brandes D, et al: Extrapulmonary silicosis: A clinical, morphologic, and ultrastructural study. *Hum Pathol* 16:393–412, 1985.

567. Carmichael GP, Targoff C, Pintar K, et al: Hepatic silicosis. *Am J Clin Pathol* 73:720–722, 1980.

568. Yao-Chang L, Tomashefski J, McMahon JT, et al: Mineral-associated hepatic injury: A report of seven cases with x-ray microanalysis. *Hum Pathol* 22:1120–1127, 1991.

569. Christoffersen P, Braendstrup O, Juhl E, et al: Lipogranulomas in human liver biopsies with fatty changes. *Acta Pathol Microbiol Scand* 79:150–158, 1971.

570. Leevy CM, Zinke MR, White TJ, et al: Clinical observations on the fatty liver. *Ann Intern Med* 92:527–541, 1953.

571. Petersen P, Christoffersen P: Ultrastructure of lipogranulomas in human fatty liver. *Acta Pathol Scand* 87:45–49, 1979.

572. Belladetsima JK, Horn T, Poulsen H: Portal area lipogranulomas in liver biopsies. *Liver* 7:9–17, 1987.

573. Landing BH, Shirkey HS: A syndrome of recurrent infection and infiltration of viscera by pigmented lipid histiocytes. *Pediatrics* 20:431–438, 1957.

574. Bridges RA, Berendes H, Good RA: A fatal granulomatous disease of childhood. *J Dis Child* 97:387–408, 1959.

575. Carson MJ, Chadwick DL, Brubaker CA, et al: Thirteen boys with progressive septic granulomatosis. *Pediatrics* 35:405–412, 1965.

576. Good RA, Quie PG, Windhorst DB, et al: Fatal (chronic) granulomatous disease of childhood: A hereditary defect of leucocyte function. *Semin Hematol* 5:215–254, 1968.

577. Emile J-F, Fraitag S, Leborgne M, et al: Langerhans' cell histiocytosis cells are activated Langerhans' cells. *J Pathol* 174:71–76, 1994.

578. Thompson HH, Pitt HA, Lewin KJ, et al: Sclerosing cholangitis and histiocytosis X. *Gut* 25:526–530, 1984.

579. Conception W, Esquivel CO, Terry A, et al: Liver transplantation in Langerhans' cell histiocytosis (histiocytosis X). *Semin Oncol* 18:24–28, 1991.

580. Zandi P, Panis Y, Debray D, et al: Pediatric liver transplantation for Langerhans' cell histiocytosis. *Hepatology* 21:129–133, 1995.

581. Brincker H: Epithelioid-cell granulomas in Hodgkin's disease. *Acta Pathol Microbiol Scand* 78:19–32, 1970.

582. Kadin ME, Donaldson SS, Dorfman RF: Isolated granulomas in Hodgkin's disease. *N Engl J Med* 283:859–861, 1970.

583. O'Connell MJ, Schimoff SC, Kirschner RH, et al: Epithelioid granulomas in Hodgkin's disease. *JAMA* 233:886–889, 1975.

584. Pak HY, Friedman NB: Pseudosarcoid granulomas in Hodgkin's disease. *Hum Pathol* 12:832–837, 1981.

585. Skovsgaard T, Brinckmeyer LM, Vesterager L, et al: The liver in Hodgkin's disease—II. Histopathologic findings. *Eur J Cancer Clin Oncol* 18:429–435, 1982.

586. Aderka D, Kraus M, Avidor I, et al: Hodgkin's and non-Hodgkin's lymphomas masquerading as "idiopathic" liver granulomas. *Am J Gastroenterol* 79:642–644, 1984.

587. Johnson LN, Iseri O, Knodell RG: Caseating hepatic granulomas in Hodgkin's lymphoma. *Gastroenterology* 99:1837–1940, 1990.

588. Delsol G, Pellegrin M, Voigt JJ, et al: Diagnostic value of granuloma with fibrinoid ring (letter). *Am J Clin Pathol* 73:289, 1980.

589. Saito K, Nakanuma Y, Ogawa S, et al: Extensive hepatic granulomas associated with peripheral T-cell lymphoma. *Am J Gastroenterol* 86:1243–1246, 1991.

590. Deleted in proof.

591. Chagnac A, Gal R, Kimche D, et al: Liver granulomas: A possible paraneoplastic manifestation of hypernephroma. *Am J Gastroenterol* 80:989–992, 1985.

592. Neuberger J, Portmann B, Nunnerley HB, et al: Oral-contraceptive–associated liver tumors: Occurrence of malignancy and difficulties in diagnosis. *Lancet* 1:273–276, 1980.

593. Malatgalian DA, Graham CH: Liver adenoma with granulomas. *Arch Pathol Lab Med* 106:244–246, 1982.

594. Le Bail B, Jouhanole H, Dengnier Y, et al: Liver adenomatosis with granulomas in two patients on long-term oral contraceptives. *Am J Surg Pathol* 16:982–987, 1992.

595. Yano K, Nishida M, Yamamot T, et al: A case of hepatocellular carcinoma with tuberculoma within tumor tissue. *J Hepatobiliary Pancr Surg* 1:294–296, 1994.

596. Mahida Y, Palmer KR, Lovell D, et al: Familial granulomatous hepatitis: A hitherto unrecognized entity. *Am J Gastroenterol* 83:42–45, 1988.

597. Nakanuma Y, Ohat G, Doishita K, et al: Granulomatous liver disease in the small hepatic and portal veins. *Arch Pathol Lab Med* 104:456–458, 1980.

598. Simon HB, Wolff SM: Granulomatous hepatitis and prolonged fever of unknown origin: A study of 13 patients. *Medicine (Baltimore)* 52:1–21, 1973.

599. Telenti A, Hermans PE: Idiopathic granulomatosis manifesting as fever of unknown origin. *Mayo Clin Proc* 66:44–50, 1989.

600. Zoutman DE, Ralph ED, Frei JV: Granulomatous hepatitis and fever of unknown origin. *J Clin Gastroenterol* 13:69–75, 1991.

601. Holtz T, Moseley RH, Scheiman JM: Liver biopsy in fever of unknown origin: A reappraisal. *Clin Gastroenterol* 17:29–32, 1993.

Antineutrophil Cytoplasmic Autoantibodies: Discovery, Specificity, Disease Associations, and Pathogenic Potential

J. Charles Jennette, M.D.

Professor of Pathology and Medicine, School of Medicine, University of North Carolina, Chapel Hill, North Carolina

Ronald J. Falk, M.D.

Associate Professor of Medicine, School of Medicine, University of North Carolina, Chapel Hill, North Carolina

DISCOVERY

Antineutrophil cytoplasmic autoantibodies (ANCAs) are specific for protein antigens in the granules of neutrophils and the peroxidase-positive lysosomes of monocytes. They are useful diagnostic serologic markers for a variety of inflammatory diseases, especially certain types of small-vessel vasculitis, and may be directly involved in the pathogenesis of these diseases.

Antineutrophil cytoplasmic antibodies were first observed when normal human neutrophils were being used as a substrate for detecting antinuclear antibodies (ANAs). In 1982, Davies and his associates were the first to publish an account of the detection of autoantibodies that bound to antigens in the cytoplasm of neutrophils.[1] While using neutrophils as a substrate to detect ANAs, they observed cytoplasmic staining of the neutrophils by serum samples from eight patients who were found by renal biopsy to have glomerulonephritis with necrosis and crescents but no immune deposits. Most of these patients also had evidence for extrarenal inflammatory disease such as arthralgias, myalgias, pulmonary infiltrates, and hemoptysis. Hall et al. confirmed Davies and associates' observation in a 1984 report of four patients with arthralgias and pulmonary disease accompanied by necrotizing glomerulonephritis (three patients), cutaneous vasculitis (two patients), and gastrointestinal complaints (two patients).[2]

These first two reports indicated a strong association between ANCAs and vascular inflammation in the kidney, lungs, skin, and gut, but these seminal publications received very little attention. The first

Advances in Pathology and Laboratory Medicine, vol. 8
© 1995, Mosby–Year Book, Inc.

widespread recognition of this class of autoantibodies resulted from a 1985 publication by van der Woude and his collaborators, who reported a high frequency of ANCAs in patients with active Wegener's granulomatosis and a lower frequency in patients in a quiescent phase of the disease.[3] They suggested that ANCAs were a sensitive and specific diagnostic serologic marker for Wegener's granulomatosis and could be used to monitor disease activity. This publication generated considerable excitement about ANCAs and was a prelude to a period of rapid advances in the understanding of ANCAs, their utility as diagnostic and prognostic markers, and their potential role in the pathogenesis of small-vessel vasculitides. In the decade since their recognition, there have been over 500 publications dealing with ANCAs.

ANTIGEN SPECIFICITY

Although, by definition, all ANCAs have specificity for autoantigens in the cytoplasm of neutrophils, there are different subtypes of ANCAs with different antigen specificities. This is analogous to subtypes of ANAs that have specificity for different antigens, such as DNA, histones, Smith antigen, and ribonucleoproteins. Antinuclear antibodies with different antigen specificities produce different patterns of nuclear staining by indirect immunofluorescence microscopy, such as homogeneous, rim, speckled, and nucleolar. In an analogous fashion, ANCAs with different antigen specificities produce different neutrophil staining patterns.

The standard indirect immunofluorescence assay for ANCAs uses alcohol-fixed normal human neutrophils as a substrate for detecting the autoantibodies in patient serum. Falk and Jennette observed that this technique resulted in two patterns of neutrophil staining when sera from patients with small-vessel vasculitis or necrotizing glomerulonephritis were tested.[4] One pattern is the typical cytoplasmic staining described originally by Davies et al. (Fig 1, A), and the second is a perinuclear or nuclear pattern of neutrophil staining (Fig 1, B). Antineutrophil cytoplasmic antibodies that produce the cytoplasmic pattern are called C-ANCAs, and those that produce the perinuclear pattern are called P-ANCAs.

The nuclear staining of alcohol-fixed neutrophils results from the diffusion of some proteins from the cytoplasm and adherence to nuclei during substrate preparation. This artifactual diffusion is prevented by formalin fixation, which fixes the cytoplasmic proteins in place and results in cytoplasmic staining by both C-ANCAs and P-ANCAs.[5] Autoantibodies that produce a P-ANCA staining pattern can be distinguished from ANAs by their failure to stain tissue cell nuclei or HEp2 cells, cytoplasmic staining of formalin-fixed neutrophils, and specific immunochemical reaction with purified antigens.

Although the name implies that ANCAs react only with neutrophils, the target antigens for ANCAs are also in the cytoplasm of monocytes but not marcophages.[5] The ability of ANCAs to react with both neutrophils and monocytes is especially significant if ANCAs are pathogenic, as will be suggested later in this review.

More precise determination of ANCA antigen specificity is obtained by immunochemical assays such as enzyme-linked immunosorbent assay (ELISA), radioimmunoassay, Western blot, and immunoprecipitation.

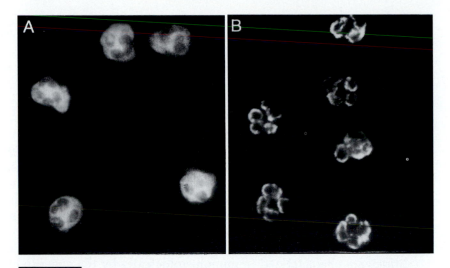

FIGURE 1.

Indirect immunofluorescence microscopy on alcohol-fixed normal human neutrophils demonstrating the cytoplasmic staining pattern of C-ANCA **(A)** and the perinuclear staining pattern of P-ANCA **(B).** (From Jennette JC, Wilkman AS, Falk RJ: *Am J Pathol* 135:921–930, 1989. Used by permission.)

In 1988, Falk and Jennette reported the first recognized antigen specificity for ANCAs.[4] They observed that both C-ANCAs and P-ANCAs from patients with vasculitis and glomerulonephritis reacted with proteins in the primary (azurophilic) granules of neutrophils and that most P-ANCAs but not C-ANCAs were specific for myeloperoxidase (MPO). The same conclusion was reported by Goldschmeding et al. in 1989.[6]

Goldschmeding et al. also observed that most C-ANCAs reacted with a 29-kD serine proteinase found in neutrophil primary (azurophilic) granules,[6] and the same conclusion was published almost simultaneously by Niles et al.[7] This observation was further confirmed by Ludemann et al.[8] and Jennette et al.[9] The biochemical properties of the serine proteinase indicated that it was a previously identified neutrophil elastinolytic enzyme called proteinase 3 (PR3).[9]

In patients with vasculitis, PR3-ANCAs and MPO-ANCAs account for over 80% of the ANCAs; however, several minor specificities have been reported. For example, some P-ANCAs are specific for elastase[6] and some C-ANCAs are specific for bactericidal permeability-increasing protein (BPI), which is also called 57-kD cationic protein.[10]

Greater than 90% of the ANCAs in patients with vasculitis can be shown to be specific for PR3, BPI, MPO, or elastase by currently available assay systems. The specificity of ANCAs that occur in patients with inflammatory bowel disease (IBD) and a variety of rheumatologic conditions such as Felty syndrome, however, remains poorly defined or unknown.[11]

DISEASE ASSOCIATIONS

Antineutrophil cytoplasmic antibodies are most frequent in patients with necrotizing small-vessel vasculitides and no immunohistologic evidence for vascular immunoglobulin deposition such as Wegener's granulomatosis, microscopic polyangiitis, and Churg-Strauss syndrome[12-16] and in patients with certain types of inflammatory bowel and hepatic disease such as ulcerative colitis, primary sclerosing cholangitis, and autoimmune hepatitis[11] (Table 1).

SMALL-VESSEL VASCULITIDES

The basic histologic appearance of the vascular lesions of ANCA-associated small-vessel vasculitis is similar in arteries, arterioles, capillaries, venules, and veins and is characterized in the acute phase by focal fibrinoid necrosis, often accompanied by neutrophil infiltration and leukocytoclasia. With progression of the lesions, the neutrophils are replaced by mononuclear leukocytes and the fibrinoid necrosis disappears and may evolve into fibrosis.

Antineutrophil cytoplasmic antibody–associated small-vessel vasculitides are characterized immunohistologically by the absence of vascular deposits of immunoglobulin. This feature distinguishes them from histologically identical small-vessel vasculitides that do have vascular immune deposits such as cryoglobulinemic vasculitis, serum sickness vasculitis, Henoch-Schönlein purpura, and anti–basement membrane antibody (GBM) mediated disease.

TABLE 1.

Approximate Frequency of Antineutrophil Cytoplasmic Antibodies in Patients With Various Active Untreated Diseases*

Disease	ANCA	C-ANCA	P-ANCA
Vasculitides			
Wegener's granulomatosis	90†	85	5
Microscopic polyangiitis	90	40	50
Churg-Strauss syndrome	75	15	60
Inflammatory bowel and hepatic diseases			
Primary sclerosing cholangiitis	80	0	80
Ulcerative colitis	70	0	70
Autoimmune hepatitis	60	0	60
Primary biliary cirrhosis	30	0	30
Crohn's disease	20	0	20
Rheumatologic diseases			
Drug-induced lupus erythematosus	80	0	80
Systemic lupus erythematosus	15	0	15
Rheumatoid arthritis	15	0	15
Felty syndrome	60	0	60

*These values are only estimates based on our experience with several hundred patients with ANCA-associated vasculitis and over 100 with inflammatory bowel disease, as well as reports in the literature. The numbers will be refined as additional patients are evaluated, better ANCA assay systems are developed, and more discriminating diagnostic criteria are available.
†Values are percentages.

Although they share common features, ANCA-associated vasculitic lesions have somewhat distinctive appearances depending on the type of vessel involved, for example, necrotizing arteritis in a renal interlobular artery (Fig 2, A), leukocytoclastic angiitis in a dermal postcapillary venule (Fig 2, B), leukocytoclastic angiitis in renal medullary vasa recta (Fig 2, C), hemorrhagic pulmonary alveolar capillaritis (Fig 2, D), and segmental necrotizing glomerulonephritis with crescent formation (Fig 2, E).

In addition to the shared feature of necrotizing small-vessel vasculitis, the ANCA-associated vasculitides can be subdivided by the presence or absence of other clinical and pathologic features.[15, 16] In an ANCA-positive patient with small-vessel vasculitis, the presence of necrotizing granulomatous inflammation (Fig 2, F) in the absence of eosinophilia or asthma warrants a diagnosis of Wegener's granulomatosis, whereas the presence of necrotizing inflammation along with eosinophilia and asthma warrants a diagnosis of Churg-Strauss syndrome. The absence of granu-

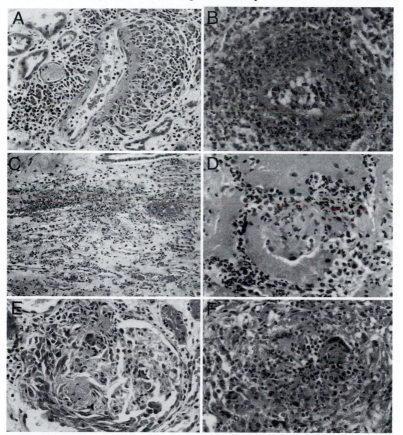

FIGURE 2.

Antineutrophil cytoplasmic antibody–associated lesions. **A,** necrotizing arteritis in an interlobular renal artery. **B,** leukocytoclastic angiitis in a dermal postcapillary venule. **C,** leukocytoclastic angiitis in renal medullary vasa recta. **D,** pulmonary alveolar capillaritis. **E,** necrotizing glomerulonephritis with crescent formation. **F,** pulmonary necrotizing granulomatous inflammation. (From Jennette JC, Falk RJ: *Am J Kidney Dis* 15:517–529, 1990, and Jennette JC: *Am J Kidney Dis* 18:164–170, 1991. Used by permission.)

lomatous inflammation, eosinophilia, or asthma in a patient with ANCA-associated small-vessel vasculitis supports a diagnosis of microscopic polyangiitis or microscopic polyarteritis. The former term is preferable to the latter because many patients with ANCA-associated small-vessel vasculitis do not have involvement of arteries.[15]

The distribution of vascular involvement by the ANCA-associated vasculitides considerably overlaps that of other types of vasculitis[15] (Fig 3). Because of this, histologic evaluation alone is not sufficient to distinguish an ANCA-associated vasculitis from other types of vasculitis with similar light microscopic features. For example, the histologic finding in a skin biopsy specimen of dermal leukocytoclastic angiitis and the resultant clinical finding of palpable purpura can be caused by ANCA-associated vasculitis (i.e., Wegener's granulomatosis, Churg-Strauss syndrome, and microscopic polyangiitis), as well as immune complex–mediated vasculitis (e.g., Henoch-Schönlein purpura, cryoglobulinemic vasculitis, and serum sickness vasculitis). Differentiation among these diagnostic possibilities would require additional data such as serologic or immunohistologic data. Similarly, a patient with pulmonary hemorrhage and crescentic glomerulonephritis (i.e., pulmonary-renal vasculitic syndrome) could have disease secondary to ANCAs, anti–basement membrane antibodies, or immune complexes that could not be differentiated by light microscopy alone but would require serology or immunohistology for an accurate pathologic diagnosis.

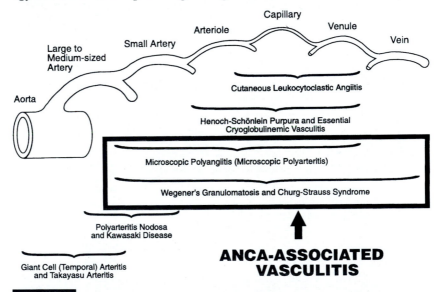

FIGURE 3.

Predominant range of vascular involvement by vasculitides as defined by the Chapel Hill Consensus Conference on the Nomenclature of Systemic Vasculitis. Note the substantial overlap among diseases. Large artery refers to the aorta and the largest branches directed toward major body regions (e.g., to the extremities and the head and neck); medium-sized artery refers to the main visceral arteries (e.g., renal, hepatic, coronary, and mesenteric arteries), and small artery refers to the distal arterial radicals that connect with arterioles. *ANCA* = antineutrophil cytoplasmic antibody. (Adapted from Jennette JC, Falk RJ, Andrassy K, et al: *Arthritis Rheum* 37:187–192, 1994.)

Although most patients with ANCA-associated vasculitis have involvement of multiple organs, some patients have disease limited to a single site, for example, Wegener's granulomatosis confined to the respiratory tract or ANCA-associated glomerulonephritis without extrarenal vasculitis. Patients with ANCA-associated vasculitis confined to a single location, however, are at risk for greater dissemination later in the course of the disease.

For pathologists in particular, it is important to realize that the typical acute inflammatory lesions of ANCA-associated vasculitis evolve into chronic sclerosing lesions over time, which expands the histologic spectrum of changes that can raise the suspicion of ANCA-associated disease. For example, in the lungs, the acute inflammatory injury can be transformed into a pattern of diffuse interstitial fibrosis that is indistinguishable from the chronic phases of other types of diffuse alveolar damage.[17] It is also important to note that the pulmonary inflammatory injury can be either vasocentric or bronchocentric and that when the latter affects small airways, it can lead to bronchiolitis obliterans.[17]

Antineutrophil cytoplasmic antibodies are sensitive diagnostic markers for active untreated systemic Wegener's granulomatosis, Churg-Strauss syndrome, and microscopic polyangiitis (defined as systemic necrotizing small-vessel vasculitis with no immunoglobulin deposits). Approximately 90% of patients with ANCA-associated small-vessel vasculitis will have either anti-MPO or anti-PR3 antibodies. Dual specificity for MPO and PR3 is very rare. The antigen specificity of the ANCA correlates to a degree with the subtype of vasculitis.

Over 90% of the patients with active systemic Wegener's granulomatosis are ANCA-positive. Precise frequencies of antigen specificities among the different types of ANCA-associated vasculitis are difficult to determine because of the problem with definitively differentiating between Wegener's granulomatosis, Churg-Strauss syndrome, and microscopic polyangiitis. In our experience, 80% to 90% of the patients with a clinical diagnosis of Wegener's granulomatosis and histologic confirmation of granulomatous inflammation have C-ANCAs with an approximately 90% specificity for PR3. Fewer than 10% have MPO-specific P-ANCAs.

Although PR3-ANCAs (C-ANCAs) are far more frequent than MPO-ANCAs (P-ANCAs) in patients with Wegener's granulomatosis, MPO-ANCAs (P-ANCAs) are more frequent than PR3-ANCAs (C-ANCAs) in patients with microscopic polyangiitis, Churg-Strauss syndrome, or ANCA-associated crescentic glomerulonephritis with no extrarenal disease.

The frequency of various types of ANCA-associated vasculitis and therefore the frequency of different ANCA antigen specificities that a given physician observes is substantially influenced by the nature of the patients evaluated in that physician's practice. For example, a pulmonary pathologist would see specimens from patients with a much higher frequency of PR3-specific C-ANCAs, whereas a renal pathologist would see specimens from patients with a higher frequency of MPO-specific P-ANCAs.

For example, Figure 4 represents the relative frequency of ANCA positivity and ANCA antigen specificity among patients with crescentic glo-

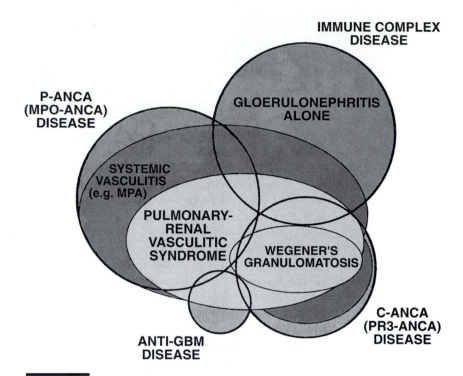

FIGURE 4.

Relationship between clinicopathologic expressions of disease *(ovals* and *shaded areas)* and immunopathologic categories *(circles)* in patients with crescentic glomerulonephritis. (Adapted from Jennette JC: *Am J Kidney Dis* 18:164–170, 1991.)

merulonephritis evaluated by a renal pathologist.[12] Antineutrophil cytoplasmic antibody–associated glomerulonephritis is the most common type of crescentic glomerulonephritis and accounts for over half of all patients with rapidly progressive glomerulonephritis.[17] Note in Figure 4 that patients with Wegener's granulomatosis very often have PR3-ANCAs (C-ANCAs) but that all patients with PR3-ANCAs (C-ANCAs) do not have Wegener's granulomatosis. Some patients with PR3-ANCAs have pulmonary-renal vasculitic syndrome with alveolar capillaritis rather than granulomatous inflammation (i.e., microscopic polyangiitis affecting the lungs), systemic small-vessel vasculitis without granulomatous inflammation (i.e., microscopic polyangiitis), or glomerulonephritis with no extrarenal vasculitis (i.e., ANCA-associated crescentic glomerulonephritis). Also note that a given clinicopathologic manifestation, such as pulmonary-renal vasculitic syndrome, can be caused by different immunopathogenic mechanisms and that a minority of patients have evidence for overlapping immunopathologic processes, such as concurrent ANCAs and anti-GBM antibodies.

Nomenclature of Vasculitides

The pathologic and clinical diagnosis of ANCA-associated vasculitis as well as other forms of necrotizing vasculitis has been complicated by the lack of a standardized nomenclature for vasculitides. Over the almost half century since the publication of Zeek's review of necrotizing vasculitis,[18] many approaches to vasculitis categorization have been published,[19-24] but none have been widely adopted, and until recently our understanding of ANCAs was not factored into the classification approaches.

An approach to classifying vasculitides was recently published by the American College of Rheumatology (ACR).[24] Their stated goal, however, was to develop criteria for classifying patients into relatively homogeneous categories for entry into clinical trials. The ACR criteria, therefore, were not designed to be optimum criteria for the clinical or pathologic diagnosis of disease, although they are being widely used for this purpose. Unfortunately, the ACR criteria are not adequate for diagnosing the different clinicopathologic expressions of ANCA-associated vasculitis. For example, a 20-year-old patient with ANCA-associated vasculitis who has (1) cutaneous purpura, (2) a skin biopsy specimen demonstrating leukocytoclastic angiitis, (3) nephritis with hypertension and renal insufficiency, and (4) mononeuritis multiplex would fulfill the ACR criteria for three different categories of vasculitis, i.e., hypersensitivity vasculitis, Henoch-Schönlein purpura, and polyarteritis nodosa. In our opinion, none of these diagnostic designations are appropriate for ANCA-associated vasculitis.

"Polyarteritis nodosa" is not an appropriate term for ANCA-associated vasculitis because many ANCA-positive patients have vasculitic lesions only in vessels smaller than arteries, i.e., arterioles, capillaries, and postcapillary venules, and those patients who do have arteritis often have involvement of predominantly small arteries that do not cause grossly discernible inflammatory nodules. In addition, patients with classic polyarteritis nodosa who do not have small-vessel involvement are usually ANCA-negative.

The term "hypersensitivity vasculitis" is inappropriate for ANCA-associated disease because ANCA-associated vasculitis is an autoimmune phenomenon rather than an allergic response. Zeek originally preferred the term "hypersensitivity angiitis" because she was aware of some patients who had small-vessel vasculitis secondary to allergic responses to horse serum or sulfonamides and she presumed that this was the basis for most small-vessel vasculitis.[18] Although hypersensitivity responses can certainly cause some examples of small-vessel vasculitis, there is no evidence that allergy has a role in the induction of ANCA-associated vasculitis.

The term "Henoch-Schönlein purpura" defines a clinically and pathogenetically uniform category of patients only if it is restricted to those patients, usually children, who have vascular inflammation induced by IgA-dominant immune complexes and do not have ANCAs. Patients with clinically and histologically identical small-vessel vasculitis have very different prognoses depending on whether they have IgA-dominant immune complex–mediated vasculitis (i.e., Henoch-Schönlein purpura) or ANCA-associated vasculitis with no immune deposits. For example, a patient with purpura caused by dermal leukocytoclastic angiitis, abdominal pain caused by arteriolitis in the gut, and hematuria caused by glomerulonephritis who is negative for ANCAs and has IgA-dominant immune complexes in skin vessels indicative of Henoch-Schönlein purpura has a good chance of spontaneous resolution of the vasculitis, whereas a patient with the same signs and symptoms of vasculitis who is positive for ANCAs and has no immune deposits in the skin is at risk for the development of life-threatening organ injury such as renal failure or massive pulmonary hemorrhage if not treated with aggressive immunosuppression.

Recently, an international consensus conference was convened in Chapel Hill to develop a proposal for standardizing the names and definitions of some of the more common forms of vasculitis, including those observed in patients with ANCAs[15] (Table 2 and Fig 3). The categories in Table 2 that are associated with ANCAs are microscopic polyangiitis (microscopic polyarteritis), Wegener's granulomatosis, and Churg-Strauss syndrome. As depicted in Figure 3, ANCA-associated vasculitis can affect a wide range of the vascular tree, and this involvement overlaps with other types of vasculitis. Therefore, clinical and even histologic criteria are not adequate for accurately differentiating among pathogenetically distinct types of vasculitis. Additional parameters such as serologic assay for ANCAs and cryoglobulins and immunohistologic analysis for vascular immune deposits are required.

TABLE 2.

Names and Definitions of Vasculitis Adopted by the Chapel Hill Consensus Conference on the Nomenclature of Systemic Vasculitis*

Name	Definition
Large-vessel vasculitis†	
Giant cell (temporal) arteritis	Granulomatous arteritis of the aorta and its major branches, with a predilection for the extracranial branches of the carotid artery. *Often involves the temporal artery. Usually occurs in patients older than 50 and is often associated with polymyalgia rheumatica*
Takayasu arteritis	Granulomatous inflammation of the aorta and its major branches. *Usually occurs in patients younger than 50*
Medium-vessel vasculitis†	
Polyarteritis nodosa (classic polyarteritis nodosa)	Necrotizing inflammation of medium-sized or small arteries without glomerulonephritis or vasculitis in arterioles, capillaries, or venules
Kawasaki disease	Arteritis involving large, medium, and small arteries and is associated with mucocutaneous lymph node syndrome. *Coronary arteries are often involved. Aorta and veins may be involved. Usually occurs in children*
Small-vessel vasculitis†	
Wegener's granulomatosis‡	Granulomatous inflammation involving the respiratory tract and necrotizing vasculitis affecting small to medium-sized vessels, e.g., capillaries, venules, arterioles, and arteries. *Necrotizing glomerulonephritis is common*

Churg-Strauss syndrome‡	Eosinophil-rich and granulomatous inflammation involving the respiratory tract and necrotizing vasculitis affecting small to medium-sized vessels and is associated with asthma and blood eosinophilia
Microscopic polyangiitis (microscopic polyarteritis)‡	Necrotizing vasculitis with few or no immune deposits affecting small vessels, i.e., capillaries, venules, or arterioles. *Necrotizing arteritis involving small and medium-sized arteries may be present. Necrotizing glomerulonephritis is very common. Pulmonary capillaritis often occurs*
Henoch-Schönlein purpura	Vasculitis with IgA-dominant immune deposits affecting small vessels, i.e., capillaries, venules, or arterioles. *Typically involves skin, gut, and glomeruli and is associated with arthralgias or arthritis*
Essential cryoglobulinemic vasculitis	Vasculitis with cryoglobulin immune deposits affecting small vessels, i.e., capillaries, venules, or arterioles, and is associated with cryoglobulins in serum. *Skin and glomeruli are often involved*
Cutaneous leukocytoclastic angiitis	Isolated cutaneous leukocytoclastic angiitis without systemic vasculitis or glomerulonephritis

*Adapted from Jennette JC, Falk RJ, Andrassy K, et al: *Arthritis Rheum* 37:187–192, 1994.
†Large vessel refers to the aorta and the largest branches directed toward major body regions (e.g., to the extremities and the head and neck); medium vessel refers to the main visceral arteries (e.g., renal, hepatic, coronary, and mesenteric arteries), and small vessel refers to the distal arterial radicals that connect with arterioles. Note that some small- and large-vessel vasculitides may involve medium-sized arteries but large- and medium-vessel vasculitides do not involve vessels smaller than arteries.
‡Strongly associated with antineutrophil cytoplasmic autoantibodies.

INFLAMMATORY BOWEL AND HEPATIC DISEASES

Autoantibodies that react with neutrophil nuclei but not nuclei in other tissues were first identified in patients with rheumatologic diseases and IBDs approximately 30 years ago by Faber and Elling, who called them "leukocyte-specific antinuclear factors."[25] Nielson et al. reported the same phenomenon in patients with IBD and designated the autoantibodies granulocyte-specific ANAs (GS-ANAs).[26] It now appears that most if not all GS-ANAs in patients with IBD are a type of P-ANCA with antigen specificity different from that in patients with vasculitis.

The ANCAs in patients with inflammatory bowel and hepatic disease (IBD-ANCAs) produce a slightly different staining pattern of alcohol-fixed neutrophils that is characterized by a very well defined staining at the periphery of the nucleus. As would be expected if the autoantibodies are directed against cytoplasmic rather than nuclear antigens, IBD-ANCAs stain the cytoplasm of formalin-fixed neutrophils.

As shown in Table 1, a variety of inflammatory bowel and hepatic diseases are associated with P-ANCAs (IBD-ANCAs).[11, 27–37] Although there are differences in frequency among the diseases, there is so much overlap of positivity that ANCA determinations are not very useful for differential diagnosis. In addition, ANCA positivity and titer do not correlate well with disease activity.

Inflammatory bowel disease ANCAs are not specific for the antigens commonly recognized by ANCAs in patients with vasculitides; for example, IBD-ANCAs do not react with PR3, MPO, or elastase. A number of candidate IBD-ANCA antigens have been proposed, including lactoferrin, lactoperoxidase, cathepsin G, and various unnamed polypeptides,[36 37] but there is no consensus on which if any of these are important target antigens.

RHEUMATOLOGIC DISEASES

The association of ANCAs with rheumatologic diseases such as rheumatoid arthritis and systemic lupus erythematosus is relatively poorly understood. This is in part because of the difficulty in distinguishing ANCAs from ANAs and GS-ANAs (if they exist) and the many other autoantibodies that occur in these disorders. There is reasonable evidence, however, that ANCAs are among the autoantibody repertoire of at least some patients with these diseases (see Table 1).

A relationship between GS-ANAs and rheumatoid arthritis, especially Felty syndrome, was recognized in the 1960s.[25] At least some investigators now consider these antibodies to be a special type of P-ANCA.[37–39] The antigen specificity of ANCAs in patients with rheumatoid arthritis and Felty syndrome has not been conclusively determined; however, Mulder et al. have evidence that at least some ANCAs in these patients react with lactoferrin or several distinct polypeptides,[39] which is similar to the specificity of IBD-ANCAs.

Only a minority of patients with systemic lupus erythematosus appear to have ANCAs, but most patients with drug-induced lupus syndrome have P-ANCAs with specificity for MPO, elastase, or both.[30, 40–43] Hydralazine and propylthiouracil are the best known drugs that are capable of inducing a high level of ANCAs.

Although patients with so-called drug-induced lupus have both ANAs and P-ANCAs, the vasculitis and glomerulonephritis that occur in these patients resemble ANCA-associated necrotizing vascular injury with no immune deposits rather than lupus-like immune complex injury. This raises the possibility that the vasculitis in these patients is mediated by ANCAs. This pathogenic potential is supported further by the observation that withdrawal of a drug that induces ANCAs and vasculitis is followed not only by a fall in ANCA titers but also by resolution of the vasculitis.[42]

PATHOGENIC POTENTIAL

There is no absolute proof that ANCAs are pathogenic; however, there is substantial circumstantial evidence that anti-MPO and anti-PR3 ANCAs participate in the mediation of vascular injury in patients with ANCA-associated vasculitides.[44] Clinically, ANCA titers correlate to a degree with disease activity. As mentioned earlier, drugs that induce ANCA formation also induce vasculitis and glomerulonephritis that resemble primary ANCA-associated vasculitis and glomerulonephritis.

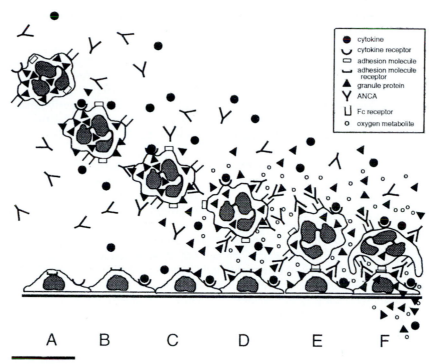

FIGURE 5.
Putative pathogenic sequence of events mediated by antineutrophil cytoplasmic antibodies (ANCA). **A,** unprimed neutrophil with ANCA antigens in the cytoplasm. **B,** neutrophil primed by cytokines, for example, as a result of a respiratory tract infection, and expressing ANCA antigens at the cell surface. **C** and **D,** ANCA binding to antigens on the neutrophil surface as well as by Fc-mediated binding of ANCA complexed with antigens in the microenvironment around the cell. **D** and **E,** neutrophil respiratory burst, degranulation, and binding to neutrophils via upregulated cell adhesion molecules and Fc receptors for ANCA bound to antigens adsorbed on endothelial surfaces. **F,** endothelial and vessel wall injury. (From Jennette JC, Falk RJ: *Lab Invest* 70:135−137, 1994. Used by permission.)

There are no clear-cut animal models of ANCA-mediated vasculitis, but there are a number of in vitro observations that support a pathogenic role for ANCAs.[44] Neutrophils that are primed with low levels of cytokines (e.g., tumor necrosis factor or interleukin-1) or microbial products (e.g., formyl peptides) express small amounts of ANCA antigens (MPO and PR3) at their surfaces that can react with ANCAs. Reaction of primed neutrophils with isolated ANCA IgG results in neutrophil degranulation and a respiratory burst that can be caused by either the Fc or F(ab′)$_2$ portions of the IgG. Antineutrophil cytoplasmic antibody−activated neutrophils bind to endothelial cells via integrin interactions and cause endothelial injury. If these in vitro events took place in vivo, vasculitis would result by the scenario depicted in Figure 5.

REFERENCES

1. Davies DJ, Moran JE, Niall JF, et al: Segmental necrotizing glomerulonephritis with antineutrophil antibody: possible arbovirus aetiology? *BMJ* 285:606, 1982.

2. Hall JB, Wadham BM, Wood CJ, et al: Vasculitis and glomerulonephritis: A subgroup with an antineutrophil cytoplasmic antibody. *Aust N Z J Med* 14:277–278, 1984.
3. van der Woude FJ, Rasmussen N, Lobatto S, et al: Autoantibodies against neutrophils and monocytes: Tool for diagnosis and marker of disease activity in Wegener's granulomatosis. *Lancet* 1:425–429, 1985.
4. Falk RJ, Jennette JC: Anti-neutrophil cytoplasmic autoantibodies with specificity for myeloperoxidase in patients with systemic vasculitis and idiopathic necrotizing and crescentic glomerulonephritis. *N Engl J Med* 318:1651–1657, 1988.
5. Charles LA, Falk RJ, Jennette JC: Reactivity of anti-neutrophil cytoplasmic autoantibodies with mononuclear phagocytes. *J Leukoc Biol* 51:65–68, 1992.
6. Goldschmeding R, van der Schoot CE, ten Bokkel Huinink D, et al: Wegener's granulomatosis autoantibodies identify a novel diisopropyl fluorophosphate-binding protein in the lysosomes of normal human neutrophils. *J Clin Invest* 84:1577–1587, 1989.
7. Niles JL, McCluskey T, Ahmad MF, et al: Wegener's granulomatosis autoantigen is a novel neutrophil serine proteinase. *Blood* 74:1888–1893, 1989.
8. Ludemann J, Utecht B, Gross WL: Anti-neutrophil cytoplasm antibodies in Wegener's granulomatosis recognize an elastinolytic enzyme. *J Exp Med* 171:357–362, 1990.
9. Jennette JC, Hoidal JH, Falk RJ: Specificity of anti-neutrophil cytoplasmic autoantibodies for proteinase 3. *Blood* 75:2263–2264, 1990.
10. Yang JJ, Becker M, Tuttle R, et al: Specificity of cytoplasmic-pattern antineutrophil cytoplasmic autoantibodies (C-ANCA) for bactericidal permeability-increasing protein (BPI). *Clin Exp Immunol,* in press.
11. Jennette JC, Falk RJ: Anti-neutrophil cytoplasmic autoantibodies in inflammatory bowel disease. *Am J Clin Pathol* 99:221–223, 1993.
12. Jennette JC: Anti-neutrophil cytoplasmic autoantibody–associated disease: A pathologist's perspective. *Am J Kidney Dis* 18:164–170, 1991.
13. Gross WL, Schmitt WH, Csernok E: ANCA and associated diseases: Immunodiagnostic and pathogenetic aspects. *Clin Exp Immunol* 91:1–12, 1993.
14. Kallenberg CGM, Brouwer E, Weening JJ, et al: Anti-neutrophil cytoplasmic antibodies: Current diagnostic and pathophysiologic potential. *Kidney Int* 46:1–15, 1994.
15. Jennette JC, Falk RJ, Andrassy K, et al: Nomenclature of systemic vasculitides: The proposal of an international consensus conference. *Arthritis Rheum* 37:187–192, 1994.
16. Jennette JC, Falk RJ: The pathology of vasculitis involving the kidney. *Am J Kidney Dis* 24:130–141, 1994.
17. Gaudin PB, Askin FB, Falk RJ, et al: The pathologic spectrum of pulmonary lesions in patients with anti-neutrophil cytoplasmic autoantibodies specific for anti–proteinase 3 and myeloperoxidase. *Am J Clin Pathol,* in press.
18. Zeek PM: Periarteritis nodosa: A critical review. *Am J Clin Pathol* 22:777–790, 1952.
19. Fauci AS, Haynes BF, Katz P: The spectrum of vasculitis. Clinical, pathologic, immunologic, and therapeutic considerations. *Ann Intern Med* 89:660–676, 1978.
20. McCluskey RT, Fienber R: Vasculitis in primary vasculitides, granulomatoses, and connective tissue diseases. *Hum Pathol* 14:305–315, 1983.
21. Lie JT: Systemic and isolated vasculitis: A rational approach to classification and pathologic diagnosis. *Pathol Annu* 24:25–114, 1989.
22. Churg J, Churg A: Idiopathic and secondary vasculitis: A review. *Mod Pathol* 2:144–160, 1989.

23. Waldherr R, Eberlein-Gonska M, Noronha IL: Histopathological differentiation of systemic necrotizing vasculitides. *APMIS Suppl* 19:17–28, 1990.
24. Hunder GG, Arend WP, Bloch DA, et al: The American College of Rheumatology 1990 criteria for the classification of vasculitis. *Arthritis Rheum* 33:1065–1067, 1990.
25. Faber V, Elling P: Leukocyte-specific antinuclear factors in patients with Felty's syndrome, rheumatoid arthritis, systemic lupus erythematosus and other diseases. *Acta Med Scand* 179:257, 1967.
26. Nielsen H, Wiik A, Elmgreen J: Granulocyte specific antinuclear antibodies in ulcerative colitis. *Acta Pathol Microbiol Immunol Scand* 91:23, 1983.
27. Snook JA, Chapman RW, Fleming K, et al: Anti-neutrophil nuclear antibody in ulcerative colitis, Crohn's disease and primary sclerosing cholangitis. *Clin Exp Immunol* 76:30–33, 1989.
28. Saxon A, Shanahan F, Landers C, et al: A distinct subset of antineutrophil cytoplasmic antibodies is associated with inflammatory bowel disease. *J Allergy Clin Immunol* 86:202–210, 1990.
29. Rump JA, Scholmerich J, Gross V, et al: A new type of perinuclear antineutrophil cytoplasmic antibody (p-ANCA) in active ulcerative colitis but not in Crohn's disease. *Immunobiology* 181:406–413, 1990.
30. Jennette JC, Hogan S, Wilkman AS, et al: Anti-neutrophil cytoplasmic autoantibody disease associations. *Am J Kidney Dis* 18:206–207, 1991.
31. Duerr RH, Targan SR, Landers CJ, et al: Anti-neutrophil cytoplasmic antibodies in ulcerative colitis. *Gastroenterology* 100:1590–1596, 1991.
32. Duerr RH, Targan SR, Landers CJ, et al: Neutrophil cytoplasmic antibodies: A link between primary sclerosing cholangitis and ulcerative colitis. *Gastroenterology* 100:1385–1391, 1991.
33. Cambridge G, Rampton DS, Stevens TRJ, et al: Anti-neutrophil antibodies in inflammatory bowel disease: Prevalence and diagnostic role. *Gut* 33:668–674, 1992.
34. Halbwachs-Mecarelli L, Nusbaum P, Noel LH, et al: Antineutrophil cytoplasmic antibodies (ANCA) directed against cathepsin G in ulcerative colitis, Crohn's disease and primary sclerosing cholangitis. *Clin Exp Immunol* 90:79–84, 1992.
35. Hardarson S, LaBrecque DR, Mitros FA, et al: Anti-neutrophil cytoplasmic antibody (ANCA) in inflammatory bowel and hepatobiliary diseases. High prevalence in ulcerative colitis, primary sclerosing cholangitis and autoimmune hepatitis. *Am J Clin Pathol* 99:277–281, 1993.
36. Mulder AH, Horst G, Haagsma EB, et al: Anti-neutrophil cytoplasmic antibodies (ANCA) in autoimmune liver disease. *Adv Exp Med Biol* 336:545–549, 1993.
37. Mulder AH, Broekroelofs J, Horst G, et al: Anti-neutrophil cytoplasmic antibodies (ANCA) in inflammatory bowel disease: Characterization and clinical correlates. *Clin Exp Immunol* 95:490–497, 1994.
38. Juby A, Johnston C, Davis P, et al: Antinuclear and anti-neutrophil cytoplasmic antibodies (ANCA) in the area of patients with Felty's syndrome. *Br J Rheumatol* 31:185–188, 1992.
39. Mulder AH, Horst G, van Leeuwen PC, et al: Anti-neutrophil cytoplasmic antibodies in rheumatoid arthritis: Characterization and clinical correlations. *Arthritis Rheum* 36:1054–1060, 1993.
40. Nassberger L, Sjoholm AG, Jonsson H, et al: Autoantibodies against neutrophil cytoplasm components in systemic lupus erythematosus and in hydralazine-induced lupus. *Clin Exp Immunol* 81:380–383, 1990.
41. Cambridge G, Wallace H, Bernstein RM, et al: Autoantibodies to myelope-

roxidase in idiopathic and drug-induced systemic lupus erythematosus and vasculitis. *Br J Rheumatol* 33:109–114, 1994.

42. Dolman KM, Gans RBO, Vervaat TJ, et al: Vasculitis and antineutrophil cytoplasmic autoantibodies associated with propylthiouracil therapy. *Lancet* 342:651–652, 1993.

43. Vogt BA, Kim Y, Jennette JC, et al: Anti-neutrophil cytoplasmic autoantibody-–positive crescentic glomerulonephritis as a complication of propylthiouracil treatment in children. *J Pediatr* 124:986–988, 1994.

44. Jennette JC, Falk RJ: Pathogenic potential of anti-neutrophil cytoplasmic autoantibodies. *Lab Invest* 70:135–137, 1994.

PCR-DNA Utilization: General Laboratory Usage for Mismatched Specimens

Darryl Shibata, M.D.
Assistant Professor of Pathology, University of Southern California School of Medicine, Los Angeles, California

MISMATCHED SPECIMENS

MIX-UPS WILL OCCUR

Despite all precautions, errors in the labeling of specimens can and do occur (Murphy's law). Once a specimen is removed from a patient, proper identification depends on its association with the correct identifying label. Inevitably, the processing of many specimens in relatively short periods of time and in close proximity with each other can lead to the disjunction between a tissue and its proper label. Errors may occur anywhere from patient identification, the operating suite, to the final labeling of microscopic slides.

Recognition of a mislabeled specimen may be immediate. For example, the loss or detachment of a label or labels from specimens may be distressingly apparent, or the tissue type may not match its description. In other instances, a mismatch may be subtle and escape recognition. In many cases, mismatches do not have immediate clinical implications since the diagnosis remains unchanged. For example, an exchange between two benign biopsy specimens has little consequence.

One major problem is the incorrect association of malignant tissue to a patient without cancer. Mislabeling may be suspected when cancer is diagnosed in a patient unlikely to have a malignancy. However, for many types of cancer, long-term survival depends on the early diagnosis and removal of in situ lesions. The emphasis on early diagnosis and higher cure rates has led to the biopsy and treatment of patients with minimal signs or symptoms of cancer. The high accuracy and tremendous faith placed by medicine on histologic diagnosis makes it difficult to ignore any tissue evidence of malignancy. The failure to obtain further malignant tissue by additional biopsies may not resolve the issue since it may be difficult to relocate occult lesions. Inappropriate actions, either the failure to act if early cancer is present or treatment if cancer is absent, are highly undesirable consequences.

Advances in Pathology and Laboratory Medicine®, vol. 8
© 1995, Mosby–Year Book, Inc.

IMMUNOHISTOCHEMICAL ANALYSIS

Once a mismatch is suspected, there are few objective criteria to correctly assign a tissue to its proper patient. Immunohistochemical detection of the major blood group antigens (A, B, O) is possible.[1] However, these antigens may not be properly expressed in tumor tissues[2, 3] and the small number of blood types reduces their ability to discriminate between individuals.

DNA ANALYSIS

Another general strategy to distinguish between individuals is by their DNA "type." There are approximately 3 billion base pairs in the human genome. Although most DNA sequences are identical between individuals, it is generally estimated that about 1 out of every 200 bases is different. Because of the large number of potential differences between individuals, anyone can be potentially uniquely identified if enough DNA sequences are analyzed.

The most common and powerful method of DNA typing is called the DNA "fingerprint." This test analyzes repetitive DNA sequences called variable numbers of tandem repeats separated on the basis of size with a Southern blot.[4] A typical fingerprint consists of 20 to 50 distinct bands. The large number of bands and their near random assortment of sizes results in DNA fingerprints that are virtually unique for every individual. Unfortunately, this fingerprint analysis requires relatively intact, high-molecular-weight DNA and generally cannot be performed on fixed tissues.

Most human tissue specimens are immediately fixed in formalin and paraffin-embedded. Although high-molecular-weight DNA can be extracted from fixed tissues,[5] the DNA is usually degraded into small fragments.[6] Therefore, analysis is generally limited to assays based on polymerase chain reaction (PCR). Polymerase chain reaction assays typically replicate only small DNA fragments and can therefore provide genetic analysis of extremely degraded or poorly handled specimens. When compared with some of the unusual specimens successfully analyzed by PCR[7] such as ancient mummies, old blood stains, insects in amber, and the unfortunate 5,000-year-old "ice man" frozen in the Alps,[8] the DNA in

TABLE 1.

Polymerase Chain Reaction and Fixed Tissues

Treatment	Outcome	
	Good	**Poor**
Fixative	10% buffered formalin	B5
	Ethanol	Bouin's
	OmniFix	Zenker's
Fixation time	<2 days	>1 wk
PCR target size	<180 base pairs	>300 base pairs

formalin-fixed, paraffin-embedded tissue is relatively and uniformly well preserved. Factors affecting the PCR analysis of formalin-fixed tissues are presented in Table 1.

EXTRACTION OF DNA FROM CLINICAL SPECIMENS

Rapid and simple DNA extraction methods are essential for clinical analysis. Because PCR can analyze very small amounts of DNA, relatively crude DNA preparations can be used since potential inhibitors can be diluted to levels nontoxic to the PCR. The ability of PCR to amplify very small amounts of DNA to easily detectable levels allows the analysis of very small tissue fragments such as tissue or needle biopsy specimens, or "floaters." Indeed, a single sperm can be genetically analyzed.[9] Typically, a fragment of the fixed tissue is placed into a microfuge tube, deparaffinized, and then extracted overnight with a tris(hydroxymethyl)aminomethane (TRIS) HCl–ethylenediaminetetraacetic acid (EDTA)–proteinase K solution.[10] Table 2 describes some of the clinical specimens that can be typed.

POLYMERASE CHAIN REACTION–BASED DNA TYPING

HLA-DQα LOCUS

Background

The HLA-DQα locus is located on chromosome 6 and consists of multiple alleles. Currently 6 alleles can be typed by an available commercial kit. The HLA locus is highly polymorphic and demonstrates mendelian inheritance, and traditional antigen-based assays have been used to distinguish between individuals. The basis for the polymorphisms are HLA alleles that differ in their DNA sequences.[11, 12] These differences are presented in Figure 1. The 6 alleles (1.1, 1.2, 1.3, 2, 3, and 4) differ from each other by 1 to 17 bases. These different alleles can be readily distin-

---

TABLE 2.

Type of Clinical Specimens Appropriate for Polymerase Chain Reaction Assay

Specimen Type	Comments
Blood	Can be stored and sent at room temperature
EDTA* lavender tubes	Only a drop is needed for analysis
Blood spots	
Paraffin blocks	Typically a single 4- to 10-μm slice is analyzed
Autopsy	
Surgical	
Biopsy	
Microscope slides	Analysis destroys the tissue
Stained	Removal of the coverslip can take several days in
Unstained	xylene

*EDTA = ethylenediaminetetraacetic acid.

ALLELE

1.1 <u>GGAGATGAGGAGTTCTACG</u>TGGA<u>CCTGGAGAGGAAGGAGAC</u>TGCCTGGCGGTGGCC<u>TGAGTTCAGCAAATTTGGAGG</u>TTTTGAC

	1.1 probe	**all but 1.3 probe**					**1 probe**	
1.2	`........C..........`							
	1.2, 1.3,4 probe							
1.3	C	`.......A.........`						
		1.3 probe						
2	C	T		T	AA	T	CT	<u>CA .G .C . .xxxA.A</u>
								2 probe
3	C	T		T	A	T	CT	<u>C. .G . . . .A . A.A</u>
								3 probe
4	C		G	T	<u>T. T. T. . . .TTC. . . .AC</u>			xxxA A
						4 probe		

FIGURE 1.

The sequence of the HLA-DQα 1.1 allele is presented. Differences between the six alleles are designated by the bases below the 1.1 sequence. The allele-specific probes used to detect these differences are presented for each allele and are immobilized on filter hybridization strips (see Fig 2). The HLA-DQα "4" allele actually represents three alleles that are all typed as "4" by the "4 probe."

guished since DNA probes (Fig 1) can be designed to specifically hybridize to sequences that differ by as little as a single base. Everyone has 2 HLA-DQα alleles (1 inherited from each parent), and therefore 21 combinations are possible from the 6 alleles.

HLA-DQα Typing With the AmpliType PCR Kit

A kit (AmpliType) that analyzes the six HLA-DQα alleles is available from Perkin-Elmer (Norwalk, Conn). This kit, originally intended for forensic use,[11, 13–15] incorporates many features that are ideal for a clinical laboratory. These features include a short turnaround time (1 to 3 days), nonisotopic detection (using a biotin, strepavidin–horseradish peroxidase system), stable reagents, and relatively easy interpretation of the final results. The AmpliType kit was originally introduced in 1989 by the now defunct Cetus corporation and is still only one of the few commercially available assays based on polymerase chain reaction.

The assay requires the mixing of just two solutions ($MgCl_2$ and the reagent mix) with the DNA specimen. The PCR primers are biotin labeled. Amplification for 32 to 37 cycles occurs over a period of 2 to 3 hours. The final PCR products are denatured into single strands at 95° C and then hybridized to allele-specific probes that are immobilized on filter strips provided in the kit. After a high-stringency wash, the specifically hybridized PCR products are detected as a blue precipitate (tetramethylbenzidine) produced by the horseradish peroxidase attached to the PCR product (Fig 2). The hybridization and detection steps require approximately 2 hours.

The primary technical disadvantage to the AmpliType kit is the use of a relatively large, 242–base pair HLA-DQα PCR target. A shorter PCR target (<200 bases) would be optimal for analysis of the degraded DNA present in most fixed specimens. However, this HLA assay is very efficient, and in my experience, greater than 90% of formalin-fixed specimens can be successfully analyzed.[16–19]

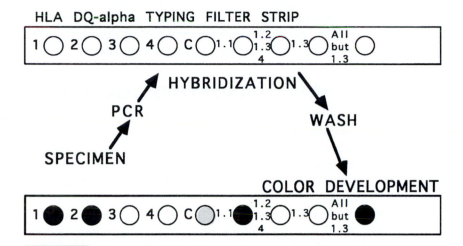

FIGURE 2.

Flow diagram for the HLA typing of a specimen with the AmpliType kit. Hybridized biotin-labeled polymerase chain reaction products complementary to HLA allele–specific probes (see Fig 1) immobilized on the provided filter strip are visualized as blue dots *(shaded)*. The patterns of the dots determines the HLA-DQα type, in this example 1.1, 2. The "C" dot represents a positive control that should always be visualized and be weaker than the dots representing the specific HLA alleles.

HLA-DQα Allelic Frequencies

The ability of the AmpliType kit to distinguish between individuals depends on the relative frequencies of the alleles in the population. The frequencies of the alleles has been empirically determined through surveys of different populations and varies between races.[11, 12] The frequencies of each allelic combination are not equal but vary between 0% and 29%, with the average being less than 10%. Therefore, more than 90% of the time two different individuals may be distinguished from each other by this test.

INCREASING THE ABILITY TO DISCRIMINATE BETWEEN INDIVIDUALS

The typing of additional DNA loci and their polymorphisms can increase the ability to discriminate between individuals. Perkin-Elmer offers another kit (AmpliType PolyMarker) similar to the HLA-DQα AmpliType kit that allows the analysis of five additional loci (three alleles of low-density lipoprotein receptor, three alleles of glycophorin A, six alleles of hemoglobin Gγ, three alleles of D7S8, and six alleles of group-specific component). Numerous other polymorphic loci can be used to further increase the ability to distinguish between individuals.

Simple repeat sequences or microsatellites are commonly used to distinguish between individuals since they are highly polymorphic in size and easily measured by PCR assays. These repetitive sequences should not be used to identify tumor tissues because in some tumors with a "mutater" phenotype,[20–22] most of these repetitive sequences differ in size between their germline sequences. Therefore microsatellite assays may yield "false" mismatches. This tumor-associated phenomenon has been observed in families with hereditary nonpolyposis colorectal cancer and sporadic colorectal, endometrial, and gastric cancers.

THEORETICAL CHANGES IN GENOTYPE ASSOCIATED WITH TUMOR TISSUES

Cancer is associated with genotypic changes responsible for the transformation of a benign cell. Typically these changes occur in tumor suppressor genes and oncogenes. Mutations in the HLA-DQα locus may rarely occur and can lead to a discordance of the HLA type between the tumor and the genotype of the individual with the tumor. This theoretical tumor-associated mutational conversion at the HLA locus leading to a "false"-negative match between tumor and normal tissue has not yet been observed. HLA antigen expression is altered in many tumors[23, 24] but generally involves class I antigens (A, B, C) because class II (D) antigens are generally not expressed on epithelial tissues or their tumors. Selective, mutational pressures on HLA-D antigens may more commonly occur in tumors (such as lymphomas, leukemias, or some melanomas[25]) that express these antigens.

In addition, many tumors demonstrate partial or total chromosomal losses, which may include the HLA locus on chromosome 6. A clonal, tumor-specific loss of one HLA allele may lead to a reduction to homozygosity and an apparent "change" in the HLA type. Fortunately, most tumors are contaminated with normal stroma cells, which should retain both HLA-DQα alleles and their germline sequences and therefore mitigate against tumor-specific HLA changes. These rare confounding possibilities must always be considered when analyzing tumor tissue.

EXAMPLES

STRATEGY OF THE APPROACH

When a mismatch is suspected, the strategy is to "round up the usual suspects" and determine and compare their DNA types. At a minimum, the suspected mismatch or unlabeled specimen and the patient in question should be typed. Ideally, all possible sources of the mismatched specimen should also be typed in order to determine the likely source of the unlabeled tissue. This strategy is outlined in Figure 3. The DNA source from a patient may be a blood specimen or, more conveniently or discretely, a tissue block known to be from a given patient.

If the DNA types differ between the "unknown" tissue and a patient, then that tissue cannot have come from that patient. If the DNA types are the same between the "unknown" and a patient, two possibilities exist. First, the unknown tissue came from the patient. Second, the unknown tissue did not come from the patient, but rather from another patient who by chance has the same DNA type. The chance of this second possibility depends on the frequency of the HLA type in the specific racial group and is typically less than 10%. The typing of all additional suspects can effectively eliminate some of the ambiguities when DNA types match.

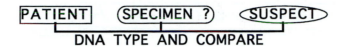

DNA TYPE AND COMPARE

SPECIMEN DOES NOT MATCH WITH PATIENT

- SPECIMEN IS NOT FROM PATIENT

SUSPECT LIKELY SOURCE
OF SPECIMEN

SUSPECT NOT SOURCE
OF SPECIMEN

-DIFFERENT SOURCE OF SPECIMEN
-POSSIBLE TUMOR SPECIFIC HLA CONVERSION

SPECIMEN MATCHES WITH PATIENT

-SPECIMEN IS FROM PATIENT OR FROM ANOTHER
PATIENT WITH THE SAME DNA TYPE

SUPPORTS CONCLUSION
THAT SPECIMEN IS
FROM PATIENT

NO CONCLUSION IS
POSSIBLE AS ALL
TYPES MATCH

FIGURE 3.
Strategy of the approach. At a minimum, the HLA type of the unknown specimen must be compared with that of the patient. If possible, suspected alternative
sources of the specimen should also be examined.

SPECIFIC EXAMPLES

The following are some of the cases examined by this method. Some of
the details have been altered to protect the innocent or highlight important aspects of this method.

The "Floater"

A series of open breast biopsies were performed. One patient suspected
of cancer had a poorly differentiated adenocarcinoma (A). However, a
much younger patient had primarily fibrocystic changes (B) except for one
fragment of tissue (2 × 2 mm) with carcinoma (C). A "floater" was suspected, but the pathologist could not confidently eliminate the possibility that the patient had cancer.

From the stained slide, the suspected "floater" (C) was microdissected
from the fibrocystic breast tissue (B). A single slice of the carcinoma (A)
was obtained from a paraffin block. All three tissues were typed (Fig 4).
The HLA type matched between the suspected "floater" (C) and the carcinoma (A) but was different between the "floater" and the fibrocystic

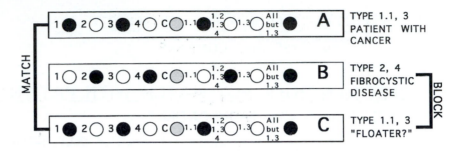

FIGURE 4.

The HLA type *(1.1, 3)* of the tumor fragment *(C)* matches with its suspected source *(A)* and not with the patient's tissue *(B)* within the same block *(2, 4)*. The tumor tissue is indeed a "floater."

breast (B). Therefore, the suspected "floater" was indeed a floater and there was no evidence that the younger women had any malignancy.

The Absentminded Surgeon

On a busy day, three hysterectomy specimens were received and processed. Afterward, an angry surgeon confronted the pathologist about his report stating that one of his hysterectomy specimens included one ovary. The surgeon insisted that he had not removed an ovary and that the pathologist had made a mistake.

Single slices from the paraffin blocks of the ovary in question (A), the uterus (B) and blood (C) of the patient, and all other uteri removed that day (D, E) were examined (Fig 5). The DNA type of the ovary (A) in question matched its uterus (B) and the patient's blood (C) but differed

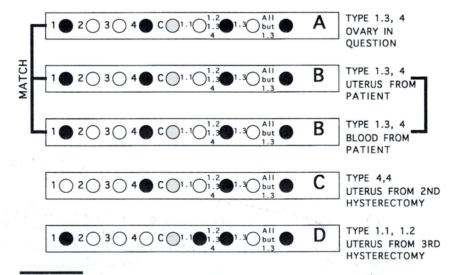

FIGURE 5.

The ovary in question *(A)* has the HLA type 1.3, 4. Comparisons between the patient's blood and other uteri removed on the same day reveals that this ovary *(A)* could have only come from the patient because its HLA type does not match the other potential hysterectomy sources.

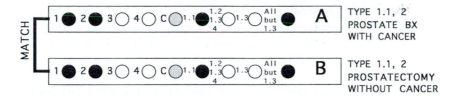

FIGURE 6.

The match between the prostate biopsy with cancer (A) and its associated prostatectomy without cancer (B) provides objective evidence that a mix-up did not occur.

from the DNA types of the other uteri (D, E). Therefore the ovary in question was most likely removed from the patient at the time of the hysterectomy. The bill was sent to the surgeon.

The Occult Tumor

A prostate needle biopsy specimen revealed unequivocal adenocarcinoma. A prostatectomy was performed. Despite cutting into the entire specimen and examining several levels, no evidence of adenocarcinoma was found. The question of a mix-up arose.

A single slice from the paraffin block of the prostate needle biopsy with adenocarcinoma (A) and from the prostatectomy specimen (B) were examined (Fig 6). The HLA types matched between the biopsy and the prostatectomy. This DNA analysis was accepted as evidence that a mix-up had not occurred.

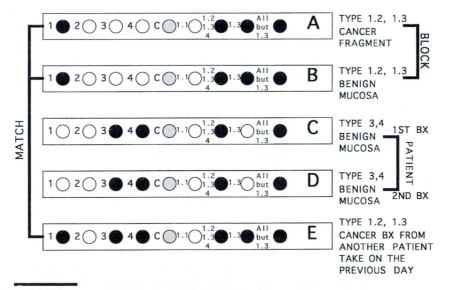

FIGURE 7.

The same HLA type was observed in both the tumor (A) and normal (B) tissue in the gastric biopsy block. This HLA type did not match the other biopsy tissues obtained at the same time (C) or at a subsequent time (D). In this case, the tumor fragment (A) is not a "floater," but rather the entire block was mislabeled. The likely source was a patient with cancer (E) who underwent biopsy on the previous day.

The Dirty Endoscope?

One day, several patients received multiple gastric biopsies. In only one relatively asymptomatic patient was carcinoma detected. Repeat biopsy failed to reveal further tissue evidence of adenocarcinoma. A mix-up was suspected.

The stained slide with the carcinoma fragment (A) was microdissected from the surrounding normal gastric mucosa (B). Single slices of normal biopsy specimens from other gastric sites taken on the day of the original biopsy (C) and subsequent biopsy (D) were analyzed (Fig 7). The DNA type of the carcinoma (A) and its surrounding normal tissue (B) matched each other. The DNA type of the other specimens (C, D) matched each other but did not match with the cancer or its surrounding tissue (A, B). It was concluded that the entire block was mislabeled and that the cancer did not come from the patient. Comparison with a gastric tumor biopsy specimen (E) taken the day before the biopsy in question revealed a match. Therefore it is likely that the tumor tissue was a carryover from the previous day. The exact mechanism of the mix-up was not determined.

CONCLUSIONS

DNA typing of fixed specimens by using PCR and appropriate polymorphisms provides objective evidence of tissue origins. The majority (>90%) of fixed specimens can be analyzed,[18] and the findings usually favor the pathologist. The relatively small number of patients who are potential sources of a mismatched specimen typically allows a definitive analysis. This application of DNA analysis represents translation of molecular biology to a critical clinical question that cannot be resolved by traditional techniques. Of note, pathologists are essential in the application of this DNA technology since they must identify when the test is needed and the tissues appropriate for analysis.

The translation of advances in molecular biology to clinical practice can be impaired at many steps. Any requirement for specially processed tissue will prevent or at least delay analysis on the majority of patients. The successful experience with DNA typing and other DNA-based assays performed on routinely obtained specimens throughout the United States suggests that many molecular tests based on PCR can be immediately applied.

Therefore the stage is set for the application of a molecular test in the clinical setting. Advances in molecular biology have provided a wealth of information, much of which has had only limited value for routine clinical diagnosis. Undoubtedly, some advances will be translated into valuable clinical information. Research involves questions and provides answers appropriate for the understanding of the pathogenesis of disease. Since pathologists understand the outstanding questions and limitations of their art better than anyone else, one of their future roles will be the recognition, selection, and translation of molecular advances into clinically relevant information.

REFERENCES

1. Ota M, Fukushima H, Akamatsu T, et al: Availability of immunostaining methods for identification of mix-up tissue specimens. *Am J Clin Pathol* 92:665–669, 1989.
2. Wolf GT, Carey TE: Tumor antigen phenotype, biologic staging, and prognosis in head and neck squamous cell carcinoma. *J Natl Cancer Inst Monogr* 13:67–74, 1992.
3. Matsumoto H, Muramatsu H, Shimotakahara T, et al: Correlation of expression of the ABH blood group carbohydrate antigens with metastatic potential in human lung carcinomas. *Cancer* 72:75–81, 1993.
4. Gill P, Jeffreys AJ, Werrett DJ: Forensic applications of DNA "fingerprints." *Nature* 318:577–579, 1985.
5. Dubeau L, Chandler LA, Gralow JR, et al: Southern blot analysis of DNA extracted from formalin-fixed pathology specimens. *Cancer Res* 46:2964–2969, 1986.
6. Greer CE, Peterson SL, Kiviat NB, et al: PCR amplification from paraffin-embedded tissues. *Am J Clin Pathol* 95:117–124, 1991.
7. Paabo S: Ancient DNA: Extraction, characterization, molecular cloning, and enzymatic amplification. *Proc Natl Acad Sci U S A* 86:1939–1943, 1989.
8. Handt O, Richards M, Trommsdorff M, et al: Molecular genetic analysis of the Tyrolean ice man. *Science* 264:1775–1778, 1994.
9. Li H, Gyllensten UB, Cui X, et al: Amplification and analysis of DNA sequences in single human sperm and diploid cells. *Nature* 355:414–417, 1988.
10. Shibata D: The polymerase chain reaction and the molecular genetic analysis of tissue biopsies, in Herrington CS, McGee JOD (eds): *Diagnostic Molecular Pathology: A Practical Approach*, vol 2. Oxford, England, IRL Press, 1992, pp 85–111.
11. *AmpliType Users Guide*, version 2. Emeryville, Calif, Cetus Corp, 1990.
12. Helmuth R, Fildes N, Blake E, et al: HLA DQa allele and genotype frequencies in various human populations, determined using enzymatic amplification and oligonucleotide probes. *Am J Hum Genet* 47:515–523, 1990.
13. Walsh PS, Fildes N, Louie AS, et al: Report of the blind trial of the Cetus AmpliType HLA DQa forensic deoxyribonucleic acid (DNA) amplification and typing kit. *J Forensic Sci* 36:1551–1556, 1991.
14. Blake E, Crim D, Mihalovich J, et al: Polymerase chain reaction (PCR) amplification and human leukocyte antigen (HLA)-DQa oligonucleotide typing on biological evidence samples: Casework experience. *J Forensic Sci* 37:700–726, 1992.
15. Saiki RK, Walsh PS, Levenson CH, et al: Genetic analysis of amplified DNA with immobilized sequence-specific oligonucleotide probes. *Proc Natl Acad Sci U S A* 86:6230–6234, 1989.
16. Shibata D, Namiki T, Higuchi R: Identification of a mis-labeled fixed specimen by DNA analysis. *Am J Surg Pathol* 14:1076–1078, 1990.
17. Shibata D, Kurosu M, Noguchi TT: Fixed human tissues: A resource for the identification of individuals. *J Forensic Sci* 36:1204–1212, 1991.
18. Shibata D: Identification of mismatched fixed specimens with a commercially available kit based on the polymerase chain reaction. *Am J Clin Pathol* 100:666–670, 1993.
19. Howard PL, Collins CC, Heintz NH: Polymerase chain reaction and allele-specific oligonucleotides in paternity testing of the deceased. *Transfusion* 31:441–442, 1991.
20. Ionov Y, Peinado MA, Malkhosyan S, et al: Ubiquitous somatic mutations in

simple repeat sequences reveals a new mechanism for colorectal carcinogenesis. *Nature* 363:558−561, 1993.

21. Aaltonen LA, Peltomaki P, Leach FS, et al: Clues to the pathogenesis of familial colorectal cancer. *Science* 260:812−815, 1993.

22. Thibodeau SN, Bren G, Schaid D: Microsatellite instability in cancer of the proximal colon. *Science* 260:816−819, 1993.

23. Tanaka K, Yoshioka T, Bieberich C, et al: Role of the major histocompatibility complex class I antigens in tumor growth and metastasis. *Annu Rev Immunol* 6:359−380, 1988.

24. Smith MEF, Marsh SGE, Bodmer JG, et al: Loss of HLA-A,B,C allele products and lymphocyte function-associated antigen 3 in colorectal neoplasia. *Proc Natl Acad Sci U S A* 86:5557−5561, 1989.

25. Natali P, Bigotti A, Cavaliere R: HLA class II antigens synthesized by melanoma cells. *Cancer Rev* 9:1−33, 1987.

The Antiphospholipid Thrombosis Syndromes: Lupus Anticoagulants and Anticardiolipin Antibodies

Rodger L. Bick, M.D.
Clinical Professor of Medicine and Pathology, University of Texas Southwestern Medical Center, and Medical Director of Hematology and Oncology, Presbyterian Comprehensive Cancer Center, Presbyterian Hospital of Dallas, Dallas, Texas

M any clinical conditions, including surgery, fractures, trauma, burns, immobility, nephrotic syndrome, malignancy, pregnancy, and many more, are associated with the development of pathologic thrombosis, often manifested as deep vein thrombosis (DVT). In 1845 Virchow recognized three major factors playing a role in thrombus formation: (1) changes in blood flow, (2) changes in the vessel wall, and (3) changes in the circulating blood.[1] Patients recognized to be at increased risk for thrombosis have loosely been termed as having a hypercoagulable state. Many blood protein and platelet defects are now known to account for hypercoagulability and thrombosis; congenital defects of blood proteins leading to thrombosis such as antithrombin, protein C and protein S, activated protein C cofactor/resistance, heparin cofactor II, plasminogen deficiency, dysfibrinogenemia, and others are generally termed the "congenital thrombophilias." Acquired blood protein defects are also associated with thrombosis, including acquired defects of protein C, protein S, or antithrombin. Acquired blood protein defects leading to thrombosis are much more common than the congenital forms. Antiphospholipid antibodies, which include the lupus anticoagulant (LA) and anticardiolipin antibodies, both of which are involved in the "antiphospholipid thrombosis (APL-T) syndrome," are also common acquired blood protein defects associated with thrombosis and are the most common of the acquired blood protein defects associated with both venous and arterial thrombosis.[2]

The APL-T syndrome consists of two closely related but distinct clinical syndromes: (1) the lupus anticoagulant thrombosis (LAT) syndrome and (2) the anticardiolipin antibody thrombosis (ACLAT) syndrome. Although the two are similar, there are distinct clinical, laboratory, and biochemical differences, especially regarding the prevalence, etiology, possible mechanisms of thrombosis,[3] clinical findings, diagnosis, and management. The ACLAT antiphospholipid syndrome is much more common

Advances in Pathology and Laboratory Medicine®, vol. 8
© 1995, Mosby–Year Book, Inc.

than the LAT antiphospholipid syndrome, the ratio being about 5 to 1.[4, 5] Both syndromes may be associated with arterial and venous thrombosis, fetal wastage, and thrombocytopenia in descending order of prevalence; however, the anticardiolipin syndrome is more commonly associated with both arterial and venous thrombosis, including typical DVT and pulmonary embolus, premature coronary artery disease, premature cerebrovascular disease, and retinal vascular disease. Lupus anticoagulant, although sometimes associated with arterial disease, is more commonly associated with venous thrombosis. Also, more predictable types of thrombosis develop in individuals with anticardiolipin syndrome than in those with LA, and management of thrombotic problems can be quite different between the two syndromes. Although both of these antiphospholipid syndromes can be seen in association with systemic lupus erythematosus (SLE), other connective tissue and autoimmune disorders, and other selected medical conditions such as lymphomas, the majority of individuals in whom either the ACLAT antiphospholipid syndrome or the LAT syndrome develops are otherwise healthy, harbor no other underlying medical condition, and are classified as having *primary* rather than *secondary* APL-T syndrome.[6] This distinction is of extreme importance because those with secondary antiphospholipid syndromes generally have heterogeneous antibodies that react with a variety of phospholipid moieties, including anticardiolipin and LA reagents, and render biological false-positive tests for syphilis, whereas those with primary antiphospholipid syndrome generally have homogeneous antibodies reacting with only one particular phospholipid moiety.[6] Thus when evaluating published studies, one must carefully scrutinize the population being studied for antiphospholipid antibodies. Studies of patients with autoimmune disorders may not necessarily be extrapolated to studies or clinical and laboratory findings in patients with primary antiphospholipid syndrome. Both of these antiphospholipid syndromes, including etiology, pathophysiology, clinical and laboratory diagnosis, and management principles, are herein discussed.

LUPUS ANTICOAGULANTS AND THROMBOSIS

Conley and Hartmann[7] in 1952 described a coagulation disorder in two patients with SLE. The patients exhibited anticoagulant activity by in vitro testing as manifested by a prolonged whole blood clotting time and prothrombin time.[7] It is now known that in patients with systemic lupus or other autoimmune diseases, an immunoglobulin may develop that has the ability to prolong phospholipid-dependent coagulation tests.[8, 9] About 10% of patients with systemic lupus harbor an LA; however, the LA is commonly seen in other conditions as well, including malignancy, lymphoproliferative disorders, and viral infections, especially human immunodeficiency virus (HIV) infection.[10–12] Most commonly the LA develops in otherwise healthy individuals (primary LAT syndrome). There is also an association with drug ingestion; commonly associated drugs include chlorpromazine, procainamide, quinidine, hydralazine, phenytoin (Dilantin), interferon, cocaine, and Fansidar.[4, 5, 13–15] A common misconception is that patients with drug-induced LA do not suffer thrombosis, but in fact these patients also have an increased risk of thrombotic disease. Most, but not all drug-induced antiphospholipid antibodies are of the IgM idiotype. The frequency of hemorrhage resulting from LAs is clearly less than 1%; however, it is important to recognize conditions that may predispose lupus patients harboring an LA to hemorrhage.[16, 17] Twenty-five percent of patients with systemic lupus have concomitant prothrombin deficiency, and more than 40% may have thrombocytopenia.[16, 18]

Of greater clinical significance, patients with LAs have an increased risk for thromboembolic disease, most commonly DVT, pulmonary emboli, and thrombosis of other large vessels.[19, 20] Thromboembolism occurs in about 10% of patients with systemic lupus; however, in patients with systemic lupus and LA, thromboembolism occurs in up to 50% of patients. Lupus anticoagulant is estimated to account for 6% to 8% of cases of thrombosis in otherwise healthy individuals. There have also been associations with recurrent fetal wastage, neuropsychiatric disorders, renal vascular thrombosis, thrombosis of dermal vessels, and thrombocytopenia.[15, 18, 21–23]

Primary LAT syndrome is much more common than the secondary type and consists of patients with LA and thrombosis who harbor no other underlying disease; secondary LAT syndrome consists of those patients with LA, thrombosis, and an underlying disease such as lupus or other autoimmune disorders, malignancy, infection, inflammation, or ingestion of drugs inducing LA.

Patients with primary LAT antiphospholipid syndrome primarily suffer venous thrombosis and pulmonary emboli. A wide variety of venous systems may be involved, including the extremities (most common finding) and the mesenteric, renal, hepatic, and portal veins and the vena cava.[6, 10] Although patients can also suffer arterial events, this is uncommon in primary LAT syndrome, as opposed to primary ACLAT syndrome, where arterial events are almost as common as venous events. This is in distinction to patients with secondary LAT syndrome, wherein patients may more commonly suffer arterial events than those with primary LAT syndrome. However, even in those with secondary LAT syndrome, the venous events are more common than arterial events. The arteries involved include the coronary, cerebral, carotid, aorta, mesenteric, and renal arteries and the extremities.[6, 10, 22, 24 26]

Purified LA inhibits the CA^{2+}-dependent binding of prothrombin and factor Xa to phospholipids, thereby inhibiting the activity of the phospholipid complex required for the conversion of prothrombin to thrombin.[9, 16] Of interest, biological false-positive tests for syphilis are seen in up to 40% of patients with systemic lupus; the number increases to 90% in patients with systemic lupus plus LA.[17, 22, 27] An abnormality often (theoretically) exists in the phospholipid-dependent coagulation reactions, including the prothrombin time, the activated partial thromboplastin time (aPTT), and Russell's viper venom time. The LA is not directed against a specific factor, but to phospholipids. The inhibitor does not exert an increasing effect upon prolonged incubation with normal plasma, and thus this simple screen can be used to distinguish the lupus inhibitor from inhibitors that neutralize specific clotting factors. Incubation of the patients' plasma with normal plasma does not cause a sensitivity of the PTT to the inhibitor's effect; one-stage assays for factors XII, XI, IX, and VII may yield low values when standard dilutions of test plasma are used. Usually further dilution of the test plasma causes the measured level of these factors to approach the normal range; an exception occurs in rare patients with a decreased concentration of prothrombin resulting from accelerated removal of prothrombin antigen-antibody complexes.[28, 29]

Multiple LA assays are currently in use.[28, 30-34] When the presence of an LA is suspected, a more definitive test, preferably the dilute Russell's viper venom time (dRVVT), should be immediately performed regardless of the PTT; detection of LA is discussed in later sections.[4, 5, 30, 31]

There is a correlation between elevated anticardiolipin antibodies and LA, especially in secondary antiphospholipid syndromes; however, the LA and anticardiolipin antibodies are two separate entities, and most of the time one occurs without the other being present, especially in the primary APL-T syndromes.[16, 35] Lupus anticoagulant has a stronger association with binding phospholipids of a hexagonal composition, such as phosphatidylcholine, or after membrane damage by infection, interleukin-1 (IL-1), or other mechanisms leading to a change from the lamellar to hexagonal form, whereas anticardiolipin antibodies have an affinity to lamellar phospholipids in a bilayer (lamellar) composition.[9, 36, 37] IgG and IgM are the most frequent idiotypes and can be detected by enzyme-linked immunosorbent assay (ELISA); IgA anticardiolipin antibodies occur slightly less frequently and are also detected by ELISA. Although LA is associated with thrombosis, the mechanism(s) whereby thrombosis occurs remains unclear. It has been proposed that there might be an interaction with the vasculature, thereby altering prostaglandin release. There may be activation of platelets and changes in prostaglandin metabolism, or the antibodies block protein C or alter phospholipid interactions with activated factor V.[38] It has also been proposed that there may be hyperactivity of the fibrinolytic system and increased levels of plasminogen activation inhibitor.[39] To date there remains no consensus on the mechanism(s) of action of LA, but many have been proposed.[4, 5, 40, 41]

Subclassification of the types of thrombosis in patients with LA and anticardiolipin antibody is important for therapy.[4, 5, 35] Patients can generally be divided into one of six subgroups. Type I syndrome includes DVT of the upper and lower extremities, inferior vena cava, and hepatic, portal, and renal veins, as well as pulmonary embolus. Type II syndrome includes patients with arterial thrombosis, including the coronary arteries, peripheral (extremity) arteries, and aorta. Type III syndrome includes patients with retinal or cerebral vascular thrombosis. Several neurologic syndromes may be seen, including transient cerebral ischemic attacks, migraine headaches, and optic neuritis.[23] Type IV syndrome includes patients with combinations of the aforementioned types of thrombosis. Like anticardiolipin antibodies, LA has been associated with a recurrent fetal wastage syndrome (FWS); this is type V. Abortion occurs frequently in the first, second, or third trimester. Placental vasculitis and vascular thrombosis may be apparent, and there may be an associated maternal thrombocytopenia.[2, 17, 42] Type VI patients are those harboring LA with no apparent disease.

Although patients with LAT syndrome can be classified similar to those with ACLAT syndrome, almost all patients with *primary* LAT syndrome will fit into type I. In secondary LAT syndrome, however, there will be more patients falling into types II and III than is seen in the primary syndrome.

The lupus inhibitor usually persists in patients with primary APL-T syndrome, although it may sometimes disappear spontaneously. In the secondary LAT antiphospholipid syndrome, treatment of the underlying autoimmune disorder frequently results in a reduction or disappearance of inhibitor activity. Corticosteroids may have a suppressive effect on LA and to a lesser degree on anticardiolipin antibodies, but they do not appear to decrease thrombotic risk. Thus there is no role for immunosuppressive therapy, including steroids, cyclophosphamide, or azathioprine, in patients with the primary LAT syndrome. When steroids or other immunosuppressive therapy is warranted in a patient with an autoimmune disease and LAT syndrome, the immunosuppression, while possibly benefiting the underlying autoimmune disorder, will generally not alleviate the propensity to thrombosis. Discovery of an LA in the absence of underlying disease and without evidence of thrombosis (type VI) does not necessarily require treatment, but current evidence suggests that these individuals may have about a 40% chance of eventually suffering thrombotic events. Thus the decision to anticoagulate an asymptomatic patient with LA requires individualization and judgment. However, patients with LA or anticardiolipin antibodies and a history of thrombosis need to be maintained on long-term anticoagulant therapy. If untreated, there is a high incidence of thromboembolic recurrence.[4, 5, 43, 44] Patients with DVT or arterial thrombosis are best managed with long-term subcutaneous porcine mucosal heparin therapy because they are notoriously resistant to warfarin therapy ($\approx$65% with type I eventually fail). In patients with retinal or cerebrovascular thrombosis, fixed low-dose warfarin (1 to 2 mg/day) plus low-dose aspirin (79 to 81 mg/day, intracranial/cerebral vessels) or pentoxiphylline (400 mg three times per day, retinal vessels) is my treatment of choice. In those with mixtures of thrombotic sites (type IV), therapy is individualized based on the predominant sites and the severity of thrombosis.[4, 5, 43] Recurrent FWS has been successfully treated and full-term delivery achieved with aspirin, low-dose heparin, intravenous immunoglobulin (IVIG), or plasma exchange; there is little role for prednisone in recurrent fetal wastage caused by LA if there is no underlying autoimmune disease.

ANTICARDIOLIPIN ANTIBODIES AND THROMBOSIS

Interest in antiphospholipids began with discovery of LA in about 10% of patients with systemic lupus in 1952,[7] and shortly thereafter it was recognized that the presence of LA was associated with thrombosis instead of bleeding.[45] It was also soon recognized that many patients without autoimmune disorders harbored LAs, and these antiphospholipid antibodies have now been reported in many conditions, including malignancy, immune thrombocytopenic purpura, leukemias, and infections; in individuals ingesting chlorpromazine, phenytoin (Dilantin), Fansidar, hydralazine, quinidine, cocaine, or procainamide (secondary APL-T syndrome); and in many otherwise normal individuals (primary APL-T syndrome).[29, 46-50] Because of a noted association between lupus, a biological false-positive test for syphilis, and the presence of LA, Harris and coworkers in 1983 devised a new test for antiphospholipids using cardiolipin.[51] This and subsequent modifications have now become known as the anticardiolipin antibody test; generally, IgG, IgA, and IgM anticardiolipin idiotypes are currently assessed.[52] Shortly after development of the anticardiolipin antibody assay, it became apparent that these antibodies were not limited to the lupus patient population, but were found in nonlupus patients as well. Of particular importance, these anticardiolipin antibodies are associated with (1) thrombosis and thromboembolus of both the arterial and venous systems,[6, 40, 53-55] (2) recurrent fetal loss,[42, 56, 57] and (3) thrombocytopenia.[58, 59] Although there is an association between LA and anticardiolipin antibodies and an association between LAs and the aforementioned syndromes, it has become clear that LA and anticardiolipin antibodies are two separate entities; most individuals with anticardiolipin antibodies do not have an LA, and most with LAs do not have anticardiolipin antibodies.[60] Also, regarding the primary APL-T syndrome, the ACLAT syndrome is at least fivefold more common than is the LAT syndrome.[4, 6] Other differences include not only differing clinical features, but also the finding that anticardiolipins are dependent on a cofactor, β_2-glycoprotein I (apolipoprotein H), in vitro, whereas in vitro LA activity appears independent of β_2-glycoprotein I, the two have markedly different isoelectric points on chromatofocusing separation, both appear to be directed against different combinations of phospholipid moieties and complexes, and purified anticardiolipin antibodies do not generally prolong any of the phospholipid-dependent coagulation tests such as the aPTT, dRVVT, phospholipid neutralization procedure (PNP), or kaolin clotting time (KCT) unless there is the concomitant presence of LA.[61, 62] Initially it was assumed that primarily IgG anticardiolipin antibody was associated with thrombosis; however, it is now clear that IgA and IgM anticardiolipin antibodies are also associated with thrombosis.[4, 5] The presence of any one anticardiolipin antibody, a combination of two, or indeed, all three together may be associated with thrombosis and thromboembolus.[63] Also, although different types of thrombosis occur, there is no apparent association between the type of thrombotic event and the type or titer of anticardiolipin antibody present.[4, 5] The mechanism of action of anticardiolipin antibodies in leading or contributing to thrombosis is unknown, but several plausible theories have been proposed. Anticardiolipin antibodies have affinity for important phospholipids involved at many points in the hemostasis system; they are directed primarily against phosphatidylserine and phosphatidylinositol, but not phosphatidylcholine, another important phospholipid in hemostasis.[64] The proposed mechanisms of action of anticardiolipin antibodies in interfering with hemostasis to induce thrombosis include (1) interference with endothelial release of prostacyclin[65]; (2) interference with activation, via thrombomodulin, of protein C or interference with protein S activity as a cofactor[66]; (3) interference with antithrombin activity[67]; (4) interaction with platelet membrane phospholipids leading to platelet activation[68]; (5) interference in prekallikrein activation to kallikrein[69]; or (6) interference with endothelial plasminogen activator release.[70] All these components of normal hemostasis are dependent on phospholipid, except possibly antithrombin activity. These concepts are reviewed elsewhere.[4, 6, 40, 41]

ANTICARDIOLIPINS AND VENOUS/ARTERIAL THROMBOSIS

Anticardiolipin antibodies are associated with many types of venous thrombotic problems, including DVT of the upper and lower extremities, pulmonary embolus, and thrombosis of the intracranial veins, inferior vena cava, hepatic vein (Budd-Chiari syndrome),[4, 5, 71] portal vein, renal vein, and retinal veins.[72–74] Arterial thrombotic sites associated with anticardiolipin antibodies have included the coronary arteries, carotid arteries, cerebral arteries, retinal arteries, subclavian and/or axillary artery (aortic arch syndrome),[75] brachial arteries, mesenteric arteries,[76] peripheral (extremity) arteries, and both the proximal and distal ends of the aorta.[77–79]

ANTICARDIOLIPINS AND CARDIAC DISEASE

In a recent study it was found that 33% of coronary artery bypass graft (CABG) patients suffering late graft occlusion (as determined by coronary angiography 12 months after CABG surgery) had preoperative anticardiolipin antibody levels over 2 SD above control values, strongly suggesting an association between graft occlusion and antiphospholipid antibodies. In 80% of the patients the anticardiolipin antibody levels rose to levels greater than the preoperative levels at some point in time. The observed increase in anticardiolipin antibody levels was greater in patients who had suffered an acute myocardial infarction than in those who had not.[80, 81] Another study has revealed that over 20% of young (less than 45 years of age) survivors of acute myocardial infarction harbor anticardiolipin antibodies; in those surviving, 61% having these antibodies experienced a later thromboembolic event. No association was found between the presence of anticardiolipin antibodies and antinuclear antibody or other clinical features that would have suggested the presence of SLE. Anticardiolipin antibodies are suggested as an indicator of increased risk for post–myocardial infarction thrombotic events and an indication for prophylactic anticoagulation or antiplatelet therapy.[82] In spite of continuous prophylactic treatment with aspirin and warfarin, acute myocardial infarction has been documented in a patient with previously documented normal coronary arteries but was treated successfully with tissue plasminogen activator.[83] In analyzing the relative frequency of acute myocardial infarction in patients with anticardiolipin antibodies, a study published in 1989 noted myocardial infarction in only 5 of 70 patients (significantly fewer than those experiencing cerebral arterial thromboses).[84] Recent studies have revealed that a very high percentage of young individuals (those under 50 years of age) who suffer acute myocardial infarction or who experience restenosis after percutaneous transluminal coronary angioplasty (PTCA) or CABG harbor anticardiolipin antibodies. Thus anticardiolipin antibodies appear to play a significant, if not major role in premature/precocious coronary artery disease.[26, 85]

Anticardiolipin antibodies are also associated with cardiac valvular abnormalities. Cardiac disease in patients with SLE has been associated with the findings of valvular vegetations, regurgitation, and stenosis. Eighty-nine percent of patients with SLE and valvular disease have been found to have antiphospholipid antibodies as compared with only 44% of patients without valvular involvement. Although only 18% of all patients with lupus have valvular disease, cardiac valvular abnormalities are found in 36% of patients with the primary antiphospholipid syndrome. The valvular abnormalities of the primary antiphospholipid syndrome are characterized by significant, irregular thickening of the mitral and aortic valves, valvular regurgitation (but not stenosis), the potential for severe hemodynamic compromise, and a surprising absence of valvular thrombi.[86] Patients with concomitant SLE and antiphospholipid antibodies have been found to have aortic and mitral valvulitis, including typical Libman-Sacks verrucous endocarditis.[87, 88] Additionally, in patients with SLE, the presence of antiphospholipid antibodies is associated with isolated left ventricular dysfunction.[89] An isolated instance has been reported of an intracardiac mass in the right ventricle, presumably resulting from the combined effects of abnormal intracardiac flow resulting from anomalous muscle bundles combined with enhanced thrombogenesis associated with antiphospholipid antibodies.[90] In view of the high incidence of valvular abnormalities in patients with antiphospholipid antibodies and arterial thromboembolism, Doppler echocardiography is recommended.[91]

CUTANEOUS MANIFESTATIONS OF ANTICARDIOLIPINS

Anticardiolipin antibodies are associated with livido reticularis, an unusual manifestation of cutaneous vascular stasis characterized by a distinctive pattern of cyanosis.[53, 92, 93] This cutaneous finding has been associated with recurrent arterial and venous thromboses, valvular abnormalities, and cerebrovascular thromboses with concomitant essential hypertension ("Sneddon syndrome").[53] Other cutaneous manifestations include a syndrome of recurrent DVT, necrotizing purpura, and stasis ulcers of the ankles.[53, 92, 93] Skin lesions of Degos' disease, a rare multisystem vasculopathy characterized pathologically by cutaneous collagen necrosis, atrophy of the epidermis, and an absence of inflammatory cells, have been linked to the other consequences of the disease such as cerebral and bowel infarction by the finding of anticardiolipin antibodies or LA.[94] Vascular thromboses may be manifested as ischemia or necrosis of entire extremities as demonstrated in association with disseminated intravascular coagulation[95] with the resultant cutaneous necrosis or more patchy, widespread demarcated areas of cutaneous necrosis (manifested as areas of painful purpura and necrosis with underlying dermal necrosis).[96] Other common cutaneous manifestations include livido vasculitis (reticularis), unfading acral microlivido, peripheral gangrene, necrotizing purpura, hemorrhage (ecchymosis and hematoma formation),[96] and crusted ulcers about the nail beds.[97] See Eng[93] for an excellent recent review of this topic.

ANTICARDIOLIPINS AND NEUROLOGIC SYNDROMES

The neurologic syndromes associated with anticardiolipin antibodies include transient cerebral ischemic attacks, small stroke syndrome, arterial and venous retinal occlusive disease, cerebral arterial and venous thrombosis, migraine headaches, Degos' disease, Sneddon syndrome,[98] Guillain-Barré syndrome,[99] chorea, seizures, and optic neuritis.[94, 100, 101] Considerable effort has been expended to link the central nervous system manifestations of SLE with the presence of antiphospholipid antibodies.[102, 103] Although it is clear that lupus patients with antiphospholipid antibodies may experience cerebrovascular thromboses, cerebral ischemia, and infarction, these events occur more commonly in patients with *primary* ACLAT syndrome and no underlying autoimmune disease. Multiple cerebral infarctions in patients with antiphospholipid antibodies may result in dementia.[104] The primary phospholipid syndrome is identified as present in patients with a constellation of concomitant arterial occlusions, strokes, transient ischemic attacks leading to multiple-infarct dementia, DVT associated with pulmonary embolization and resultant pulmonary hypertension, recurrent fetal loss, thrombocytopenia, a positive Coombs' test, and chorea.[23, 105] The primary distinction between patients with primary antiphospholipid syndrome and Sneddon syndrome is the involvement of large vessels in the former and exclusively medium-sized arteries in the latter.[98, 106, 107] Patients with antiphospholipid antibodies are more likely to experience cerebral ischemic or thrombotic events when also harboring primary hypertension or coronary disease.[108] Anticardiolipin antibodies and recurrent stroke have also been associated with thymoma.[109] The complicated topic of neurologic manifestations in APL-T syndromes has recently been reviewed.[23]

ANTICARDIOLIPINS AND COLLAGEN VASCULAR DISEASE

Although much of the initial research and many early reports of antiphospholipid antibodies resulted from investigation of LA, antiphospholipid antibodies occur in patients without SLE more frequently than in those with lupus or other autoimmune disorders. In patients with lupus, the presence of livido reticularis may represent an important cutaneous marker for their presence or the later development of antiphospholipid antibodies.[92] Antiphospholipid antibodies may occur with increased frequency in individuals with other autoimmune disorders and have been reported in patients with mixed connective tissue disease, rheumatoid arthritis,[96] Sjögren syndrome,[88] Behçet syndrome (possible role in the pathogenesis of the multisystem manifestations of this syndrome),[110] and autoimmune thrombocytopenic purpura.[58] Most patients with ACLAT syndrome, however, have the primary syndrome with no such underlying autoimmune disorder. The clinical manifestations can be varied and substantial.[22, 107]

ANTICARDIOLIPINS AND OBSTETRIC SYNDROMES

Anticardiolipin antibodies are associated with a high incidence of fetal wastage; the characteristics of this syndrome are frequent abortion in the first trimester, recurrent fetal wastage in the second and third trimesters, placental thrombosis/vasculitis, and maternal thrombocytopenia. This is especially likely in the presence of moderate or high IgG anticardiolipin levels.[111] This syndrome has been successfully treated to normal term by the institution of aspirin, low-dose heparin, or plasma exchange.[57, 112-114] Women harboring anticardiolipin antibodies have about a 50% to 75% chance of fetal wastage, and successful anticoagulant therapy can increase the chances of a normal term delivery to about 80%.

Optimal therapy for FWS has not yet been defined. A variety of heparin doses have been used with significant success in carrying patients to term, and most of these have been in combination with aspirin therapy. In the primary antiphospholipid syndrome (absence of an underlying autoimmune disorder such as SLE), the use of corticosteroids or other immunosuppressive therapy is not warranted and only enhances side effects. However, immunosuppressive therapy may be useful in those with anticardiolipin syndrome and lupus. Also, a variety of vigorous antibody-removing/eradicating modes of therapy have been attempted with varying degrees of success, including plasmapheresis, plasma exchange, immunoadsorption column treatment, and IVIG. Based on available reports and our own experience, the use of low-dose aspirin (about 81 mg/day) in combination with low-dose porcine mucosal heparin (5,000 units subcutaneously twice daily) appears to consistently be the most effective therapy for term delivery at the present time. My approach in treating FWS is to start a patient on low-dose aspirin (79 to 81 mg/day) at the time a diagnosis of FWS is made (i.e., the demonstration of anticardiolipin antibody or LA and a history of recurrent abortion). As soon as the woman becomes pregnant, fixed low-dose porcine mucosal heparin (5,000 units every 12 hours) is added to the aspirin and used throughout the pregnancy. The low-dose heparin need not be stopped during delivery because it is extremely unlikely to be associated with significant hemorrhage and affords peripartum and postpartum protection against thrombosis and thromboembolic disease. Thus far our success rate with this regimen has been 100%.[6, 42]

The incidence of antiphospholipid antibodies in FWS has been studied by a number of groups. Most, however, did not use control pregnant populations. Lin studied a population of 245 women with FWS and found 13.5% to have anticardiolipin antibodies.[115] Parazzini et al. studied 220 patients with two or more spontaneous abortions and found 19% to harbor anticardiolipin antibodies.[116] Grandone et al.[117] assessed 32 patients with FWS and found 28% to have anticardiolipin antibodies, and Birdsall et al.[118] studied 81 patients with FWS and found that 41% harbored anticardiolipin antibodies. Maclean and colleagues assessed 243 patients with FWS (two or more spontaneous abortions) and found 17% to have anticardiolipin antibodies, 7% to have LAs, and 2% to harbor both.[119] Howard et al. assessed 29 nonlupus patients with FWS and found 48% to have LAs.[120] Taylor et al.,[121] in a study of 189 women with unexplained miscarriage, found LAs in 7% and anticardiolipin antibodies in 15%. The only two studies assessing matched controls were those of Parke et al.[122] who found 7% of pregnant women without FWS and 16% of those with FWS to have antiphospholipid antibodies, and Parazzini et al.,[116] who found a 3% incidence of anticardiolipin antibodies in control women. Thus it appears a small population of normal pregnant females without symptoms of FWS will also harbor antiphospholipid antibodies. This, of course, raises the question of treatment in a pregnant female harboring antiphospholipid antibodies but no prior history of spontaneous miscarriage; no data to date provide adequate direction for this dilemma.

Anticardiolipin antibodies are also associated with a peculiar postpartum syndrome of spiking fevers, pleuritic chest pain, dyspnea and pleural effusion, patchy pulmonary infiltrates, cardiomyopathy, and ventricular arrhythmias. This syndrome characteristically occurs 2 to 10 days postpartum.[123] Since the majority of patients with postpartum syndrome recover spontaneously, most require no therapy other than symptomatic treatment. It is unclear whether any type of antithrombotic therapy is warranted in this population since recovery is almost always spontaneous.

MISCELLANEOUS DISORDERS AND ANTICARDIOLIPIN THROMBOSIS SYNDROME

Anticardiolipin antibodies have recently been reported in patients with HIV infection, with or without immune thrombocytopenic purpura.[124] Particularly elevated are IgG isotypes; however, there is no correlation between the antiphospholipid antibody level and disease progression or the incidence of thrombosis in spite of a correlation with the titer and presence of thrombocytopenia.[124-127] Elevations of one or more of the anticardiolipin isotypes have been observed following a number of acute infections, including ornithosis, *Mycoplasma* infection, adenovirus infection, rubella, varicella, mumps, malaria, and Lyme disease.[128] Transient asymptomatic anticardiolipin antibodies may develop in children with these infections. Abnormalities of the aPTT in patients with hepatic cirrhosis have recently been attributed to the presence of antiphospholipid antibodies.[129] Drugs associated with the development of anticardiolipin antibodies include phenytoin,[130] quinidine, Fansidar, hydralazine, procainamide, and phenothiazine (with predisposition to thrombosis).[4, 5, 131] The ACLAT syndrome can be divided into those that are primary and those that are secondary. Primary ACLAT syndrome is much more common and consists of patients with anticardiolipin antibody and thrombosis who harbor no other underlying disease; secondary ACLAT syndrome consists of those patients with anticardiolipin antibody, thrombosis, and an underlying disease such as lupus or another autoimmune disorder, malignancy, infection, inflammation, or ingestion of drugs inducing an anticardiolipin antibody.

CLASSIFICATION OF ANTIPHOSPHOLIPID THROMBOSIS SYNDROMES

The finding of anticardiolipin antibodies or LAs in association with thrombosis is referred to as the APL-T syndrome. We are herein limiting this discussion to a classification of the APL-T syndromes associated with anticardiolipin antibodies. This classification discussion is limited primarily to anticardiolipin antibodies because patients with LA tend to not have thromboses that are as predictable as those with anticardiolipin antibody; however, management principles, as far as is currently known, apply equally to both.

The APL-T syndrome *associated with anticardiolipin antibodies* can be divided into one of *six* subgroups. Type I syndrome is composed of patients with DVT and pulmonary embolus, *type II* syndrome is composed of patients with coronary artery or peripheral arterial (including aorta and carotid artery) thrombosis, *type III* syndrome is composed of patients with retinal or cerebrovascular (intracranial) thrombosis, and *type IV* patients are those with admixtures of the first three types. Type IV patients are uncommon, with most patients fitting into one of the first three types. *Type V* patients are those with FWS, and *Type VI* patients are those harboring antiphospholipid syndromes without any (as yet) clinical expression, including thrombosis. There is little overlap between these subtypes, and patients usually conveniently fit into only one of these clinical types. The types of APL-T syndromes associated with anticardiolipin antibodies are summarized in Table 1.[4, 5, 43] Al-

TABLE 1.

Syndromes of Thrombosis Associated With
Anticardiolipin Antibodies (the APL-T Syndromes)

Type I syndrome
  Deep venous thrombosis with or without pulmonary
    embolus
Type II syndrome
  Coronary artery thrombosis
  Peripheral artery thrombosis
  Aortic thrombosis
  Carotid artery thrombosis
Type III syndrome
  Retinal artery thrombosis
  Retinal vein thrombosis
  Cerebrovascular thrombosis
  Transient cerebral ischemic attacks
Type IV syndrome
  Mixtures of types I, II, and III
  Type IV patients are rare
Type V (fetal wastage) syndrome
  Placental vascular thrombosis
  Maternal thrombocytopenia (uncommon)
  Fetal wastage common in the first trimester
  Fetal wastage can occur in the 2nd and 3rd trimesters
Type VI syndrome
  Antiphospholipid antibody
  No apparent clinical manifestations

though there appears to be no correlation with the type or titer of anticardiolipin antibody and the type of syndrome (I through VI), the subclassification of patients with thrombosis and anticardiolipin antibody into these groups is important from a therapy standpoint.[4, 5, 43] Type I patients are best managed by use of long-term, fixed low-dose subcutaneous heparin therapy and commonly ($\approx$65%) fail warfarin therapy, Type II patients are also best managed with long-term, fixed low-dose subcutaneous porcine mucosal heparin therapy (usually 5,000 units every 12 hours), and type III patients are best managed by the use of fixed low-dose warfarin (1 to 2 mg/day) plus low-dose aspirin (79 to 81 mg/day, intracranial vascular thrombosis) or pentoxiphylline (400 mg three times per day, retinal vascular thrombosis), and therapy for type IV depends on the types and sites of thrombosis present.[4, 5, 43] Patients with type V (FWS) are best treated with preconception initiation of low-dose acetylsalicylic acid (ASA) (79 to 81 mg/day) as soon as the diagnosis is made and then fixed low-dose porcine mucosal heparin (5,000 units subcutaneously every 12 hours) started immediately postconception. Patients with type V syndrome are encouraged to stop the heparin following delivery but to continue long-term low-dose ASA indefinitely. The decision to continue ASA therapy after delivery in

---

TABLE 2.

Recommended Antithrombotic Regimens for Syndromes of Thrombosis Associated With Antiphospholipid Antibodies (the APL-T Syndromes)

Type I syndrome
　　IV or SC heparin followed by long-term* self-administration of SC
　　　porcine heparin
Type II syndrome
　　IV or SC heparin followed by long-term* self-administration of SC
　　　porcine heparin
Type III syndrome
　　Cerebrovascular
　　　　Long-term* low-dose warfarin (1–2 mg/day) plus low-dose ASA
　　　　　(81 mg/day)
　　Retinal
　　　　Pentoxiphylline* at 400 mg three times daily
Type IV syndrome
　　Therapy is dependent on the type(s) and site(s) of thrombosis, as per
　　　the above recommendations
Type V (fetal wastage) syndrome
　　Low-dose ASA (81 mg/day) preconception and add fixed low-dose
　　　porcine heparin at 5,000 units every 12 hr immediately
　　　postconception
Type VI syndrome
　　No clear indications for antithrombotic therapy

---

*Antithrombotic therapy should not be stopped unless the anticardiolipin antibody has been absent for the preceding 4 to 6 months.

these patients is somewhat empirical but might ward off other thrombotic manifestations of the APL-T syndrome.

Obviously, patients with thrombosis and anticardiolipin antibodies require long-term anticoagulant therapy, and treatment should only be stopped if the anticardiolipin antibody is persistently absent for at least 6 months before considering cessation of anticoagulation.[4, 5, 43] After persistent absence of antiphospholipid antibody for at least 6 months, I usually discuss the risks and benefits of continuing antithrombotic therapy and encourage patients to take one low-dose ASA tablet (79 to 81 mg/day) in the hope that the antibody and thrombosis will not return. Obviously, patients with types I, II, or IV APL-T syndrome who are going to receive long-term, fixed low-dose porcine mucosal heparin therapy should have initial bone density studies and should be cautioned about heparin-induced thrombocytopenia, mild alopecia, mild allergic reactions, osteoporosis, and the development of benign eosinophilia. I monitor patients with weekly heparin levels (anti-Xa method) and complete blood count/platelet count for the first month of therapy and monthly thereafter; this also applies to patients with type V syndrome. Table 2 outlines suggested anticoagulant regimens based on the type of ACLAT syndrome. Also, since many patients with type I ACLAT syndrome fail warfarin therapy, the clinician should always suspect and search for anticardiolipin antibodies when evaluating a patient for warfarin failure.

CLINICAL FINDINGS

It is becoming increasingly clear that with more experience in using the anticardiolipin assay in clinical practice, antiphospholipid syndromes are much more common than suspected. Diagnostic evaluation of a patient to determine the etiology of a wide variety of thrombotic problems must now include assays for anticardiolipin antibodies and LA. Although it is appropriate to suspect anticardiolipin antibodies in virtually any clinical problem complicated by thrombosis, certain findings are stronger indicators than others.

In patients with type I disease, a strong index of suspicion is appropriate, particularly in individuals with DVT unaccompanied by a potential risk factor such as exogenous estrogen administration, surgery, prolonged immobility, malignancy, or another hypercoagulable state. Likewise, patients may have recurrent DVT with or without a significant risk factor. As is frequently observed in clinical practice, patients may only be referred for evaluation after a second episode of thrombosis. The initial thrombotic event may have appeared to result from a recognizable predisposing problem, only later proven to be present concomitantly with anticardiolipin antibodies. Although the severity or location (iliofemoral, popliteal calf vein, or other sites) or thrombosis or the presence of pulmonary embolization does not correlate with the presence of anticardiolipin antibodies, recurrent thromboembolic events or multiple sites of thrombosis should strongly suggest an anticardiolipin antibody. Another very common situation is a patient referred because of failing warfarin therapy. The failure of seemingly adequate doses of warfarin should immediately alert the physician to strongly consider APL-T syndrome.

Patients with type II disease frequently have catastrophic illness. A

TABLE 3.
Drugs Associated With
the Antiphospholipid
Thrombosis Syndromes*

Phenytoin
Fansidar
Quinidine
Quinine
Hydralazine
Procainamide
Phenothiazines
Interferon-α
Cocaine

*Most are IgM and are associated with thrombosis.

history of myocardial infarction at a young age, recurrent myocardial infarction, early graft occlusion following CABG surgery, and early reocclusion after transluminal angioplasty are typical. Aorta, subclavian, mesenteric, femoral, or other large vessel thrombosis may be characterized by complete occlusion and acute symptoms of ischemia and threatened limb loss. Emergent diagnosis and appropriate therapy may be lifesaving.

Type III patients may be referred for a variety of problems. Acute loss or distortion of vision may lead to ophthalmologic confirmation of retinal artery thrombosis. Focal neurologic symptoms may suggest the presence of cerebrovascular thrombosis and result in symptoms of stroke or transient ischemic attack. Alternatively, multiple-infarct dementia may be manifested more gradually, without clearly defined acute strokes. Early diagnosis is critical in type III patients since failure to treat may result in irreversible cerebral injury.

Type IV patients, who have a mixture of the aforementioned types, are extremely rare and account for only about 1% of patients with ACLAT syndrome. A strong index of suspicion is required for the diagnosis, and therapy must be individualized depending on the particular combination of thromboses.

Type V patients are usually those with one or more spontaneous miscarriages and are most often referred by obstetricians or high-risk fertilization experts. Most women relate a history of spontaneous miscarriage in the first trimester (most commonly the 6th to 12th week), but some also spontaneously miscarry in the second and third trimesters.

Drugs associated with APL-T syndromes are listed in Table 3.

PREVALENCE OF THE ANTIPHOSPHOLIPID THROMBOSIS SYNDROME

Unfortunately, very little information is available on the prevalence of LAs or anticardiolipin antibodies, especially in asymptomatic individuals. Additionally, nothing is known about the potential propensity for the development of thrombosis or other clinical manifestations when seemingly healthy individuals are found to harbor these antibodies. Only two recent studies have addressed this issue. The first such study was the Montpellier Antiphospholipid (MAP) study,[132] wherein 1,014 patients (488 males and 526 females) admitted to a general internal medicine department for a variety of reasons were assessed for IgG, IgA, and IgM anticardiolipin antibodies. Lupus anticoagulant assays were not performed. Of the patients tested, 72 (7.1%) were positive for at least one idiotype. When assessing these 72 patients, 20 (28%) were determined to have clinical manifestations of the APL-T syndrome. Fifty-two patients, when questioned, had not yet demonstrated any manifestations of APL-T syndrome, which suggests a false-positive incidence of 5.1%. However, long-term follow-up of the thus far asymptomatic patients has not occurred, and a follow-up report of the MAP study will be awaited with interest. In another recent study,[133] 552 healthy blood donors were screened for study; IgG and IgM idiotypes and LAs were assessed. It was found that 6.5% (28 donors) of the population harbored IgG and 9.4% (38 donors) of the population harbored IgM anticardiolipin antibodies, with 5 donors having both idiotypes. No donor was positive for LA. The donors were followed for 12 months; during the follow-up time, in no anticardiolipin antibody–positive patient did a thrombotic event develop. However, none of the anticardiolipin antibody–positive donors had a positive family history for thrombosis, and 3 of the anticardiolipin antibody–positive donors had a history of unexplained miscarriage.[133]

CHARACTERISTICS OF 105 CONSECUTIVE PATIENTS WITH PRIMARY ANTICARDIOLIPIN THROMBOSIS SYNDROME

We have evaluated, treated, and followed 105 patients with thrombosis and found on evaluation to harbor anticardiolipin antibodies. Excluding patients with FWS, there were 51 males and 31 females in the group, a male-to-female ratio of 1.64:1, quite different from the male-to-female ratio usually noted for LAs. The mean age at diagnosis was 44.8 years for males and 48.5 years for females. Of the 105 patients, 39 (37%) had DVT or pulmonary embolus (type I syndrome). In this group there were 23 males and 16 females with a mean age of 41 years. Thirteen had isolated IgG anticardiolipin antibodies, 5 had isolated IgA anticardiolipin antibodies and 6 had isolated IgM anticardiolipin antibodies. Fifteen had mixtures of idiotypes. The characteristics and idiotype distribution for type I patients when initially seen is given in Table 4. An inordinate number of these patients were referred because of coumarin failure. All of these type I patients have been treated with low-dose subcutaneous heparin, and none have yet failed treatment. I have elected to maintain patients on this therapy as long as anticardiolipins can be demonstrated and only stop long-term therapy if anticardiolipin antibody has been persistently absent for 6 months. In a recent survey of 100 consecutive patients with DVT or pulmonary embolus, 24% of the patients were found to have anticardiolipin antibodies.[134] It is suggested that anticardiolipin antibodies are common in patients with unexplained DVT or pulmonary embolism, and certainly any patient with unexplained DVT or pulmonary embolism should be evaluated for the presence of anticardiolipin antibodies.

Of the 105 patients, 23 (22%) had the type II syndrome of coronary artery thrombosis, or large peripheral arterial thrombosis (renal, aorta, carotid, etc.). There were 19 males and 4 females in this group with a mean age of 47.4 years at diagnosis. All of these patients have also been treated with long-term low-dose porcine heparin therapy; only 1 has failed treatment (recurrent femoral artery thrombosis). Like the previous group, all of these patients continue on therapy as long as the presence of anticardiolipin antibody is demonstrated. In this group, 7 patients initially had isolated IgG anticardiolipin antibody, 2 initially had isolated IgA, and 8 had isolated IgM initially. Eight patients had admixtures of idiotypes. The characteristics and anticardiolipin antibody idiotypic distribution for this group are summarized in Table 5.

Twenty of the 105 patients (19%) had the type III syndrome of cerebrovascular or retinal thrombosis. There were 9 males and 11 females in this group with a mean age of 54.2 years. Patients with cerebrovascular thrombosis have been treated with low-dose coumarin plus low-dose aspirin or intrapulmonary heparin (investigational protocol), and patients with type III syndrome and retinal vascular thrombosis have been treated with oral pentoxiphylline. None of the patients have failed treatment with intrapulmonary heparin or pentoxiphylline; 2 patients failed low-dose coumarin plus ASA and were then successfully controlled (no recurrence as yet) with intrapulmonary heparin given as 10,000 to 20,000 units/wk by ultrasonic nebulizer.[135] As in the other types, I have elected to continue therapy as long as the anticardiolipin antibody persists. In this group, 12 patients had isolated IgG, 2 patients had isolated IgA, and 1 patient had isolated IgM anticardiolipin antibody when initially seen. Five patients had admixtures of idiotypes. The characteristics and idiotypic distribution of anticardiolipin antibodies for this group is summarized in Table 6.

Of the 105 patients, 29 (27.6%) had FWS. The mean age of these women was 34.4 years. Twenty had isolated IgG, 2 had isolated IgA, and 6 had isolated IgM anticardiolipin antibodies. Only 1 had more than one idiotype. The characteristics of these FWS patients are summarized in Table 7. Only 9 of the 105 patients (8.6%) had clinical crossover from the type of thrombotic disease (type IV patients) present when first seen; these are summarized in Table 8.

The importance of measuring all three idiotypes of anticardiolipin antibody (IgG, IgA, IgM) cannot be overemphasized. In our studies of these 105 patients with anticardiolipin antibody and thrombosis it was found that 27.6% have mixtures of anticardiolipin antibodies and 72.3% have a *single* idiotype of anticardiolipin antibody. Of those patients having only a single anticardiolipin antibody, 47% have isolated IgG, 10.4% have isolated IgA, and 15.2% have isolated IgM. Although most women with FWS appear, in our experience, to have an isolated IgG idiotype, we have also seen numerous women with singular IgA or IgM, which makes it imperative to always measure all three idiotypes. The titer of anticardiolipin antibody is not related to the incidence of thrombosis, and lowering of the titer with immunosuppressive therapy does not abort thrombotic events; thus there is no role for immunosuppressive therapy in patients with pri-

TABLE 4.
Characteristics of Patients With Type I Antiphospholipid Thrombosis Syndrome

Patient No.	Age	Sex	Type Thrombosis No. 1	Type Thrombosis No. 2	IgG	IgA	IgM	Type	Other Laboratory Findings
1	22	F	DVT*	None	P	P	N	I	None
2	31	F	DVT	None	P	N	N	I	+LA
3	31	F	DVT	None	P	N	N	I	None
4	35	F	DVT	PE	N	P	N	I	None
5	38	F	DVT—bilateral legs	None	P	N	N	I	+LA
6	38	F	PE	None	P	P	N	I	None
7	38	F	DVT	PE	P	P	N	I	None
8	42	F	DVT	None	P	N	N	I	None
9	43	F	DVT	PE	P	N	N	I	None
10	46	F	DVT	IVC	N	N	N	I	None
11	51	F	DVT—bilateral arms	None	P	P	P	I	None
12	57	F	DVT	None	P	N	N	I	None
13	68	F	DVT	None	P	P	N	I	None
14	77	F	DVT	None	N	P	P	I	None
15	79	F	DVT	None	N	N	P	I	None
16	90	F	DVT	PE	N	P	N	I	Antithrombin deficiency
17	5	M	DVT	DIC	P	P	N	I	Homocyteinuria
18	32	M	DVT	None	P	N	N	I	None

19	34	M	DVT	None	P	P	P	I	Protein S deficiency
20	38	M	DVT	None	P	N	N	I	None
21	43	M	DVT	PE × 2	P	P	N	I	None
22	44	M	DVT	PE	P	P	N	I	None
23	47	M	DVT	None	N	N	P	I	Protein S deficiency
24	47	M	DVT	PE	P	P	N	I	None
25	54	M	DVT	PE	P	P	P	I	None
26	57	M	DVT	None	P	N	P	I	None
27	61	M	DVT	None	P	P	P	I	+LA
28	64	M	DVT	None	N	N	P	I	None
29	68	M	DVT—bilateral legs	None	P	N	N	I	None
30	68	M	DVT—arm	SVC	P	N	N	I	None
31	69	M	DVT	None	N	N	P	I	+LA
32	71	M	DVT	None	N	P	N	I	Protein S deficiency
33	72	M	DVT	None	P	N	N	I	None
34	76	M	DVT	PE	N	N	N	I	None
35	76	M	DVT	PE	P	N	N	I	None
36	37	M	DVT/PE	CAD/femoral artery thrombosis	P	P	P	I and II	+LA
37	65	M	DVT	PE/CAD	N	N	P	I and II	None
38	66	M	DVT	PE/CAD/vasculitis	P	N	P	I and II	Protein S deficiency
39	49	M	DVT	MI	P	P	P	II and I	HC-II deficiency

*DVT = deep venous thrombosis; P = positive; N = negative; LA = lupus anticoagulant; PE = pulmonary embolus; IVC = intravascular coagulation; DIC = disseminated intravascular coagulation; SVC = systemic vascular coagulation; CAD = coronary artery disease; MI = myocardial infarction; HC-II = heparin cofactor II.

TABLE 5.
Characteristics of Patients With Type II Antiphospholipid Thrombosis Syndrome

Patient No.	Age	Sex	Type Thrombosis No. 1	Type Thrombosis No. 2	IgG	IgA	IgM	Type	Other Laboratory Findings
1	37	M	CAD*/Femoral artery thrombosis	DVT/PE	P	P	P	II and I	+LA
2	65	M	CAD/PE	DVT	N	N	P	II and I	None
3	66	M	CAD/vasculitis/PE	DVT	P	N	P	II and I	Protein S deficiency
4	49	M	MI	DVT	N	P	P	II and I	HC-II deficiency
5	22	M	MI	DVT	N	P	N	II and I	Protein S deficiency
6	30	F	Mesenteric artery	None	N	P	N	II	SPS
7	33	F	MI	None	P	P	P	II	+LA
8	67	F	CAD	Failed graft and angioplasty	P	P	P	II	High LPA
9	32	M	MI	None	N	N	P	II	None
10	36	M	MI	Failed PTCA	N	N	P	II	None
11	41	M	MI	None	N	N	P	II	None
12	41	M	CVT	Carotid—bilateral	P	N	N	II	None
13	42	M	Renal artery	None	N	N	P	II	None
14	51	M	MI	None	P	N	N	II	None
15	52	M	Renal artery	Femoral artery	P	N	N	II	+LA
16	53	M	MI	None	P	N	N	II	High fibrinogen
17	55	M	MI	Aorta—distal	P	P	P	II	None
18	61	M	MI	Failed CABG	P	P	N	II	Protein C deficiency
19	67	M	MI	Failed CABG	P	P	P	II	None
20	71	M	MI	Femoral artery	N	N	N	II	None
21	71	M	MI	None	P	N	P	II	None
22	36	F	Forearm artery	CVT	P	N	N	II and III	None
23	76	M	Carotid—right	CVT	N	P	P	II and III	None

*CAD = coronary artery disease; DVT = deep venous thrombosis; PE = pulmonary embolus; P = positive; LA = lupus anticoagulant; N = negative; MI = myocardial infarction; HC-II = heparin cofactor II; PTCA = percutaneous transluminal coronary angioplasty; CVT = cerebrovascular thrombosis; CABG = coronary artery bypass.

TABLE 6.
Characteristics of Patients With Type III Antiphospholipid Thrombosis Syndrome

Patient No.	Age	Sex	Type Thrombosis No. 1	Type Thrombosis No. 2	IgG	IgA	IgM	Type	Other Laboratory Findings
1	27	F	Retinal—right	Retinal—left	P*	P	N	III	None
2	29	F	CVT	TIA	P	N	N	III	None
3	33	F	CVT	None	P	N	N	III	None
4	37	F	Retinal artery—bilateral	None	P	N	N	III	None
5	40	F	CVT	None	P	N	N	III	None
6	50	F	CVT	None	P	N	P	III	ANA and +LA
7	61	F	Retinal—right	None	P	N	N	III	None
8	68	F	CVT	None	P	N	N	III	Antithrombin deficiency
9	77	F	CVT	None	P	N	N	III	+LA
10	82	F	CVT	None	P	P	N	III	+LA
11	43	M	Retinal—bilateral	None	N	N	P	III	None
12	44	M	CVT	None	P	N	N	III	None
13	51	M	CVT	TIA	P	N	N	III	None
14	56	M	Retinal artery—right	None	P	N	P	III	None
15	68	M	Retinal artery	None	P	N	N	III	None
16	68	M	Retinal artery	None	P	N	N	III	None
17	69	M	Retinal artery—bilateral	None	N	P	N	III	None
18	70	M	CVT	None	N	P	N	III	None
19	36	F	CVT	Forearm artery	P	N	N	III + II	None
20	76	M	CVT	Carotid—right	N	P	P	III + II	None

*P = positive; N = negative; CVT = cerebrovascular thrombosis; TIA = transient ischemic attack; ANA = antinuclear antibody; LA = lupus anticoagulant.

TABLE 7.
Characteristics of Patients With Type V Antiphospholipid Thrombosis Syndrome (Fetal Wastage Syndrome)

Patient No.	Age	Dx*	No. of Abs	IgG	IgA	IgM	Type	Other Dxs
1	27	FWS	Ab × 2	P	N	N	V	None
2	29	FWS	Ab × 1	P	N	N	V	None
3	29	FWS	Ab × 3	P	N	N	V	DIC—abruption
4	30	FWS	Ab × 2	N	N	P	V	None
5	30	FWS	Ab × 1	P	N	N	V	None
6	30	FWS	Ab × 3	P	N	N	V	None
7	31	FWS	Ab × 4	P	N	N	V	None
8	32	FWS	Ab × 1	N	P	N	V	None
9	32	FWS	Ab × 1	P	N	N	V	None
10	32	FWS	Ab × 3	P	N	N	V	None
11	33	FWS	Ab × 2	N	N	P	V	None
12	33	FWS	Ab × 5	N	N	P	V	None
13	33	FWS	Ab × 2	P	N	N	V	None
14	33	FWS	Ab × 2	P	N	N	V	None
15	34	FWS	Ab × 1	P	N	N	V	HEELP/+ANA
16	35	FWS	Ab × 3	N	N	P	V	None
17	35	FWS	Ab × 3	P	N	N	V	None
18	35	FWS	Ab × 3	P	N	N	V	None
19	37	FWS	Ab × 3	N	N	P	V	None
20	37	FWS	Ab × 3	P	N	N	V	None
21	38	FWS	Ab × 3	P	N	N	V	None
22	39	FWS	Ab × 9	N	P	N	V	None
23	39	FWS	Ab × 2	P	N	N	V	None
24	39	FWS	Ab × 6	P	N	N	V	None
25	41	FWS	Ab × 3	N	N	P	V	None
26	35	FWS	Ab × 3	P	N	N	V and I	DVT
27	49	FWS	Ab × 2	P	N	N	V and II	DVT/PE
28	35	FWS	Ab × 1	P	N	P	V and II	DVT/PE
29	37	FWS	Ab × 4	P	N	N	V and III	Retinal thrombosis

*Dx = diagnosis; Ab = abortion; FWS = fetal wastage syndrome; P = positive; N = negative; DIC = disseminated intravascular coagulation; ANA = antinuclear antibody; DVT = deep venous thrombosis; PE = pulmonary embolus.

mary ACLAT syndrome. It is of interest that only 10 (9.5%) of these 105 patients with anticardiolipin antibodies also harbored LA, which again demonstrates that in primary APL-T syndrome, the antibodies tend to be quite homogeneous.

LABORATORY DIAGNOSIS OF ANTIPHOSPHOLIPID SYNDROMES

DETECTION OF ANTICARDIOLIPIN ANTIBODIES

The detection of anticardiolipin antibodies is straightforward, and there is general agreement that solid-phase ELISA is the method of

TABLE 8.
Characteristics of Patients With Type IV Antiphospholipid Thrombosis Syndrome (Mixtures)

Patient No.	Age	Sex	Type Thrombosis No. 1	Type Thrombosis No. 2	IgG	IgA	IgM	Types	Other Laboratory Findings
1	37	M	DVT/PE*	CAD/Femoral artery thrombosis	P	P	P	I and II	+LA
2	65	M	DVT/PE	CAD	N	N	P	I and II	None
3	66	M	DVT/PE	CAD/vasculitis	P	N	P	I and II	Protein S deficiency
4	36	F	CVT	DVT of arm shunt	P	N	N	III + II	None
5	76	M	CVT	Carotid—right	N	P	P	III + II	None
6	35	F	FWS/Ab × 3	DVT	P	N	N	V and II	None
7	35	F	FWS/Ab × 1	DVT/PE	P	N	P	V and II	None
8	35	F	FWS/Ab × 1	DVT/PE	P	N	P	V and II	None
9	49	F	FWS/Ab × 2	DVT/PE	P	N	N	V and II	None

*DVT = deep venous thrombosis; PE = pulmonary embolus; CAD = coronary artery disease; P = positive; LA = lupus anticoagulant; N = negative; CVT = cerebrovascular thrombosis; FWS = fetal wastage syndrome.

choice.[136, 137] In the past, only IgG and IgA idiotypes have been assayed; however, with the current recognition that IgM idiotypes, whether primary or secondary (especially drug induced), are also associated with thrombosis, most laboratories are or should be assaying all three idiotypes. Some have advocated assaying more specific "anticardiolipin" idiotypes by ELISA, such as antiphosphotidylinositol or antiphosphotidylserine, but there is no evidence these subtypes are of clinical significance and they are rarely present in primary APL-T or ACLAT syndromes.[138] However, commercial interests and exploitation have convinced many credible clinical laboratories to offer these "more sensitive" subtype assays. Also, it is known that the in vitro ELISA assays for anticardiolipin antibodies are dependent on a plasma cofactor, β_2-glycoprotein I (apolipoprotein H), but the in vivo clinical significance of this phenomenon remains unclear.[30] Thus the appropriate assay for detecting ACLAT syndrome is a solid-phase ELISA measuring all three (IgG, IgA, and IgM) idiotypes.[27, 31]

DETECTION OF LUPUS ANTICOAGULANTS

In the presence of LA, an abnormality exists in the phospholipid-dependent coagulation reactions, including the prothrombin time, the aPTT, and Russell's viper venom time.[5, 9] The lupus anticoagulant is not directed against a specific factor, but to phospholipids. The inhibitor does not exert an increasing effect upon prolonged incubation with normal plasma, and thus this simple screen can be used to distinguish the lupus inhibitor from inhibitors that neutralize specific clotting factors. Incubation of the patients' plasma with normal plasma does not cause a sensitivity of the PTT to the inhibitor's effect, and one-stage assays for factors XII, XI, IX, and VII may yield low values when standard dilutions of test plasma are used.[9] Usually, further dilution of the test plasma causes the measured level of these factors to approach the normal range; an exception occurs in rare patients with a decreased concentration of prothrombin resulting from accelerated removal of prothrombin antigen-antibody complexes, sometimes seen in patients with SLE.

Multiple LA assays are currently in use. Sensitivity of the aPTT to the presence or absence of LA is highly dependent on the reagents used. Many patients with thrombosis and LA have normal aPTTs, even with the newer, allegedly more "sensitive" reagents; thus the aPTT is not a reliable screening test for LA and should not be used for this purpose.[5, 9, 30, 31, 139–141] When the presence of LA is suspected, a more definitive test, preferably the dRVVT, should be immediately performed regardless of the aPTT. The lupus inhibitor is identified by the ability to bind phospholipid and inhibit phospholipid-dependent coagulant reactions. The assays available are based on the use of limiting amounts of phospholipid and therefore sensitized in platelet-poor plasma. Initially, a prothrombin time was performed with dilute tissue thromboplastin and a reduced number of platelets in the mixture; however, IgM inhibitors were missed. Subsequently, a "modified" Russell's viper venom time was developed in which the venom is diluted to give a "normal" time of 23 to 27 seconds, and the phospholipid is then diluted down to a minimal level that continues to support this range. Prolongation of this system will not be corrected with a mixture of patient and normal plasma; this system detects both IgG and IgM LAs.[32] This assay, generally known as the dRVVT, appears to be the most sensitive of all assays for LA.[142] The KCT has also been modified to assay for LA inhibitor. In the KCT, platelet-poor plasma is mixed with varying proportions of test plasma and normal plasma. Kaolin is added and the time required for clotting determined.[9] The KCT is then plotted against proportions of patients' plasma with normal plasma; an inhibitor is assumed to be present when a small portion of test plasma, in comparison with normal plasma, prolongs the assay. A kaolin aPTT with rabbit brain phospholipid in a standard and fourfold-increased "high" lipid concentration to normalize or "out-inhibit" the abnormal "standard" aPTT has also been used in the diagnosis of lupus inhibitor.[9] This is known as the rabbit brain neutralization procedure and, although specific (due to rabbit brain neutralization), lacks sensitivity comparable to the dRVVT. The best test to detect LA at present is the dRVVT; if this test is prolonged, confirmation of a lupus inhibitor by noting correction of the prolonged dRVVT after the addition of phospholipid in some form (unfortunately often platelet membrane derived) is required, especially if the patient is receiving warfarin or heparin therapy. Both heparin and warfarin are capable of also prolonging the dRVVT. Confirmation of an LA in the aforementioned assays is by phospholipid neutralization (shortening) of the prolonged test.[5, 9, 142] As a practical matter, most clinicians and laboratories are asked to evaluate patients for LA after anticoagulant therapy has been started. Both heparin and warfarin prolong most of the aforementioned tests, including the most sensitive test, the dRVVT. If the patient is receiving warfarin and the dRVVT is prolonged and then neutralized by phospholipid, LA is confirmed.[5, 9] However, if the patient is receiving heparin and the dRVVT is prolonged, neutralization by platelet-derived phospholipid is not confirmatory because large amounts of platelet-derived platelet factor 4 may inhibit the heparin effect to correct the test. For example, commercially available platelet extract for the platelet neutralization procedure (Bio-Data Corporation) contains about 100 IU/mL of platelet factor 4, and normal male freeze-thaw platelet extract, commonly prepared for "platelet or phospholipid neutralization procedures" in the clinical laboratory, contains about 95 IU/mL of platelet factor 4, enough to neutralize heparin, shorten a prolonged clotting test, and render a false-positive result in the dRVVT or platelet neutralization procedure for LA.[5, 9, 143] As a practical matter, therefore, use of the dRVVT offers the most sensitive assay for detection of LA, and neutralization of this test by a non–platelet-derived phospholipid, in particular, cephalin (Bell-Alton extract),[144] which contains no platelet factor 4, makes this test the most specific as well.

Because of marked heterogeneity of antiphospholipid antibodies, especially in the secondary antiphospholipid syndromes, there is a correlation between elevated anticardiolipin antibodies and LA in secondary APL-T syndromes. However, the LA and anticardiolipin antibodies are two separate entities, and most of the time one occurs without the other being present, especially in the primary APL-T syndromes.[4] Lupus anti-

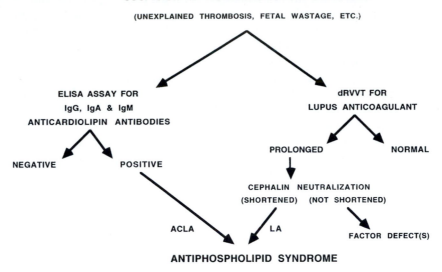

SUSPICION OF ANTIPHOSPHOLIPID SYNDROME

(UNEXPLAINED THROMBOSIS, FETAL WASTAGE, ETC.)

ELISA ASSAY FOR
IgG, IgA & IgM
ANTICARDIOLIPIN ANTIBODIES

dRVVT FOR
LUPUS ANTICOAGULANT

NEGATIVE   POSITIVE

PROLONGED   NORMAL

CEPHALIN NEUTRALIZATION
(SHORTENED)   (NOT SHORTENED)

ACLA   LA   FACTOR DEFECT(S)

ANTIPHOSPHOLIPID SYNDROME

FIGURE 1.

Laboratory diagnosis of antiphospholipid syndromes. *ELISA* = enzyme-linked immunosorbent assay; *dRVVT* = dilute Russell's viper venom test; *ACLA* = anticardiolipin antibody; *LA* = lupus anticoagulant.

coagulant has a stronger association with binding phospholipids of a hexagonal composition such as phosphatidylcholine or after membrane damage by infection, IL-1, or other mechanisms leading to a change from the lamellar to hexagonal form, whereas anticardiolipin antibodies have an affinity to lamellar phospholipids in a bilayer (lamellar) composition. Although stronger avidity of LA to hexagonal phospholipids is noted in vitro, the clinical significance of this remains unclear.[145] Thus the ordering of or purchase of LA assays by "hexagonal configuration" is of more benefit to commercial interests than to patient care at present.[31] Laboratory diagnosis of the APL-T syndromes is simple and summarized in Figure 1.

SUMMARY

Anticardiolipin antibodies and LA are strongly associated with thrombosis and appear to be the most common of the acquired blood protein defects causing thrombosis. Although the precise mechanism(s) whereby antiphospholipid antibodies alter hemostasis to induce a hypercoagulable state remain unclear, several theories, as previously discussed, have been advanced. The most common thrombotic events associated with anticardiolipin antibodies are DVT and pulmonary embolus (type I syndrome), coronary or peripheral artery thrombosis (type II syndrome), or cerebrovascular/retinal vessel thrombosis (type III syndrome); occasionally patients have mixtures (type IV syndrome). Type V patients are those with antiphospholipid antibodies and FWS. It is as yet unclear how many seemingly normal individuals in whom manifestations of antiphospholipid syndrome (type VI) may never develop harbor asymptomatic antiphospholipid antibodies. The relative frequency of anticardiolipin antibodies in association with arterial and venous thrombosis strongly suggests that these should be looked for in any individual with unexplained thrombosis; all three idiotypes (IgG, IgA, and IgM) should be assessed. Also, the type of syndrome (I through VI) should be defined if possible because this may dictate both the type and duration of immediate and long-term anticoagulant therapy. Unlike those with anticardiolipin antibodies, patients with primary LAT syndrome usually suffer venous thrombosis. Since the aPTT is unreliable in patients with LA (prolonged in only about 40% to 50% of patients) and is not usually prolonged in patients with anticardiolipin antibodies, definitive tests (ELISA for anticardiolipin antibodies and the dRVVT for lupus anticoagulant) should be immediately ordered when antiphospholipid syndrome is suspected or in individuals with otherwise unexplained thrombotic or thromboembolic events.

REFERENCES

1. Virchow R: Phlogose und Thrombose, in Virchow R (ed): *Gesammelte Abhandlungen zur Wissenschaflichen Medicin.* Frankfurt, Germany, Van Meidlinger Sohn, 1856, pp 458–636.
2. Bick RL: Hypercoagulability and thrombosis. *Med Clin North Am* 78:635, 1994.
3. Oosting JD, Derksen RH, Bobbink IWG: Antiphospholipid antibodies directed against a combination of phospholipids with prothrombin, protein C or protein S: An explanation for their pathogenic mechanism? *Blood* 81:2618, 1993.
4. Bick RL, Baker WF: Anticardiolipin antibodies and thrombosis. *Hematol Oncol Clin North Am* 6:1287, 1992.
5. Bick RL: Lupus anticoagulants and anticardiolipin antibodies. *Biomed Prog* 6:35, 1993.
6. Bick RL, Baker WF: The antiphospholipid and thrombosis syndromes. *Med Clin North Am* 78:667, 1994.
7. Conley CL, Hartmann RC: A hemorrhagic disorder caused by circulating anticoagulant in patients with disseminated lupus erythematosus. *J Clin Invest* 31:621, 1952.
8. Criel A, Collen D, Masson PL: A case of IgM antibodies which inhibit the contact activation of blood coagulation. *Thromb Res* 12:833, 1978.
9. Kunkel L: Acquired circulating anticoagulants. *Hematol Oncol Clin North Am* 6:1341, 1992.
10. Coller BS, Hultin MB, Hoyer LW: Normal pregnancy in a patient with a prior postpartum factor VIII inhibitor: With observations on pathogenesis and prognosis. *Blood* 58:619, 1981.
11. LeFrere JJ, Gozin D, Lerable J: Circulating anticoagulant in asymptomatic persons seropositive for human immunodeficiency virus. *Ann Intern Med* 108:771, 1988.
12. Tailan B, Roul C, Fuzibet JG: Circulating anticoagulant in patients seropositive for human immunodeficiency virus. *Ann Intern Med* 87:238, 1989.
13. Davis S, Furie B, Griffin JH: Circulating inhibitors of blood coagulation associated with procainamide-induced lupus anticoagulants. *Am J Hematol* 4:401, 1978.
14. Jeffrey RF: Transient lupus anticoagulant with Fansidar therapy. *Postgrad Med J* 62:893, 1986.
15. Morgan M, Downs K, Chesterman CN, et al: Clinical analysis of 125 patients with the lupus anticoagulant. *Aust N Z J Med* 23:148, 1993.

16. Bick RL, Ucar K: Hypercoagulability and thrombosis. *Hematol Oncol Clin North Am* 6:1421, 192.

17. Schleider MA, Nachman RL, Jaffe EA: A clinical study of the lupus anticoagulant. *Blood* 48:499, 1976.

18. Regan MG, Lackner H, Karpatkin S: Platelet function and coagulation profile in lupus erythematosus. *Ann Intern Med* 81:462, 1974.

19. Mueh JR, Herbst KD, Rapaport SI: Thrombosis in patients with the "lupus"-type circulating anticoagulant. *Ann Intern Med* 92:156, 1980.

20. Shapiro SS, Siegel JE: Hemorrhagic disorders associated with circulating anticoagulants, in Ratnoff OD, Forbes CD (eds): *Disorders of Hemostasis*. Philadelphia, WB Saunders, 1991, p 245.

21. Bick RL, Ancypa D: The antiphospholipid and thrombosis (APL-T) Syndromes: Clinical and laboratory correlates, in *Clinics and Laboratory medicine: Thrombosis and Hemostasis for the Clinical Laboratory, Part II*. Philadelphia, WB Saunders, 1995, p 63.

22. Kampe CE: Clinical syndromes associated with lupus anticoagulants. *Semin Thromb Hemost* 20:16, 1994.

23. Hinton RC: Neurological syndromes associated with antiphospholipid antibodies. *Semin Thromb Hemost* 20:46, 1994.

24. Kleinknecht D, Bobrie G, Meyer O, et al: Recurrent thrombosis and renal vascular disease in a patient with lupus anticoagulant. *Nephrol Dial Transplant* 4:854, 1989.

25. Pope JM, Canny CL, Bell DA: Cerebral ischemic events associated with endocarditis, retinal vascular disease and lupus anticoagulant. *Am J Med* 90:299, 1991.

26. Baker WF, Bick RL: Antiphospholipid antibodies in coronary artery disease. *Semin Thromb Hemost* 20:27, 1994.

27. Reyes H, Dearing L, Shoenfeld Y: Antiphospholipid antibodies: A critique of their heterogeneity and hegemony. *Semin Thromb Hemost* 20:89, 1994.

28. Kaczor NA, Bickford NN, Triplwett DA: Evaluation of different mixing study reagents and dilution effect in lupus anticoagulant testing. *J Clin Pathol* 95:408, 1991.

29. Shapiro SS, Thagarajan P: Lupus anticoagulants. *Prog Hemost Thromb* 6:263, 1982.

30. Ko J, Guaglianone P, Wolin M, et al: Variation in the sensitivity of an activated thromboplasin time reagent to the lupus anticoagulant. *Am J Clin Pathol* 99:333, 1993.

31. Bick RL: The antiphospholipid-thrombosis syndromes: Fact, fiction, confusion, and controversy. *Am J Clin Pathol* 100:477, 1993.

32. Thiagarajan P, Pengo V, Shapiro SS: The use of the dilute Russel viper venom time for the diagnosis of lupus anticoagulants. *Blood* 68:869, 1986.

33. McGehee WG, Patch MJ, Lingao JU: Detection of the lupus anticoagulant: A comparison of the kaolin clotting time with the tissue thromboplastin inhibition test (abstract). *Blood* 62(suppl):276, 1983.

34. Rosove MH, Ismail M, Koziol BJ: Lupus anticoagulants: Improved diagnosis with a kaolin clotting time using rabbit brain phospholipid in standard and high concentrations. *Blood* 68:472, 1986.

35. Bick RL: Hypercoagulability and thrombosis, in *Disorders of Thrombosis and Hemostasis: Clinical and Laboratory Practice*. Chicago, American Society of Clinical Pathologists, 1992, p 261.

36. Harris EN: Immunology of antiphospholipid antibodies, in Lahita R (ed): *Systemic Lupus Erythematosus*, ed 2. New York, Churchill Livingstone, 1992, p 305.

37. Rauch J, Janoff AS: The nature of antiphospholipid antibodies. *J Rheumatol* 19:1782, 1992.

38. De Castellarnau C, Vila CL, Sancho MJ: Lupus anticoagulant, recurrent abortion, and prostacyclin production by cultured smooth muscle cells. *Lancet* 2:1137, 1983.

39. Felippo MJ, Drayann CJ: Prekallikrein inhibition associated with the lupus anticoagulant: A mechanism for thrombosis. *Am J Clin Pathol* 77:275, 1982.

40. Bick RL, Baker WF: Antiphospholipid and thrombosis syndromes. *Semin Thromb Hemost* 20:3, 1994.

41. Roubey RAS: Autoantibodies to phospholipid-bonding plasma proteins: A new view of lupus anticoagulants and other "antiphospholipid" antibodies. *Blood* 84:2854, 1994.

42. Bick RL, Cohen BM, Staub AJ, et al: Coagulation protein defects associated with fetal wastage syndrome: Diagnosis and management. *Blood* 84:82, 1994.

43. Bick RL: The Antiphospholipid thrombosis (APL-T) syndromes: Characteristics and recommendations for classification and treatment. *Am J Clin Pathol* 96:424, 1991.

44. Rosove MH, Brewer PMC: Antiphospholipid thrombosis: Clinical course after the first thrombotic event in 70 patients. *Ann Intern Med* 117:303, 1992.

45. Bowie EJW, Thompson JH, Pascuzzi CA: Thrombosis in systemic lupus erythematosus despite circulating anticoagulant. *J Lab Clin Med* 62:416, 1963.

46. Bell WR, Boss GR, Wolfson JS: Circulating anticoagulant in the procainamide-induced lupus syndrome. *Arch Intern Med* 137:1471, 1977.

47. Bick RL: Circulating anticoagulants, in *Disorders of Thrombosis and Hemostasis: Clinical and Laboratory Practice.* Chicago, American Society of Clinical Pathologists, 1992, p 223.

48. Espinoza LR, Hartmann RC: Significance of the lupus anticoagulant. *Am J Hematol* 22:331, 1986.

49. Manoussakis MN, Tzioufas AG, Silis MP: High prevalence of anticardiolipin and other autoantibodies in a healthy elderly population. *Clin Exp Immunol* 69:557, 1987.

50. Zarrabi MH, Zucker S, Miller F: Immunologic and coagulation disorders in chlorpromazine-treated patients. *Ann Intern Med* 91:914, 1979.

51. Harris EN, Gharavi AE, Boey ML: Anticardiolipin antibodies: Detection by radioimmunoassay and association with thrombosis in systemic lupus erythematosus. *Lancet* 2:1211, 1983.

52. Weidmann CE, Wallace D, Peter J: Studies of IgG, IgM and IgA antiphospholipid antibody isotypes in systemic lupus erythematosus. *J Rheumatol* 15:74, 1988.

53. Asherson RA, Harris EN: Anticardiolipin antibodies: Clinical associations. *Postgrad Med J* 62:1081, 1986.

54. Hughes GVR, Harris EN, Gharavi AE: The anticardiolipin syndrome. *J Rheumatol* 13:486, 1986.

55. Triplett DA: Clinical significance of antiphospholipid antibodies. *Hemost Thromb* 10:1, 1988.

56. Derue G, Englert H, Harris E: Fetal loss in systemic lupus: Association with anticardiolipin antibodies. *Br J Obstet Gynaecol* 5:207, 1985.

57. Lubbe WF, Palmer SJ, Butler WS: Fetal survival after prednisolone suppression of maternal lupus anticoagulant. *Lancet* 1:1361, 1983.

58. Harris EN, Gharavi AE, Hedge U: Anticardiolipin antibodies in autoimmune thrombocytopenia purpura. *Br J Haematol* 59:231, 1985.

59. Harris EN, Asherson RA, Gharavi AE: Thrombocytopenia in SLE and related autoimmune disorders: Association with anticardiolipin antibodies. *Br J Haematol* 59:227, 1985.

60. Rosove MH, Brewer P, Runge A: Simultaneous lupus anticoagulant and an-

ticardiolipin assays and clinical detection of antiphospholipids. *Am J Hematol* 32:148, 1989.

61. McNeil HP, Chesterman CN, Krilis SA: Anticardiolipin antibodies and lupus anticoagulants comprise separate antibody subgroups with different phospholipid binding characteristics. *Br J Haematol* 73:506, 1989.

62. Shi BS, Chong BH, Chesterman CN: Beta-2-glycoprotein I is a requirement for anticardiolipin antibodies binding to activated platelets: Differences with lupus anticoagulants. *Blood* 81:1255, 1993.

63. Harris EN, Hughes GRV, Gharavi AE: Antiphospholipid antibodies: An elderly statesman dons new garments. *J Rheumatol* 14:208, 1987.

64. Gharavi AE, Harris EN, Asherson RA: Anticardiolipin antibodies: Isotype distribution and phospholipid specificity. *Ann Rheum Dis* 46:1, 1987.

65. Carreras L, Manchin S, Deman R: Arterial thrombosis, intrauterine death and lupus anticoagulant: Detection of immunoglobulin interfering with prostacyclin formation. *Thromb Haemost* 57:374, 1987.

66. Cariou R, Tobelem G, Bellucci S: Effect of lupus anticoagulant on antithrombogenic properties of endothelial cells: Inhibition of thrombomodulin-dependent protein C activation. *Thromb Haemostas* 60:54, 1988.

67. Cosgriff TM, Martin BA: Low functional and high antigenic antithrombin III level in a patient with the lupus anticoagulant. *Arthritis Rheum* 24:94, 1981.

68. Khamashta MA, Harris EN, Gharavi AE: Immune mediated mechanism for thrombosis: Antiphospholipid antibody binding to platelet membranes. *Ann Rheum Dis* 47:849, 1988.

69. Sanfelippo MJ, Drayna CJ: Prekallikrein inhibition associated with the lupus anticoagulant. *Am J Clin pathol* 77:275, 1982.

70. Angeles-Cano E, Sultan Y, Clauvel JP: Predisposing factors to thrombosis in systemic lupus erythematosus. Possible relationship to endothelial cell damage. *J Lab Clin Med* 94:312, 1979.

71. Ginsburg KS, Liang MH, Newcomer L, et al: Anticardiolipin antibodies and the risk for ischemic stroke and venous thrombosis. *Ann Intern Med* 117:997, 1992.

72. Boey ML, Colaco CB, Gharavi AE: Thrombosis in SLE: Striking association with the presence of circulating "lupus anticoagulant." *BMJ* 287:1021, 1983.

73. Elias M, Eldor A: Thromboembolism in patients with the "lupus-like" circulating anticoagulant. *Arch Intern Med* 144:510, 1984.

74. Hall S, Buettner H, Luthra HS: Occlusive retinal vascular disease in systemic lupus erythematosus. *J Rheumatol* 11:96, 1984.

75. Asherson RA, Harris EN, Gharavi AE: Arterial occlusions associated with antibodies to anticardiolipin (abstract). *Arthritis Rheum* 28(suppl):89, 1985.

76. Hamilton ME: Superior mesenteric artery thrombosis associated with antiphospholipid syndrome. *West J Med* 155:174, 1991.

77. Asherson RA, Harris EN, Gharavi AE: Aortic arch syndrome associated with anticardiolipin antibodies and the lupus anticoagulant. *Arthritis Rheum* 28:94, 1985.

78. Asherson RA, Morgan SH, Harris EN: Arterial occlusion causing large bowel infarction: A reflection of clotting diathesis in SLE. *Clin Rheumatol* 5:102, 1986.

79. Asherson RA, MacKay IR, Harris EN: Myocardial infarction in a young male with systemic lupus erythematosus, deep vein thrombosis and antiphospholipid antibodies. *Br Heart J* 56:910, 1986.

80. Gavaghan TP, Krilis SA, Daggard GE: Anticardiolipin antibodies and occlusion of coronary artery bypass grafts. *Lancet* 2:977, 1987.

81. Morton KT, Gavaghan S, Krilis G: Coronary artery bypass graft failure: An autoimmune phenomenon? *Lancet* 1:1353, 1986.

82. Hamsten A, Norberg R, Bjorkholm M: Antibodies to cardiolipin in young survivors of myocardial infarction: An association with recurrent cardiovascular events. *Lancet* 1:113, 1986.

83. Harpaz D, Sidi Y: Successful thrombolytic therapy for acute myocardial infarction in a patient with the antiphospholipid antibody syndrome. *Am Heart J* 122:1492, 1991.

84. Asherson RA, Khamashta MA, Ordi-Ros J: The "primary" antiphospholipid syndrome: Major clinical and serological features. *Medicine (Baltimore)* 68:366, 1989.

85. Bick RL, Ismail Y, Baker WF: Coagulation abnormalities in patients with precocious coronary artery thrombosis and patients failing coronary artery bypass grafting and percutaneous transcoronary angioplasty. *Semin Thromb Hemost* 19:411, 1993.

86. Galve E, Ordi J, Barquinero J: Valvular heart disease in the primary antiphospholipid syndrome. *Ann Intern Med* 116:293, 1992.

87. Chartash EK, Lans DM, Paget SA: Aortic insufficiency and mitral regurgitation in patients with systemic lupus erythematosus and the antiphospholipid syndrome. *Am J Med* 86:407, 1989.

88. Chartash EK, Paget SA, Lockshin MD: Lupus anticoagulant associated with aortic and mitral valve insufficiency. *Arthritis Rheum* 29:95, 1986.

89. Leung WH, Wong KL, Wong CK: Association between antiphospholipid antibodies and cardiac abnormalities in patients with systemic lupus erythematosus. *Am J Med* 89:411, 1990.

90. Coppock MA, Safford RE, Danielson GK: Intracardiac thrombosis, phospholipid antibodies, and two-chambered right ventricle. *Br Heart J* 60:455, 1988.

91. Reisner SA, Blumenfeld Z, Brenner B: Cardiac involvement in patients with primary antiphospholipid syndrome. *Circulation* 82(suppl 3):398, 1990.

92. Weinstein C, Miller M, Axtens R: Livido reticularis associated with increased titers of anticardiolipin antibodies in systemic lupus erythematosus. *Arch Dermatol* 123:596, 1987.

93. Eng AM: Cutaneous expressions of antiphospholipid syndromes. *Semin Thromb Hemost* 20:71, 1994.

94. Englert H, Hawkes C, Boey M: Dagos' disease: Association with anticardiolipin antibodies and the lupus anticoagulant. *BMJ* 289:576, 1984.

95. Bird AG, Iendrum R, Asherson RA: Disseminated intravascular coagulation, antiphospholipid antibodies, and ischemic necrosis of extremities. *Ann. Rheum Dis* 46:251, 1987.

96. Wolf P, Peter-Soyer H, Auer-Grumbach P: Widespread cutaneous necrosis in a patient with rheumatoid arthritis associated with anticardiolipin antibodies. *Arch. Dermatol* 127:1739, 1991.

97. Ingram SB, Goodnight SH, Bennett RM: An unusual syndrome of a devastating noninflammatory vasculopathy associated with anticardiolipin antibodies: Report of two cases. *Arthritis Rheum* 30:1167, 1987.

98. Levine SR, Langer SL, Albers JW: Sneddon's syndrome: An antiphospholipid antibody syndrome? *Neurology* 38:798, 1988.

99. Frampton G, Winer JB, Cameron JS: Severe Guillain-Barré syndrome: An association with IgA anti-cardiolipin antibody in a series of 92 patients. *J Neuroimmunol* 19:133, 1988.

100. Levine S, Welch K: The spectrum of neurologic disease associated with anticardiolipin antibodies. *Arch Neurol* 44:876, 1987.

101. Oppenheimer S, Hoffbrand B: Optic neuritis and myelopathy in systemic lupus erythematosus. *Can J Neurol Sci* 13:129, 1986.

102. Harris EN, Gharavi AE, Asherson RA: Cerebral infarction in systemic lupus: Association with anticardiolipin antibodies. *Clin Exp Rheumatol* 2:47, 1984.

103. Williams RC: Cerebral infarction in systemic lupus: Association with anti-cardiolipin antibodies *Clin Exp Rheumatol* 2:3, 1984.

104. Coull BM, Bourdette DN, Goodnight SH: Multiple cerebral infarctions and dementia associated with anticardiolipin antibodies. *Stroke* 18:1107, 1987.

105. Asherson RA, Khamashta MA, Hughes GRV: Sneddon's syndrome. *Neurology* 39:1138, 1989.

106. Moral A: Sneddon's syndrome with antiphospholipid antibodies and arteriopathy. *Stroke* 22:1327, 1991.

107. Sohngen D, Wehmeier A, Specker C: Antiphospholipid antibodies in systemic lupus erythematosus and Sneddon's syndrome. *Semin Thromb Hemost* 20:55, 1994.

108. Levine SR, Brey RL, Joseph CLM: Risk of recurrent thromboembolic events in patients with focal cerebral ischemia and antiphospholipid antibodies. *Stroke* 23(suppl 1):29, 1992.

109. Levine SR, Diaczok IM, Deegan MJ: Recurrent stroke associated with thymoma and anticardiolipin antibodies. *Arch Neurol* 44:678, 1987.

110. Hull RD, Harris N, Gharavi AE: Anticardiolipin antibodies: Occurrence in Behçet's syndrome. *Ann Rheum Dis* 43:746, 1984.

111. Harris NE, Spinnato JA: Should anticardiolipin tests be performed in otherwise healthy pregnant women? *Am J Obstet Gynecol* 165:1272, 1991.

112. Buchanan NM, Khamashta MA, Morton KE, et al: A study of 100 high-risk lupus pregnancies. *Am J Reprod Immunol* 28:192, 1992.

113. Editorial: Anticardiolipin antibodies: A risk factor for venous and arterial thrombosis. *Lancet* 1:912, 1985.

114. Kwak JY, Gilman-Sachs A, Beaman KD, et al: Reproductive outcome in women with recurrent spontaneous abortions of alloimmune and autoimmune causes: Preconception versus postconception treatment. *Am J Obstet Gynecol* 166:1787, 1992.

115. Lin QD: Investigation of the association between autoantibodies and recurrent abortions. *Chin J Obstet Gynecol* 28:674, 1993.

116. Parazzini F, Acaia B, Faden D: Antiphospholipid antibodies and recurrent abortion. *Obstet Gynecol* 77:854, 1991.

117. Grandone E, Margaglione M, Vecchione G: Antiphospholipid antibodies and risk of fetal loss: A pilot report of a cross-sectional study. *Thromb Haemost* 69:597, 1993.

118. Birdsall M, Pattison N, Chamley L: Antiphospholipid antibodies in pregnancy. *Aust N Z J Obstet Gynaecol* 32:328, 1992.

119. Maclean MA, Cumming GP, McCall F: The prevalence of lupus anticoagulant and anticardiolipin antibodies in women with a history of first trimester miscarriages. *Br J Obstet Gynaecol* 101:103, 1994.

120. Howard MA, Firkin BG, Healy DL: Lupus anticoagulant in a woman with multiple spontaneous miscarriage. *Am J Hematol* 26:175, 1987.

121. Taylor M, Cauchi MN, Buchanan RRC: The lupus anticoagulant, anticardiolipin antibodies, and recurrent miscarriage. *Am J Reprod Immunol* 23:33, 1990.

122. Parke AL, Wilson D, Maier D: The prevalence of antiphospholipid antibodies in women with recurrent spontaneous abortion, women with successful pregnancies, and women who have never been pregnant. *Arthritis Rheum* 34:1231, 1991.

123. Kochenour NK, Branch DW, Rote NS: A new postpartum syndrome associated with antiphospholipid antibodies. *Obstet Gynecol* 69:460, 1987.

124. Intrator L, Oksenhendler E, Desforges L: Anticardiolipin antibodies in HIV infected patients with or without immune thrombocytopenic purpura. *Br J Haematol* 67:269, 1988.

125. Canoso RT, Zon LI, Groopman JE: Anticardiolipin antibodies associated with HTLV-III infection. *Br J Haematol* 65:495, 1987.
126. Panzer S, Stain C, Hartl H: Anticardiolipin antibodies are elevated in HIV-1 infected haemophiliacs but do not predict for disease progression. *Thromb Haemost* 61:81, 1989.
127. Stimmler MM, Quismorio FP, McGehee WG: Anticardiolipin antibodies in acquired immunodeficiency syndrome. *Arch Intern Med* 149:1833, 1989.
128. Vaarala O, Palosuo T, Kleemola M: Anticardiolipin response in acute infections. *Clin. Immunol Immunopathol* 41:8, 1986.
129. Violi F, Ferro D, Quintarelli C: Dilute aPTT prolongation by antiphospholipid antibodies in patients with liver cirrhosis. *Thromb Haemost* 63:183, 1990.
130. Harrison RL, Alperin JB, Kumar D: Concurrent lupus anticoagulants and prothrombin deficiency due to phenytoin use. *Arch Pathol Lab Med* 111:719, 1987.
131. Lillicrap DP, Pinto M, Benford K: Heterogeneity of laboratory test results for antiphospholipid antibodies in patients treated with chlorpromazine and other phenothiazines. *Am J Clin Pathol* 93:771, 1990.
132. Schved JF, Dupuy-Fons C, Biron C: A prospective epidemiological study on the occurrence of antiphospholipid antibody: The Montpellier Antiphospholipid (MAP) Study. *Haemostasis* 24:175, 1994.
133. Vila P, Hernandez MC, Lopez-Fernandez MF: Prevalence, follow-up and clinical significance of the anticardiolipin antibodies in normal subjects. *Thromb Haemost* 72:209, 1994.
134. Bick RL, Baker WF: Deep vein thrombosis: Prevalence of etiologic factors and results of management in 100 consecutive patients. *Semin Thromb Hemost* 18:267, 1992.
135. Bick RL, Ross EL: Clinical use of intrapulmonary heparin. *Semin Thromb Hemost* 11:217, 1985.
136. Falcon CR, Hoffer AM, Forastiero RR, et al: Clinical significance of various ELISA assays for detecting antiphospholipid antibodies. *Thromb Haemost* 64:21, 1990.
137. Loizou S, McCrea JD, Rudge AC, et al: Measurement of anti-cardiolipin antibodies by an enzyme-linked immunosorbent assay (ELISA): Standardization and quantitation of results. *Clin Exp Immunol* 62:738, 1985.
138. Falcon CR, Hoffer AM, Carreras LO: Antiphosphatidylinositol antibodies as markers of the antiphospholipid syndrome. *Thromb Haemost* 63:321, 1990.
139. Triplett DA: Laboratory evaluation of circulating anticoagulants, in Bick RL, Bennett RM, Brynes RK, et al (eds): *Hematology: Clinical and Laboratory Practice*. St Louis, Mosby, 1993, pp 1539–1548.
140. Mannucci PM, Canciani MT, Mari D, et al: The varied sensitivity of partial thromboplastin and prothrombin time reagents in the demonstration of the lupus-like inhibitor. *Scand J Haematol* 22:423, 1979.
141. Bick RL, Pascoe HR, Laughlin WR: Efficacy of four common activated thromboplastin times in screening for the lupus anticoagulant. *Blood* 84:82, 1994.
142. Saxena R, Saraya AK, Kotte VK, et al: Evaluation of four coagulation tests to detect plasma lupus anticoagulants. *Am J Clin Pathol* 96:755, 1991.
143. Exner T, Triplett DA, Taberner D, et al: Guidelines for testing and revised criteria for lupus anticoagulants. *Thromb Haemost* 65:320, 1991.
144. Bell HG, Alton HG: A brain extract as a substitute for platelet suspensions in the thromboplastin generation test. *Nature* 174:880, 1954.
145. Rauch J, Tannenbaum M, Janoff AS: Distinguishing plasma lupus anticoagulants from anti-factor antibodies using hexagonal (II) phase phospholipids. *Thromb Haemost* 62:892, 1989.

Testicular Biopsy in the Evaluation of Male Infertility

John E. Tomaszewski, M.D.

Associate Professor of Pathology and Laboratory Medicine, Department of Pathology and Laboratory Medicine, University of Pennsylvania Medical Center, Philadelphia, Pennsylvania

Male infertility contributes to a failure to conceive in about 50% of cases.[1] Thus the classification and study of male infertility represent major considerations in the care of infertile couples. The conditions associated with male infertility have been variously classified depending on the interests and orientation of the author. Clinicians will tend to stratify infertile men according to the results of the physical examination, endocrine evaluation, and semen analysis. Wong and Horvath[2] have taken an anatomic approach and divided conditions associated with male infertility into causes localized to pretesticular conditions, primary gonadal damage, and post-testicular factors. For pathologists who are responsible for the interpretation of testicular biopsies, a logical approach to the classification of conditions associated with male infertility is to attach differential diagnostic possibilities to the histopathologic patterns seen on biopsy. This is the method that will be adopted in this review.

APPROACH TO THE INFERTILE MALE AND INDICATIONS FOR TESTICULAR BIOPSY

The initial approach to evaluating fertility potential in men includes a complete history and physical examination. Pertinent historical points include elucidation of the presence or absence of cryptorchidism, orchitis, occupational hazards, drugs, toxins, medical diseases (in particular diabetes[3]), previous surgery, potency, ejaculatory competency, and sexual awareness. The physical examination should be thorough. Particular attention should be given to the distribution of body hair, gynecomastia, penile curvature, location of the urethral meatus, epididymal texture, epididymal cysts or masses, vasal nodularity, varicoceles, and hydroceles. Testicular size and consistency must be described. Since the seminiferous tubules are the major contributor to testicular mass, a decrease in testicular volume is a sensitive indicator of diminished spermatogenesis.

Semen analysis is the second step in the standard evaluation of male fertility. Semen analysis is not a test for fertility. Fertility is a couple-related phenomenon that takes a number of factors into account. Semen analysis does provide important laboratory data that may act as a point

Advances in Pathology and Laboratory Medicine®, vol. 8

of departure for further evaluation. A number of factors are evaluated in routine semen analysis.[4, 5]

1. Coagulation.—Fresh semen coagulates on emission. Seminal fructose, which is produced solely by the seminal vesicle, provides the substrate for coagulation. Failure to coagulate is evidence for absent seminal vesicles.

2. Liquification.—Ejaculates should liquify within 5 to 25 minutes under the action of prostatic proteolytic enzymes. Failure to liquify and increased viscosity may limit sperm mobility.

3. Sperm concentration.—The minimal standard of adequacy is 20×10^6/mL. Fertility is less likely with counts below this concentration.

4. Volume.—The minimal standard of adequacy is 1.5 to 5.0 mL.

5. Motility.—This is defined as the percentage of sperm moving in ten random high-power fields. The minimum standard of adequacy is 60%.

6. Progression.—This is a measure of the quality of movement exhibited by the majority of sperm. Straight motion at good speed is preferred. Progression can be estimated by semiquantitative scoring, or it may be measured directly.

7. Morphology.—The morphologic examination of any particular patient's semen is relatively constant, and deviations from baseline usually indicate some new insult. Sperm can usually be categorized into one of five groups: normal, amorphous, tapered, duplicated, and immature. Immature forms should not exceed 4%. Tapered forms should not exceed 10%. Overall, a minimal standard of adequacy is greater than 60% normal forms.

8. Agglutination.—Increased clumping of sperm during a motility examination may suggest an inflammatory or immunologic process. No significant agglutination should be present.

9. Pyospermia.—White cells should not be present.

Endocrine-related infertility can sometimes be apparent from the history and physical examination; however, serum evaluation for luteinizing hormone (LH), follicle-stimulating hormone (FSH), and testosterone are powerful tools in screening for endocrine causes of infertility. The nature of the underlying defect(s) in the hypothalamic-pituitary-gonadal axis in men with endocrine-related oligospermia is varied.[6] Primary testicular failure, where the defect is localized gonadal pathology, is characterized by an elevation in LH and FSH levels. Patients with isolated damage to the germinal epithelial compartment will often have elevated FSH but normal LH levels. Luteinizing hormone pulse frequency is also increased in primary testicular failure.[7] In men with idiopathic oligospermia and elevated LH and FSH values, there is also an increased LH pulse frequency, which suggests that a common mechanism may be reflected in abnormal androgen feedback on gonadotrophs in both circumstances.[8] On the other hand, most patients with secondary testicular failure have impaired secretion of LH and FSH, and they usually have pangonadal insufficiency, including both androgen deficiency and infertility. The pathogenetic mechanisms and the extent of the gonadotropin defect will vary with the specific condition.

Two schools of thought exist as to the utility of testicular biopsy in the evaluation of an infertile male. Biopsy may be used effectively in azospermic men to differentiate primary testicular failure from obstruction.[9] Others advocate biopsy as a guide to diagnosis, prognosis, and the choice of treatment in oligospermic as well as azospermic men.[10] In addition to the evaluation of fertility potential in obstruction, testicular biopsy may be indicated in azospermic/oligospermic men with normal testicular size and normal FSH levels, including those men who may have primary spermatogeneic defects. In these latter instances, the purpose of the biopsy would be to help establish the fertility potential and prognosis.

BIOPSY TECHNIQUES

Classically, testicular biopsy is performed in the context of a formal scrotal exploration in order to properly evaluate not only the testis but also the epididymis, vas deferens, and accessory genital structures. The best results are obtained with an open surgical incision. The biopsy incision should be large enough to permit an examination of about 100 seminiferous tubules. Bouin's fixative or another good nuclear fixative is necessary to preserve the fine chromatin structure. Fixation in cold 2% glutaraldehyde, postfixation in osmium tetroxide, embedding in epon, and sectioning at 0.5 to 1.0 μm are the steps of a special preparative method that is particularly useful if differential cell counts are required for research. Huff et al.[11] have used this method to great advantage in the evaluation of pediatric cryptorchid testes.

Fine needle aspiration (FNA) has recently been used as an alternative, less invasive biopsy approach. Adequate material can be obtained in about 80% of cases. In the evaluation of hypospermatogenesis, Mellidis and Baker[12] have found full agreement with open biopsy in 56% and partial agreement in 38% of cases. Gottschalk-Sabag et al.[13] found good correlation between FNA and biopsy in 87% of a small cohort. At present, FNA is an investigative technique that holds promise for the analysis of germinative cells. Information as to architectural malorganization, matrix components, and the interstitial compartment is lost with this biopsy method.

Wet preparations of fresh testicular tissue have been advocated by Jow et al.[14] These authors have found that when complete sperm with tails and motility are found on a testicular biopsy specimen, obstruction is almost certain. This novel finding could help direct immediate exploration and reconstructive surgery.

METHODS OF ANALYSIS

QUALITATIVE ANALYSIS

Qualitative analysis of testicular biopsy tissue is a rapid and fairly efficient approach to biopsy interpretation. In qualitative analysis, the pathologist, after review of all the available seminiferous tubules, assigns the predominant pattern of pathologic change. Meinhard et al. have outlined one easily adoptable classification.[15] Under this system, testicular biopsy specimens may have one or more patterns of damage (see later), and one pattern often predominates. The use of qualitative classifications permits rapid identification of those patients who are unlikely to benefit from therapy. Those patients with severe hypoplasia, Sertoli cell–only tubules, or tubular hyalinization are unlikely to regain fertility from surgical therapy. Although qualitative analysis provides a very utilitarian approach, it is subjective and difficult to standardize.

SEMIQUANTITATIVE ANALYSIS

Scoring systems can be applied to the evaluation of testicular biopsy specimens to rate the level of spermatogenesis of each seminiferous tubule. These data are collected and expressed as a modal value, a mean, or a histogram. The most widely used scoring system is that of Johnsen.[16] In this method, each seminiferous tubule is assigned a value corresponding to the pattern of damage and the extent of loss of germinative epithelium. All the tubular profiles in the best section of the specimen are evaluated. The scores range from 1 to 10, with values representing the histopathologic patterns enumerated in Table 1. The compiled values across all of the seminiferous tubules in a biopsy specimen may be displayed as a modal number, a mean and standard deviation, or a histogram. Johnsen found that in normal men at least 60% of the tubules are at score 10. Table 2 shows the Johnsen scores in some pathologic conditions. By surveying the entire biopsy specimen and categorizing the entire range of histopathologic change, the Johnsen scoring system takes into account the inherent variability present in human spermatogenesis. The maturation of spermatogonia to spermatozoa is not a uniform process even in a normal testis. Clermont has shown six patterns of cellular association within human germ cell elements.[17] Recently this organization has been shown to form a helical pattern with the helices contracted conically toward the lumen of the seminiferous tubule.[18, 19] Under the Johnsen scoring system,

---

TABLE 1.
Johnsen Scoring System*

---

1. No cells in tubular sections
2. No germ cells. Only Sertoli cells present
3. Spermatogonia are the only germ cells present
4. Only few spermatocytes (<5) and no spermatids or spermatozoa present
5. No spermatozoa, no spermatids, but several or many spermatocytes present
6. No spermatozoa and only few spermatids present (<5–10)
7. No spermatozoa but many spermatids present
8. Only few spermatozoa present (<5–10)
9. Many spermatozoa present but germinal epithelium disorganized with marked sloughing
10. Complete spermatogenesis with many spermatozoa

---

*From Johnsen SG: *Hormone* 1:2–25, 1970. Used by permission.

TABLE 2.

Modal and Mean Johnsen Scores in Various Disease Categories*

Modal Score(s)	Mean Score ± SD	Diagnosis
10	9.38 ± 0.24	Normal
		Defined etiology
3	3.80 ± 1.80	Hypogonadotropic eunuchoidism
3–9	6.09 ± 2.25	Acquired adult hypopituitarism
1–2	1.25 ± 0.28	Klinefelter syndrome
2–8	4.43 ± 2.30	Cryptorchid testes
		Unrecognized etiology
2	2.0 ± 0.03	Sertoli cell–only
2–8	5.32 ± 2.13	"Severe" hypospermatogenesis
7–10	7.80 ± 1.26	"Moderate" hypospermatogenesis

*Adapted from Johnsen SG: Hormone 1:2–25, 1970.

certain conditions can be seen to be very homogeneous in their seminiferous tubular pathology. For example, classic Klinefelter and Sertoli cell–only syndromes show an almost uniform lack of germ cells. Other conditions such as "hypospermatogenesis" are much more variable in their morphologic expression. Maturation arrest can be recognized by a nearly complete failure to progress past a certain score. An inspection of the Johnsen scores can quickly help highlight these facts.

QUANTITATIVE ANALYSIS

Quantitative analysis of testicular biopsy tissue has long been a research method in the study of male infertility. Early methods of quantitative analysis have been labor-intensive and tedious. Such techniques have included the following:

1. Categorizing each tubule for germ cell type and expressing counts as cells per unit of tubular wall length[20]
2. Enumerating germ cells and stereologically determining tubular cross-sectional areas[21]
3. Establishing a total germ cell–Sertoli cell ratio by counting at least 20 tubular cross sections[22]

All of these methods are somewhat difficult to apply in a busy diagnostic laboratory.

One quantitative method that we have found to be rather efficient is that of Silber and Rodriguez-Rigau.[23] Here, only the oval spermatids with dark, densely stained chromatin are counted. At least 20 tubular profiles are evaluated. This count is expressed as spermatids per tubular profile and is believed by its authors to correlate well with postoperative sperm counts. In the absence of obstruction, the correlations between spermatids per tubular profile on biopsy and sperm count on postoperative semen analysis are listed in Table 3. The mature spermatid count correlates with the sperm count because the rate of spermatogenesis is a rela-

TABLE 3.
Correlation Between
Spermatids/Tubular Cross
Section and Postoperative
Sperm Counts

Spermatids per Tubular Cross Section	Sperm Counts
45	85×10^6
40	45×10^6
20	10×10^6
6–10	3×10^6

tive constant in man and lowered sperm counts are a result of decreased cell numbers and not a decreased rate of maturation per cell. This quantitative method allows one to compare the sperm count with the amount of spermatogenesis predicted by the biopsy. Discrepancies suggest an obstructive component to the patient's azospermia or oligospermia. Thus this method allows some estimation of what postoperative sperm counts might be after surgical therapy. In our hands, this method has been a time-efficient method of quantitative analysis.

Flow Cytometry

Another quantitative method in the evaluation of testicular biopsies is flow cytometry (FCM). Cytometric evaluation of testicular biopsy tissue has the advantages of being quantitative and reproducible. In this method, the biopsy material is obtained by either standard open technique or needle aspiration and disaggregated by a combination of mechanical shearing and protease digestion. The resulting cell suspension may be stained with either propridium iodide[24] or acridine orange (AO).[25] Acridine orange staining provides the advantage of permitting the simultaneous analysis of both DNA and RNA content. Samples are analyzed for the percentage of cells that are haploid, diploid, or tetraploid. Spermatozoa and spermatids are haploid (1N) or near haploid. The peak for spermatozoa appears before that for spermatids because the chromatin is more densely packed and is less susceptible to staining. Diploid (2N) cells include Sertoli cells, Leydig cells, secondary spermatocytes, and spermatogonia. Tetraploid cells (4N) are primary spermatocytes in various stages of development. Additionally, haploid cells can be further separated into round spermatids, elongated spermatids, and spermatozoa by using AO staining[26] or differential DNA staining based on progressive condensation of chromatin among these cell types, which makes the DNA less accessible to the DNA dyes as sperm maturation proceeds.[27]

Studies employing FCM as a diagnostic method in the evaluation of infertility are relatively few. Abyholm and Clausen[28] found normal DNA distribution patterns on FCM in azospermic men with normal gonadotropic levels. Kaufman and Nagler[29] correlated FCM with qualitative biopsy analysis. Flow cytometry of testicular aspirates has also been correlated with sperm concentrations of the electrostimulated ejaculates of men with spinal cord injuries.[30, 31] Recently Hirsch et al.[32] have compared ploidy values with quantitative biopsy parameters, including the mean concentration of late spermatids, the mean spermatid-to–Sertoli cell ratio per tubular profile, and the mean tubular wall thickness to the percentage of haploid cells in a limited number of conditions. Correlations were good for spinal cord injury and obstruction. Other conditions were difficult to evaluate because of the low numbers.

Despite the promise, there are a number of unresolved issues in the routine application of FCM to the analysis of testicular biopsies. First, more clinical material will need to be examined by this method in order to establish a more robust database that can be compared with standard histopathologic methods. Second, with FCM there may be difficulty in making important distinctions such as the separation of maturation arrest from Sertoli cell–only patterns. Third, FCM concentrates exclusively on the cellular content of testicular biopsies. Important features may not be addressed if FCM is the sole modality employed in the analysis of testicular biopsy material. Some of these features include the frequency of global sclerosis, the amount and type of matrix content in the tunica propria and interstitium, the integrity of the interstitial vessels, and the identification of unexpected cell types (including unsuspected neoplastic infiltrates). In this author's opinion, the likely future role of FCM in testicular biopsies will be adjunctive in that it will provide a powerful independent quantitative analysis that can be integrated into standard histopathologic analysis.

MEIOTIC CHROMOSOMAL ANALYSIS

Testicular biopsy material may be used for the karyotypic analysis of chromosomes in meiosis. Aberrations not seen in somatic cell meiotic chromosome analysis can be found by this method. Asynapsis, desynapsis, low chiasma content, and dissociation of the X and Y chromosomes can be found with this technique.[33]

PATTERNS OF DAMAGE

The basic patterns of damage that can be found on the histopathologic examination of testicular biopsy tissue from men with infertility are listed in Table 4.

Damage may not be uniform across all tubules, and more than one pattern may be found within one biopsy specimen. Damage may also differ between the two gonads, and bilateral biopsies may be indicated when there is a suspicion of asymmetrical disease.[34] Despite these limitations, the damage patterns listed in Table 4 represent the fundamental qualitative descriptors that stratify gonadal damage. The results of testicular biopsy can significantly narrow the differential diagnostic possibilities as to etiology, and when coupled with quantitative analysis, the biopsy can also provide a statement as to the prognosis for fertility. The discussions that follow will outline the salient features of the histopathologic alter-

TABLE 4.
Histologic Patterns of Damage*

Normal histology
Immature testes
Sloughing of immature cells
Hypospermatogenesis
Maturation arrest
Sertoli cell—only pattern
Peritubular fibrosis and tubular hyalinization

*Adapted from Rudy F: Male infertility, in Hill GS (ed):
Uropathology. New York, Churchill Livingstone, 1989.
Used by permission.

ations under each of the categories in Table 4. Although space limitations
do not permit a discussion of every etiologic association, an attempt will
be made to highlight the associations that are most frequently seen with
each pattern.

INFERTILITY ASSOCIATED WITH NORMAL HISTOLOGY

The morphology is that seen in a normal postpubertal testis (Fig 1 and
Table 5). There are no abnormalities in either the type or organization of
germinative cells. A normal histologic pattern is most often seen with obstructive azospermia.[35]

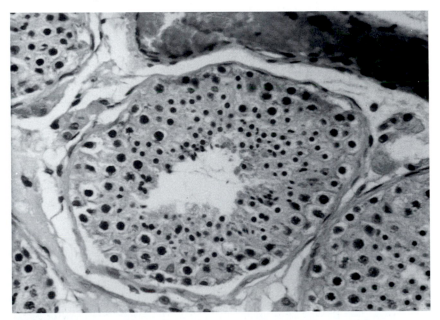

FIGURE 1.
Seminiferous tubule showing normal spermatogenesis with a full range of orderly
maturation from spermatogonia to spermatocytes to spermatids (hematoxylin =
eosin [HE], original magnification × 160).

TABLE 5.

Infertility Associated With Normal Histology*

Ductal obstruction
  Congenital
  Acquired
Impaired sperm motility
  Immotile cilia syndrome
Seminiferous tubule hypercurvature and branching
Hyperabsorption of sperm by the epididymis
Varicocele
Inadequate sampling
Idiopathic

*Adapted from Rudy F: Male infertility, in Hill GS (ed): *Uropathology*. New York, Churchill Livingstone, 1989. Used by permission.

Ductal obstruction may be congenital or acquired. The most common congenital lesion of the ductal system is atresia of the tail of the epididymis and proximal portions of the vas deferens.[36] A variety of partial or complete deficiencies in the efferent ducts and epididymal duct connections can occur. In some instances these are inherited as an autosomal recessive trait.[37] Absence or atresia of the vasa accounts for about 1% of azospermia in the general population, but it is the dominant cause for azospermia in patients with cystic fibrosis.[38]

Forty percent to 50% of cases with obstructive azospermia have an infectious etiology. This frequency may vary with the population.[39] Inflammation of the epididymis can resolve with scarring and blockage of the epididymis and vas. Before the days of antibiotics, the most common infectious cause of acute epididymitis was gonococcal. Today, an infectious etiology for acute epididymitis can be identified in 80% of cases. In men older than 35 years, *Escherichia coli* is the predominant pathogen, whereas *Neisseria gonorrhoeae* and *Chlamydia trachomatis* are more common in men younger than 35. Other organisms may include *Pseudomonas*, *Klebsiella*, *Ureaplasma urealyticum*, *Trichomonas vaginalis*, *Haemophilus influenza*, *Neisseria meningitidis*, staphylococci, streptococci, and viruses such as mumps. Organisms may reach the epididymis through hematogenous, canalicular, lymphatic, or direct routes. Iatrogenic surgical trauma may account for 1% to 6% of cases (without urinary infection). Acute epididymitis has been associated with drugs, including amiodarone and interferon-α.[40, 41]

Vasectomy, a common form of contraception, represents another cause of infertility clearly due to acquired ductal obstruction. Controversy exists as to the testicular changes following obstruction, and the histopathologic changes following vasectomy are particularly disputed. Some authors maintain that vasectomy in the absence of infection or ischemia produces no adverse effects on the germinal epithelium or the Leydig cells.[42] Others have described marked degeneration of the germinal epithelium (with maturation arrest at the spermatocyte level), thickening of tubular basement membranes, and increased interstitial connective tissue 1 month postvasectomy while failing to find significant changes at 2 to 3 years.[43] Still other investigators have described reduced spermatogenesis, maturation arrest, germinal cell vacuolization, thickening of the tubular basement membranes, interstitial edema, and fibrosis years after vasal interruption.[44]

Impaired sperm motility is often seen in conjunction with oligospermia, but in a small subset of infertile men, impaired motility is present as an isolated finding. The "immotile cilia syndrome" refers to a collection of abnormalities in ciliary function and ultrastructure in patients who have infertility and often histories of respiratory infection. The best known of these defects is Kartagener syndrome, in which infertility is associated with situs inversus, chronic infection, sinusitis, and bronchiectasis. The spermatozoa as well as respiratory cilia defects in the dynein arms on the peripheral microtubular doublets. Other defects are now also considered as part of the immotile cilia syndrome, such as abnormalities of the radial spokes, transposition of one pair of peripheral microtubules to the center of the axoneme, and absence of the central sheath.[45, 46] Because subtle partial defects in these structures are also described, the term "dyskinetic cilia syndrome" has been offered as an alternative term.[47] Three variants are recognized: type 1 with defective dynein arms, type 2 with defective radial spokes, and type 3 with microtubule translocation. The genes that control the ciliary structure of spermatozoa and respiratory mucosa may not, however, be identical; extended heterogeneity in this area is to be expected in the future.

INFERTILITY ASSOCIATED WITH AN IMMATURE TESTIS IN AN ADULT

In a small percentage of infertile adult men, the testes are histologically identical to prepubertal testes (Table 6). Seminiferous tubules are small and lumenless and lined by immature Sertoli cells and germ cells that have not progressed beyond the stage of spermatogonia or primary spermatocytes (Fig 2). The specialized Sertoli cell junctional complexes that form the blood/testis barrier are absent. Peritubular elastic fibers that form under the influence of pituitary gonadotropins at puberty are absent. Mature Leydig cells are not present; however, immature Leydig cell precursors resembling undifferentiated mesenchyme may be seen.

A number of conditions are associated with this pattern. The common denominator among all of the conditions is prepubertal *diminished or absent gonadotropin secretion.*

Organic lesions that may result in panhypopituitarism include tumors, cysts, or trauma in the sella or suprasellar areas. Patients with such lesions are characterized by sexual infantilism, lack of somatic growth, and varying degrees of thyroid and adrenal hypofunction. At the level of the hypothalamus, the lesions may include trauma, infiltrative diseases (e.g., sarcoid), tuberculosis, fungal infections, histiocytosis X, or neoplasms (such as craniopharyngioma or metastatic tumor). Among these, craniopharyngioma is the most common cause for organic gonadotropin

TABLE 6.

Infertility Associated With
an Immature Testis in an Adult*

Prepubertal panhypopituitarism
  Congenital
  Acquired
Hypogonadotropic eunuchoidism
  Kallman syndrome
  Laurence-Moon-Biedl syndrome
  Prader-Willi syndrome
Prepubertal androgen excess
  Androgen-producing tumor
  Adrenogenital syndrome
  Exogenous androgen administration

*Adapted from Rudy F: Male infertility, in Hill
GS (ed): *Uropathology.* New York, Churchill
Livingstone, 1989. Used by permission.

releasing hormone (GnRH) deficiency. This tumor, usually seen before the
age of 15, commonly exhibits suprasellar calcifications and produces anterior pituitary failure and diabetes insipidus in addition to GnRH deficiency—related gonadal failure.

    Hypogonadotropic eunuchoidism is a collection of congenital defi-
ciencies of LH and/or FSH in adult patients who give a history of never

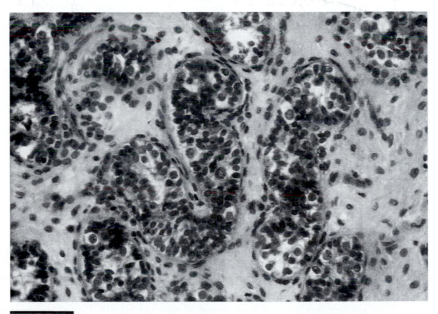

FIGURE 2.

Immature testis in an adult with hypogonadotropic hypogonadism. There is no
progression of maturation beyond the level of spermatogonia. The overall appearance is that of a prepubertal testis (HE, original magnification × 100).

having undergone normal puberty. In contrast to patients with organic pituitary/hypothalamic lesions, these men are typically tall with a eunuchoid habitus, small testes, and absent ejaculations. The classic hypogonadotropic eunuch has deficiencies in both FSH and LH. The primary abnormality may lie in the hypothalamus[48, 49] with faulty secretion of GnRH. Spratt et al.[50] have described a spectrum of abnormal patterns of GnRH secretion in men with idiopathic hypogonadotropic hypogonadism. In this study, men with no detectable LH or FSH pulsations and no history of puberty had small testes and a prepubertal appearance of the seminiferous tubules on biopsy. Gonadotropin levels were markedly decreased, and anosmia (see later) was frequent in this group. A second set of men, also apulsatile for LH and FSH, had a history of partial or complete sexual maturation. In these men the testicular volumes were larger and the testicular histology variable despite the depressed gonadotropin levels. The sense of smell was intact in this group.

Variants include isolated deficiencies of LH ("the fertile eunuch") and isolated FSH deficiencies. The "fertile eunuch," or Pasqualini syndrome,[51] refers to a group of individuals with variable virilization and often gynecomastia. The cause appears to be a partial LH deficiency in which there is adequate LH to stimulate intratesticular testosterone levels sufficient for spermatogenesis but insufficient to promote virilization. These variants do not demonstrate the histology of a prepubertal testis in adult patients, but testicular biopsies show either hypospermatogenesis or maturation arrest.

Kallman syndrome is hypogonadotropic eunuchoidism secondary to a congenital defect in GnRH secretion by the hypothalamus. The defect is inherited in an autosomal dominant manner with incomplete penetrance. Patients have anosmia, cleft lip and palate, cryptorchidism, microphallus, and craniofacial asymmetry in addition to the hypogonadism. Anosmia and hypogonadism may be related because of a failure of GnRH-releasing neurons to migrate from the olfactory placode to the hypothalamus during development.[52] Absent GnRH appears to be etiologic because GnRH administration will stimulate the release of both LH and FSH in these patients.[53]

Laurence-Moon-Biedl syndrome is a familial syndrome characterized by growth retardation, mental deficiency, polydactyly, obesity, diabetes insipidus, retinitis pigmentosa, and hypogonadotropic hypogonadism. Cryptorchidism, abnormalities of the external genitalia, and renal disease are also common.

In the *Prader-Willi syndrome*, small, usually cryptorchid testes and hypogonadotropism are accomplished by mental retardation, neonatal muscle hypotonia, hyperphagia with massive obesity, infantile external genitalia, and impaired temperature regulation. The pituitary response to a single bolus of GnRH is subnormal, and the hypogonadism is thought to be due to hypothalamic dysfunction since it is often associated with low gonadotropin and low gonadal steroid levels. Cryptorchidism, micropenis, and scrotal hypoplasia are recognized in 80% to 100% of affected males during the neonatal period. Prader-Willi syndrome is associated with an interstitial deletion of the long arm of chromosome 15 (usually of paternal origin) in 50% of patients.[54] Testicular biopsy may show an immature testis; however, normal histology, tubular atrophy, hyaliniza-tion, and absence of germinal epithelium have also been reported.

Androgen excess will have a negative feedback on the pituitary and hypothalamus and suppress gonadotropin release. *Prepubertal excess an-drogens* are usually secondary to tumor, i.e., androgen-producing tumors of the adrenal cortex, or a variant of the adrenogenital syndrome.

The most common form of the *adrenogenital syndrome* associated with excess androgen production is a deficiency of 21-hydroxylase. The gene for this defect is located on the short arm of chromosome 6 and is HLA linked.[55] Carroll et al.[56] mapped this gene to the major histocom-patibility class III locus. There is one functional gene, CYP21A2, and one pseudogene, CYP21A1P.[57] Since 21-hydroxylase is responsible for the conversion of 17α-hydroxyprogesterone to 11-desoxycortisol, a blockade at this step will result in decreased cortisol, increased adrenocorticotropic hormone (ACTH) production, and increased adrenal androgen produc-tion. This condition has also been termed *congenital adrenal hyperpla-sia* (CAH). There are several deletions and gene conversions described in CAH.[57] Excess androgen in a prepubertal genetic male will cause prema-ture development of secondary sex characteristics, however, the testes do not mature normally. They remain in the prepubertal state because the excess androgens suppress the gonadotropin secretion necessary for go-nadal development. A deficiency in FSH leads to impaired spermatogen-esis, and a deficiency in LH leads to abnormal Leydig cell development. The degree of impaired spermatogenesis may vary in each case; however, the trend is toward an adult morphotype resembling an immature prepu-bertal testis. In those men with less severe CAH, the degree of testicular damage may include varying degrees of hypospermatogenesis.[58] The tes-tes of patients with CAH may have interstitial tumoral nodules composed of cells that histologically simulate Leydig cell tumor. Whether these cells represent intratesticular adrenal rests that become hyperplastic or Leydig cells that are "captured" by the excess ACTH effect is a matter of debate.

Prepubertal androgen excess secondary to Leydig cell tumor, viriliz-ing adrenal cortical adenoma/adenocarcinoma, or exogenous androgen may cause the same picture.

INFERTILITY ASSOCIATED WITH SLOUGHING OF IMMATURE CELLS

In this histologic pattern, the orderly pattern of maturation is lost and the germinative epithelium has a jumbled appearance. The centers of the tubules contain numerous desquamated cells (Fig 3) and appear hyper-cellular in comparison to the periphery. Immature germ cells, including primary spermatocytes, are commonly found in the tubular lumina. Peri-tubular and interstitial fibrosis is usually mild. The Leydig cells are nor-mal. Only cases with more than 50% sloughing should be placed into this category; minor degrees of sloughing may represent an inconsistent arti-fact.

Varicoceles are tortuosities and dilatations of the pampiniform plexus within the spermatic cord that are commonly associated with a pattern of sloughing on testicular biopsy (Table 7). Varicoceles are thought to be secondary to vascular reflux as a consequence of incompetent or absent

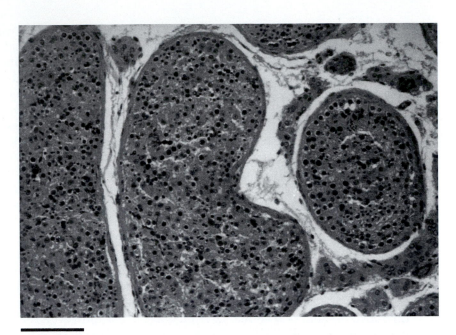

FIGURE 3.

Sloughing of immature germ cells into tubular lumina. The overall appearance is that of disorganization and misplacement of the immature germinative epithelium into the tubular lumina (HE, original magnification × 60).

venous valves. Grades can be assigned according to the size of the varicocele: grade 1, palpable scrotal varicosity less than 1.0 cm; grade 2, a pronounced varicocele mass 1 to 2 cm in diameter, and grade 3, a venous mass filling the hemiscrotum that is easily visible at a distance and larger than 2.0 cm in diameter.[59] Fertility indices have been reported to be lower for men with grade 3 varicoceles.[60] The left side is affected in 70% of cases. Varicocele is reported in 21% to 41% of men being evaluated for infertility. One large international study investigating 9,034 men evaluated as partners of infertile couples found varicocele in 24.4% of the men with abnormal semen as compared with 11.7% of the men with

TABLE 7.

Infertility Associated
With Sloughing of
Immature Cells*

Varicocele
Prior vasectomy
Mumps orchitis
Idiopathic

*Adapted from Rudy F: Male infertility, in Hill GS (ed): *Uropathology*. New York, Churchill Livingstone, 1989. Used by permission.

normal semen.[61] Varicocelectomy improves semen quality in 50% to 80% of cases and is associated with subsequent paternity in 24% to 39% of men.[62] The role of varicoceles as a cause for infertility is still debated. Several hypotheses have been proposed to explain the postulated negative effect on spermatogenesis. These include (1) hyperthermia, (2) reflux of renal and adrenal blood into the testis with the delivery of metabolic products toxic to the germ cells, (3) altered testicular steroidogenesis mediated by a slower venous outflow of testosterone, (4) hypoxia, and (5) mechanical compression. None of these mechanisms has been proved to dominate. On biopsy the testes may be affected bilaterally. In addition to germ cell sloughing, hypospermatogenesis, tubular fibrosis, hyalinization of small interstitial vessels, and Leydig cell hyperplasia can also be seen; the Leydig cell hyperplasia may be associated with a reduced paternity rate.[63]

INFERTILITY ASSOCIATED WITH HYPOSPERMATOGENESIS

The histologic feature in this pattern consists of seminiferous tubules that are normal to slightly decreased in diameter. All of the germinative elements are present in approximately normal proportions. The numbers of germ cells are, however, reduced, which gives an overall appearance of thinning of the germinative epithelium (Fig 4) with luminal enlargement. In extreme cases of hypospermatogenesis, the changes may approximate a Sertoli cell–only pattern (see later). The tunica propria of the seminiferous tubules and the Leydig cells are usually normal.

Hypospermatogenesis is a common finding in a variety of conditions (Table 8). *Chemotherapy* for malignant neoplasms imposes a severe toxic

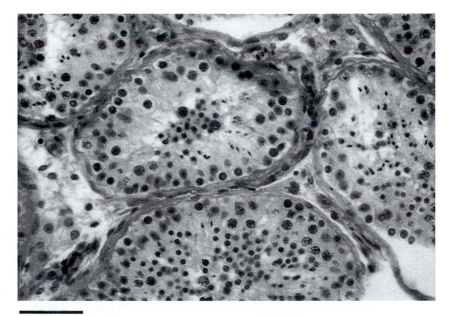

FIGURE 4.

Mild hypospermatogenesis. All of the germ cell elements are present, and there is orderly maturation; however, there is an overall thinning of the germinative epithelium (HE, original magnification × 100).

TABLE 8.
Infertility Associated with
Hyperspermatogenesis*

Environmental
  Malnutrition
  Excessive heat exposure
  Antecedent febrile illness
  Toxic chemicals/chemotherapy
Genetic
  Advancing age
  Down syndrome
  Fertile eunuch syndrome
Endocrine
  Glucocorticoid excess
  Hypothyroidism
  Hyperthyroidism
  Hyperprolactinemia
  Adrenogenital syndrome
Ductal obstruction
Idiopathic

*Adapted from Rudy F: Male infertility,
in Hill GS (ed): *Uropathology.* New York,
Churchill Livingstone, 1989. Used by
permission.

stress on the germinative epithelium, and hypospermatogenesis is a frequent finding in biopsy specimens of infertile men who have undergone prior therapy for malignancies. With the improved survival statistics achieved by modern chemotherapy, issues of long-term fertility have become pertinent. Cytoreductive chemotherapy causes profound temporary damage, and the long-term outcomes have varied with the therapeutic protocol. Single-agent chemotherapy with alkylating agents such as nitrogen mustard, chlorambucil, cyclophosphamide, and procarbazine are toxic to the testis; however, in general these agents, when used alone, are more likely to be associated with recovery of fertility.[64] On the other hand, multidrug chemotherapy (using a combination of agents) has a low frequency of recovery of germ cell damage during the years immediately following therapy.[65] The intensity and duration of therapy are also likely to play important roles in fertility outcome. With increasing time after cessation of chemotherapy, however, fertility may improve. In a recent study of adult men who had undergone therapy for childhood acute lymphoblastic leukemia, Wallace et al. found that only 6 of 37 men had conclusive evidence of persistent germ cell damage.[66] Chemotherapy is toxic to the germinative epithelium, and post-therapy serum FSH levels are almost always elevated.[67] Leydig cell damage is less, and serum LH levels are mildly elevated. The serum testosterone concentration is usually normal. The histopathologic changes are variable. Hypospermatogenesis of varying degrees of severity is common; however, maturation arrest, Sertoli cell–only, and complete tubular hyalinization patterns may also be seen.

Toxic chemicals in the environment may produce effects similar to chemotherapy; however, the changes are generally less severe and more difficult to document. Chronic exposure to the nematocide dibromochloropropane can be associated with near-total loss of spermatocytes and spermatogonia.[68] Battery plant workers with long-term exposure to lead compounds may have oligospermia and reduced fertility due to the direct toxicity of lead on germinative epithelium.[69] The list of substances suspected of causing infertility in the workplace is quite long.[70-72]

The effect of *heat* on fertility is discussed under in the section on varicocele. A variety of stressful events such as *acute febrile illness*, major surgery, burns, etc., may also be associated with temporary depressions in semen quality. Serum testosterone levels decrease, FSH and LH increase shortly after the event, and semen quality diminishes about 70 days later, a reflection of germinative maturation time.

Endocrine conditions associated with hypospermatogenesis include hyperprolactinemia, glucocorticoid excess, hypothyroidism and hyperthyroidism, and "testicular toxicosis." *Excess prolactin* is found in approximately 3% of men with oligospermia and 13% of men with azospermia.[73, 74] Hyperprolactinemia can cause sexual dysfunction with impotence as well as reproductive failure. Hyperprolactinemia may be associated with either pituitary macroadenoma or microadenoma. Men with macroadenomas may have visual field abnormalities and headache. Although prolactin levels vary, levels over 200 ng/mL are most suggestive of macroadenoma. Other symptoms of pituitary adenoma may include loss of libido, impotence, galactorrhea, and gynecomastia in addition to depressed spermatogenesis. In addition to pituitary adenoma, other causes of hyperprolactinemia may include hypothalamic tumors, craniopharyngiomas, dopamine antagonists, hypothyroidism, and excess estrogen. Hyperprolactinemia inhibits gonadotrope secretion by inhibiting GnRH release; men with prolactinomas respond to an infusion of GnRH with an increase in LH.[75] Prolactin may also have a direct effect on the pituitary response to GnRH, a direct effect on the testis, and/or a direct effect on the central nervous system. Men with elevated prolactin levels who are given androgens may not have an improvement in libido as long as prolactin levels are elevated. The gonadal changes associated with hyperprolactinemia are also diverse and include hypospermatogenesis and, with severe prolactin elevation, Sertoli cell–only patterns (see later). By ultrastructural examination, seminiferous tubules show thickening of the lamina propria and basal lamina with focal invagination.[76] Sertoli cells show degeneration along their luminal aspect or an absence of normal junctions with maturing spermatids.

Excess glucocorticoids may be associated with oligospermia. The source of the steroids may be either endogenous or exogenous. Patients with Cushing syndrome may have decreased libido and impotence in addition to abnormal testicular function. Levels of serum testosterone, LH, and FSH are low. On testicular biopsy, hypospermia or maturation arrest may be seen.[77, 78] Removing the cause for the excess steroid may restore fertility. Abnormalities of thyroid function are rare causes of male infertility and represent only 0.6% of cases.[79] *Hypothyroidism* ranging from mild to marked may be associated with hypospermatogenesis on biopsy.[80] The effect of hypothyroidism on male fertility may be related to excess prolactin secondary to the elevated thyroid releasing hormone (TRH) levels. Treatment with thyroid hormone replacement can improve fertility. Juvenile hypothyroidism, although not a cause for infertility, can be associated with precocious testicular maturation, presumably through the effect of high levels of GnRH. Patients with *hyperthyroidism*, particularly thyrotoxicosis, have decreased sperm counts on semen analysis; testicular biopsies show varying degrees of hypospermatogenesis or incomplete maturation arrest.[81, 82] The mechanisms of infertility in hyperthyroidism are not well understood. Stress or increased temperature has been suggested, and endocrine factors are believed to play an important role since hyperthyroidism is associated with increased testosterone, estradiol, testosterone-binding globulin, and gonadotropin levels. The increased testosterone-binding globulin concentrations decrease the free testosterone, thus stimulating gonadotropins. Hudson and Edwards[83] have shown a decreased free testosterone/free estradiol ratio. Increased conversion of androgens to estrogens, partial Leydig cell failure, and subtle alterations in the sensitivity of the hypothalamus to feedback inhibition by sex steroids may also play roles.

"Testicular toxicosis" refers to familial gonadotropin-independent male sexual precocity, which is inherited as an autosomal dominant trait. The gonads of affected boys show hyperplasia of Leydig cells without Reinke crystals.[84, 85] Despite the prepubertal chronology, germ cells at all stages of maturation are seen, but with disorganization, degeneration, and abnormal spermatids. Sertoli cells show early development of tight junctions. Basement membrane and peritubular collagen may be increased. In adult patients with this syndrome there is marked oligospermia, and in the rare adult undergoing biopsy for infertility, degenerative changes in the germinative epithelium are accompanied by germ cell disorganization, peritubular fibrosis, and Leydig cell hyperplasia without Reinke crystals.[86]

INFERTILITY ASSOCIATED WITH MATURATION ARREST

Maturation arrest is present in 12% to 35% of testicular biopsy specimens in infertile men. In this pattern, spermatogenesis abruptly stops at an early stage, which is usually the primary spermatocyte level (Fig 5). The arrested cells may be increased in number and can be found sloughed into tubular lumina. No abnormalities of Sertoli cells, tunica propria, or Leydig cells are seen. When maturation occurs at the primary spermatocyte stage, degenerative chromatin changes may be seen.[87]

A wide variety of conditions may be associated with maturation arrest (Table 9), and a thorough clinical evaluation is required to identify the cause.

Occupational exposure to pesticides (particularly dibromochloropropane), heavy metals, and vinyl chloride, can be associated with this pat-

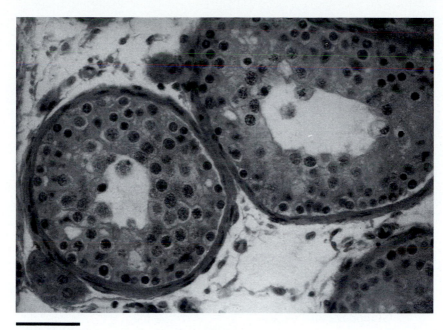

FIGURE 5.

Maturation arrest. In these seminiferous tubules, there is an abrupt cessation of maturation at the level of the primary spermatocyte (HE, original magnification × 160).

tern. Wong et al.[88] identified maturation arrest in several men with industrial exposure to petroleum products or lead fumes.

Down syndrome, or trisomy 21, is associated with a variety of testicular changes. During gestation, midterm fetuses show a decrease in the number of spermatogonia.[89] In adults, a variety of patterns can be found, with the most common histologic pattern being a mild decrease in the germinative epithelium with maturation arrest at the level of the primary spermatocyte. Other patterns may be seen, including hypospermatogenesis, Sertoli cell—only, and tubular hyalinization. Leydig cell abnormalities are not found. During spermatogenesis, the extra chromosome 21 associates with the XY complex, perhaps interfering with meiosis.[90]

An isolated deficiency of FSH is a very rare cause of hypogonadotropic infertility. The clinical manifestation is severe oligospermia or azospermia. The testes are of normal size and serum LH is normal, but serum FSH levels are low. Gonadotropin replacement may improve fertility, but FSH levels do not respond to GnRH infusion, thus suggesting a deficiency in hypothalamic releasing hormone specific for FSH.[91, 92]

INFERTILITY ASSOCIATED WITH SERTOLI CELL—ONLY SYNDROME

Absence of germinal epithelium without damage to Sertoli or Leydig cells is termed the "Sertoli cell—only" syndrome, also known as germinal aplasia or del Castillo syndrome. This is seen in 7% of cases with azospermia. The tubules are small in size and lined exclusively by elongated Sertoli cells arranged perpendicular to the basement membrane (Fig 6). The

TABLE 9.
Infertility Associated With Maturation Arrest*

Environmental
    Exposure to noxious chemicals
    Excessive heat exposure
    Chemotherapy
Genetic
    XYY
    Cystic fibrosis
    Adrenogenital syndrome
    Isolated follicle-stimulating hormone deficiency
    Sickle cell disease
Metabolic
    Uremia
Infection
    Mumps orchitis
Endocrine
    Glucocorticoid excess
    Postpubertal gonadotropin deficiency
Trauma
    Spinal cord injury, varicocele, vasectomy

*Adapted from Rudy F: Male infertility, in Hill GS (ed): *Uropathology*. New York, Churchill Livingstone, 1989. Used by permission.

basement membranes and tunica propria are usually normal. The number of Leydig cells is variable.

This histologic picture has been associated with the wide variety of conditions listed in Table 10. Generally, histology is not helpful in distinguishing the possibilities except that when the Sertoli cell–only pattern is associated with basement membrane thickening and Leydig cell hyperplasia, the adrenogenital syndrome may be suggested.[93] Idiopathic Sertoli cell–only syndrome has been considered to be a failure of primitive germ cells to migrate from the yolk sac to the developing gonadal primordia. Since many conditions can cause this pattern, it seems likely that this explanation holds for only a fraction of the idiopathic cases.

INFERTILITY ASSOCIATED WITH PERITUBULAR FIBROSIS AND TUBULAR HYALINIZATION

Generalized peritubular fibrosis is associated with a variety of clinical conditions (Table 11), but it almost always signifies a reduction in fertility. In these cases, the germinal epithelium is damaged by fibrosis interposed between it and the blood supply. Peritubular fibrosis may be caused by a proliferation of myofibroblasts of the tunica propria, by a dense band of collagen laid down between the basement membrane and the myofibroblasts of the tunica propria (Fig 7), by basement membrane thickening, or by a combination of these change. Fibrosis may be localized or

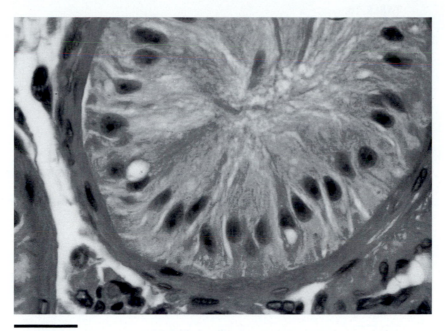

FIGURE 6.
Sertoli cell–only pattern. This tubule is lined only by Sertoli cells with prominent single nucleoli and abundant filigree cytoplasm. There is also some thickening of the tubular basement membrane (HE, original magnification × 160).

widespread, and the extent of sclerosis roughly parallels the impairment
in fertility. Men in whom these changes are present in more than 10% of
the tubules are hypofertile.[94] As the sclerosing process proceeds, the germinal epithelium is lost first, followed by the Sertoli cells, and at the end
stage the entire tubule is filled with collagen (Fig 8). Elastic fibers are usually present and indicate prior gonadotropin stimulation in puberty. Leydig cells are variable in number.

Exposure of a postpubertal testis to excess estrogen initially leads to
a failure of germ cell maturation, followed by progressive hypospermatogenesis, decreased diameter of the seminiferous tubules, and thickening
of the tunica propria. Eventually, if the estrogen exposure is continuous,
there is complete tubular sclerosis and Leydig cells become atrophic or
show vacuolization. Long-term exposure to excess estrogen inhibits the
hypothalamus and pituitary and causes decreased pituitary gonadotropin
secretion and subsequent testicular failure. Excess estrogen may come
from either endogenous or exogenous sources. A common cause of endogenous hyperestrinism is adrenocortical neoplasm, including adrenocortical adenoma carcinoma. Sertoli or Leydig cell tumors can secrete
both estradiol as well as estrogen. A relative excess of estrogen to androgen is seen in liver cirrhosis. Male-to-female transsexual patients are
chronically exposed to exogenous estrogens. The testes of the hyper-
estrinemic patients are small and atrophic at surgery. The histologic appearance of these gonads shows severe hypospermatogenesis with only
occasional residual spermatogonia, Sertoli cells, and tubular hyalinization.

Klinefelter syndrome, a relatively frequent cause of hypogonadism,

TABLE 10.
Infertility Associated With Sertoli Cell–Only Syndrome*

Environmental
  Chemotherapy
  Irradiation
Genetic
  Klinefelter syndrome with mosaicism
  XYY
  Down syndrome
Endocrine
  Adrenogenital syndrome
  Isolated follicle-stimulating hormone deficiency
Hyperprolactinemia
Metabolic
  Uremia
Infection
  Mumps orchitis
Varicocele
Idiopathic

*Adapted from Rudy F: Male infertility, in Hill GS (ed): *Uropathology*. New York, Churchill Livingstone, 1989. Used by permission.

TABLE 11.
Infertility Associated With Peritubular Fibrosis
and Tubular Hyalinization*

Environmental
  Chemotherapy
  Irradiation damage
  Alcoholism
Genetic
  Klinefelter syndrome
  Adrenogenital syndrome
  XYY
  Reifenstein syndrome
  Myotonic muscular dystrophy
  Cystic fibrosis
Endocrine
  Postpubertal androgen or estrogen excess
  Postpubertal hypopituitarism
  Androgen insensitivity in otherwise normal men
  Hypoprolactinemia
Mumps orchitis
Trauma
Vascular sclerosis (diabetes)
Varicocele
Idiopathic

*Adapted from Rudy F: Male infertility, in Hill GS (ed): *Uropathology*. New York, Churchill Livingstone, 1989. Used by permission.

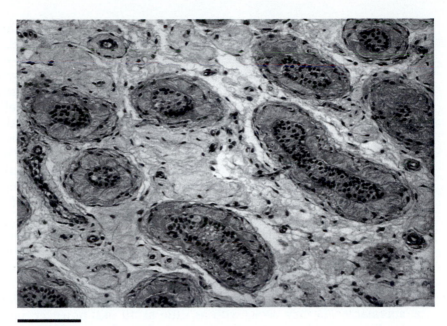

FIGURE 7.
Peritubular fibrosis. This testis is undergoing atrophy secondary to exogenous estrogen administration. There is marked peritubular fibrosis (HE, original magnification × 60).

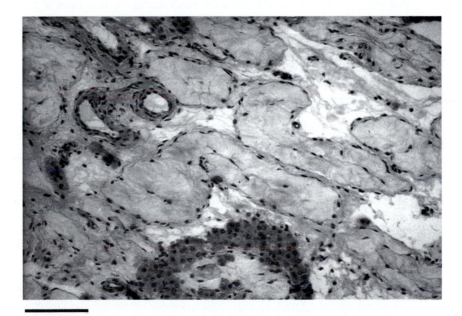

FIGURE 8.
Complete tubular hyalinization. This end-stage testis shows complete occlusion of tubular lumina by fibrosis. Aggregates of residual Leydig cells are seen in the interstitium (HE, original magnification × 60).

occurs in 0.2% of the general population. The classic genetic abnormality is a 47XXY chromosome complement that is thought to be the result of nondisjunction during meiosis. Other genetic abnormalities can also produce the Klinefelter phenotype. Some men with Klinefelter syndrome have a 46XX karyotype; these individuals express the H-Y antigen.[95] Patients with Klinefelter syndrome may also have a mosaicism of cells, with some having a normal 46XY complement and others the abnormal 46XXY karyotype. Adults with Klinefelter syndrome have small, firm testes usually measuring no more than 2 cm in maximum dimension. These patients have tall stature with a eunuchoid habitus. Cognitive function may be decreased. Virilization is variable, and gynecomastia is seen in 50% to 80% of cases. Mean serum testosterone levels are about 50% of normal, although there is great variability. Since this is a condition of primary testicular failure, FSH and LH levels are elevated. Azospermia is most common. Testicular damage is thought to be progressive, beginning in puberty and leading to a pattern of complete hyalinization, the most common pattern seen in adult patients with Klinefelter syndrome.

Radiation may also cause a pattern of peritubular fibrosis. Damage to spermatogonia may occur with as little as 10 rad; however, permanent sterility probably requires doses of more than 600 rad.[96] Acute changes include vacuolization and necrosis of spermatogonia; the spermatocytes and spermatids are relatively radioresistant. Since spermatogenesis takes about 70 days, hypofertility may not be present for many weeks after exposure. Chronic changes include thickening of the tunica propria and basement membranes, tubular atrophy, and loss of germ cells, eventually leaving tubules that are lined only by Sertoli cells or completely sclerosed. Leydig cells are usually preserved.

REFERENCES

1. Swerdloff RS, Wang C, Kandeel FR: Evaluation of the infertile couple. *Endocrinol Metab Clin North Am* 17:301–337, 1988.
2. Wong TW, Horvath KA: Pathological changes of the testis in infertility, in Gondos B, Riddick DH (eds): *Pathology of Infertility.* New York, Thieme Medical, 1987, pp 265–289.
3. Garcia-Diez LC, Corrales Hernandez JJ, Hernandez-Diaz J, et al: Semen characteristics and diabetes mellitus: Significance of insulin in male infertility. *Arch Androl* 26:119–127, 1991.
4. Adelman MM, Cahill EM: Atlas of Sperm Morphology Chicago, ASCP Press, 1989.
5. Bar-Charma N, Lamb DJ: Evaluation of sperm function: What is available in the modern andrology laboratory? *Urol Clin North Am* 21:433–446, 1994.
6. McClure RD: Male infertility: endocrine investigation and therapy. *Urol Clin North Am* 14:471–488, 1987.
7. Winters SJ, Sherins RJ, Loriaux DL: Studies on the role of sex steroids in the feedback control of gonadotropin concentrations in men. III. Androgen resistance and primary gonadal failure. *J Clin Endocrinol Metab* 48:553–558, 1979.
8. Bennet A, Bujan L, Plantavid M, et al: Luteinizing hormone pulse frequency and in vitro bioactivity in male idiopathic infertility. *Fertil Steril* 55:612–618, 1991.

9. Charny CW: Reflections on testicular biopsy. *Fertil Steril* 14:610, 1963.
10. Coburn M, Wheeler T, Lipshultz LI. Testicular biopsy: Its use and limitations. *Urol Clin North Am* 14:551–561, 1987.
11. Huff DS, Haadziselimovic F, Snyder H, et al: Histologic maldevelopment of unilaterally cryptorchid testes and their descended partners. *Eur J Pediatr* 152(suppl):10–14, 1993.
12. Mellidis C, Baker HW: Fine needle aspiration biopsy of the testis. *Fertil Steril* 61:367–375, 1994.
13. Gottschalk-Sabag S, Glick T, Weiss DB: *Acta Cytol* 37:67–72, 1993.
14. Jow WW, Steckel J, Schlegel PN, et al: Motile sperm in human testis specimens. *J Androl* 14:194–198, 1993.
15. Meinhard E, McRae CU, Chisholm GD: Testicular biopsy in evaluation of male infertility. *BMJ* 3:577–581, 1973.
16. Johnsen SG: Testicular biopsy score count—a method for registration of spermatogenesis in human testes: Normal values and results in 335 hypogonadal males. *Hormones* 1:2–25, 1970.
17. Clermont Y: Kinetics of spermatogenesis in mammals: Seminiferous epithelium cycle and spermatogonial renewal. *Physiol Rev* 52:198–236, 1972.
18. Schulze W, Rehder U: Organization and morphogenesis of the human seminiferous epithelium. *Cell Tissue Res* 237:395–407, 1984.
19. Schulze W, Reimer M, Rehder U, et al: Computer-aided three dimensional reconstructions of the arrangements of primary spermatocytes in human seminiferous tubules. *Cell Tissue Res* 244:1–8, 1986.
20. Steinberger E, Tjioe DY: A method for quantitative analysis of human seminiferous epithelium. *Fertil Steril* 19:959–961, 1968.
21. Weissbach L, Ibach B: Quantitative parameters for light microscopic assessment of the tubuli seminiferi. *Fertil Steril* 27:836–847, 1976.
22. Skakkebaek NE, Heller CG: Quantification of human seminiferous epithelium. I. Histological studies in twenty-one fertile men with normal chromosome complements. *J Reprod Fertil* 32:379–389, 1973.
23. Silber SJ, Rodriguez-Rigau LJ: Quantitative analysis of testicular biopsy: Determination of partial obstruction and prediction of sperm count after surgery for obstruction. *Fertil Steril* 36:480–485, 1981.
24. Zimmermann A, Truss F: The prognostic power of flow-through cytophotometric DNA determinations for testicular diseases. *Anal Quant Cytol* 2:247–251, 1980.
25. Evenson DP: Male germ cell analysis by flow cytometry: Effects of cancer, chemotherapy, and other factors on testicular function and sperm chromatin structure. *Ann N Y Sci* 468:350–367, 1986.
26. Evenson DP, Melamed MR: Rapid analysis of normal and abnormal cell types in human semen and testis biopsies by flow cytometry. *J Histochem Cytochem* 31(suppl 1A):248–253, 1983.
27. Evenson DP, Darzynkiewicz Z, Jost L, et al: Changes in accessibility of DNA to various fluorochromes during spermatogenesis. *Cytometry* 7:45–53, 1986.
28. Abyholm T, Clausen OPF: Clinical evaluation of DNA flow cytometry of fine needle aspirates from testis of infertile men. *Int J Androl* 4:505–514, 1981.
29. Kaufman DG, Nagler HM: Aspiration flow cytometry of the testes in the evaluation of spermatogenesis in the infertile male. *Fertil Steril* 48:287–291, 1987.
30. Hellstrom WJG, Stone AR, Deitch AD, et al: The clinical application of aspiration deoxyribonucleic acid flow cytometry to neurologically impaired men entering an electroejaculation program. *J Urol* 142:309–312, 1989.
31. Hirsch IH, Kulp-Hughes D, McCue P, et al: The value of quantitative testicular biopsy and deoxyribronucleic acid flow cytometry in predicting sperm recovery from electrostimulated ejaculates. *J Urol* 149:1345–1349, 1993.

32. Hirsch IH, McCue P, Kulp-Hughes D, et al: Validation of flow cytometric analysis in the objective assessment of spermatogenesis: Comparison to the quantitative testicular biopsy. *J Urol* 150:342–346, 1993.

33. Wong TW, Horvath KA, Kao NL: Chromosome abnormalities and male infertility, in Gondos B, Riddick DH (eds): *Pathology of Infertility*. New York, Thieme Medical, 1987, pp 243–263.

34. Ibrahim AA, Awad HA, El-Haggar S, et al: Bilateral testicular biopsies in men with varicocele. *Fertil Steril* 28:663–667, 1977.

35. Wong TW, Straus FH, Warner NE: Testicular biopsy in the study of male infertility. II. Post-testicular causes of infertility. *Arch Pathol* 95:160–164, 1973.

36. Lipschulz LI, Cunningham GR, Howard SS: Differential diagnosis of male infertility, in Lipschulz LI, Howards SS (eds): *Infertility in the Male*. New York, Churchill Livingstone, 1983, p 249.

37. Schellen TM, van Straaten A: Autosomal recessive hereditary congenital aplasia of the vasa deferencia in four siblings. *Feril Steril* 34:401–404, 1980.

38. Kaplan E, Schwachman H, Perlmutter AD, et al: Reproductive failure in males with cystic fibrosis. *N Engl J Med* 279:65, 1958.

39. Yeboah ED, Wadhwani JM, Wilson JB: Etiological factors of male infertility in Africa. *Int J Fertil* 37:300–307, 1992.

40. Gasparich JP, Mason JT, Greene HL, et al: Non-infectious epididymitis associated with amiodarone therapy. *Lancet* 2:1211–1212, 1984.

41. Bevan PC: Interferon induced parotitis and epididymitis. *Lancet* 1:561, 1985.

42. Gupta AS, Kothari LK, Bapna RB: Surgical sterilization by vasectomy and its effect on the structure and function of the testis in man. *Br J Surg* 62:59–63, 1975.

43. Jenkins IL, Muri VY, Blacklock NJ, et al: Consequences of vasectomy: An immunological and histological study related to subsequent fertility. *Br J Urol* 51:406–410, 1979.

44. Jarow JP, Budin RE, Dym M, et al: Quantitative pathologic changes in the human testis after vasectomy. *N Engl J Med* 313:1252–1256, 1985.

45. Eliasson R, Mossberg B, Camner P, et al: The immotile cilia syndrome: A congenital ciliary abnormality as an etiologic factor in chronic airway infections and male sterility. *N Engl J Med* 297:1–6, 1977.

46. Afzelius BA, Eliasson R: Flagellar mutants in man: On the heterogeneity of the immotile-cilia syndrome. *J Ultrastruct Res* 69:43–52, 1979.

47. Rossman CM, Forrest JB, Lee RM, et al: The dyskinetic cilia syndrome. Abnormal ciliary motility in association with abnormal ciliary ultrastructure. *Chest* 80:860–865, 1981.

48. Snoep MC, de Lange WE, Sluiter WJ, et al: Differential response of serum LH in hypogonadotropic hypogonadism and delayed puberty to LH-RH stimulation before and after clomiphene citrate administration. *J Clin Endocrinol Metab* 44:603–606, 1977.

49. Yoshimoto Y, Modidera K, Imura H: Restoration of a normal pituitary gonadotropin reserve by administration of luteinizing-hormone releasing hormone in patients with hypogonadotropic hypogonadism. *N Engl J Med* 292:242–245, 1975.

50. Spratt DI, Carr DB, Merriam GR, et al: The spectrum of abnormal patterns of gonadotropin-releasing hormone secretion in men with idiopathic hypogonadotropic hypogonadism: Clinical laboratory correlations. *J Clin Endocrinol Metab* 64:283–291, 1987.

51. Faiman C, Hoffman DL, Ryan RL, et al: The "fertile eunuch" syndrome: Demonstration of isolated luteinizing hormone deficiency by radioimmunoassay technique. *Mayo Clin Proc* 43:661–667, 1968.

52. Schwanzel-Fukuda M, Pfaff DW: Origin of luteinizing hormone–releasing hormone neurons. *Nature* 338:161–164, 1989.

53. Hoffman AR, Crowley WF: Induction of puberty in men by long-term pulsatile administration of low-dose gonadotropin-releasing hormone. *N Engl J Med* 307:1237–1241, 1982.

54. Butler MG: Prader-Willi syndrome: Current understanding of cause and diagnosis. *Am J Med Genet* 35:319–332, 1990.

55. Levine LS, Zachmann M, New MI, et al: Genetic mapping of the 21-hydroxylase deficiency gene within the HLA linkage group. *N Engl J Med* 299:911–915, 1979.

56. Carroll MC, Campbell RD, Porter RR: Mapping of steroid 21-hydroxylase genes to complement component C4 genes in HLA, the major histocompatibility locus in man. *Proc Natl Acad Sci U S A* 82:521–525, 1985.

57. Morel Y, Miller WL: Clinical and molecular genetics of congenital adrenal hyperplasia due to 21-hydroxylase deficiency. *Adv Hum Genet* 20:1–68, 1991.

58. Bonaccorsi AC, Adler I, Figueiredo JG: Male infertility due to congenital adrenal hyperplasia: Testicular biopsy findings, hormonal evaluation, and therapeutic results in three patients. *Fertil Steril* 47:664–670, 1987.

59. Steeno O, Knops J, Declerck L, et al: Prevention of fertility disorders by detection and treatment of varicocele at school and college age. *Andrologia* 8:47–53, 1976.

60. Steckel J, Dicker AP, Goldstein M: Relationship between varicocele size and response to varicocelectomy. *J Urol* 149:769–771, 1993.

61. World Health Organization: The influence of varicocele on parameters of fertility in a large group of men presenting to infertility clinics. *Fertil Steril* 57:1289–1293, 1992.

62. Pryor JL, Howards SS: Varicocele. *Urol Clin North Am* 14:499–513, 1987.

63. McFadden MR, Mehan DJ: Testicular biopsies in 101 cases of varicocele. *J Urol* 119:372–374, 1978.

64. Lentz RD, Bergstein J, Steffes MW, et al: Postpubertal evaluation of gonadal function following cyclophosphamide therapy before and during puberty. *J Pediatr* 91:385–394, 1977.

65. Quigely C, Cowell C, Jimenez M, et al: Normal or early development of puberty despite damage in children treated for acute lymphoblastic leukemia. *N Engl J Med* 321:143–151, 1989.

66. Wallace WHB, Shalet SM, Lendon M, et al: Male fertility in long-term survivors of childhood acute lymphoblastic leukemia. *Int J Androl* 14:312–319, 1991.

67. Chapman RM, Sutcliffe SB, Rees LH, et al: Cyclical combination chemotherapy and gonadal function. *Lancet* 1:285–289, 1979.

68. Biava CG, Smuckler EA, Whorton D: The testicular morphology of individuals exposed to dibromochloropropane. *Exp Mol Pathol* 29:448–458, 1978.

69. Lancranjan I, Popescu HI, Gavanescu O, et al: Reproductive ability of workmen occupationally exposed to lead. *Arch Environ Health* 30:396–401, 1975.

70. Steeno OP, Pangkahila A: Occupational influences on male fertility and sexuality. *Andrologia* 16:5–22, 1984.

71. Paul M, Himmelstein J: Reproductive hazards in the workplace: What the practitioner needs to know about chemical exposures. *Obstet Gynecol* 71:921–938, 1988.

72. Keck O, Bergmann M, Ernst E, et al: Autometallographic detection of mercury in testicular tissue of an infertile man exposed to mercury vapor. *Reprod Toxicol* 7:469–475, 1993.

73. Wong TW, Jones TM: Hyperprolactinemia and male infertility. *Arch Pathol Lab Med* 108:35–39, 1984.

74. Micic S, Micic M, Ilic V, et al: Hyperprolactinemia: Histological and meiotic analyses in azoospermic men. *Arch Androl* 8:217–220, 1982.

75. Carter JN, Tyson JE, Tolis G, et al: Prolactin secreting tumors and hypogonadism in 22 men. *N Engl J Med* 299:847–852, 1978.

76. Cameron DF, Murray FT, Drylie DD: Ultrastructural lesions in testes from hyperprolactinemic men. *J Androl* 5:283–293, 1984.

77. Mancini RE, Lavieri JC, Muller F, et al: Effect of prednisolone upon normal and pathologic human spermatogenesis. *Fertil Steril* 17:500–513, 1966.

78. Gabrilove JL, Nicols GL, Sohval AR: The testis in Cushing's syndrome. *J Urol* 112:95–99, 1974.

79. Dubin L, Amelar RD: Etiologic factors in 1294 consecutive cases of male infertility. *Fertil Steril* 22:469–474, 1971.

80. Wong TW, Straus FH, Warner NE: Testicular biopsy in the study of male infertility. III. Pretesticular causes of infertility. *Arch Pathol* 98:1–8, 1974.

81. Clyde HR, Walsh PC, English RW: Elevated plasma testosterone and gonadotropin levels in infertile males with hyperthyroidism. *Fertil Steril* 27:662–666, 1976.

82. Kidd GS, Glass AR, Vigersky RA: The hypothalamic-pituitary-testicular axis in thyrotoxicosis. *J Clin Endocrinol Metab* 48:798–802, 1979.

83. Hudson RW, Edwards AL: Testicular function in hyperthyroidism. *J Androl* 13:117–124, 1992.

84. Schedewie HK, Reiter EO, Beitins IZ, et al: Testicular Leydig cell hyperplasia as a cause of familial sexual precocity. *J Clin Endocrinol Metab* 52:271–278, 1981.

85. Gondos B, Egli CA, Rosenthal SM, et al: Testicular changes in gonadotropin-independent familial male sexual precocity. *Arch Pathol Lab Med* 109:990–995, 1985.

86. Gondos B: Development of the testis and associated disorders, in Gondos B, Riddick DH (eds): *Pathology of Infertility*. New York, Thieme Medical, 1987, pp 238–239.

87. Soderstrom KO, Suominen J: Histopathology and ultrastructure of miotic arrest in human spermatogenesis. *Arch Pathol Lab Med* 104:476–482, 1980.

88. Wong TW, Straus FH, Warner NE: Testicular biopsy in the study of male infertility. *Arch Pathol* 95:151–159, 1973.

89. Coerdt W, Rehder H, Gausmann I, et al: Quantitative histology of human fetal testes in chromosomal disease. *Pediatr Pathol* 3:245–259, 1985.

90. Johannison R, Gropp A, Winking H, et al: Down's syndrome in the male. Reproductive pathology and meiotic studies. *Hum Genet* 63:132–138, 1983.

91. Maroulis GB, Parlow AF, Marshall JR: Isolated follicle-stimulating hormone deficiency in man. *Fertil Steril* 28:818–822, 1977.

92. Al-Ansari AA, Khalil TH, Kelani Y, et al: Isolated follicle-stimulating deficiency in men: Successful long-term gonadotropin therapy. *Fertil Steril* 42:618–626, 1984.

93. Craig JM: The pathology of infertility. *Pathol Annu* 10:299, 1975.

94. Nelson WO: Interpretation of testicular biopsies. *JAMA* 151:449, 1953.

95. Wachtel SS, Koo GC, Breg WR, et al: Serologic detection of a Y-linked gene in XX males and XX true hermaphrodites. *N Engl J Med* 295:750–754, 1976.

96. Lushbaugh CC, Casaret GW: The effects of gonadal irradiation in clinical radiation therapy: A review. *Cancer* 37(suppl):1111–1125, 1976.

Diagnosis of Gastrointestinal Diseases in AIDS

Jan Marc Orenstein, M.D., Ph.D.
Professor of Pathology, Department of Pathology, George Washington University
Medical Center, Washington, D.C.

G astrointestinal diseases are exceedingly common worldwide complications of human immunodeficiency virus (HIV) infection and present a challenge to clinicians and pathologists alike.[1-16] Chronic diarrhea and wasting are frequent acquired immunodeficiency syndrome (AIDS)-defining diagnoses that all too often go unexplained. Even the most experienced of gastrointestinal pathologists are confronted with an array of processes that they may rarely if ever have encountered firsthand before. Many of the opportunistic gastrointestinal pathogens have been heretofore distinctly uncommon, whereas others had not been previously identified, even in patients with other forms of immunosuppression. The gastrointestinal tract in HIV disease is the target of a full range of viral, fungal, and protozoal pathogens. Coinfections are particularly common and occur simultaneously at both the same and different levels of the alimentary tract. Infectious and proliferative/neoplastic processes occur throughout the alimentary tract, from the mouth to the anus. Symptoms include dysfunction, diarrhea, wasting, malabsorption, pain, bleeding, bloating, and obstruction.

Whether HIV is a direct enteric pathogen in its own right is a controversial issue.[17-22] There is little if any HIV infection of enterocytes, but lamina propria and intraepithelial mononuclear cells are infected at all levels of the gastrointestinal tract. As more pathogens are identified and fewer patients are left without a specific diagnosis after adequate workup, HIV is less frequently invoked as the explanation for patients' gastrointestinal symptoms and histopathology.

Not only is the compromised immune state responsible for the opportunism, but it also helps explain the confounding cellular responses.[23] Inflammatory bowel disease is common in the HIV-infected age group and, presumably because of the patient's altered immune state, can present a diagnostic and therapeutic challenge. Furthermore, processes can mimic one another, e.g., CMV infection of the ileum can resemble Crohn's disease.

Since others have surveyed gastrointestinal diseases in HIV infection, the approach taken here is to emphasize the diagnostic evaluation of gastrointestinal biopsy specimens.[1, 13, 14]

How will this area of diagnostic pathology fare in this age of managed health care? Of course no one can be sure, but if the criteria are clini-

Advances in Pathology and Laboratory Medicine®, vol. 8
© 1995, Mosby–Year Book, Inc.

cal utility, patient care, and cost containment, the rapid and accurate diagnosis of gastrointestinal diseases in HIV-infected patients should logically fare well. Many of the pathogens are treatable, whereas others are the subject of intense drug development, some with promising preliminary results.

DIAGNOSTIC CONSIDERATIONS

Poor-quality hematoxylin-eosin–stained sections are unfortunately much too often the cause of missed diagnoses. Small, fragile, endoscopic gastrointestinal biopsy specimens are particularly sensitive to mishandling, the introduction of artifacts during processing, poor slide preparation, and misinterpretation. Taking into consideration the patient and his or her symptoms, the gastroenterologist must decide on the most appropriate diagnostic evaluation. As regards the specimen, the pathologist must decide on the most appropriate approach for arriving at the diagnosis.

In most situations, stool studies should come first, except perhaps when gastrointestinal bleeding is prominent.[14, 24] If a potential pathogen is detected in the stool, it should be appropriately treated. If no potential etiologic agent is identified or if the therapy fails, endoscopy should logically ensue. However, one must always consider the patient's condition (e.g., whether endoscopy can be tolerated) and whether nonspecific treatment (e.g., antidiarrheal agents) may be more appropriate under the circumstances. An inherent problem with this stool-first approach lies in the adequacy of the evaluation of the stool specimen. A typical stool analysis includes *Clostridium difficile* toxin studies; cultures for *Salmonella, Shigella,* and *Campylobacter* species; and ova and parasite studies for *Cryptosporidium, Isospora,* and *Giardia.*[7, 25, 26] Viral studies are problematic, not just because of their difficulty but also in interpreting their clinical relevance, e.g., identification of cytomegalovirus (CMV) in stool.[11] The sensitivity and accuracy of standard stool studies in HIV-infected patients are unknown and, as with interpretation of biopsy specimens, probably vary, especially when comparing laboratories in the epicenters of the HIV epidemic with those in emerging areas. At this time, microbiology laboratories should also be able to identify the spores of microsporidia and cyclospora cayetanensis in stool, as well as the organisms described earlier. The modified trichrome chromotrope 2R[27–29] and the fluorescence chitin spore stains[30] have revolutionized the stool diagnosis of microsporidiosis.[31] Stool studies should also screen for adenovirus,[32, 33] enteropathogenic *Escherichia coli,*[34, 35] and spirochetes,[36] which are all potentially important pathogens.

The argument becomes progressively less tenable for those who maintain that since many of the gastrointestinal pathogens in HIV disease are not treatable, nonspecific therapy should be initiated and endoscopy omitted.[37, 38] A negative stool is only the first diagnostic step since some infections may be harder to diagnose by stool examination, e.g., isosporiasis, small intestinal cryptosporidiosis, *Mycobacterium avium* complex (MAC), and giardiasis. Promising drugs for treating *Cryptosporidium* (e.g., paromomycin) are being tested, and one of the two diarrheogenic species of microsporidia, *Septata intestinalis,* responds completely to albendazole.[39–42] Precise diagnoses are of increasing importance for patients; endoscopy provides specimens not only for diagnostic microscopic analyses but also for culture and molecular analysis, as well as for clinical and basic research. It is important to appreciate that drug development depends on comprehensive diagnoses and follow-up. In addition to the biopsy specimen, intestinal (duodenal and colonic) aspirates should be obtained since not only are they easily acquired during endoscopy but, because of the relatively high concentration of organisms and low background, they are excellent for identifying ova and parasites and for culture as well.

All patients with diarrhea are not the same. Some suffer from malabsorption, wasting, and voluminous diarrhea, typical of small-bowel disease. Others have a more irritable, colonic-type diarrhea with frequent small stools. Still others have both manifestations. Some gastroenterologists choose to perform upper and lower endoscopy at the same diagnostic session, others seem to consistently start with colonoscopy (sigmoidoscopy is inadequate) followed by upper endoscopy if the lower gastrointestinal study is negative, and still others perform colonoscopy and include ileal biopsy. Whichever the endoscopic approach, it should ultimately be comprehensive if tolerated by the patient.

WHAT IS AN ADEQUATE BIOPSY SPECIMEN?

The answer relates to the patient's symptoms, the endoscopic findings, and the level of the gastrointestinal tract examined. Whereas a biopsy of the base of an esophageal ulcer may readily disclose CMV (because it preferentially infects endothelium in the gastrointestinal tract), it is much less likely to reveal herpes simplex virus (HSV) or *Candida* (which particularly involve the epithelium)[43–49] (Fig 1). The best approach to an esophageal ulcer is to include samplings of the base and epithelial margins of any ulcer, as well as samplings of superficial erosions and exophytic lesions.[44–52] Whereas the endoscopist may clearly visualize an esophageal lesion, such is not necessarily the case elsewhere in the bowel, where gross changes may be subtle at best. However, even an apparently normal-appearing esophagus may reveal CMV endotheliitis in the lamina propria and/or superficial epithelial candidiasis. A grossly normal-appearing intestine may harbor virtually any known pathogen.[53–55] In general, random biopsies, as well as samples of gross lesions, are warranted and can be surprisingly productive. To perform endoscopy and not take biopsy specimens is insupportable unless there is a bleeding diathesis, and in that case, duodenal and colonic aspirates and mucosal cytobrush specimens are excellent diagnostic alternatives.[56–60]

WHAT LEVELS OF THE GASTROINTESTINAL TRACT SHOULD BE EVALUATED?

An examination limited to the esophagus (Table 1) may be all that seems warranted in response to odynophagia or dysphagia (unless the lesion extends into the stomach). However, evaluation of the stomach (Table 2) and duodenum (Table 3) in the same patient may reveal pathology (gross and microscopic) obscured by the esophageal complaints (and vice versa).

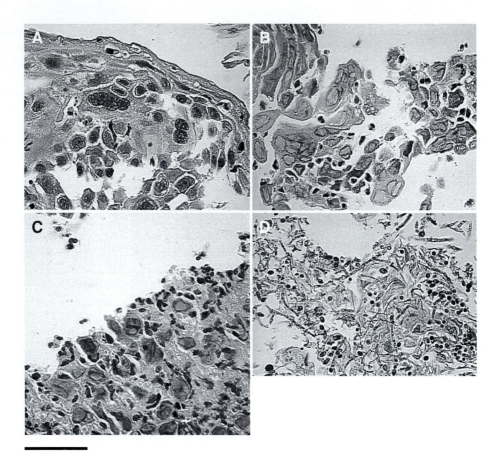

FIGURE 1.

A, dissociating squamous cells contain multinucleated cells that lack the characteristic ground glass appearance of HSV seen in the free multinucleated squamous cells **(B)** and in mono and binucleate macrophages in an ulcer base **(C)** (HE, original magnification ×640). **D,** esophageal epithelial debris mixed with hyphae and spores of *Candida albicans* and mixed bacteria infection (HE, original magnification ×40). (See also color plate.)

Gastrointestinal biopsy specimens have given the first indication of infection (or dissemination) by CMV, *Mycobacterium*, *Cryptococcus*, *Histoplasma*, and Pneumocystis carinii, as well as identified unsuspected microsporidia, *Cryptosporidium*, and *Giardia* infections[1, 61, 62] (Figs 2 and 3). Thus upper gastrointestinal endoscopy in an HIV-infected patient should routinely include examination and sampling of the esophagus, stomach, and duodenum.

Chronic diarrhea, malabsorption, and epigastric or left upper quadrant pain are symptoms that should lead to an upper endoscopy with evaluation of the esophagus, stomach, distal portion of the duodenum, and (according to some) the proximal segment of the jejunum. Lesional and random biopsy samples from all of these sites are warranted. Unless unfeasible, small-bowel evaluation should never stop at the proximal portion of the duodenum; the distal end of the duodenum (third and fourth portions) and, when possible, the proximal portion of the jejunum should

TABLE 1.
Esophagus

Pathogen*	Infected Cell(s)	Diagnostic Site†	Histopathology	HE‡, Section	Special Stains/Procedures
CMV	Endothelium >>> macs and mesenchyme, not epithelium	Lamina propria	NSHA through ulcers	Large purple INI, red granular ICI	IHC, ISH, PCR
HSV	Epithelium>> macs	Ulcer edge >> base	Ulcers, many macs	Glassy gray INI, multinucleated epithelium, mononucleated and binucleated macs. No ICI	IHC, ISH, PCR
Candida	Epithelium	Surface	Invasion of the surface through ulcers. Bacterial overgrowth	Oval purple spores, nonseptated pink hyphae. Larger *C. tropicalis*	GMS, PAS; fragments of hyphae and debris

*Rare infections by Epstein-Barr virus, herpes zoster, human papillomavirus, papovavirus, *Actinomyces*, *Aspergillus*, *Cryptococcus*, Kaposi sarcoma, *mycobacterium avium complex* (MAC), *Pneumocystis carinii*, *Cryptosporidium*, and *Penicillium chrysogenum*.
†Must be included in the specimen.
‡HE = hematoxylin-eosin; CMV = cytomegalovirus; >, >>, >>> = increasing degree of difference/frequency; macs = macrophages; mesenchyme = smooth muscle cells, fibroblasts; NSHA = no specific histologic abnormality; INI = intranuclear inclusion; ICI = intracytoplasmic inclusion; IHC = immunohistochemistry; ISH = in situ hybridization; PCR = polymerase chain reaction; HSV = herpes simplex virus; GMS = Gomori methenamine silver stain; PAS = periodic acid–Schiff stain.

TABLE 2.
Stomach*

Pathogen†	Infected Cell(s)	Diagnostic Site‡	Histopathology	HE, Section	Special Stains/Procedures
CMV	Endothelium >>> macs and mesenchyme, rare epithelium	Lamina propria	NSHA through rare ulcers	Large purple INI, red granular ICI; epithelial INI, rare ICI	IHC, ISH, PCR
Cryptosporidium	Epithelium, surface and glands	Mucosa	Atrophy, disarray, dilated glands, ± PMNs§	Small round bodies "in" brush border	Giemsa, darker blue
Helicobacter pylori	Associated with surface and glandular epithelium	Mucosa	NSHA through dilated glands, ± PMNs	Small undulating pink bacteria on surface	WS, Giemsa

*See Table 1 for abbreviations.
†Rare infections by *Treponema pallidum, Candida, Aspergillus*.
‡Must be included in the specimen.
§PMN = polymorphonuclear neutrophil; WS = Warthin-Starry stain.

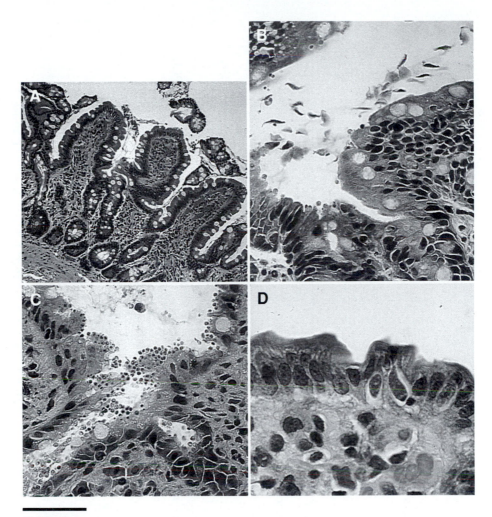

FIGURE 2.

A, a relatively well-oriented small bowel biopsy displaying the nonspecific pleomorphic villi and elongated crypts which can be seen in cryptosporidiosis, microsporidiosis, and giardiasis, which this is (HE, original magnification ×160). **B,** comma– and horseshoe crab–shaped *Giardia lamblia* organisms adjacent to the brush border. The areas of epithelial disarray seem to be more closely associated with the *Cryptosporidium* coinfection (HE, original magnification ×640). **C,** innumerable cryptosporidia stud the small bowel surface and crypt epithelium. Note the epithelial disarray, cytoplasmic vesiculation, and cell and nuclear pleomorphism (HE, original magnification ×640). **D,** isospora schizonts infecting two adjacent small bowel surface epithelial cells. This parasite develops within loose parasitophorous vacuoles usually near the basement membrane (HE, original magnification ×1,000). (See also color plate.)

be sampled (e.g., *Enterocytozoon bieneusi* appears to prefer the more distal of these sites)[63] (Fig 4,A–C).

The large bowel, from the cecum to the rectum, should be thoroughly examined and sampled (collected in separately labeled containers) in patients complaining of symptoms compatible with a lower gastrointestinal origin (Table 4). Enteropathogenic bacterial infections appear to preferentially involve the right colon; adenovirus is more common in biopsy

TABLE 3.
Small Intestine*

Pathogen†	Infected Cells(s)	Diagnostic Site‡	Histopathology	HE, Section	Special Stains/Procedures
Cryptosporidium	Enterocytes of villi and crypts. Brunner's glands and ducts	Mucosa (villi and crypts)	Subtle through severe atrophy. V/V§ ± PMNs. Cryptitis, crypt abscesses	2- to 3-μm intracellular extracytoplasmic bodies in BB	Giemsa, darker blue. Not acid-fast, IHC
CMV	Endothelium >>> macs and mesenchyme. Rare Brunner's gland epithelium	Lamina propria	NSHA through moderate epithelial damage, PMNs in lamina propria and epithelium. Ileal ulcers, crypt mitoses and apoptosis	Large purple INI, red granular ICI	IHC, ISH, PCR
Giardia lamblia	None, near BB	Intervillus area	Mild damage, V/V, atrophy	Bluish horseshoe crab to comma shaped, 1–2 nuclei	Giemsa, blue to purple

Isospora belli	Epithelium, rare macs	Villus surface	Mild disarray	Parasite stages in vacuole near basement membrane	Giemsa, dark blue
Enterocytozoon bieneusi	Enterocytes, distal villus	Tips of villi	Shedding cells, cell and villus atrophy, disarray, V/V, IELs	Supranuclear blue bodies ± clear clefts and cupped nuclei, refractile spores in shed cells	B&B & WS, polarize
Septata intestinalis	Enterocytes, distal villus >> crypts, plus macs	Villi and lamina propria	Cell and villus atrophy, IELs, disarray, V/V	Clusters of supranuclear refractile bodies, pseudo-Gaucher macs	B&B & WS, polarize
Mycobacterium avium complex	Macrophages	Lamina propria	Blunting, epithelial disarray	Gaucher-like gray filamentous cytoplasm	AF, GMS, PAS

*Abbreviations as in Tables 1 and 2.

†Also Whipple's disease-like pathogens: Mycobacterium kansasii (longer, beaded, crook shaped), Histoplasma capsulatum (midwest United States budding yeast). Mycobacterium tuberculosis is rarely found in the gastrointestinal tract of persons infected with human immunodeficiency virus. Candida is rare outside the esophagus.

‡Must be included in the specimen.

§V/V = vesiculation and vacuolization; BB = brush border; IEL = intraepithelial lymphocyte; B&B & WS = Brown-Brenn and Warthrin-Starry modified for microsporidia; AF = acid-fast stain.

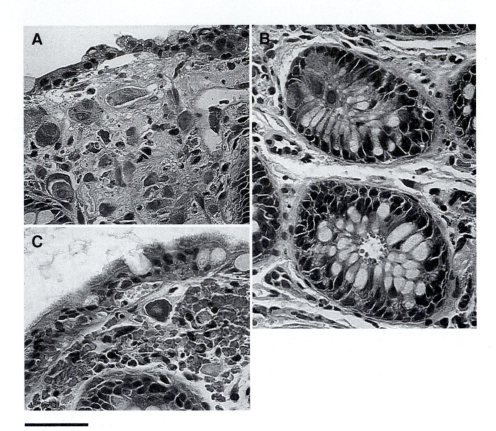

FIGURE 3.

A, colon biopsy with innumerable CMV-infected endothelial cells and lamina propria macrophages. The intranuclear inclusions are ill-defined and more purple-staining than the granular red intracytoplasmic inclusions. Note the fragile sloughing epithelium (HE, original magnification ×640). **B,** a purple-staining intranuclear inclusion in a CMV-infected colonic crypt epithelial cell. The surface blebs in the adjacent crypt can be mistaken for *Cryptosporidium* (HE, original magnification ×640). **C,** a dual spirochete:CMV-infected rectal biopsy specimen. The spirochetes appear as a fine purplish surface fuzz. The CMV-infected endothelial cell has a deep purple intranuclear inclusion and fills a capillary lumen near damaged epithelium (HE, original magnification ×640). (See also color plate.)

specimens of the distal end of the colon and rectum, CMV is more abundant in the right colon and *Cryptosporidium* burden can vary widely[1, 34, 35, 64–67] (Figs 3 and 5). Since the ileum is a "window" on small-bowel infections and may reveal microsporidiosis, giardiasis, and cryptosporidiosis, it should be sampled during colonoscopy if possible.

HOW MANY PIECES OF TISSUE ("BITES") CONSTITUTE AN ADEQUATE BIOPSY SPECIMEN?

Although this issue has never been critically evaluated, personal experience suggests that at least three bites is warranted. Pathologic processes can vary considerably from bite to bite in a specimen. Experienced gastroenterologists incur no greater rate of complications when taking multiple bites at each level, e.g., six to ten bites, than after removing a single piece of tissue (something that is seen all too frequently). These six to ten bites allow for light microscopy (LM) (three to six), transmission elec-

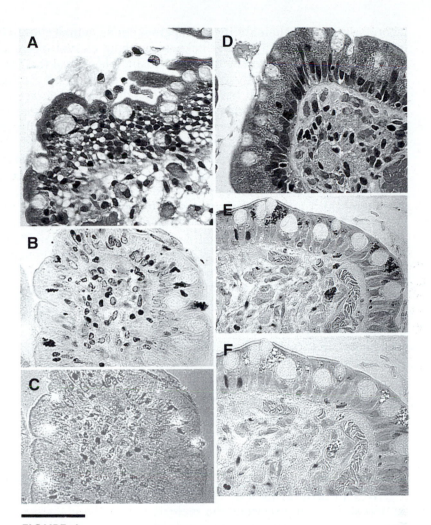

FIGURE 4.

A, a tell-tale sign of *Enterocytozoon bieneusi* infection is the shedding of pyknotic epithelial cells containing small white refractile spores. Plasmodia appear as purple supranuclear bodies, some with clear clefts. Note the apparent piling-up of epithelial cells, the intraepithelial lymphocytes, and the disarray (HE, original magnification ×640). **B** and **C,** spores of *E. bieneusi* stained with the modified Warthin-Starry stain appear as oval black bodies on a yellow background and polarize a yellow-white (HE, original magnification ×640). **D,** *S. intestinalis* appears as collections of bluish supranuclear bodies in epithelial cells. Note the molding of the apical nuclear pole. Infected lamina propria macrophages have a clear granular cytoplasm (HE, original magnification ×640). **E** and **F,** modified Brown-Brenn–stained *S. intestinalis* appear as aggregates of small red to blue structures on a yellow background. Note the positive lamina propria macrophages. The organisms polarize white on a yellow background (HE, original magnification ×640). (See also color plate.)

tron microscopy (TEM) (one or two), culture (one or two), and freezing (one or two).

It is not unusual to see intestinal biopsy specimens extensively stripped of their surface epithelium. This may result from intrinsic tissue fragility (e.g., due to CMV infection), a heavy biopsy hand, or suboptimal specimen handling following biopsy (see Fig 3). Histopathology laboratories vary in their ability to prepare sections, which should be uniformly cut, about 4 to 5 μm in thickness, without chatter or cracks, and stained with well-balanced hematoxylin-eosin. It is critical that the specimen be transferred directly from the endoscope (e.g., by toothpick or needle) to the fixative and never be put in saline or in contact with absorbent materials. A specimen stripped of its epithelium is no impediment to identifying CMV-infected lamina propria endothelial cells, but the CMV burden may be so low that not all pieces of tissue have identifiable inclusions at all specimen levels. On the other hand, having the superficial epithelium intact is critical for diagnosing microsporidiosis since these protozoal parasites almost exclusively infect only distal villus enterocytes[55] (see Fig 4). *Cryptosporidium* organisms may be confined to either small intestinal villi or crypts (see Fig 2),[67] and *Isospora* is usually found in scattered superficial enterocytes. Mycobacterial infections may be very focal and subtle, and enteropathogenic bacteria and adenovirus are typically focal (see Figs 2,D and Fig 5). These are all reasons why it is necessary for a specimen to include several bites and for the specimen to be handled and prepared well.

WHEN SHOULD SAMPLES BE TAKEN FOR OTHER THAN ROUTINE PARAFFIN-SECTION LIGHT MICROSCOPY?

Those skilled in ultrastructural diagnosis believe that samples (lesional and random) for TEM should be taken routinely.[68] Semithin plastic section LM often obviates the need for paraffin section special stains by clearly demonstrating infections by *Mycobacterium*, *Giardia*, *P. carinii*, *Histoplasma*, *Cryptococcus*, and microsporidia of either species. The major drawback to plastic sections (no matter whether stained with toluidine blue or the combined methylene blue, azure II, and basic fuchsin stains) is in identification of viral inclusions (e.g., CMV, HSV, and adenovirus). In plastic sections the inclusions lack the characteristic tinctorial properties that make them stand out in hematoxylin-eosin–stained sections.[68, 69] Practically speaking (in terms of laboratory resources), plastic embedding for LM (and correspondingly, TEM evaluation) may not currently be readily available and may be less so in the future. It may be hoped that there will continue to be electron microscopy laboratories, e.g., in academic medical centers, that can provide assistance for TEM, either as part of research interests or as a diagnostic service.

It is important to reiterate that in all fields of pathology, appreciation of ultrastructural and plastic section histology greatly enhances LM diagnosis and especially so in the setting of opportunistic infections.[68] With experience, one finds that TEM and even plastic section LM will be called upon less frequently as a diagnostic aid, save for perhaps with coinfections, a low pathogen burden, and/or unexplained or unusual LM findings. One finds that well-prepared hematoxylin-eosin–stained paraffin sections will be more than adequate to diagnose the majority of gastrointestinal pathogens.[70–72]

Formalin-fixed specimens are perfectly adequate for TEM; the interval between biopsy and fixation is much more important than whether the fixative is glutaraldehyde or formalin. Thus a small fraction of any

TABLE 4.
Large Intestine*

Pathogen†	Infected Cell(s)	Diagnostic Site‡	Histopathology	HE, Section	Special Stains/Procedures
Cryptosporidium	Endothelium >>> macs and mesenchyme >> crypt epithelium	Mucosa	Subtle through erosions and cryptitis, crypt abscesses, PMNs	Small round bodies in BB	Giemsa, darker blue
Mycobacterium avium complex	Lamina propria, macs	Lamina propria	Subtle through moderate	Gaucher-like cells, bluish gray filamentous cytoplasm	AF, GMS, PAS
Escherichia coli	Surface epithelium	Mucosa	Focal damage, defects, cobblestone, shedding	Bacilli, coccobacilli, coat defects, shedding cells	Gram (−), Giemsa (+)
Spirochetes	Surface into crypt mouth	Mucosa	Mild focal damage	Undulating bluish fuzz replacing BB	WS
Adenovirus	Surface epithelium	Mucosa	Focal damage, cell debris	Amphophilic goblet cell nuclei, basal orientation	¼ to full-moon INI, IHC
CMV	Endothelium >>> macs and mesenchyme >> crypt epithelium	Lamina propria and crypts	Subtle through ulcers, fragile surface	Large purple INI, granular red ICI	IHC, ISH, PCR

* Abbreviations as in Tables 1 to 3.
†Rare infections by herpes simplex virus, cryptoccocosis, leishmaniasis, toxoplasmosis, *Histoplasma capsulatum* (midwest United States), and Whipple's disease−like pathogens.
‡Must be included in the specimen.

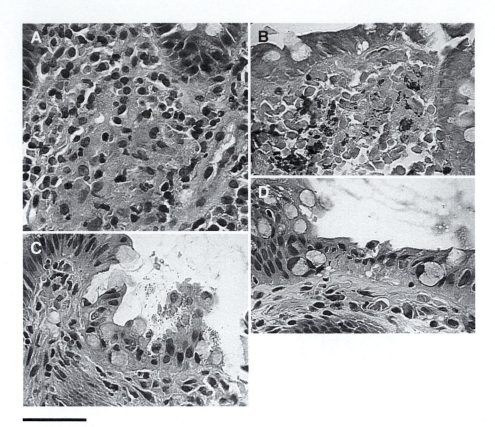

FIGURE 5.

A and **B,** a subtle collection of macrophages with abundant pink fibrillar cytoplasm (HE stain) located deep in the colonic lamina propria **(A).** Ziehl-Neelsen,
acid fast stain (same biopsy, different area) reveals red-staining bacilli in macrophage cytoplasm **(B)** (HE, original magnification ×640). **C,** colonic epithelium
damaged by attaching and effacing bacilli which appear as small blue rods coating epithelial defects and shedding cells (HE, original magnification ×640). **D,**
adenovirus-infected colorectal goblet cells with purple-staining 1/4− to 1/2−
moon-shaped intranuclear inclusions. Note the damaged epithelium and that the
mucin is lateral to or beneath the infected nuclei (HE, original magnification
×640). (See also color plate.)

biopsy specimen (trimmed off with a fresh scalpel blade) received in formalin can be transferred to buffered glutaraldehyde and set aside for potential TEM. One strategy (employed at our institution) is to use enough
of the TEM specimen (sampling all pieces of tissue and grossly different
areas in larger specimens) to yield eight plastic blocks (0.5 to 1.0 mm
each) and to save the rest in glutaraldehyde. Finally, even a
glutaraldehyde-fixed specimen can be processed into paraffin (although
there is some minor difference in staining results and immunohistochemistry can be problematic).

HOW SHOULD THE PATHOLOGIST HANDLE THE BIOPSY SPECIMEN?

As with any specimen submitted to pathology, it is important to know
the relevant clinical history, e.g., symptoms, HIV status, AIDS, known op-

portunistic infections and malignancies, latest CD4 cell count, and previous gastrointestinal history, including specimens and diagnoses. It is not necessary to orient gastrointestinal biopsy specimens for diagnostic evaluation, particularly if the number of bites is adequate and the tissue has been properly embedded for sectioning of its long axis. Sections should be cut from three levels of the block (from half of the total block: first "full" tissue face and 25% and 50% into the block, respectively). This preserves tissue for histochemical stains and retrieval for TEM if necessary. There should be three to five sections on each slide. For esophageal biopsy tissue, it is a distinct advantage to have multiple levels and sections for diagnosing CMV, *Candida*, and HSV esophagitis (see Table 1). In the stomach, *Cryptosporidium*, CMV, and *Helicobacter pylori* infections are often quite focal (see Table 2). Multiple levels in small-bowel specimens are important for CMV and *Isospora* detection but tend to be less critical for the identification of microsporidia, *Cryptosporidium*, and *Giardia* (Table 3). In the large bowel (Table 4), multiple levels and sections are more important for detecting CMV, adenovirus, mycobacteria, and enteropathogenic bacteria than *Cryptosporidium*.

The evaluation scheme often depends on the source of the specimen and what is observed in the very first section examined. *Candida* hyphae and spores and HSV-infected cells may be found only in small fragments of the specimen and may only be in one level. A recommended approach is to scrutinize every piece of tissue (even the tiniest fragments) in at least one section of each level with 4× to 40× objectives. An oil-immersion lens (63× or 100×) is rarely necessary except perhaps for photography. If one begins with examination of the middle section (second of three or third of five), one has the option of examining a suspicious area in adjacent sections. If necessary, each section on a slide may be examined, but perhaps only with a 20× lens.

It seems logical to not only render a diagnosis but also convey some estimate (albeit semiquantitative) of the severity of the process, e.g., pathogen burden, histopathology (erosions and ulcers), and crypt vs. surface epithelial involvement.[67] This information can be helpful for clinicopathologic correlation, e.g., whether the findings adequately explain the symptoms and the endoscopic findings, and for comparison with follow-up specimens.

Before placing the slide on the microscope stage, one should note the number of pieces of tissue and their relative size. All specimens are then screened with a 4× lens (10× eyepieces) to evaluate for overall architecture, state of the specimen, and features that require closer scrutiny, e.g., ulcers/erosions, villus flattening, and crypt loss and distortion. The lamina propria, crypts, and surface epithelium should be consciously and systematically examined separately at progressively higher magnifications up to 40×. With this approach one is less likely to overlook a few CMV-infected endothelial cells, a small collection of mycobacteria-infected lamina propria macrophages, several *Cryptosporidium*-infected crypt epithelial cells, or a few *Giardia* organisms between villi (see Figs 2, 3, and 5). Disciplined examination is important because the cellular response in an immunocompromised HIV-infected patient may be of little help since it generally reflects more the degree of immunodeficiency than the pathogen.

Architectural abnormalities of any degree should initiate a search for an explanation. A "normal-appearing" specimen with, for example, long delicate villi, short tight crypts, tall columnar epithelial cells with "identical" basal nuclei, homogeneously stained cytoplasm, and a crisp brush border, rarely harbors a pathogen, let alone a symptomatic one. However, it is possible to find a rare, CMV-infected endothelial cell in a specimen that otherwise appears normal. Finding a few CMV-infected endothelial cells in otherwise normal tissue may indicate that there is a more significant CMV infection elsewhere in the gastrointestinal tract or body or that the patient has a "generalized" CMV endotheliitis. Parenthetically, the intranuclear inclusions of CMV are surprisingly easy to identify in a well-balanced hematoxylin-eosin–stained section, even with a 10× or 20× objective. There are few things that mimic the cytologic appearance of CMV; these include the large purple-staining activated macrophage (common in ulcers), which has a smaller and bluer nucleus with a prominent central reddish purple nucleolus and a prominent nuclear membrane, and the lighter-staining ganglion cell nucleus, which also has a prominent central nucleolus.[43, 69, 73]

Knowledge of the range of possible pathogens common to each gastrointestinal location, their characteristic histopathology, and their appearance under different staining conditions, together with an intense curiosity, is a critical asset to approaching gastrointestinal specimens.

One should look for histologic features that break the monotonous pattern characteristic of normal bowel tissue. An explanation should be sought for shortened/atrophied/blunted and pleomorphic villi which are usually associated with elongated crypts (normal ratio of 3 or 5 to 1) and for distorted or dilated crypts or distorted Brunner glands. Evaluation of the inflammatory response should include a search for collections of lamina propria neutrophils or histiocytes, increased intraepithelial lymphocytes, and epithelial infiltrates of neutrophils and eosinophils. Indications of increased cell turnover include cellular debris in the epithelium, sloughing of individual cells or strips of cells, crypt mitoses, and apoptotic cells. Individual features worthy of note are enterocyte atrophy (cuboidal, flattened, pleomorphic), inhomogeneous enterocyte staining, enlarged or pleomorphic nuclei, change in goblet cell distribution, and cytoplasmic vesiculation/vacuolization.

It goes without saying that pathologists are at their best when analyzing a specimen that has been properly obtained, handled, and prepared. Ultimately, faults in the system are costly to everyone, especially the patient. Sections from intestinal biopsy specimens submitted from some very experienced institutions in epicenters of the HIV epidemic have been surprisingly poor (torn, crushed, folded, variably stained, too thick, and full of chatter and cracks). Hematoxylin-eosin stains may be unbalanced, either too pink (eosinophilic) or too blue (basophilic). Since most, if not all diagnoses will be made by hematoxylin-eosin section (with experience), a consistent and reliable routine hematoxylin-eosin–stained section is vital and automated staining devices are helpful. Diagnosing microsporidiosis, adenovirus infection, and isosporiasis are particularly difficult in a poor specimen. Giardiasis, cryptosporidiosis, mycobacteria, and candidiasis are somewhat easier but will more likely require special stains for verification if the initial hematoxylin-eosin sections are not good.[74]

Since coinfections are common in the gastrointestinal tract of HIV-infected patients, conscientious examination of the material must be carried out to its completion, regardless of what is found partway through the examination. Coinfections are especially problematic since the histopathology induced by one pathogen may obfuscate the identification of another pathogen and obscure evidence of its presence. One should be particularly suspicious if a pathogen, e.g., a few CMV-infected endothelial cells, does not seem to explain the degree of histopathologic change.

WHEN SHOULD HISTOCHEMICAL STAINS BE PERFORMED?

The need for special stains varies with the biopsy site and with the pathologist's experience. Standard procedures vary among laboratories, not only as to the number of levels and sections routinely prepared but also as to whether and when to perform special stains. Cost, time, and diagnostic accuracy are considerations. Experience suggests that there is in general a limited need for "automatic" special stains for gastrointestinal biopsy specimens from HIV-infected patients. The possible exceptions are Gomori methenamine silver (GMS) and/or periodic acid–Schiff (PAS) stains of esophageal biopsy specimens for diagnosing esophageal candidiasis (especially with few organisms present) and an acid-fast stain for identifying subtle atypical mycobacterial infections, especially in the colon. Although small numbers of Gaucher-like macrophages containing mycobacteria (MAC or *Mycobacterium kansasii*) may be overlooked by hematoxylin-eosin staining, scattered bacilli that do not "stuff" macrophages are more likely to be overlooked without acid-fast stains. How often this occurs and the significance for the patient (except as a first indication of a mycobacterial infection) is unclear, but in one case an unexplained esophageal ulcer was found to contain *M. kansasii* after staining with silver and acid-fast stains for what were apparently the wrong reasons, i.e., smooth muscle cells in the base of the ulcer that were misinterpreted as spindle Gaucher-like cells. In general, special stains should be ordered after viewing the hematoxylin-eosin–stained section, and then only judiciously.

At present, special stains are probably needed by most pathologists to diagnose microsporidiosis (see Fig 4). The best techniques appear to be the Armed Forces Institute of Pathology (AFIP) modification of the Brown-Brenn stain and the Warthin-Starry stain modified for microsporidia.[75, 76] Spores stain red to blue on a yellow background and black on a light brown background, respectively. The Brown-Brenn stain has the advantage since one can see the diagnostic central band of microsporidia spores. The Warthin-Starry stain is less specific (the central band cannot be visualized) but is more sensitive since it stains more than just mature spores and enhances their size. Spores in both specimens polarize brightly (pink and white, respectively), which can be extremely helpful. Special stains play an initial role in building experience and confidence.

Eventually, their limited role may be for detection of a low microsporidia burden, for revealing a second (or third) obscured pathogen, and for research.

Immunohistochemistry, in situ hybridization (ISH), and polymerase chain reaction (PCR) technology have unproven diagnostic roles for identifying gastrointestinal pathogens, especially as routine procedures. They may give a better appreciation of the true proportion of virus-infected cells (e.g., CMV) but may not add any CMV diagnoses not made with routine hematoxylin-eosin–stained sections. Since clinical CMV and HSV infections are considered to result from reactivation of virus, PCR and ISH may reveal carrier states rather than active infections of clinical importance. These analyses may prove to have a role in revealing (and classifying) new pathogens, disclosing preclinical infections that should be prophylactically treated, and identifying particularly difficult coinfections.[73, 77–82]

Finally, there are gastrointestinal pathogens that because of their geographic variability may be overlooked in nonendemic areas. Whereas CMV, *Cryptosporidium*, and microsporidia appear to be relatively common worldwide pathogens, *Isospora* and *Histoplasma* have regional distribution. There are also potential gastrointestinal pathogens that we know little about because they have only been reported infrequently in gastrointestinal specimens, e.g., *Leishmania*, *Toxoplasma*, *Treponema pallidum*, *Penicillium chrysogenum*, *Actinomyces*, papovavirus, and Epstein-Barr virus (EBV).[50–52, 83–86]

PROLIFERATIVE AND NEOPLASTIC DISEASES

Except for the central nervous system (CNS), Kaposi sarcoma is seen regularly in every organ or tissue of the body in patients with AIDS, including the alimentary tract.[15] Kaposi sarcoma lacks features of a true neoplasia, e.g., clonality and metastatic potential, and more resembles a de novo HIV and immunodeficiency-related granulation tissue–like proliferative process of perhaps other viral origin, e.g., herpes-like virus.[87] Depending on the size and location of the gastrointestinal Kaposi sarcoma lesions, symptoms may include pain, hemorrhage, obstruction, and dysfunction. The histology of visceral Kaposi sarcoma is essentially identical anywhere it is encountered and need not be accompanied or preceded by cutaneous lesions. The endoscopist may suspect a Kaposi sarcoma lesion on the basis of the patient's history, symptoms (bleeding), and the erythematous (possibly raised) appearance of the lesions. However, subtle, deeper lesions may be revealed only by histologic evaluation of a biopsy specimen. The Kaposi sarcoma may simply elicit architectural changes in the form of villus blunting and crypt distortion or displacement in the presence of a totally intact epithelium. Since Kaposi sarcoma lesions most resemble granulation tissue, they could potentially be confused with an ulcer base. Close scrutiny will reveal atypical, reactive spindle and endothelial cells, slit-like vessels leaking red blood cells (RBCs), fragmented RBCs, hemosiderin, and mononuclear cells, all characteristics of Kaposi sarcoma.

Lymphomas, already relatively common in HIV disease, are increasing in incidence as patients live progressively longer. Typically, HIV-related lymphomas are extranodal (e.g., CNS, gastrointestinal tract) and, because of their mass effect, are not usually difficult to diagnose in the intestinal tract. Although Hodgkin's disease and T-cell lymphomas are increased in incidence, high-grade non-Hodgkin's B-cell lymphomas are especially associated with HIV disease anywhere in the body, including the gastrointestinal tract.[15]

Mucosal-associated lymphoid tissue (MALT) in toto represents the largest lymphoid organ in the body. It is not unusual to see diffuse and organized lymphoid elements (follicles with germinal centers) in gastrointestinal biopsy specimens from HIV-infected patients, especially in ileal (Peyer patches) and rectal biopsy tissue. This process may correlate with persistent generalized lymphadenopathy, but this has not been studied. Hyperplasia of MALT can have direct clinical implications.[88] Preliminary studies of specimens from HIV-infected patients and simian immunodeficiency virus (SIV)-infected primates show similar histopathologic processes in the MALT and peripheral lymph nodes, that is, follicular hyperplasia and involution, lymphocyte depletion, and sclerosis.[89, 90] Human immunodeficiency virus is identified by in situ hybridization for HIV mRNA, by immunohistochemical stains for HIV proteins, and by TEM (association of virions with follicular dendritic cells). Multinucleated lymphocytes of the Warthin-Finkeldey type, which may be seen in hyperplastic lymph nodes, are more common in intestinal follicles, as well as in diffuse lymphoid areas; they are generally larger than those seen in lymph nodes. In HIV infection, the lamina propria undergoes a progressive hypocellularity, especially of T cells (starting with CD4 helper cells), and is eventually composed of varying numbers of plasma cells, plasmacytoid cells, eosinophils, and macrophages. The appearance of symptomatic opportunistic gastrointestinal infections correlates with the CD4 count (usually less than 100 and especially less than 50) in the peripheral blood and in the mucosa of the gastrointestinal tract.[91]

UNANSWERED QUESTIONS

Many issues concern students of gastrointestinal disease in HIV infection. What is the significance of an apparently low "pathogen" burden (e.g., rare CMV-infected endothelial cell) in a biopsy specimen from a symptomatic patient? The presence of replicating virus indicates an active rather than a latent infection. Explanations include (1) a failure to appreciate the true pathogen burden by the methods employed (hematoxylin-eosin staining vs. immunohistochemistry or ISH), (2) diagnostic inexperience, and (3) more significant pathogens at other sites that are not included in the specimen.

Why is there often (especially at lower pathogen burden) a lack of correlation between histopathology and pathogen burden? *Giardia intestinalis* is an example of an enteric pathogen that can cause severe diarrhea with only minimal contact with the epithelium and associated with relatively little apparent histopathology (see Figs 2,A and B). It may be that functional damage to cells in HIV disease (which would be better appreciated by TEM) may occur without a significant inflammatory response.

How does a particular pathogen cause symptoms/disease? *Cryptosporidium,* which clearly reduces the brush border absorptive area, has also had a possible cytotoxin implicated, although not proved. Bacteria can be seen attached firmly to the cell, effacing the brush border and directly associated with histopathologic change, but this may be only a part of its effect since many bacteria have been shown to secrete toxins. The bacteria need not be histologically apparent to be pathogenic.[34, 35] Does CMV cause disease by specifically impinging on the blood supply to the surface epithelium, by causing the infected endothelial cell to release cytokines directly into the vessels that supply the epithelium, or by killing the endothelial cell?

There are many basic questions that relate to targets of pathogens. For example, CMV variably targets selected cells along the gastrointestinal tract, different from the target cells in other organs and tissues. Other herpesviruses, e.g., HSV, have another pattern of infection. Adenovirus has a striking preference for goblet cells of the large bowel. Microsporidia prefer distal villus enterocytes, and one species *(S. intestinalis)* also infects macrophages and disseminates whereas the other species *(E. bieneusi)* does not.

HISTOPATHOLOGY IN SEARCH OF AN ETIOLOGY

It is not unusual in a gastrointestinal biopsy specimen from an HIV-infected patient to detect histopathologic change without an apparent etiology or to see a pathogen not associated with obvious pathology. "Mild, nonspecific enteritis (or colitis)" is still all too frequently the final diagnosis. Students of gastrointestinal diseases in HIV infection still consider themselves on the incline of the learning curve; undoubtedly, there are more surprises in store for all of us.

What is the meaning of the numerous, even aggregated lamina propria macrophages that are foamy and rich in secondary lysosomes of varying sizes and shapes (e.g., round, angular)? Is there more significance than simply the state of host immunodeficiency to the particular cellular pattern of the lamina propria? Why is interepithelial and lamina propria edema also a common finding? Lipid accumulation in small intestinal mucosa is relatively common and has recently been shown to correlate with fat malabsorption, for which the etiology and pathophysiology are unclear.[92]

Pseudomembranous colitis is surprisingly uncommon in HIV-infected individuals, a patient population that is heavily exposed to antibiotics. Since inflammatory bowel disease is seen in HIV-infected patients (even when only some of the usual diagnostic features are detected), it must be considered when all studies fail to reveal a possible infectious etiology. It remains to be seen whether HIV-infected patients with inflammatory bowel disease clinically respond to the therapeutic regimens used for non–HIV-infected patients.

Are any of these features due to the patient's bowel preparations, to the diarrhea itself, to the wide range of medicines (traditional and nontraditional) used by HIV-infected patients, or to sexually related practices? There is so much to learn that each specimen should be considered a new challenge and the one that may provide the answers long sought.

REFERENCES

1. Rotterdam H, Tsang P: Gastrointestinal disease in the immunocompromised patient. *Hum Pathol* 25:1123–1140, 1994.
2. Feczko PJ: Gastrointestinal complications of human immunodeficiency virus (HIV) infection. *Semin Roentgenol* 3:275–287, 1994.
3. Gazzard BG: Diarrhea in human immunodeficiency virus antibody–positive patients. *Semin Liver Dis* 12:154–166, 1992.
4. Lubeck DP, Bennett CL, Mazonson PD, et al: Quality of life and health service use among HIV-infected patients with chronic diarrhea. *J Acquir Immune Defic Syndr* 6:478–484, 1993.
5. Lewis LG, Cohen MB: Gastrointestinal infection in children. *Curr Opin Pediatr* 5:573–579, 1993.
6. Thea DM, St Louis ME, Atido U, et al: A prospective study of diarrhea and HIV-1 infection among 429 Zairian infants. *N Engl J Med* 329:1696–1702, 1993.
7. Wittner M, Tanowitz HB, Weiss LM: Parasitic infections in AIDS patients. *Parasitic Dis* 7:569–586, 1993.
8. Greenson J, Belitsos P, Yardley J, et al: AIDS enteropathy: Occult enteric infections and duodenal mucosal alterations in chronic diarrhea. *Ann Intern Med* 114:366–372, 1991.
9. Kotloff KL, Johnson JP, Nair P, et al: Diarrheal morbidity during the first 2 years of life among HIV-infected infants. *JAMA* 271:448–452, 1994.
10. Sanchez-Mejorada G, Ponce-de-Leon S: Clinical patterns of diarrhea in AIDS: Etiology and prognosis. *Rev Invest Clin* 46:187–196, 1994.
11. Grohmann GS, Glass RI, Pereira HG, et al: Enteric viruses and diarrhea in HIV-infected patients. *N Engl J Med* 329:14–20, 1993.
12. Tanowitz HB, Simon G, Wittner M: Gastrointestinal manifestations. *Med Clin North Am* 76:45–62, 1992.
13. Schwarz ED, Greene JB: Diagnostic considerations in the human immunodeficiency virus–infected patient with gastrointestinal or abdominal symptoms. *Semin Liver Dis* 12:142–153, 1994.
14. Bartlett JG, Belitsos PC, Sears CL: AIDS enteropathy. *Clin Infect Dis* 15:726–735, 1992.
15. Herndier BG, Friedman SL: Neoplasms of the gastrointestinal tract and hepatobiliary system in acquired immunodeficiency syndrome. *Semin Liver Dis* 12:128–138, 1992.
16. Rene E, Marche C, Regnier B: Intestinal infections in patients with acquired immunodeficiency syndrome: A prospective study in 132 patients. *Dig Dis Sci* 34:773–780, 1989.
17. Kotler DP, Reka S, Borcich A, et al: Detection, localization, and quantification of HIV-associated antigens in intestinal biopsies from patients with HIV. *Am J Pathol* 139:823–830, 1991.
18. Ullrich R, Zeitz M, Heise W, et al: Small intestinal structure and function in patients infected with human immunodeficiency virus (HIV): Evidence for HIV-induced enteropathy. *Ann Intern Med* 111:15–21, 1989.

19. Batman PA, Miller AR, Forster SM, et al: Jejunal enteropathy associated with HIV infection: Quantitative histology. *J Clin Pathol* 42:275–281, 1989.

20. Kotler DP, Reka S, Orenstein JM, et al: Chronic idiopathic esophageal ulceration in AIDS. *J Clin Gastroenterol* 15:284–290, 1992.

21. Fox CH, Kotler DP, Tierney AR, et al: Detection, localization, and quantitation of HIV-associated antigens in intestinal biopsies from HIV-infected patients. *J Infect Dis* 159:467–471, 1989.

22. Smith PD, Eisner MS, Manischewitz JF, et al: Esophageal disease in AIDS is associated with pathologic processes rather than mucosal human immunodeficiency virus type 1. *J Infect Dis* 167:547–552, 1993.

23. Smith PD, Mai UE: Immunopathophysiology of gastrointestinal disease in HIV infection. *Gastroenterol Clin North Am* 21:331–345, 1992.

24. Donowitz M, Kokke FT, Saidi R: Evaluation of patients with chronic diarrhea. *N Engl J Med* 332:725–729, 1995.

25. Berger BJ, Hussain F, Roistacher K: Bacterial infections in HIV-infected. *Infect Dis Clin North Am* 8:449–465, 1994.

26. Mannheimer SB, Soave R: Protozoal infections in patients with AIDS: Cryptosporidiosis, isosporiasis, cyclosporiasis, and microsporidiosis. *Infect Dis Clin North Am* 8:483–498, 1994.

27. Weber R, Bryan R, Owen R, et al: Improved light-microscopical detection of microsporidia spores in stool and duodenal aspirates. *N Engl J Med* 326:161–166, 1992.

28. Ryan NJ, Sutherland G, Coughlan K, et al: A new trichrome-blue stain for detection of microsporidial species in urine, stool, and nasopharyngeal specimens. *J Clin Microbiol* 31:3264–3269, 1993.

29. Kokoskin E, Gyorkos T, Camus A, et al: Modified technique for efficient detection of microsporidia. *J Clin Microbiol* 32:1074–1075, 1994.

30. van Gool T, Snijders F, Reiss P, et al: Diagnosis of intestinal and disseminated microsporidial infections in patients with HIV by a new rapid fluorescence technique. *J Clin Pathol* 46:694–699, 1993.

31. Weber R, Bryan RT, Schwartz DA, et al: Human microsporidial infections. *Clin Microbiol Rev* 7:426–461, 1994.

32. Janoff EN, Orenstein JM, Manischewitz JF, et al: Adenovirus colitis in the acquired immunodeficiency syndrome. *Gastroenterology* 100:976–979, 1991.

33. Maddox A, Francis N, Moss J, et al: Adenovirus infection of the large bowel in HIV positive patients. *J Clin Pathol* 45:684–688, 1992.

34. Kotler DP, Giang TT, Thiim M, et al: Chronic bacterial enteropathy in patients with AIDS. *J Infect Dis* 171:552–558, 1995.

35. Orenstein JM, Kotler DP: Diarrheogenic bacterial enteritis in acquired immunodeficiency syndrome: A light and electron microscopy study of 52 cases. *Hum Pathol* 26:481–492, 1995.

36. Surawicz CM, Roberts PL, Rompalo A, et al: Intestinal spirochetosis in homosexual men. *Am J Med* 82:587–592, 1987.

37. Rabeneck L: Diagnostic workup strategies for patients with HIV-related chronic diarrhea. *J Clin Gastroenterol* 16:245–250, 1993.

38. Johanson JF, Sonnenberg A: Efficient management of diarrhea in the acquired immunodeficiency syndrome (AIDS). *Ann Intern Med* 112:942–948, 1990.

39. Bissuel F, Cotte L, Rabodonirina M, et al: Paromomycin: An effective treatment for cryptosporidial diarrhea in patients with AIDS. *Clin Infect Dis* 18:447–449, 1994.

40. Dieterich D, Lew E, Orenstein JM, et al: Divergence between clinical and histologic responses during treatment for *Enterocytozoon bieneusi* infection. *AIDS* 7(suppl 3):43–44, 1993.

41. Dieterich DT, Lew EA, Kotler DP, et al: Treatment with albendazole for in-

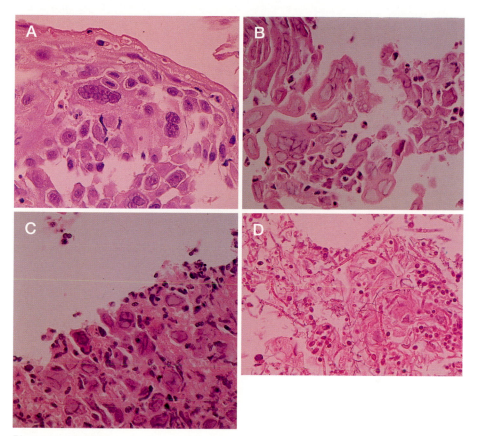

Plate I (see p. 458).

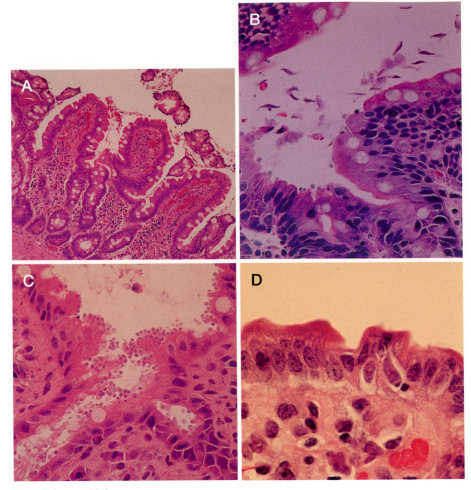

Plate II (see p. 461).

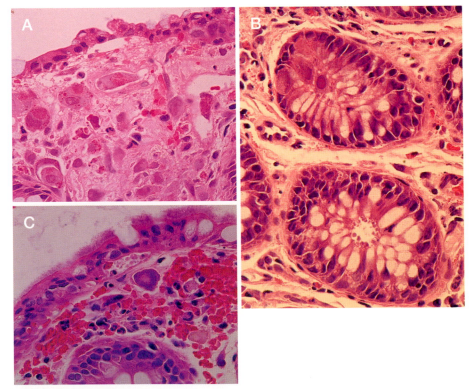

Plate III (see p. 464).

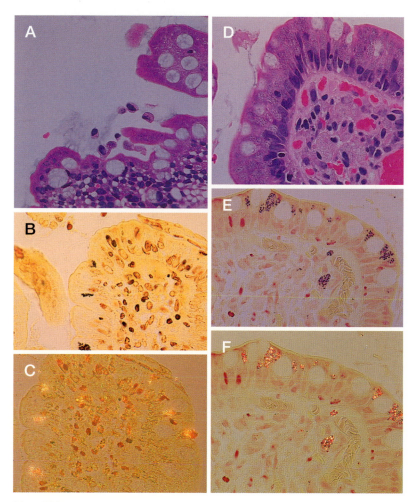

Plate IV (see p. 465).

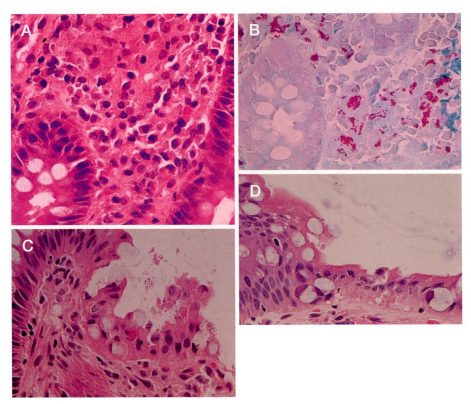

Plate V (see p. 468).

testinal disease due to *Enterocytozoon bieneusi* in patients with AIDS. *J Infect Dis* 169:178–183, 1994.

42. Orenstein JM, Dieterich DT, Lew EA, et al: Albendazole as a treatment for intestinal and disseminated microsporidiosis due to *Septata intestinalis* in AIDS patients: A report of four patients. *AIDS* 7(suppl 3):40–42, 1993.

43. Schwartz DA, Wilcox CM: Atypical cytomegalovirus inclusions in gastrointestinal biopsy specimens from patients with the acquired immunodeficiency syndrome: Diagnostic role of in situ nucleic acid hybridization. *Hum Pathol* 23:1019–1026, 1992.

44. Wilcox CM, Diehl DL, Cello JP, et al: Cytomegalovirus esophagitis in patients with AIDS—A clinical, endoscopic, and pathologic correlation. *Ann Intern Med* 113:589–593, 1990.

45. Wilcox CM: Esophageal disease in the acquired immunodeficiency syndrome: Etiology, diagnosis, and management. *Am J Med* 92:412–421, 1992.

46. Wilcox CM, Straub RF, Schwartz DA: Prospective endoscopic characterization of cytomegalovirus esophagitis in AIDS. *Gastrointest Endosc* 40:481–484, 1994.

47. Greenson JK, Beschorner WE, Boitnott JK, et al: Prominent mononuclear cell infiltrate is characteristic of herpes esophagitis. *Hum Pathol* 22:541–549, 1991.

48. Bonacini M, Young T, Laine L: The causes of esophageal symptoms in human immunodeficiency virus infection. A prospective study of 110 patients. *Arch Intern Med* 151:1567–1572, 1991.

49. Lopez-Dupla M, Sanz PM, Garcia VP, et al: Clinical, endoscopic, immunologic, and therapeutic aspects of oropharyngeal and esophageal candidiasis in HIV-infected patients: A survey of 114 cases. *Am J Gastroenterol* 87:1171–1176, 1992.

50. Kitchen VS, Helbert M, Francis ND, et al: Epstein-Barr virus associated oesophageal ulcers in AIDS. *Gut* 31:1223–1225, 1990.

51. Schechter M, Pannain VLN, de Oliveira AV: Papovavirus-associated esophageal ulceration in a patient with AIDS. *AIDS* 5:238, 1991.

52. Poles MA, McMeeking AA, Scholes JV, et al: Actinomyces infection of a cytomegalovirus esophageal ulcer in two patients with acquired immunodeficiency syndrome. *Am J Gastroenterol* 89:1569–1572, 1994.

53. Yi ES, Powell HC: Adenovirus infection of the duodenum in an AIDS patient: An ultrastructural study. *Ultrastruct Pathol* 18:549–551, 1994.

54. Comin CE, Santucci M: Submicroscopic profile of Isospora belli enteritis in a patient with acquired immune deficiency syndrome. *Ultrastruct Pathol* 18:473–482, 1994.

55. Orenstein JM: Microsporidiosis in the acquired immunodeficiency syndrome. *J Parasitol* 77:843–864, 1991.

56. Silverman JF, Levine J, Finley JL, et al: Small intestinal brushing cytology in the diagnosis of cryptosporidiosis in AIDS. *Diagn Cytopathol* 6:193–196, 1990.

57. Medoza ML, Martin-Rabadan P, Carrion I, et al: *Helicobacter pylori* infection. Rapid diagnosis with brush cytology. *Acta Cytol* 37:181–185, 1993.

58. Teot LA, Ducatman BS, Geisinger KR: Cytologic diagnosis of cytomegaloviral esophagitis: A report of three acquired immunodeficiency syndrome–related cases. *Act Cytol* 37:93–96, 1993.

59. Geisinger KR: Endoscopic biopsies and cytologic brushings of the esophagus are diagnostically complementary. *Am J Clin Pathol* 103:295–299, 1995.

60. Orenstein JM, Lew E, Poles MA, et al: The endoscopic brush cytology specimen in the diagnosis of intestinal microsporidiosis. *AIDS*, in press.

61. Dieterich DT, Lew EA, Bacon DJ, et al: Gastrointestinal pneumocystosis in

HIV-infected patients on aerosolized pentamidine: Report of five cases and literature review. *Am J Gastroenterol* 87:1763–1770, 1992.

62. Clarkston WK, Bonacini M, Peterson I: Colitis due to *Histoplasma capsulatum* in the acquired immune deficiency syndrome. *Am J Gastroenterol* 86:913–916, 1991.

63. Orenstein JM, Tenner M, Kotler DP: Localization of infection by the microsporidian *Enterocytozoon bieneusi* in the gastrointestinal tract of AIDS patients with diarrhea. *AIDS* 6:195–197, 1992.

64. Rene E, Marche C, Chevalier T, et al: Cytomegalovirus colitis in patients with acquired immunodeficiency syndrome. *Dig Dis Sci* 33:741–750, 1988.

65. Genta RM, Chappell CL, White AC, et al: Duodenal morphology and intensity of infection in AIDS-related intestinal cryptosporidiosis. *Gastroenterology* 105:1769–1775, 1993.

66. Goodgame RW, Genta RM, White AC, et al: Intensity of infection in AIDS-associated cryptosporidiosis. *J Infect Dis* 167:704–709, 1993.

67. Clayton F, Heller T, Kotler DP: Variation in the enteric distribution of cryptosporidia in acquired immunodeficiency syndrome. *Am J Clin Pathol* 102:420–425, 1994.

68. Orenstein JM: Ultrastructural pathology of human immunodeficiency virus infection. *Ultrastruct Pathol* 16:179–210, 1992.

69. Francis ND, Boylston AW, Roberts AHG, et al: Cytomegalovirus infection in gastrointestinal tracts of patients infected with HIV-1 or AIDS. *J Clin Pathol* 42:1055–1064, 1989.

70. Kotler CP, Giang TT, Garro ML, et al: Light microscopic diagnosis of microsporidiosis in patients with AIDS. *Am J Gastroenterol* 89:540–544, 1994.

71. Orenstein JM, Chiang J, Steinberg W, et al: Intestinal microsporidiosis as a cause of diarrhea in human immunodeficiency virus–infected patients: A report of 20 cases. *Hum Pathol* 21:475–481, 1990.

72. Rijpstra AC, Canning EU, Van Ketel RJ, et al: Use of light microscopy to diagnose small-intestinal microsporidiosis in patients with AIDS. *J Infect Dis* 157:827–831, 1988.

73. Wu G-D, Shintaku IP, Chien K, et al: A comparison of routine light microscopy, immunohistochemistry, and in situ hybridization for the detection of cytomegalovirus in gastrointestinal biopsies. *Am J Gastroenterol* 84:1517–1520, 1989.

74. Randhawa VS, Sharma VK, Malhotra V, et al: Human giardiasis. *Arch Pathol Lab Med* 18:891–894, 1994.

75. Field AS, Hing MC, Milliken ST, et al: Microporidia in the small intestine of HIV-infected patients. A new diagnostic technique and a new species. *Med J Aust* 158:390–394, 1993.

76. Orenstein JM: Intestinal microsporidiosis. *Adv Anat Pathol,* in press.

77. Goodgame RW, Genta RM, Estrada R, et al: Frequency of positive tests for cytomegalovirus in AIDS patients: Endoscopic lesions compared with normal mucosa. *Am J Gastroenterol* 88:338–343, 1993.

78. Roberts WH, Hammond S, Sneddon JM, et al: In situ DNA hybridization for cytomegalovirus in colonoscopic biopsies. *Arch Pathol Lab Med* 112:1106–1109, 1988.

79. Roberts WH, Sneddon JM, Waldman J, et al: Cytomegalovirus infection of gastrointestinal endothelium demonstrated by simultaneous nucleic acid hybridization and immunohistochemistry. *Arch Pathol Lab Med* 113:461–464, 1989.

80. Smith MA, Brennessel DJ: Cytomegalovirus. *Infect Dis Clin North Am* 8:927–939, 1994.

81. Cotte L, Drouet E, Bissuel F, et al: Diagnostic value of amplification of hu-

man cytomegalovirus DNA from gastrointestinal biopsies from human immunodeficiency virus–infected patients. *J Clin Microbiol* 31:2066–2069, 1993.

82. Strickler JG, Manivel JC, Copenhaver CM, et al: Comparison of in situ and immunohistochemistry for detection of cytomegalovirus and herpes simplex virus. *Hum Pathol* 21:443–448, 1990.

83. Laguna F, Garcia-Samaniego J, Morento V, et al: Prevalence of gastrointestinal leishmaniasis in Spanish HIV-positive patients with digestive symptoms. *Am J Gastroenterol* 89:1606, 1994.

84. Garcia LW, Hemphill RB, Marasco WA, et al: Acquired immunodeficiency syndrome with disseminated toxoplasmosis presenting as an acute pulmonary and gastrointestinal illness. *Arch Pathol Lab Med* 115:459–463, 1991.

85. Hoffman M, Bash E, Berger SA, et al: Fatal necrotizing esophagitis due to *Penicillium chrysogenum* in a patient with acquired immunodeficiency syndrome. *Eur J Clin Microbiol Infect Dis* 11:1158–1160, 1992.

86. Kasmin F, Reddy S, Mathur-Wagh U, et al: Syphilitic gastritis in an HIV-infected individual. *Am J Gastroenterol* 87:1820–1822, 1992.

87. Chang Y, Cesarman E, Pessin MS, et al: Identification of herpesvirus-like DNA sequences in AIDS-associated Kaposi's sarcoma. *Science* 206:1865–1869, 1995.

88. Levendoglu H, Rosen Y: Nodular lymphoid hyperplasia of gut in HIV infection. *Am J Gastroenterol* 87:1200–1202, 1992.

89. Heise C, Miller CJ, Lackner A, et al: Primary acute simian immunodeficiency virus infection of intestinal lymphoid tissue associated with gastrointestinal dysfunction. *J Infect Dis* 169:1116–1120, 1994.

90. Heise C, Vogel P, Miller CJ, et al: Simian immunodeficiency virus infection of the gastrointestinal tract in Rhesus macaques: Functional, pathological, and morphological changes. *Am J Pathol* 142:1759–1771, 1993.

91. Ullrich R, Zeitz M, Riecken EO: Enteric immunologic abnormalities in human immunodeficiency virus infection. *Semin Liver Dis* 12:167–174, 1992.

92. Benhamou Y, Hilmarsdottir I, Desportes-Livage I, et al: Association of lipid accumulation in small intestinal mucosa with decreased serum triglyceride and cholesterol levels in AIDS. *Dig Dis Sci* 39:2163–2169, 1994.

PART III

Mechanisms of Disease

Evolution in Concepts of the Molecular Pathogenesis of Colon Cancer

Amy E. Noffsinger, M.D.

Assistant Professor, Department of Pathology and Laboratory Medicine, University of Cincinnati College of Medicine, Cincinnati, Ohio

Cecilia M. Fenoglio-Preiser, M.D.

MacKenzie Professor and Director, Department of Pathology and Laboratory Medicine, University of Cincinnati College of Medicine, Cincinnati, Ohio

C arcinomas usually evolve through a series of well-defined histologic steps, eventually culminating in metastatic spread of the disease and death of the patient. Accompanying this series of histologic changes are molecular genetic alterations that underlie the phenotypic changes visible through the microscope. Such molecular genetic alterations fall into two basic categories: (1) deregulation of cell proliferation through overexpression or amplification of oncogenes and mutation or deletion of tumor suppressor genes and (2) deregulation of programmed cell death.

The fact that many cancers appear to have an inherited or genetic basis has been known for over a century. Real evidence implicating a genetic factor, however, was not available until Rous demonstrated in 1911 that a cell-free filtrate from a chicken sarcoma could induce sarcomas in chickens.[1] It was not until nearly 60 years later that the Rous sarcoma virus transforming gene, v-src, was identified.[2, 3] Since the discovery of the src oncogene, more than 60 other oncogenes have been identified, some of which play critical roles in human cancers.

Oncogenes are characterized by their positive effects in transforming cells to the malignant phenotype. Introduction of an oncogene into cells in culture results in transformation characterized by increased cell proliferation and impaired differentiation.

For many years it was also thought that a second class of genes existed that were important in the genesis of cancer, so-called tumor suppressor genes. In 1971, Knudson[4] proposed his "two-hit" hypothesis for the development of retinoblastoma. In this hypothesis he proposed that patients with the hereditary form of retinoblastoma inherited an inactivating germline mutation in one allele of the responsible gene. When a second, somatic mutation occurs in a cell within the retina, a retinoblastoma will subsequently form. Sporadic retinoblastomas, on the other hand, occur only after two somatic mutations affect the same retinal cell. This hypothesis was later confirmed when the RB1 gene on chromosome

Advances in Pathology and Laboratory Medicine®, vol. 8
© 1995, Mosby–Year Book, Inc.

13 was found to be inactivated in the inherited form of retinoblastoma.[5, 6] These studies provided strong evidence for the existence of tumor suppressor genes.

Because tumor suppressor genes are cancer genes that achieve their oncogenic effects by inactivation of both normal alleles, it is possible to identify potential tumor suppressor gene loci through studies of loss of heterozygosity (LOH). Such studies take advantage of the fact that a mutation in a tumor suppressor locus is usually accompanied by loss of the second, normal allele. Loss of specific allelic markers in tumor tissue, as compared with normal tissue from the same patient, suggests that the lost DNA sequences encode functions vital to maintenance of the non-neoplastic state. Through such studies of allelic loss, a number of putative tumor suppressor genes have been identified in recent years.

Numerous factors make colorectal neoplasia a useful system to investigate the molecular genetic changes that accompany carcinogenesis. First, colorectal neoplasia is an extremely common disease, especially in Western countries. It is a major health concern in the United States. According to surveillance, epidemiology, and end results (SEER) data collected between the years 1973 and 1987, the incidence of adenocarcinoma of the colon was 33.7 per 100,000.[7] Second, a well-defined histologic continuum from normal to carcinoma exists. Finally, a number of hereditary colon cancer syndromes are recognized, including familial adenomatous polyposis coli (FAP) and hereditary nonpolyposis colon cancer (HNPCC), or Lynch syndrome.

THE HISTOLOGIC CONTINUUM

It is generally accepted that most colonic adenocarcinomas arise from a benign precursor lesion, the adenoma. Adenomas show abnormalities of both epithelial cell differentiation and maturation. Even small adenomas are neoplastic, clonal populations of colonic epithelial cells, whereas normal colonic epithelium is polyclonal.[8] This suggests that adenomas arise from a single, abnormal precursor stem cell.[9] Although we have developed an understanding of the steps that occur in the transition from adenoma to carcinoma, our understanding of the transition from normal mucosa to adenoma is less well established. It is thought that adenomas probably do not arise directly from normal epithelium, but instead from areas of mucosal hyperproliferation.[10, 11]

Some but not all adenomas ultimately progress through a series of histologically defined stages to frankly invasive carcinoma over a period of years to decades. The histologic spectrum of changes along this continuum is as follows: small adenoma with minimal atypia, larger adenoma with high-grade dysplasia or in situ carcinoma, adenoma with intramucosal carcinoma, and finally, invasive cancer (Fig 1).

The notion of an adenoma-carcinoma sequence is supported by the frequent observation of a direct transition from adenoma to carcinoma in tissues examined pathologically.[12-15] In addition, patients with FAP, whose colons are typically carpeted with hundreds to thousands of adenomatous polyps, have a nearly 100% lifetime chance of colorectal carcinoma developing if a prophylactic colectomy is not performed. Additional evidence supporting the adenoma-carcinoma continuum is summarized in Table 1.

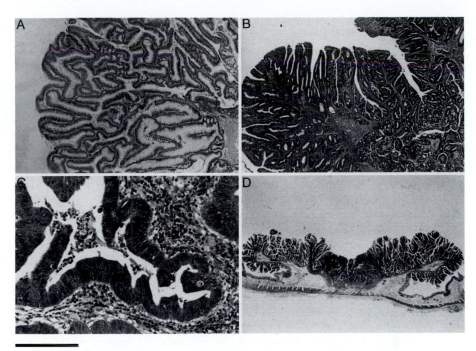

FIGURE 1.

Histologic progression in the adenoma-carcinoma sequence. **A,** small tubular adenoma without significant dysplasia. **B,** larger adenoma with high-grade dysplasia. **C,** higher-power view of the polyp shown in **B.** The glands are lined by stratified, disorganized cells with pleomorphic nuclei and clumped chromatin. **D,** low-power view of a sessile adenoma containing a central focus of invasive adenocarcinoma.

Although most sporadic colon carcinomas arise in the setting of typical, pre-existing adenoma, there are several circumstances in which this is not the case. Patients with long-standing ulcerative colitis are known to have an increased risk of developing adenocarcinomas of the colon. Dysplasia of the colonic mucosa is a precursor to the development of car-

TABLE 1.

Evidence in Favor of the Adenoma-Carcinoma Sequence

The distribution of adenomas and carcinomas is similar.
The frequency of carcinomas is increased in patients with adenomas.
Adenomas occur with increased frequency in colons containing carcinomas.
Removal of adenomas reduces the expected incidence of carcinoma.
Patients who refuse treatment (removal) of adenomas are later treated for carcinoma at the same site.
Colonic adenocarcinomas almost universally develop in patients with familial polyposis if untreated.
Areas of direct transition from adenoma to carcinoma are often identifiable.
Growth of adenomatous cells in culture results in cell populations that acquire features of carcinoma in situ or invasive carcinoma.
There is a progressive accumulation of molecular genetic changes in the continuum from adenoma to carcinoma.

cinoma. Like the adenoma-carcinoma sequence, the dysplasia-carcinoma sequence in ulcerative colitis consists of a series of histologically identifiable steps beginning with low-grade dysplasia and progressing to invasive carcinoma.

The other condition in which colorectal carcinoma is not preceded by typical adenomas is HNPCC. Although it was initially thought that no adenomas preceded the development of carcinomas in this syndrome, it is now clear that HNPCC-related carcinomas arise from flat, sometimes inverted adenomas. The molecular genetic mechanisms underlying carcinogenesis in this syndrome appear to be different from those operative in other settings. These changes will be discussed in a separate section.

THE MOLECULAR GENETIC CONTINUUM

The dramatic technological advances that have occurred in the field of molecular genetics over the last decade have allowed us to begin to understand the molecular changes that accompany the histologic steps in the progression of cancers arising in a number of sites. Perhaps because colon carcinoma is a common disease that progresses through a definable histologic continuum and is characterized by lesions readily accessible to the endoscopist, it has become the best characterized neoplasm from a molecular genetic point of view. In addition, many investigations into the genetic basis of colorectal cancer development took advantage of the existence of a number of hereditary syndromes characterized by an increased susceptibility to colon carcinoma. Such syndromes include FAP, Gardner syndrome, and HNPCC.

Through the efforts of numerous investigators it is now clear that colon cancer occurs through an accumulation of molecular genetic changes. Some alterations appear early in the progression, whereas others are necessary for development of the invasive phenotype. Still others are responsible for allowing cells to implant and survive in sites distant from the primary tumor during the process of metastasis. The principal changes that are significant in the development of colon carcinoma include ab-

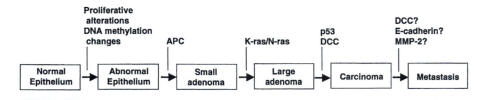

FIGURE 2.

Diagrammatic representation of the timing of the molecular genetic events known to be significant in the development of colon cancer. The earliest changes involve alterations in proliferation and DNA methylation. Mutation and/or allelic loss in the *APC* (adenomatous polyposis coli) gene probably plays a role in the transition from hyperproliferative mucosa to adenoma. Mutations of the *ras* gene are thought to play a role in the growth and progression of adenomas. *p53* and *DCC* (deleted in colon cancer) gene mutations are late events in neoplastic progression. Less is known about factors important in the development of malignancy, but cell adhesion molecules and metalloproteinases *(MMP-2)* have been implicated.

normalities in the pattern of cell proliferation and DNA methylation, as well as alterations in the *APC* (adenomatous polyposis coli), *ras*, *DCC* (deleted in colon cancer), *p53*, and other oncogenes and tumor suppressor genes. In addition, colon carcinomas display abnormalities in programmed cell death. The timing of these alterations with the histologic changes in neoplastic progression are summarized in Figure 2. We will discuss these changes in more detail in the remainder of this review.

EARLY CHANGES IN THE ADENOMA-CARCINOMA SEQUENCE

ALTERATIONS IN CELL PROLIFERATION

In the normal colon, cell proliferation occurs mainly in the lower two thirds of the crypts[16] (Fig 3). Cells then migrate from the base of the crypt upward toward the mucosal surface where they ultimately slough into the gut lumen. In adenomas, the proliferative compartment is expanded, often reaching the mucosal surface (Fig 4). The proliferative index progressively increases from normal mucosa, to adenoma with low-grade dysplasia, and finally to adenoma with high-grade dysplasia. Adenomas with high-grade dysplasia have a proliferative profile essentially identical to that of invasive carcinoma.[17] In addition, a number of studies have demonstrated increased proliferative activity in the non-neoplastic mucosa of patients with familial polyposis and HNPCC syndromes.[18-20] These findings support the hypothesis that carcinoma results from a progressive deregulation of the cell cycle characterized by increasingly uncontrolled proliferative activity.

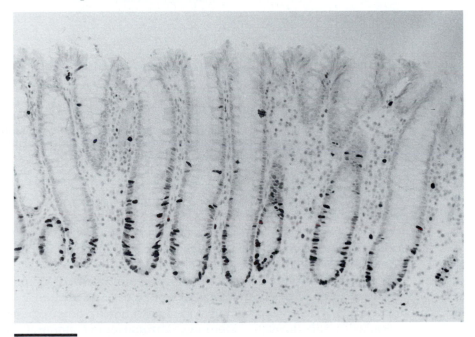

FIGURE 3.
Immunohistochemical stain of normal colon with antibodies against the proliferation-associated antigen Ki-67. Note that the positive immunoreactivity is restricted to the lower half of the colonic glands.

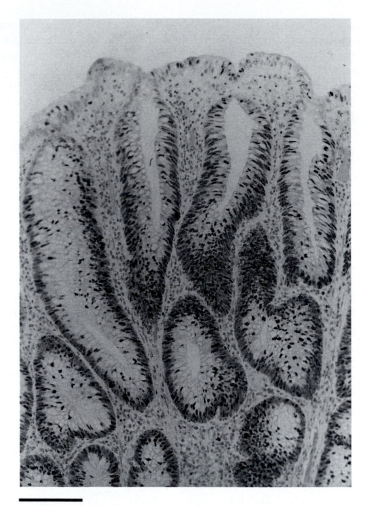

FIGURE 4.

In this adenoma, Ki-67 immunoreactivity is present in cells not only in the bases of the crypts but also in the more superficial cells. Even cells on the mucosal surface demonstrate positive staining. This pattern is characteristic of the deregulated proliferation that exists in colonic adenomas.

ALTERATIONS IN DNA METHYLATION

Overall DNA hypomethylation occurs in many forms of cancer. In the colon, DNA hypomethylation appears to be an early step in the neoplastic progression. Examination of DNA from even small adenomas shows loss of methyl groups in approximately one third of the regions that are methylated in non-neoplastic colonic epithelial cells.[21, 22] Diets deficient in folate and methionine, both of which are required for DNA methylation, are associated with an increased risk of colorectal adenomas and carcinomas. DNA hypomethylation may contribute to genetic instability in neoplastic cells through inhibition of chromosome condensation,[23] alterations in DNA stability,[24] alterations in DNA protein binding patterns,[25, 26] and increased fragile site instability.[27]

Although colonic neoplasms demonstrate overall hypomethylation of DNA, a few specific regions are hypermethylated.[28] In normal cells, areas of decreased DNA methylation are seen in so-called CpG islands. Demethylation of these regions presumably makes genes in these regions available for transcription. These CpG islands are often hypermethylated in cancer cells. Transcripts of DNA methyltransferase, an enzyme that acts to methylate CpG islands, are increased 15-fold over normal in the non-neoplastic mucosa of patients with colonic neoplasia, up to 60-fold in colonic adenomas, and greater than 200-fold in carcinomas.[29] DNA hypermethylation in cancer cells is a phenomenon that may be significant in preventing the transcription of genes important in promoting differentiation.[30]

THE *APC* GENE

Familial adenomatous polyposis is an autosomal dominantly inherited disease characterized by the development of hundreds of adenomatous polyps within the colon, usually before the age of 20 or 30 (Fig 5). Adenocarcinoma of the colon is almost certain to develop in untreated patients with FAP, often before the age of 40. Familial adenomatous polyposis appears to be a generalized disorder of cell proliferation. In addition to colonic adenomas, adenomas also develop in the small intestine, especially the duodenum, and the stomach. These patients have a propensity for extraintestinal neoplasms as well, some of which may be malignant. These extraintestinal neoplasms include desmoid tumors, osteomas, thyroid tumors, liver and bile duct tumors, brain tumors, and adrenocortical tumors.

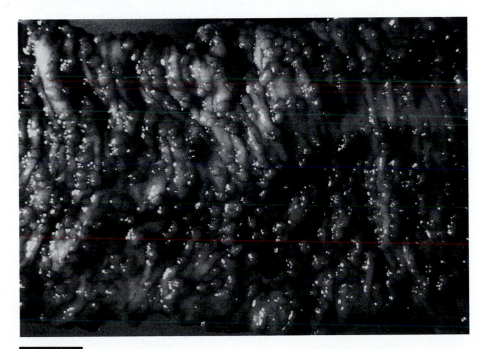

FIGURE 5.
Gross photograph of a segment of colon from a patient with familial adenomatous polyposis. The mucosal surface is carpeted with large numbers of adenomas of varying size.

The gene associated with FAP was first mapped to chromosome 5q21 through linkage analysis[31, 32] and was cloned in 1991.[33, 34] Mutation of the APC gene is a consistent finding in the germline of patients with FAP.[33–35] In addition, somatic mutations of APC are common in cells derived from sporadic colorectal carcinomas.[36] Loss of heterozygosity of chromosome 5q is commonly demonstrated in tumors occurring in both patients with FAP and those with sporadic colorectal carcinomas.[31, 32, 37–41] In patients with FAP, the allele that is lost is almost always the wild-type allele.[42] The finding that neoplasia is preceded by functional loss of both copies of the normal gene suggests that APC functions as a tumor suppressor in the classic sense.

Alterations at the APC locus on chromosome 5 in colorectal neoplasms appears to be a phenomenon that in many cases occurs early in the neoplastic progression toward malignancy. APC mutations occur in small adenomas, and the frequency of their occurrence does not increase in carcinomas.[36, 43] Tsao and Shibata[43] microdissected eight colonic adenomas and analyzed their components separately for the presence of APC mutations. In these neoplasms, APC abnormalities were found in adenomatous epithelium, but not in the non-neoplastic epithelium of the stalks of adenomas, which suggests that mutations in this gene are directly related to adenoma formation. At the present time it is not known whether inactivation of a single APC allele has any effect on cell proliferation, although some studies suggest that this may be the case.[10] Therefore, APC inactivation may have the overall effect of increasing cell proliferation rather than promoting a malignant phenotype per se.[44] This increase in proliferation might then predispose the cells to the development of subsequent genetic abnormalities, thereby increasing the likelihood of malignant transformation.

The mechanism by which APC affects these early neoplastic changes is at present unknown. The protein product of the APC gene is 2,843 amino acids in length, but the normal function of the protein is not known. In most cases, mutations result in truncation of the carboxy-terminus of the APC-encoded protein,[36, 45–49] which suggests that this portion of the protein is most important in mediating its growth suppressor effects. The APC protein is known to associate with α- and β-catenin, proteins that are associated with the cell adhesion molecule E-cadherin. Further evidence suggests that the wild-type, but not the mutant, APC gene product associates with cytoskeletal microtubules and promotes their assembly in vitro.[50, 51] It has been suggested that the protein may somehow act to relay extracellular signals from cell adhesion molecules such as E-cadherin to the cytoskeleton.[50] Alternatively, its apparent role in microtubule assembly may have an effect on cell growth and division, processes known to be associated with coordinated assembly and disassembly of microtubular structures.[51] In addition, microtubule depolymerization may play a role in directly promoting DNA synthesis.[52]

THE ras GENE

The ras family of oncogenes functions in normal cell growth and differentiation.[53] The ras gene–encoded protein, referred to as p21, functions as a G protein and participates in signal transduction from growth factor receptors on the cell membrane. The role of the p21 protein in this signal transduction pathway is outlined in Figure 6. Point mutations in *ras* genes result in proteins that cannot be inactivated[53-56] and consequently autonomous cell growth and proliferation.

Mutations of *ras* occur most frequently in codons 12, 13, and 61 of the K-, N-, and H-*ras* oncogenes in human cancers. In colorectal neoplasia, *ras* mutations seem to occur early in the adenoma-carcinoma sequence. Vogelstein et al.[57] identified *ras* mutations in only 9% of adenomas less than 1 cm in diameter. In contrast, 58% of the adenomas greater than 1 cm and 47% of the adenocarcinomas contained mutated *ras* genes. Burmer and Loeb[58] report similar findings. They identified *ras* mutations in 75% of the adenomas and 65% of the carcinomas of the colon. These findings suggest that *ras* mutations may be instrumental in promoting the growth of small adenomas into larger lesions. In addition, these data suggest that *ras* probably does not directly affect conversion of adenomatous cells to a frankly malignant phenotype.

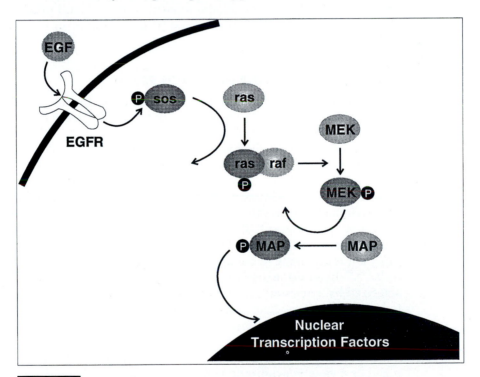

FIGURE 6.

Simplified representation of the signal transduction pathway involving the protein encoded by the *ras* gene. The cascade is initiated when epidermal growth factor (EGF) or transforming growth factor α binds to the epidermal growth factor receptor (EGFR). Binding of the ligand results in receptor dimerization and phosphorylation of the product of the *sos* oncogene. Next, inactive *ras*-GDP is converted to activated *ras*-GTP, which acts to affect phosphorylation of MEK followed by MAP kinase. MAP kinase activates a number of transcription factors within the nucleus, thereby triggering DNA replication.

ABNORMALITIES IN PROGRAMMED CELL DEATH

Perhaps the best characterized regulator of programmed cell death to date is the proto-oncogene bcl-2. The bcl-2 gene encodes a 26-kD protein known to block apoptosis.[59-62] The gene was initially identified through its involvement in a 14;18 translocation in follicular lymphoma.[63] The bcl-2 protein is now known to play a critical role in lymphomagenesis.

The role of abnormalities in programmed cell death, or apoptosis, has not been extensively studied in colorectal neoplasia. There has been one recent study that examined expression of bcl-2 in gastrointestinal neoplasia.[64] In this study the authors examined bcl-2 expression in a variety of gastrointestinal lesions with the use of immunohistochemistry. They found no increase in bcl-2 expression in non-neoplastic or inflammatory lesions in various sites within the gastrointestinal tract. In contrast, bcl-2 expression was increased in the majority of adenomas of all sizes, areas of flat dysplasia, and adenocarcinomas. In addition, altered expression was noted in nondysplastic epithelium adjacent to neoplastic lesions, which suggests that bcl-2 alterations may precede the development of neoplasia. Clearly, the role of abnormalities in bcl-2 and other regulators of programmed cell death need to be further defined in colorectal neoplasia.

ABNORMALITIES IN DNA MISMATCH REPAIR

The HNPCC syndrome was initially described by Lynch in the 1960s.[65] The carcinomas that arise in patients with HNPCC were observed to be somewhat different from those arising sporadically.[66-68] These lesions have a tendency to be right sided, with approximately 70% of cases arising proximal to the splenic flexure. They tend to arise at a younger age and are often multiple. There is an increased risk for the development of extracolonic neoplasms as well, most notably carcinomas of the endometrium, stomach, small intestine, biliary tract, ovary, and urinary tract.[68-70]

Colon carcinomas that arise in patients with HNPCC have histologic differences as well when compared with sporadic colorectal carcinomas. They are more likely to be mucinous and poorly differentiated than controls.[68, 71] In addition, carcinomas associated with HNPCC are often characterized by a marked host-lymphocytic response. Despite their tendency to be poorly differentiated, many studies have suggested that they behave indolently[72] and have improved survival relative to sporadic carcinomas.[73]

Hereditary nonpolyposis colon cancer became unequivocally recognized as a genetic syndrome when linkage studies demonstrated that the disease segregated with markers on chromosome 2p.[74] A short time later, a second linked locus was noted on chromosome 3p in other HNPCC kindreds.[75]

The real clue to understanding the underlying abnormality in this syndrome came when several groups identified the presence of microsatellite instability in tumors from patients with HNPCC.[76-78] Microsatellites are dinucleotide and trinucleotide repeat sequences scattered throughout the genome and are widely altered in neoplastic tissues from patients with HNPCC. This suggested that HNPCC was associated with malfunction of a factor that might be involved in regulating the fidelity of DNA replication.

This hypothesis soon proved to be correct. Genes on chromosome 2p (*hMSH2*) and 3p (*hMLH1*) have both now been identified and cloned, and it is now known that they represent homologues to bacterial mismatch repair genes.[79-82] Both *hMSH2* and *hMLH1* act essentially as tumor suppressor genes, with loss of both copies of the gene resulting in abnormalities in DNA mismatch repair and a resultant high rate of somatic mutation. The normal function of these mismatch-repaired genes is well established in bacteria and outlined in Figure 7.

Tumors exhibiting microsatellite instability are said to be replication error—positive (RER+). The RER+ phenotype is not restricted to carcinomas arising in the setting of HNPCC, but has been reported in 10% to 15% of sporadic colorectal carcinomas[76-78, 83, 84] and has been identified in neoplastic lesions in patients with ulcerative colitis.[85] Like their

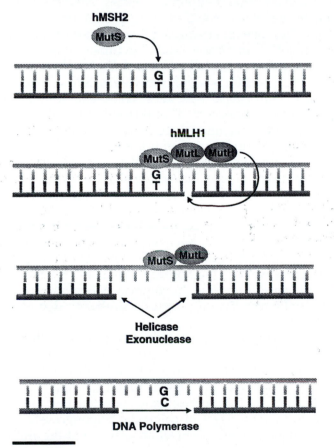

FIGURE 7.

Diagrammatic representation of DNA mismatch repair in bacteria. The human homologue of the bacterial *MutS* (*hMSH2*) and the homolog of the bacterial *MutL* (*hMLH1*) are known to be mutated in hereditary nonpolyposis colon cancer. In bacteria, these proteins act to recognize mismatched nucleotide pairs. The MutH protein induces a nick in the DNA molecule near the mismatch site. This abnormal area is then excised with the aid of a DNA helicase and an exonuclease. DNA polymerase then fills in the gap.

HNPCC counterparts, these lesions tend to occur on the right side of the colon and are usually mucinous, poorly differentiated, and DNA diploid. Patients with sporadic RER+ tumors also have increased survival when compared with those whose tumors are RER−.[83]

Whether the RER+ phenotype develops early or late in the adenoma-carcinoma sequence in sporadic carcinomas is still unclear. Shibata et al.[86] demonstrated RER+ adenomas in colons from patients with RER+ carcinomas, which suggests that this change may occur early. Further studies will certainly shed light on this issue.

LATER CHANGES IN THE ADENOMA-CARCINOMA SEQUENCE

THE *DCC* GENE

Allelic loss contributes to carcinogenesis by unmasking either somatic or germline mutations in tumor suppressor genes. Allelic loss of the long arm of chromosome 18 was noted to occur commonly in colorectal carcinomas, and it was therefore suspected that a tumor suppressor gene resided in this area.[41, 57] In 1990 a candidate tumor suppressor gene was identified in the region of 18q21 and termed *DCC* (deleted in colon cancer).[87] *DCC* gene expression is significantly decreased in many colorectal carcinomas and colon cancer cell lines, consistent with its presumed function as a tumor suppressor.[87−89] In line with these data is the observation that the addition of a normal chromosome 18 in COKFu colon carcinoma cells results in suppression of tumorigenicity.[90]

Loss of *DCC* function appears to be a relatively late occurrence in colorectal carcinogenesis. Loss of heterozygosity involving 18q has been noted in approximately 75% of colonic adenocarcinomas, 47% of adenomas containing foci of carcinoma, and only 13% of adenomas without carcinoma.[41] Interestingly, absence of *DCC* expression has been noted in colon cancers metastatic to the liver but was uncommon in neoplasms that did not metastasize.[91] In addition, allelic loss of *DCC* in patients with stage II colon cancer worsens their prognosis so that it resembles that seen in patients with stage III disease. In contrast, patients with stage II cancers without allelic loss have a prognosis similar to that of stage I patients.[92]

The *DCC* gene is now known to encode a protein with homology to the family of neural cell adhesion molecules.[87] These molecules function in the normal mediation of cell adhesion and cell recognition.[93] However, very little is known at the present time regarding the actual function of the DCC protein. It is interesting to speculate that the loss of *DCC* bears fruition in the late stages of colorectal tumorigenesis, perhaps affecting invasiveness, properties of cell adhesion, and the ability of cells to metastasize.

THE *p53* GENE

The *p53* gene is the most frequently mutated gene identified to date in human cancers and is now widely recognized as a tumor suppressor gene[94] whose deletions and/or mutations are oncogenic. Its involvement in carcinogenesis is likely since it is mutated in many cancers, including approximately 50% of all types of lung cancer,[95, 96] 70% of all colon cancers,[97, 98] and 36% of breast cancers.[99] In addition, p53 mutations have been reported in hepatocellular,[100] pancreatic,[101] gastric,[102] esophageal,[102] head and neck,[103] and ovarian carcinomas.[104]

The p53 gene is located on the short arm of chromosome 17 and, as its name implies, encodes a 53-kD phosphoprotein 393 amino acids in length.[105] Structural studies have indicated that p53 consists of several separate functional domains, each of which contributes to its regulation. The N-terminal domain functions as a transcriptional activator and is a substrate for phosphorylation.[106] The central third of the protein contains four exons that are evolutionarily conserved, which suggests that they are essential for normal protein function.[98] The physiologic importance of this portion of the molecule is emphasized by the fact that murine mutations in this region cause transformation. In addition, most mutations in human tumors cluster in this area as well.[107] The central portion of the molecule is a proline-rich, hydrophobic region responsible for determining the conformation of the protein as well as its sequence-specific DNA binding properties.[108] This region also contains the site bound by the SV40 large T antigen.[109] The carboxy-terminal portion of the p53 protein is required for oligomerization, a function required for DNA binding and transactivation.[110–112] Phosphorylation sites are present in this region as well.

The p53 protein appears to play numerous roles within the cell. It has been implicated in control of cell proliferation and differentiation, DNA repair and synthesis, and programmed cell death.[94, 106, 113–119] Because it affects cell cycle arrest in the G_1 phase in response to DNA damage, p53 has been referred to as the "guardian of the genome."[105] This presumably allows the injured cell time to repair the alterations in its DNA before entering the S phase of the cell cycle. Loss of this checkpoint control could potentially result in replication of damaged DNA and the generation of genomic instability in affected cells.[106, 120–122] In addition, p53 has a role in directing cells into a pathway of programmed cell death, presumably in cases in which DNA damage is too severe to be repaired.[123, 124]

The p53 gene was initially believed to be an oncogene because it cooperated with ras to transform cells in culture.[125, 126] The wild-type protein, however, was found to have a tumor suppressor function in that it could block the transformation of cultured cells by oncogenes.[127, 128] Consistent with its putative function as a tumor suppressor, introduction of a wild-type p53 gene into cancer cells in culture results in growth suppression.[129] Loss of the normal growth regulatory activity of the wild-type protein provides cells with a selective growth advantage, promotes genetic instability, and contributes to the development of cancer. However, p53 mutations alone are probably not sufficient to initiate a cancer. Instead, mutations at additional tumor suppressor or oncogene loci are necessary for complete malignant transformation of a cell.[113]

The types of p53 mutations most frequently identified in carcinomas are missense mutations involving the DNA sequence-specific binding region.[130, 131] This region of the gene spans exons 4 to 9 and is known to include highly conserved sequence blocks.[132] Alterations in p53 range from complete deletion of the gene resulting in no p53 synthesis at all to a variety of different point mutations that retain the synthesis of full-length, albeit mutant, p53 proteins. In fact, missense point mutations resulting in faulty p53 proteins are the most prevalent type of p53 alteration in human tumors.[113]

Although the wild-type p53 acts as a tumor suppressor, mutant p53 in some circumstances may exert a dominant negative effect.[133–135] The polypeptides of mutated p53 have a longer half-life than the wild-type protein. As a result, they tend to accumulate to high levels in cancer cells. They have been shown to form oligomeric protein complexes with wild-type p53 subunits, thereby functionally inactivating them.[133, 134, 136, 137] Therefore, p53 mutations may result in complete or near complete loss of normal p53 function, although the normal allele has not been lost.

Recent studies have also suggested that mutations in p53 not only induce a loss of function but may represent "gain-of-function" mutations. This hypothesis has been tested directly through the introduction of mutated p53 genes into cultured cells that completely lack wild-type p53.[138, 139] In such a system, any alteration in cell function can be attributed to the action of the mutant p53. Such cells become tumorigenic in nude mice, which suggests that mutant p53 not only acts to inactivate wild-type p53 but also has some intrinsic transforming properties of its own. Some studies have demonstrated that mutant p53 is able to promote transcription of the multiple drug resistance gene whereas wild-type p53 cannot.[138] In this way, mutant p53 may contribute directly to the malignant phenotype.

A number of studies have provided evidence that p53 mutation and allelic loss are late events in colorectal carcinogenesis. Chromosome 17p allelic deletions are infrequent in adenomas, affecting fewer than 10%.[41, 140] In contrast, p53 mutation and associated LOH are relatively common in colorectal carcinomas (Fig 8). Mutation of p53 occurs in approximately 42% to 64% of carcinomas, and LOH is present in from 48% to 76%.[41, 140–143] In some adenomas harboring carcinomas, alterations in the APC, ras, and DCC genes can be demonstrated in both the adenomatous and carcinomatous tissue, but p53 mutation and allelic loss are observed only in the carcinoma.[144]

When 17p allelic loss does occur, it is often associated with mutation in the retained p53 allele.[97, 98, 142, 145, 146] Baker et al.[144] found p53 mutations in 2 of 19 colorectal adenomas without evidence of LOH and in 4 of 6 adenomas that did exhibit LOH. Overall, 17p allelic loss was identified in 7 of 66 adenomas. In carcinomas, p53 mutation was detected in 86% of the tumors with LOH and in 17% of the tumors without LOH. Therefore, allelic loss appears to be preceded in most cases by p53 gene mutation.

In some settings, however, loss of p53 may not be a late event in the neoplastic progression in the colon. Several studies have suggested that unlike the situation in sporadic colorectal cancers, p53 mutation and allelic loss occur early in carcinogenesis associated with ulcerative colitis (Fig 9). Such p53 alterations have been identified in the earliest recognizable dysplastic lesions in this setting.[147–149] This finding supports the concept that development of the malignant phenotype is dependent on

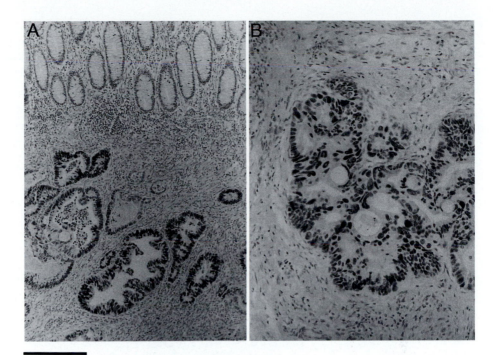

FIGURE 8.

Immunohistochemical stain using antibodies directed against the p53 protein. **A,** numerous positively staining cells are noted in this colonic adenocarcinoma. Note that the overlying, non-neoplastic epithelium does not stain. **B,** a higher-power view of the tumor demonstrates intranuclear p53 staining. The p53 antibody recognizes both wild-type and mutant p53, but the half-life of the wild-type protein is so short that it is not readily detected. Mutant protein has a longer half-life and accumulates in the cell, thus making it detectable with immunohistochemistry.

the total accumulation of genetic abnormalities rather than the sequence in which such abnormalities are acquired.

OTHER TUMOR SUPPRESSOR GENES

The retinoblastoma gene (Rb) lies on chromosome 13 at position q14.2. As its name suggests, this gene was first identified in association with both hereditary and sporadic retinoblastomas in children.[150–154] Since that time, loss of Rb has been demonstrated in a variety of other human malignancies.[152, 154–159] A number of studies have examined the role of Rb in colorectal neoplasia. Allelic loss of chromosome 13 is uncommon in colon cancer.[160] In fact, increased allelic copy numbers from chromosome 13 have been reported in 30% to 50% of colon carcinomas.[160–162] In addition, increased levels of Rb mRNA are observed in many tumors.[161] Although none of these findings rule out the possibility of mutation in the Rb gene, they do suggest that Rb is not lost or inactivated in colon carcinoma. These findings also do not rule out the possibility that overexpression of Rb somehow plays a role in carcinogenesis in the colon, perhaps through effects on cell cycle regulation.

Allelic loss in colorectal carcinoma has additionally been reported at sites on the short arms of chromosomes 1 and 8.[163–166] The putative tu-

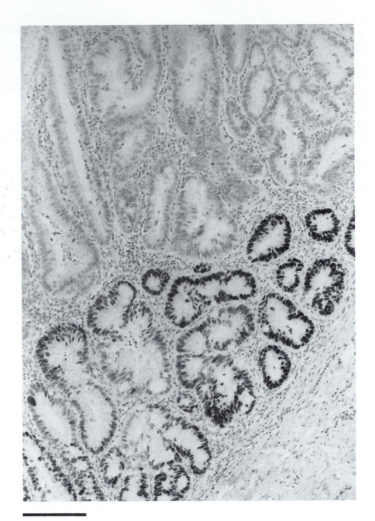

FIGURE 9.

Immunohistochemical stain for p53 in ulcerative colitis. Numerous strongly positive cells are present in this area of low-grade dysplasia (*right*). On the *left* is an area with a similar histology but negative for p53, which suggsts that the p53-positive clone probably arose after the initial development of dysplasia. The frequent identification of p53 abnormalities in low-grade dysplasia in ulcerative colitis is cited as evidence that *p53* mutations are important early in colorectal carcinogenesis in this setting.

mor suppressor genes located on these chromosomes have not yet been identified. Changes in chromosome 1p were observed in early adenomas and in one instance in non-neoplastic mucosa, thus suggesting that alterations in this putative tumor suppressor gene may occur early in the neoplastic progression.[164] Chromosome 8p losses, on the other hand, have been associated with late clinicopathologic stage in colon carcinomas.[166]

OTHER ONCOGENES

A number of studies have examined the role of the *myc* oncogene in colorectal neoplasia. Many studies have reported increased expression of c-*myc* in colorectal carcinomas[167–169] but no evidence of amplification or rearrangements of the gene.[167] In many cases, this increase in c-*myc* expression is probably a reflection of increased proliferative activity (DNA synthesis) in neoplastic cells.[167, 170] Therefore, c-*myc* probably does not play a direct role in neoplastic progression in the colon.

CHANGES ASSOCIATED WITH THE METASTATIC PHENOTYPE

The most lethal characteristic of any malignant tumor is its ability to metastasize. However, despite the obvious clinical importance of metastatic potential, the molecular genetic changes accompanying the acquisition of this phenotype are not yet well understood. In order to invade and metastasize, cancer cells must acquire a number of characteristics. They must be able to leave the primary tumor, invade local host tissues, gain access to the circulation, arrest at a distant site, leave the vascular system and enter the tissues, and finally proliferate at the target site.[171]

Clearly, metastasis is not a simple process; it presumably requires the combined action of multiple host-tumor interactions. There are many factors that have been implicated in the metastatic process. These include alterations in the properties of cell adhesion molecules, proteolytic enzymes, and angiogenic factors, as well as loss of putative "antimetastasis" genes. The role of these factors in late progression of colorectal cancer is still poorly understood, and much of the data is conflicting.

In one study of E-cadherin expression in colorectal carcinomas, the authors demonstrated loss of this cell adhesion molecule with increasing degrees of dedifferentiation.[172] In addition, they reported that metastasis to regional lymph nodes was more frequent in tumors that were E-cadherin−negative. In addition, E-cadherin expression was strongly correlated with stage, with Dukes' stage C and D carcinomas displaying significantly less E-cadherin than stage A and B tumors. Other studies have found that loss of E-cadherin expression does not correlate with stage.[173]

Several studies have examined the role of metalloproteinases in colorectal neoplasia. The metalloproteinases represent a group of enzymes that have the ability to degrade the extracellular matrix and are therefore thought to be important in tumor invasion and metastasis.[171, 174] Type IV collagenase (MMP-2) is detectable in cells derived from colorectal carcinomas and adenomas.[175, 176] In addition, MMP-2 is strongly expressed in desmoplastic stroma surrounding invading tumor cells, which suggests that there is an important contribution to invasive potential made not only by tumor cells but by stromal cells as well.[175] Increased activity of MMP-2 has been localized to areas of tumor invasion as compared with matched normal epithelium from the same patients.[176] How metalloproteinase activity correlates with tumor behavior is not yet known.

The role played by the putative metastasis suppressor gene *nm23* in colon carcinogenesis is controversial. The *nm23* gene was first identified because its expression was increased in nonmetastatic murine melanoma cells.[177] Transfection of *nm23* into cell lines with a high degree of metastatic potential inhibits this activity.[178] The human homologues of the murine *nm23* gene have now been identified and are referred to as *nm23-H1* and *nm23-H2*.[179]

Allelic deletions of *nm23-H1* have been identified in colon carcinomas,[180] and Cohn et al.[181] found that such allelic losses were associated with the development of distant metastases. Other studies have found increased levels of *nm23-H1* mRNA in colorectal neoplasms and have demonstrated that these levels are similar in metastatic and nonmetastatic tumors.[182, 183] Further studies are clearly needed to sort out the role of this gene in the development of metastatic carcinoma of the colon.

CONCLUSION

Our understanding of the molecular genetic changes that accompany neoplastic progression has improved markedly in the last decade primarily because of the numerous technological advancements that have recently been made. Many of the new insights we have gained have come from work done in the area of colorectal carcinogenesis. These studies have firmly established the notion that cancers arising in the colon, or for that matter at any site, develop as a result of the accumulation of multiple, sequential genetic abnormalities. Although these changes often occur in a relatively consistent, site-specific sequence, it is the total sum of the genetic changes that determine the phenotype of the malignant cell.

Although tremendous advances have been made in our understanding of colon cancer biology, there is probably still much more to be discovered. There are certainly additional oncogenes and tumor suppressor genes yet to be identified that play important roles in colorectal carcinogenesis. The changes that enhance metastatic potential in colon carcinoma cells also require further elucidation. Finally, few of the new insights gained in the molecular biology of colorectal neoplasia have yet been translated into routine clinical usage. In the future, molecular biological factors will undoubtedly contribute to the diagnosis, determination of prognosis, and treatment of human malignancies.

REFERENCES

1. Rous P: A sarcoma of the fowl transmissible by an agent separable from the tumour cells. *J Exp Med* 13:397–411, 1911.
2. Martin GS: Rous sarcoma virus: A function required for the maintenance of the transformed state. *Nature* 227:1021–1023, 1970.
3. Stehlin D, Varmus HE, Bishop JM, et al: DNA related to the transforming gene(s) of avian sarcoma viruses is present in normal avian DNA. *Nature* 260:170–173, 1976.
4. Knudson AG: Mutation and cancer: Statistical study of retinoblastoma. *Proc Natl Acad Sci U S A* 68:820–828, 1971.
5. Hansen MF, Cavenee WK: Genetics of cancer predisposition. *Cancer Res* 47:5518–5527, 1987.
6. Stanbridge EJ, Cavenee WK: Heritable cancer and tumor suppressor genes: A tentative connection, in Weinberg RA (ed): *Oncogenes and the Molecular Origins of Cancer*. Cold Spring Harbor, NY, Cold Spring Harbor Laboratory, 1989, pp 281–306.
7. Thomas RM, Sobin LH: Gastrointestinal cancer. *Cancer* 75:154–170, 1995.
8. Fearon ER, Hamilton SR, Vogelstein B: Clonal analysis of human colorectal tumors. *Science* 238:193–197, 1987.
9. Ponder BAJ, Wilkinson MM: Direct examination of the clonality of

carcinogen-induced colonic epithelial dysplasia in chimeric mice. *J Natl Cancer Inst* 77:967–976, 1986.

10. Lipkin M: Biomarkers of increased susceptibility of gastrointestinal cancer: New application to studies of cancer prevention in human subjects. *Cancer Res* 48:235–245, 1988.

11. Tudek WR, Bird RP, Bruce WR: Foci of aberrant crypts in the colon of mice and rats exposed to carcinogens associated with foods. *Cancer Res* 49:1236–1240, 1989.

12. Fenoglio CM, Pascal RR: Colorectal adenomas and cancer: Pathologic relationships. *Cancer* 50(suppl 11):2601–2608, 1982.

13. Helwig EB: Adenomas and the pathogenesis of cancer of the colon and rectum. *Dis Colon Rectum* 2:5–7, 1959.

14. Kozuka S: Premalignancy of the mucosal polyp in the large intestine: I. Histologic gradation of the polyp on the basis of epithelial pseudostratification and glandular branching. *Dis Colon Rectum* 18:483–493, 1975.

15. Kozuka S, Nogaki M, Ozeki T, et al: Premalignancy of the mucosal polyp in the large intestine: II. Estimation of the periods required for malignant transformation of mucosal polyps. *Dis Colon Rectum* 18:494–500, 1975.

16. Maskens AP, Deschner EF: Tritiated thymidine incorporation into epithelial cells of normal-appearing colorectal mucosa of cancer patients. *J Natl Cancer Inst* 58:1221–1224, 1977.

17. Risio M, Coverlizza S, Ferrari A, et al: Immunohistochemical study of epithelial cell proliferation in hyperplastic polyps, adenomas, and adenocarcinomas of the large bowel. *Gastroenterology* 94:899–906, 1988.

18. Terpstra TO, van Blankenstein J, Dees J, et al: Abnormal pattern of cell proliferation in the entire colonic mucosa of patients with familial adenomas or colon cancer. *Gastroenterology* 92:704–708, 1987.

19. Lipkin M, Blattner WE, Fraumeni JF, et al: Tritiated thymidine labeling distribution as a marker for hereditary predisposition to colon cancer. *Cancer Res* 43:1899–1904, 1983.

20. Deschner EE, Lipkin M: Proliferation patterns in colonic mucosa in familial polyposis. *Cancer* 35:413–418, 1975.

21. Goelz SE, Vogelstein B, Hamilton SR, et al: Hypomethylation of DNA from benign and malignant human colon neoplasms. *Science* 228:187–190, 1985.

22. Feinberg AP, Gehrke CW, Kuo KC, et al: Reduced genomic 5-methylcytosine content in human colonic neoplasia. *Cancer Res* 48:1159–1161, 1988.

23. Schmid M, Haaf T, Grunert D: 5-Azacytidine–induced undercondensations in human chromosomes. *Hum Genet* 67:257–263, 1984.

24. Hausheer FH, Rao SN, Gamcsik MP, et al: Computational analysis of structural and energetic consequences of DNA methylation. *Carcinogenesis* 10:1131–1137, 1989.

25. Antequera F, Macleod D, Bird AP: Specific protection of methylated CpGs in mammalian nuclei. *Cell* 58:509–517, 1989.

26. Meehan RR, Lewis JD, McKay S, et al: Identification of a mammalian protein that binds specifically to DNA containing methylated CpGs. *Cell* 58:499–507, 1989.

27. Laird C, Jaffe E, Karpen G, et al: Fragile sites in human chromosomes as regions of late-replicating DNA. *Trends Genet* 3:274–281, 1987.

28. Silverman AL, Park JG, Hamilton SR, et al: Abnormal methylation of the calcitonin gene in human colonic neoplasms. *Cancer Res* 49:3468–3473, 1989.

29. El-Diery WS, Nelkin BD, Celano P, et al: High expression of the DNA methyltransferase gene characterizes human neoplastic cells and progression stages of colon cancer. *Proc Natl Acad Sci U S A* 88:3470–3474, 1991.

30. Antequera F, Boyes J, Bird A: High levels of de novo methylation and altered chromatin structure at CpG islands in cell lines. *Cell* 62:503–514, 1990.

31. Bodmer WF, Bailey CJ, Bodmer J, et al: Localization of gene for familial adenomatous polyposis on chromosome 5. *Nature* 328:614–616, 1987.

32. Leppert M, Dobbs M, Scambeler P, et al: The gene for familial polyposis coli maps to the long arm of chromosome 5. *Science* 238:1411–1413, 1987.

33. Groden J, Thliveris A, Samowitz W, et al: Identification and characterization of the familial adenomatous polyposis gene. *Cell* 66:589–600, 1991.

34. Kinzler KW, Nilbet M, Su L-K, et al: Identification of the FAP locus genes from chromosome 5q21. *Science* 253:661–664, 1991.

35. Nishisho I, Nakamura Y, Miyoshi Y, et al: Mutations of the chromosome 5q21 genes in FAP and colorectal patients. *Science* 253:665–669, 1991.

36. Powell SM, Zilz N, Beazer-Barclay Y, et al: APC mutations occur early during colorectal tumorigenesis. *Nature* 359:235–237, 1992.

37. Okamoto M, Sasaki M, Sugio K, et al: Loss of constitutional heterozygosity in colon carcinoma from patients with familial polyposis coli. *Nature* 331:273–277, 1988.

38. Sasaki M, Okamoto M, Sato C, et al: Loss of constitutional heterozygosity in colorectal tumors from patients with familial polyposis coli and those with nonpolyposis colorectal carcinoma. *Cancer Res* 49:4402–4406, 1989.

39. Rees M, Leigh SEA, Delhanty JDA, et al: Chromosome 5 allele loss in familial and sporadic colorectal adenomas. *Br J Cancer* 59:361–365, 1989.

40. Solomon E, Voss R, Hall V, et al: Chromosome 5 allele loss in human colorectal carcinomas. *Nature* 328:616–619, 1987.

41. Vogelstein B, Fearon ER, Hamilton SR, et al: Genetic alterations during colorectal-tumor development. *N Engl J Med* 319:525–532, 1988.

42. Miyaki M, Seki M, Okamoto M, et al: Genetic changes and histopathological types in colorectal tumors from patients with familial adenomatous polyposis. *Cancer Res* 50:7166–7173, 1990.

43. Tsao J-I, Shibata D: Further evidence that one of the earliest alterations in colorectal carcinogenesis involves APC. *Am J Pathol* 145:531–534, 1994.

44. Fearon ER, Jones PA: Progressing toward a molecular description of colorectal cancer development. *FASEB J* 6:2783–2790, 1992.

45. Nakatsuru S, Yanagisawa A, Ichii S, et al: Somatic mutation of the APC gene in gastric cancer: Frequent mutations in very well differentiated adenocarcinoma and signet-ring cell carcinoma. *Hum Mol Gen* 1:559–563, 1992.

46. Miyoshi Y, Ando H, Nagase H, et al: Germ-line mutations of the APC gene in 53 familial adenomatous polyposis patients. *Proc Natl Acad Sci U S A* 89:4452–4456, 1992.

47. Smith KJ, Johnson KA, Bryan TM, et al: The APC gene product in normal and tumor cells. *Proc Natl Acad Sci U S A* 90:2846–2850, 1993.

48. Su L-K, Johnson KA, Smith KJ, et al: Association between wildtype and mutant APC products. *Cancer Res* 53:2728–2731, 1993.

49. Miyaki M, Konishi M, Kikuchi-Yanoshita R, et al: Characteristics of somatic mutation of the adenomatous polyposis coli gene in colorectal tumors. *Cancer Res* 54:3011–3020, 1994.

50. Smith KJ, Levy DB, Maupin P, et al: Wild-type but not mutant APC associates with the microtubule cytoskeleton. *Cancer Res* 54:3672–3675, 1994.

51. Munemitsu S, Souza B, Muller O, et al: The APC gene product associates with microtubules in vivo and promotes their assembly in vitro. *Cancer Res* 54:3676–3681, 1994.

52. Crossin KL: Evidence that microtubule depolymerization early in the cell cycle is sufficient to initiate DNA synthesis. *Cell* 23:61–71, 1981.

53. Barbacid M: ras Genes. *Annu Rev Biochem* 56:779–827, 1987.

54. Yoshida T, Sakamoto H, Terada M: Amplified genes in cancer of the upper digestive tract. *Semin Cancer Biol* 4:33–49, 1993.
55. Bos JL: ras Oncogenes in human cancer: A review. *Cancer Res* 49:4682–4689, 1989.
56. McCormick F: ras GTPase activating protein: Signal transmitter and signal terminator. *Cell* 56:5–8, 1989.
57. Vogelstein B, Fearon ER, Kern SE, et al: Allelotype of colorectal carcinomas. *Science* 244:207–211, 1989.
58. Burmer GC, Loeb LA: Mutations in the KRAS2 oncogene during progressive stages of human colon carcinoma. *Proc Natl Acad Sci U S A* 86:2403–2407, 1989.
59. Hockenbery DM, Nunez G, Milliman C, et al: Bcl-2 is an inner mitochondrial membrane protein that blocks programmed cell death. *Nature* 348:334–336, 1990.
60. Korsmeyer SJ: Bcl-2 initiates a new category of oncogenes: Regulators of cell death. *Blood* 80:879–886, 1992.
61. Vaux DL: Toward an understanding of the molecular mechanisms of physiological cell death. *Proc Natl Acad Sci U S A* 90:786–789, 1993.
62. Reed JC: Bcl-2 and the regulation of programmed cell death. *J Cell Biol* 124:1–6, 1993.
63. Tsujimoto Y, Croce CM: Analysis of the structure, transcripts and protein products of bcl-2, the gene involved in human follicular lymphoma. *Proc Natl Acad Sci U S A* 83:5214–5218, 1986.
64. Bronner MP, Culin C, Reed JC, et al: The bcl-2 proto-oncogene and the gastrointestinal epithelial tumor progression model. *Am J Pathol* 146:20–26, 1995.
65. Lynch HT, Shaw MW, Magnuson CW, et al: Hereditary factors in two large midwestern kindreds. *Arch Intern Med* 117:206–212, 1966.
66. Vasen HFA, Hartog-Jager FCA, Menko FH, et al: Screening for hereditary non-polyposis colorectal cancer: A study of 22 kindreds in the Netherlands. *Am J Med* 86:278–281, 1989.
67. Cameron BH, Fitzgerald GWN, Cox J: Hereditary site-specific colon cancer in a Canadian kindred. *Can Med Assoc J* 140:41–45, 1989.
68. Lynch HT, Smyrk TC, Watson P, et al: Genetics, natural history, tumor spectrum in pathology of hereditary nonpolyposis colorectal cancers, an updated review. *Gastroenterology* 104:1535–1549, 1993.
69. Vasen HFA, Offerhaus DJA, Den Hartog FCA, et al: The tumor spectrum in hereditary nonpolyposis colorectal cancer: A study of 24 kindreds in the Netherlands. *Int J Cancer* 46:31–34, 1990.
70. Mecklin JP, Jarvinen HJ: Tumor spectrum in cancer family syndrome (hereditary nonpolyposis colorectal cancer). *Cancer* 68:1109–1112, 1991.
71. Mecklin JP, Sipponen P, Jarvinen HJ: Histopathology of colorectal carcinomas and adenomas in cancer family syndrome. *Dis Colon Rectum* 29:849–853, 1986.
72. Albano WA, Recebaren JA, Lynch HT, et al: Natural history of hereditary cancer of the breast and colon. *Cancer* 50:360–363, 1982.
73. Love RR: Small bowel cancers, B-cell lymphatic leukemia and six primary cancers with metastases and prolonged survival in the cancer family syndrome of Lynch. *Cancer* 55:499–502, 1985.
74. Peltomaki P, Aaltonen L, Sistonen P, et al: Genetic mapping of a locus predisposing to human colorectal cancer. *Science* 260:810–812, 1993.
75. Lindblom A, Tannergard P, Werelius B, et al: Genetic mapping of a second locus predisposing to hereditary non-polyposis colon cancer. *Nat Genet* 5:279–282, 1993.

76. Thibodeau SN, Bren G, Schaid D: Microsatellite instability in cancer of the proximal colon. *Science* 260:816–819, 1993.
77. Aaltonen LA, Peltomaki P, Leach FS, et al: Clues to the pathogenesis of familial colorectal cancer. *Science* 260:812–816, 1993.
78. Ionov YM, Peinado A, Malkhosyan S, et al: Ubiquitous somatic mutation in simple repeated sequences reveals a new mechanism for colonic carcinogenesis. *Nature* 363:558–561, 1993.
79. Fishel R, Lescoe MK, Rao MRS, et al: The human mutator gene homolog MSH2 and its association with hereditary nonpolyposis colon cancer. *Cell* 75:1027–1038, 1993.
80. Leach FS, Nicolaides NC, Papadopoulos N, et al: Mutations of a mutS homolog in hereditary nonpolyposis colorectal cancer. *Cell* 75:1215–1225, 1993.
81. Papadopoulos N, Nicolaides NC, Wei YF, et al: Mutation of a mutL homolog in hereditary colon cancer. *Science* 263:1625–1628, 1993.
82. Bronner CE, Baker SM, Morrison PT, et al: Mutation in the DNA mismatch repair gene homologue hMLH1 is associated with hereditary nonpolyposis colon cancer. *Nature* 368:258–261, 1994.
83. Lothe RA, Peltomaki P, Meling GI, et al: Genomic instability in colorectal cancer: Relationship to clinicopathologic variables and family history. *Cancer Res* 53:5849–5852, 1993.
84. Kim H, Jen J, Vogelstein B, et al: Clinical and pathological characteristics of sporadic colorectal carcinomas with DNA replication errors in microsatellite sequences. *Am J Pathol* 145:148–156, 1994.
85. Suzuki H, Harpaz N, Tarmin L, et al: Microsatellite instability in ulcerative colitis–associated colorectal dysplasias and cancers. *Cancer Res* 54:4841–4844, 1994.
86. Shibata D, Peinado MA, Ionov Y, et al: Genomic instability in repeated sequences is an early somatic event in colorectal tumorigenesis that persists after transformation. *Nat Genet* 6:273–280, 1994.
87. Fearon ER, Cho KR, Nigro JM, et al: Identification of a chromosome 18q gene that is altered in colorectal cancers. *Science* 247:49–56, 1990.
88. Kikuchi-Yanoshita R, Konishi M, Fukunari H, et al: Loss of expression of the DCC gene during progression of colorectal carcinomas in familial adenomatous polyposis and non-familial adenomatous polyposis patients. *Cancer Res* 52:3801–3803, 1992.
89. Itoh F, Hinoda Y, Ohe M, et al: Decreased expression of DCC mRNA in human colorectal cancers. *Int J Cancer* 53:260–263, 1993.
90. Tanaka K, Oshimura M, Kikuchi R, et al: Supression of tumorigenicity in human colon carcinoma cells by introduction of normal chromosome 5 or 18. *Nature* 389:340–342, 1991.
91. Zetter BR: Adhesion molecules in tumor metastasis. *Semin Cancer Biol* 4:219–229, 1993.
92. Jen J, Kim H, Piantadosi S, et al: Allelic loss of chromosome 18q and prognosis in colorectal cancer. *N Engl J Med* 331:213–221, 1994.
93. Edelman GM: Morphoregulatory molecules. *Biochemistry* 27:3533–3543, 1988.
94. Hollstein M, Sidransky D, Vogelstein B, et al: p53 mutations in human cancers. *Science* 253:49–53, 1991.
95. Suzuki H, Takahashi T, Kuroishi T, et al: p53 mutations in non–small cell cancer in Japan: Association between mutations and smoking. *Cancer Res* 52:734–736, 1992.
96. Kishimoto Y, Murakami Y, Shiraishi M, et al: Aberrations of the p53 tumor suppressor gene in human non–small cell carcinomas of the lung. *Cancer Res* 52:4799–4804, 1992.

97. Baker S, Fearon E, Nigro J, et al: Chromosome 17 deletions and p53 gene mutations in colorectal carcinomas. *Science* 244:217–221, 1989.

98. Nigro JM, Baker SJ, Preisinger AC, et al: Mutations in the p53 gene occur in diverse human tumour types. *Nature* 342:705–708, 1988.

99. Runnebaum IB, Nagarajan M, Bowman M, et al: Mutations in p53 as potential molecular markers for human breast cancer. *Proc Natl Acad Sci U S A* 88:10657–10661, 1991.

100. Nose H, Imazeki F, Ohto M, et al: p53 gene mutations and 17p allelic deletions in hepatocellular carcinoma from Japan. *Cancer* 72:355–360, 1993.

101. Scarpa A, Capelli P, Mukai K, et al: Pancreatic adenocarcinomas frequently show p53 gene mutations. *Am J Pathol* 142:1534–1543, 1993.

102. Imazeki F, Omata M, Nose H, et al: p53 gene mutations in gastric and esophageal cancers. *Gastroenterology* 103:892–896, 1992.

103. Brachman DG, Graves D, Vokes E, et al: Occurrence of p53 gene deletions and human papilloma virus infection in human head and neck cancer. *Cancer Res* 52:4832–4836, 1992.

104. Tsao S-W, Mok C-H, Oike K, et al: Involvement of p53 gene in the allelic deletion of chromosome 17p in human ovarian tumors. *Anticancer Res* 11:1975–1982, 1991.

105. Lane DP: p53, guardian of the genome. *Nature* 358:15–16, 1992.

106. Vogelstein B, Kinzler KW: p53 function and dysfunction. *Cell* 70:523–526, 1992.

107. Greenblatt MS, Bennett WP, Hollstein M, et al: Mutations in the p53 tumor suppressor gene: Clues to cancer etiology and molecular pathogenesis. *Cancer Res* 54:4855–4878, 1994.

108. Srinivasan R, Roth JA, Maxwell SA: Sequence-specific interaction of a conformational domain of p53 with DNA. *Cancer Res* 53:5361–5364, 1993.

109. Ruppert JM, Stillman B: Analysis of a protein-binding domain of p53. *Mol Cell Biol* 13:3811–3820, 1993.

110. Cho Y, Gorina S, Jeffrey P, et al: Crystal structure of a p53 tumor suppressor–DNA complex: A framework for understanding how mutations inactivate p53. *Science* 265:346–355, 1994.

111. Tarunina M, Jenkins JR: Human p53 binds DNA as a protein homodimer but monomeric variants retain full transcription transactivation activity. *Oncogene* 8:3165–3173, 1993.

112. Pietenpol JA, Tokino T, Thiagalingam S, et al: Sequence-specific transcriptional activation is essential for growth suppression by p53. *Proc Natl Acad Sci U S A* 91:1998–2002, 1994.

113. Levine AJ, Momand J, Finlay CA: The p53 tumour suppressor gene. *Nature* 351:453–456, 1991.

114. Rotter V, Prokocimer M: p53 and human malignancies. *Adv Cancer Res* 57:257–272, 1991.

115. Oren M: p53: The ultimate tumor suppressor gene? *FASEB J* 6:3169–3176, 1992.

116. Caron de Fromentel C, Soussi T: TP53 tumor suppressor gene: A model for investigating human mutagenesis. *Genes Chromosom Cancer* 4:1–15, 1992.

117. Montenarh M: Biochemical properties of the growth suppressor/oncoprotein p53. *Oncogene* 7:1673–1680, 1992.

118. Dutta A, Ruppert JM, Aster JC, et al: Inhibition of DNA replication factor RPA by p53. *Nature* 365:79–82, 1993.

119. Pietenpol JA, Vogelstein B: No room at the p53 inn. *Nature* 365:17–18, 1993.

120. Hartwell L: Defects in a cell cycle checkpoint may be responsible for the genomic instability of cancer cells. *Cell* 71:543–546, 1992.

121. Livingston LR, White A, Sprouse J, et al: Altered cell cycle arrest and gene

amplification potential accompany loss of wild type p53. *Cell* 70:923–935, 1992.

122. Yin Y, Tainsky MA, Bischoff FZ, et al: Wild type p53 restores cell cycle control and inhibits gene amplification in cells with mutant p53 alleles. *Cell* 70:937–948, 1992.

123. Clarke AR, Purdie CA, Harrison DL, et al: Thymocyte apoptosis induced by p53 dependent and independent pathways. *Nature* 362:849–852, 1993.

124. Lowe SW, Schmitt EM, Smith SW, et al: p53 is required for radiation-induced apoptosis in mouse thymocytes. *Nature* 362:847–849, 1993.

125. Eliyahu D, Raz A, Gruss P, et al: Participation of p53 cellular tumour antigen in transformation of normal embryonic cells. *Nature* 312:646–649, 1984.

126. Parada L, Land H, Weinberg RA, et al: Cooperation between gene encoding p53 tumour antigen and ras in cellular transformation. *Nature* 312:649–651, 1984.

127. Finlay CA, Hinds PW, Levine AJ: The p53 proto-oncogene can act as a suppressor of transformation. *Cell* 57:1083–1093, 1989.

128. Eliyahu D, Michalovitz D, Eliyahu S, et al: Wild-type p53 can inhibit oncogene-mediated focus formation. *Proc Natl Acad Sci U S A* 86:8763–8767, 1989.

129. Matozaki T, Sakamoto C, Suzuki T, et al: p53 gene mutations in human gastric cancer: Wild-type p53 but not mutant p53 suppresses growth of human gastric cancer cells. *Cancer Res* 52:4335–4341, 1992.

130. Bodner SM, Minna JD, Jensen SM, et al: Expression of mutant p53 proteins in lung cancer correlates with the class of p53 gene mutation. *Oncogene* 7:743–749, 1992.

131. Chiba I, Takahashi T, Nau MM, et al: Mutations in the p53 gene are frequent in primary, resected non–small cell lung cancer. *Oncogene* 5:1603–1610, 1990.

132. Soussi T, Caron de Fromentel C, May P: Structural aspects of the p53 protein in relation to gene evolution. *Oncogene* 5:945–952, 1990.

133. Milner J, Medcalf EA: Cotranslation of activated mutant p53 with wild type drives the wild type p53 protein into the mutant conformation. *Cell* 65:765–774, 1991.

134. Milner J: A conformation hypothesis for the suppressor and promoter function of p53 in cell growth control and cancer. *Proc R Soc Lond B Biol Sci* 245:139–145, 1991.

135. Srivastava S, Wang S, Tong YA, et al: Dominant negative effect of a germline mutant p53: A step fostering tumorigenesis. *Cancer Res* 53:4452–4455, 1993.

136. Kern S, Pietenpol JA, Thiagalingam S, et al: Oncogenic forms of p53 inhibit p53-regulated gene expression. *Science* 256:827–832, 1992.

137. Farmer GE, Bargonetti J Zhu H, et al: Wild-type p53 activates transcription in vitro. *Nature* 358:83–86, 1992.

138. Chin KV, Ueda K, Pastan I, et al: Modulation of activity of the promoter of the human MDR1 gene by ras and p53. *Science* 255:459–462, 1992.

139. Hsaio M, Low J, Dorn E, et al: Gain-of-function mutations of the p53 gene induce lymphohematopoietic metastatic potential and tissue invasiveness. *Am J Pathol* 145:702–714, 1994.

140. Ohue M, Tomita N, Monden T, et al: A frequent alteration of p53 gene in *carcinoma in adenoma* of colon. *Cancer Res* 54:4798–4804, 1994.

141. Lothe RA, Fossli T, Danielsen HE, et al: Molecular genetic studies of tumor suppressor gene regions on chromosomes 13 and 17 in colorectal tumors. *J Natl Cancer Inst* 84:1100–1108, 1992.

142. Shaw P, Tardy S, Benito E, et al: Occurrence of Ki-ras and p53 mutations in primary colorectal tumors. *Oncogene* 6:2121–2128, 1991.
143. Cunningham J, Lust JA, Schaid DJ, et al: Expression of p53 and 17p allelic loss in colorectal carcinoma. *Cancer Res* 52:1974–1980, 1992.
144. Baker SJ, Preisinger AC, Jessup JM, et al: p53 gene mutations occur in combination with 17p allelic deletions as late events in colorectal tumorigenesis. *Cancer Res* 50:7717–7722, 1990.
145. Takahashi T, Nau MM, Chiba I, et al: p53: A frequent target for genetic abnormalities in lung cancer. *Science* 246:491–494, 1989.
146. Menon AG, Anderson KM, Riccardi VM, et al: Chromosome 17p deletions and p53 gene mutations associated with the formation of malignant neurofibrosarcomas in von Recklinghausen neurofibromatosis. *Proc Natl Acad Sci U S A* 87:5435–5439, 1990.
147. Yin J, Harpaz N, Tong Y, et al: p53 point mutations in dysplastic and cancerous ulcerative colitis lesions. *Gastroenterology* 104:1633–1639, 1993.
148. Burmer GC, Crispin DA, Killi VR, et al: Frequent loss of a p53 allele in carcinomas and their precursors in ulcerative colitis. *Cancer Commun* 3:167–172, 1991.
149. Burmer GC, Rabinovitch PS, Haggitt RC, et al: Neoplastic progression in ulcerative colitis: Histology, DNA content, and loss of a p53 allele. *Gastroenterology* 103:1602–1610, 1992.
150. Cavanee WK, Dryja TP, Phillips RA, et al: Expression of recessive alleles by chromosomal mechanisms in retinoblastoma. *Nature* 305:779–784, 1983.
151. Dryja TP, Rapaport JM, Joyce JM, et al: Molecular detection of deletions involving bank q14 of chromosome 13 in retinoblastoma. *Proc Natl Acad Sci U S A* 83:7391–7394, 1986.
152. Friend SH, Bernards R, Rogelj S, et al: A human DNA segment with properties of the gene that predisposes to retinoblastoma and osteosarcoma. *Nature* 323:643–646, 1986.
153. Lee WH, Bookstein R, Hong F: Human retinoblastoma susceptibility gene: Cloning, identification and sequence. *Science* 235:1394–1399, 1987.
154. Fung YKT, Murphree AL, T'Ang A, et al: Structural evidence for the authenticity of the human retinoblastoma gene. *Science* 235:1657–1661, 1987.
155. Harbour JW, Lai SL, Whang-Peng J, et al: Abnormalities in structure and expression of the human retinoblastoma gene in SCLC. *Science* 241:353–357, 1988.
156. Yokota J, Akiyama T, Fung YKT, et al: Altered expression of the retinoblastoma (RB) gene in small cell carcinoma of the lung. *Oncogene* 3:471–475, 1988.
157. Lee EYHP, To H, Shew JY, et al: Inactivation of the retinoblastoma susceptibility gene in human breast cancers. *Science* 241:218–221, 1988.
158. T'Ang A, Varley JM, Chakraborty S, et al: Structural rearrangement of the retinoblastoma gene in human breast carcinoma. *Science* 2442:263–266, 1988.
159. Horowitz JM, Yandell DW, Park SH, et al: Point mutational inactivation of the retinoblastoma antioncogene. *Science* 243:937–940, 1989.
160. Meling GI, Lothe RA, Borresen A-L, et al: Genetic alterations within the retinoblastoma locus in colorectal carcinomas: Relation to DNA ploidy pattern studied by flow cytometric analysis. *Br J Cancer* 64:475–480, 1991.
161. Gope R, Christensen MA, Thorson A, et al: Increased expression of the retinoblastoma gene in human colorectal carcinomas relative to normal colonic mucosa. *J Natl Cancer Inst* 82:310–314, 1990.
162. Muleris M, Salmon RJ, Dutrillaux AM: Characteristic chromosomal imbalances in 18 near-diploid colorectal tumors. *Cancer Genet Cytogenet* 29:289–302, 1987.

163. Reichmann A, Martin P, Levin B: Chromosomal banding patterns in human large bowel cancer. *Int J Cancer* 28:431–440, 1981.

164. Bardi G, Pandis N, Fenger C, et al: Deletion of 1p36 as a primary chromosomal aberration in intestinal tumorigenesis. *Cancer Res* 53:1895–1898, 1993.

165. Leister I, Weith A, Bruderlein S, et al: Human colorectal cancer: High frequency of deletions at chromosome 1p35. *Cancer Res* 50:7232–7235, 1990.

166. Fujiwara Y, Emi M, Ohata H, et al: Evidence for the presence of two tumor suppressor genes on chromosome 8p for colorectal carcinoma. *Cancer Res* 53:1172–1174, 1993.

167. Viel A, Maestro R, Toffoli G, et al: c-myc overexpression is a tumor-specific phenomenon in a subset of human colorectal carcinomas. *J Cancer Res Clin Oncol* 116:288–294, 1990.

168. Klimpfinger M, Zisser G, Ruhri C, et al: Expression of c-myc and c-fos mRNA in colorectal carcinoma in man. *Virchows Arch B Cell Pathol Incl Mol Pathol* 59:165–171, 1990.

169. Guillem JG, Levy MF, Hsieh LL, et al: Increased levels of phorbin, c-myc, and ornithine decarboxylase RNAs in human colon cancer. *Mol Carcinog* 3:68–74, 1990.

170. Rew DA, Taylor I, Cox H, et al: c-myc protein product is a marker of DNA synthesis but not of malignancy in human gastrointestinal tissues and tumours. *Br J Surg* 78:1080–1083, 1991.

171. Liotta LA, Tryggvason K, Garbisa S, et al: Metastatic potential correlates with enzymatic degradation of basement membrane collagen. *Nature* 284:67–68, 1980.

172. Dorudi S, Sheffield JP, Poulsom R, et al: E-cadherin expression in colorectal cancer: An immunohistochemical and in situ hybridization study. *Am J Pathol* 142:981–986, 1993.

173. Van der Wurff AAM, Kate JT, Van der Linden EPM, et al: L-CAM expression in normal, premalignant, and malignant colon mucosa. *J Pathol* 168:287–291, 1992.

174. Matrisian LM: Metalloproteinases and their inhibitors in matrix remodeling. *Trends Genet* 6:121–125, 1990.

175. Poulsom R, Pignatelli M, Stetler-Stevenson WG, et al: Stromal expression of 72 kda type IV collagenase (MMP-2) and TIMP-2 mRNAs in colorectal neoplasia. *Am J Pathol* 141:389–396, 1992.

176. Emmert-Buck MR, Roth MJ, Zhuang Z, et al: Increased gelatinase A (MMP-2) and cathespin B activity in invasive tumor regions of human colon cancer samples. *Am J Pathol* 145:1285–1290, 1994.

177. Steeg PS, Bevilacqua G, Kopper L, et al: Evidence for a novel gene associated with low tumor metastatic potential. *J Natl Cancer Inst* 80:200–204, 1988.

178. Leone A, Flatow U, King CR, et al: Reduced tumor incidence, metastatic potential, and cytokine responsiveness of nm23-transfected melanoma cells. *Cell* 65:25–35, 1991.

179. Stahl JA, Leone A, Rosengard AM, et al: Reduced nm23/awd protein in tumor metastasis and aberrant *Drosophila* development. *Nature* 342:177–180, 1989.

180. Leone A, McBride OW, Weston A, et al: Somatic allelic deletion of nm23 in human cancer. *Cancer Res* 51:2490–2493, 1991.

181. Cohn KH, Wang FS, DeSoto-LaPaix F, et al: Association of nm23-H1 allelic deletions with distant metastasis in colorectal carcinoma. *Lancet* 338:722–724, 1991.

182. Haut M, Steeg PS, Willson JKV, et al: Induction of nm23 gene expression in

human colonic neoplasms and equal expression in colon tumors of both high and low metastatic potential. *J Natl Cancer Inst* 83:712–716, 1991.

183. Myeroff LL, Markowitz SD: Increased nm23-H1 and nm23-H2 messenger RNA expression and absence of mutations in colon carcinomas of low and high metastatic potential. *J Natl Cancer Inst* 85:147–152, 1993.

Epithelial-Stromal Relationships in the Prostate and Their Role in Prostate Tumor Progression

Ray B. Nagle, M.D., Ph.D.
Professor of Pathology and Anatomy, University of Arizona Health Sciences Center, Tucson, Arizona

Anne E. Cress, Ph.D.
Associate Professor of Radiation Oncology, University of Arizona Health Sciences Center, Tucson, Arizona

G. Tim Bowden, Ph.D.
Professor of Radiation Oncology, University of Arizona Health Sciences Center, Tucson, Arizona

P rostate cancer has become a major public health problem in the United States. The number of newly diagnosed cases of prostate cancer now surpasses lung cancer in frequency,[1] and this neoplasm is now the second leading cause of death in men. With the increase in elderly males in the population this problem is projected to become an even greater health burden. The advent of serum prostate-specific antigen (PSA) testing has resulted in the discovery of an increasing number of men with early-stage disease and has led to extensive debate as to the appropriate treatment of these lesions. The options range from radical prostatectomy with its associated morbidity and mortality to "active surveillance." Our collective ability to select the correct management scheme for a given patient with disease confined to the prostate is severely hampered by the fact that we do not currently possess sufficient markers that accurately forecast the biological potential of prostate carcinoma.[2]

Progress in our understanding of prostate carcinoma has been slowed by a variety of factors. First, because of the gland's location it is difficult to sample and impossible to directly visualize. Almost without exception, investigations examining the expression of gene products have observed a confusing degree of heterogeneity within prostate tissues.[3] Even the morphologic heterogeneity observed by light microscopy has led to a multiplicity of terms and even classification schemes.[4] Many of the established cell lines are aneuploid and lack desirable characteristics.[5-7] The animal models currently available have also been criticized as lacking relevance to human prostate carcinoma.[8, 9]

Since we currently lack effective chemotherapeutic agents to treat dis-

Advances in Pathology and Laboratory Medicine®, vol. 8
© 1995, Mosby–Year Book, Inc.

seminated prostate disease, cures can only be ensured by surgical removal of organ-confined disease. The focus of our laboratory has been to attempt to understand the mechanism(s) of invasion and metastasis used by prostate carcinoma. According to the three-step theory of invasion and metastasis, the malignant cells must first attach to the underlying extracellular matrix (ECM), they must then digest the basal lamina, and finally, they must disassociate from their neighbors and migrate into the surrounding interstitium.[10] A peculiarity of prostate carcinoma is the proclivity of the malignant cells to migrate along the perineural spaces of the perineal nerve tracts as they perforate the capsule.[11] Eventually they enter lymphatic spaces and disseminate to local lymph nodes and preferentially to bone. In this chapter we will review our current understanding of the ECM, adhesion molecules, and proteases of the prostate and their involvement in prostate carcinogenesis.

MORPHOLOGIC CONSIDERATIONS

The human prostate is divided into four anatomic zones: central, peripheral, periurethral transition, and anterior fibromuscular stromal zones.[12] These anatomic definitions have great relevance to the pathologist since benign prostatic hyperplasia (BPH) affects primarily the transition zone whereas the peripheral zone is the major region in which carcinoma arises. Within each zone the entire duct-acinar system is lined by secretory columnar epithelium resting on a basal cell layer. The larger ducts entering the urethra are lined by a transitional-type epithelium.

EXTRACELLULAR MATRIX

The normal prostate acinus is surrounded by a thin (80-nm) basal lamina that is similar in composition to other epithelial basal laminae. With an ultrastructural approach it was our initial impression that there was progressive loss of this basement membrane with progressive histologic grade in primary carcinoma.[13] With more sensitive immunohistochemical techniques and frozen sections, it is now clear that in most carcinomas, including even high-grade cases, the carcinoma cells are surrounded by a thin, ephemeral basal lamina.[14, 15] The major components of this basal lamina are entactin, type IV collagen, and laminin. Further analysis reveals that this basal lamina contains the laminin subchains $\alpha 1$ (A), $\alpha 2$ (M), $\beta 1$ (B1), $\beta 2$ (S), and $\gamma 1$ (B2).[16, 17] We have demonstrated that the prostate cell lines DU145, PC3, and LNCaP also synthesize S laminin.[18] In addition to the proteins of the basal lamina, $\gamma 2$ (B2t) (anchoring filaments) and type VII collagen (anchoring fibrils), as well as the components of hemidesmosomes, are also present in normal basement membranes. All of these proteins are also present in the basal lamina surrounding prostatic intraepithelial neoplasia (PIN) lesions. In carcinoma, however, $\gamma 2$ (B2t) and collagen VII are lost (Fig 1).

Thus prostate cancers within the prostate are confined by a basal lamina that is similar to normal basal lamina except that it lacks essential components associated with normal cell attachment. Therefore the malignant cells must have migrated into the surrounding interstitium and then resynthesized a de novo basal lamina, or as has been suggested by

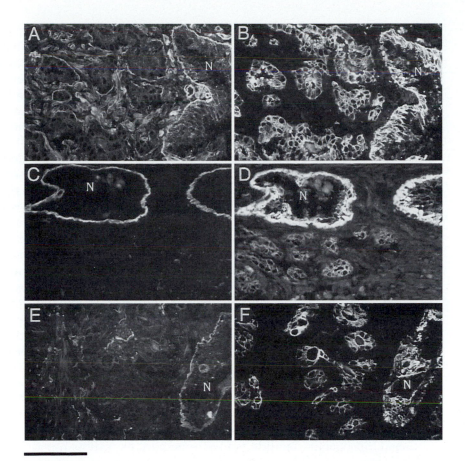

FIGURE 1.

Extracellular matrix changes in prostate carcinoma. On the *left,* **A, C,** and **E** show indirect immunofluorescence when the following primary antibodies are used: **A,** antilamini; **C,** anti–type VII collagen; **E,** anti-γ2 (B2t) subchain of laminin. On the *right,* **B, D,** and **F** are the same sections double-stained with anticytokeratin. The sections contain both normal *(N)* and invasive primary prostate carcinoma. Note that the carcinomas are surrounded by a basal lamina containing laminin **(A).** Also note that the normal glands contain type VII collagen **(C)** and the truncated form of γ2 (B2t) laminin **(E),** but that the carcinomas lack both of these structures **(C** and **E)** (original magnification, ×215).

some investigators, they have grown by out-pouching from the original basal lamina. It is generally accepted that the basal lamina in normal glands is synthesized by the basal cell. In prostate carcinoma, basal cells per se do not exist, although the tumor cells themselves form a basal lamina, perhaps suggesting that they retain certain basal cell characteristics. The presence of a confining basal lamina may explain the relatively long latency of these tumors and the fact that many remain occult and confined to the prostate.

ADHESION MOLECULES

It has been known for some time that the loss of differentiation in carcinomas is accompanied by increased migration and invasiveness, characteristics associated with reduced intercellular adhesion.[19] Intercellular adhesion in the prostate is mediated in part by E-cadherin. This is a calcium-dependent transmembrane cell adhesion molecule that has been shown to play an important role in normal growth and development. Its effects are mediated by homotypic/homophilic cell-cell interactions.[19] Interest in this molecule was accelerated when it was discovered that its gene mapped to the 16q chromosome region. Earlier studies had shown that the short arm of 16q was frequently deleted in prostate carcinoma and was therefore a possible site of tumor suppressor genes.[20] Subsequently, a study by Bergenheim et al. also reported frequent allelic loss on chromosome 16q in both primary and metastatic prostate cancer.[21] Immunohistochemical analysis demonstrated that approximately half of the cases of prostate carcinomas lacked E-cadherin, as compared with the nonmalignant prostate, which uniformly stained strongly positive.[22] The loss of E-cadherin was statistically related to tumor differentiation.[22] In a subsequent study these authors also found a significant correlation between E-cadherin expression, tumor stage, and overall survival. Sixty-three percent of tumors that extended beyond the prostate capsule had aberrant expression, as opposed to 33% of tumors confined to the prostate.[23] It has been shown that the cytoplasmic tail of the E-cadherin molecule interacts with catenins α, β, and γ, which bridge E-cadherin to the cytoskeleton. In addition, it has been demonstrated that E-cadherin function is dependent on its proper anchorage to the cytoskeleton. The role that these associated catenin molecules may play has thus far not been adequately evaluated in prostate carcinoma.[18]

A group of transmembrane heterodimer molecules known as integrins are composed of α and β units and bind cells to the ECM molecules (collagen, fibronectin, laminin, and vitronectin), as well as function in cell-cell interactions.[24] It is now known that certain α units can combine with more than one β subunit, e.g., $\alpha 6$ can couple with either the $\beta 1$ or $\beta 4$ subunit. Alterations in integrin expression on cancer cells have been correlated with increased invasiveness, tumor progression, and metastatic potential.[25-28]

Involvement of integrin $\alpha 6\beta 1$ in tumor cell invasion has been demonstrated by the ability of anti-$\alpha 6$ antibodies to block invasion. Specifically, an antibody against $\alpha 6$ was able to inhibit the invasion of chemically transformed cells through a reconstituted basal lamina and inhibit the experimental metastasis of melanoma cells to the lung in a mouse model system.[29] A role for integrin $\alpha 6\beta 1$ in invasion is also suggested by the recent study of Witkowski et al.[30] in which four human prostatic cell lines were injected into severe combined immunodeficient (SCID) mice. The two cell lines that formed invasive tumors expressed $\alpha 6$ and $\beta 1$, which led the authors to suggest that the $\alpha 6\beta 1$ heterodimer may play a role in prostate tumor progression.

Recent studies in our laboratory, as well as Bonkhoff's laboratory, have identified the $\alpha 2\beta 1$ collagen receptor, the $\alpha 3\beta 1$ epiligrin receptor, the $\alpha 4\beta 1$ fibronectin receptor, the $\alpha 6\beta 1$ laminin receptor, the $\alpha v\beta 1$ vitronectin receptor, and the $\alpha 6\beta 4$ hemidesmosome-associated laminin receptor at the basal cell/basal lamina interface in normal prostate glands.[14, 31] The $\alpha 6\beta 4$ laminin receptor is associated with the hemidesmosome and therefore interacts with the intermediate-filament cytoskeleton.[32] The remaining integrin pairs interact through vinculin and other associated proteins with the actin cytoskeleton.[24] These relationships are shown in Figure 2.

The aforementioned integrin expressions are normally maintained in PIN, a lesion in which normal basal cells are, by definition, retained.[33] This is an interesting observation since our cytometric analysis of the cells microdissected and isolated from high-grade PIN lesions show by 15 different nuclear parameters that they are indistinguishable from invasive cancer.[34] In earlier studies we have also shown that the cells making up PIN lesions differ from normal luminal cells in regard to their cytoskeleton.[35] The anticytokeratin antibody KA4,[36] which recognizes cytokeratins 14, 15, 16, and 19, normally stains the basal cells (based on their content of cytokeratin 14), but not the luminal cells. KA4 reacts strongly with the proliferating cells forming the PIN lesions. Whereas the luminal cells of normal prostate express vimentin and basal cells do not, in PIN lesions vimentin expression is lost. These phenotypic changes indicate that loss of "normal" integrin expression is a relatively late event in prostate cancer progression.

Later in the progression, where frankly invasive carcinomas are seen, there is a downregulation of integrins. The $\alpha6\beta1$ laminin receptor is retained, but the restriction to the basal part of the basal cells that is observed in a normal gland is lost and replaced by a nonpolarized cytoplasmic distribution.[14, 31] (Fig 3). The $\beta4$ integrin, which normally couples with $\alpha6$ to form part of the hemidesmosome structure,[32] is absent in carcinoma (Fig 4).[15] It is unclear whether the $\beta4$ is synthesized and then degraded or whether its transcription is down regulated.

Our recent studies have shown that hemidesmosomes are formed by

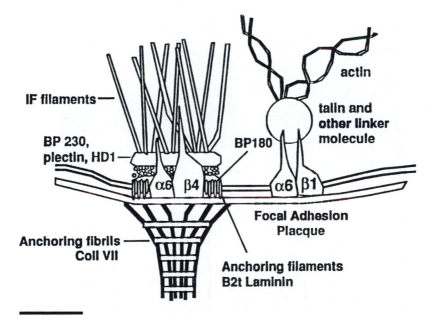

FIGURE 2.

Diagrammatic representation of the two major types of extracellular adhesions found at the basal aspect of the basal cell. On the *left* is a hemidesmosome with its associated proteins and on the right is an integrin pair, in this case $\alpha6\beta1$, the major laminin receptor.

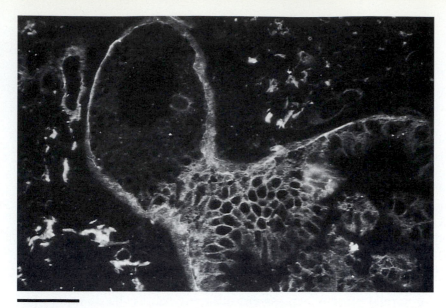

FIGURE 3.

A normal gland being invaded by carcinoma stained with anti-α6 integrin antisera. Note the distribution of α6 around the entire circumference of the malignant cells. Also note the normal distribution of α6 along the basal lamina of the uninvolved portion of the gland (×215). (From Nagle RB, Knox JD, Wolf C, et al: *J Cell Biochem* 19(suppl):236, 1994. Used by permission.)

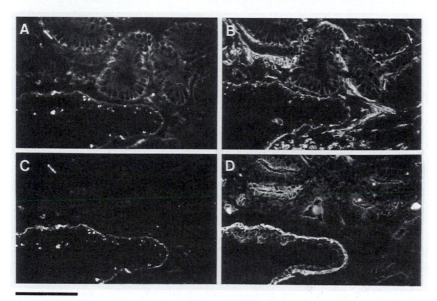

FIGURE 4.

Integrin distribution in carcinoma. Serial sections containing a normal tubular alveolar structure adjacent to carcinoma stained with anti=α6 **(A)**, anti-β1 **(B)**, and anti-β4 **(C)**. Anticytokeratin staining with the polyclonal 18A **(D)** shows a brightly staining normal structure on the lower left with emphasis on the basal cells immediately adjacent to several neoplastic acini that lack the basal cell staining pattern. Note that the neoplastic cells are stained only with α6 and β1 and that the entire circumference of the neoplastic cells is immunoreactive. In contrast, α6β1 and β4 stain only the basal aspects of the basal cells with normal tubular alveolar structure. Note also that in panel **C** the carcinoma cells totally lack staining with β4 (×215). (From Knox JD, Cress AE, Clark V, et al: *Am J Pathol* 145:167–174, 1994. Used by permission.)

the normal basal cell as it interacts with the underlying basal lamina.[37] These structures contain the α6β4 integrin pair, as well as the bullous pemphigoid 180-kD and 230-kD proteins,[38] the HD1 500-kD associated hemidesmosomal protein,[39] and plectin.[40] In addition, the truncated form of laminin γ2 (B2t),[41] a component of the anchoring filaments, is present in normal glands, as is the anchoring fibril collagen VII.[14] Therefore the hemidesmosomes of the prostate contain all the components found in the previously characterized hemidesmosome of skin.[42]

In addition to the loss of β4 integrin expression in carcinoma, there is also loss of the BP 180 antigen, the anchoring filaments γ2 (B2t), and the anchoring fibrils. In a percentage of carcinomas, the BP 230 antigen, plectin, and HD1 antigen are retained. These three proteins are thought to be associated with the internal plaque where intermediate filaments are anchored into the hemidesmosomal structure.[42, 43] The fact that these are sometimes retained along with basal cell–type cytokeratins has led us and other authors to speculate that PIN and carcinoma lesions may in fact evolve from a basal cell precursor population.[44] Recent studies by Bonkhoff et al. suggest this possibility based on double-staining studies showing coexpression of PSA (a luminal cell marker) and basal cell cytokeratins in the same cells.[45]

PROTEASES EXPRESSED IN THE PROSTATE

Numerous authors have investigated the role of various proteases in prostate carcinoma (Table 1.) Our laboratory has concentrated on the role of the metalloproteinase family of enzymes. The metalloproteinases are suspected to be important in the invasion process since they are active at neutral pH. Nine of these zinc-requiring enzymes have been identified: interstitial collagenase, neutrophil collagenase, stromelysin-1, stromelysin-2, stromelysin-3, matrilysin, gelatinase A, gelatinase B, and a newly discovered transmembrane protein designated MT-MMP.[52–57]

The metalloproteinases are secreted as proenzymes. The end-terminal portion of the enzyme is linked to the catalytic zone through a cysteine-zinc bond. When this bond is broken, the end-terminal portion of the enzyme is autocleaved, thereby forming the active enzyme. These enzymes are coordinately secreted with their specific inhibitors, TIMP-1 and

TABLE 1.

Proteases Implicated in Prostate Carcinoma Tumor Progression

Protease	Enzyme	Author
Cysteine endopeptidase	Cathepsin B	Sinha,[46] 1993
Aspartic endopeptidase	Cathepsin D	Nagle,[47] 1994
Serine endopeptidase	Plasminogen activator	Gaylis,[48] 1989
		Camiolo,[49] 1981
Metalloproteinase	Matrilysin	Siadat-Pajouh,[50] 1991
	Gelatinase A	Stearns,[51] 1993
	Gelatinase B	Nagle,[16] 1994

TIMP-2 (tissue inhibitor of metalloproteinase). Isolation of some of these enzymes usually reveals a complex of the inactive enzyme and its TIMP inhibitor.[58] It has been shown that there is a specific receptor on epithelial cells for the gelatinase A/TIMP-2 complex.[59, 60] A recent study by Sato et al. has shown that the bound enzyme is activated by a third molecule, which appears to be the first example of a transmembrane metalloproteinase.[57]

A number of investigators, including our own laboratory, have demonstrated a positive correlation between metalloproteinase expression and invasion or metastatic potential in animal models.[61-63] Transfection of DU145 cells with matrilysin converts these cells from noninvasive to invasive phenotypes in a diaphragm invasion model in SCID mice.[62] Immunohistochemistry has shown metalloproteinase expression in human neoplasms, including breast,[56, 64-66] prostate,[16, 51, 67] colon,[68, 69] gastric,[69] lung,[70] ovarian,[71] and thyroid cancers.[72]

Using Northern analysis of mRNA isolated from primary prostate carcinoma, we demonstrated that the message for gelatinase A and for matrilysin was overexpressed when compared with normal prostate.[50] Zymography identified three metalloproteinase proteins, gelatinase A and B and matrilysin,[16] in human prostate carcinoma (Fig 5). Only matrilysin was present in its active form.

Our in situ and immunohistochemical studies with matrilysin showed that both the message and the protein are expressed focally in the malignant cells (Fig 6, A and B). Interestingly, dilated "atrophic" ductal structures are also high expressers of matrilysin. The function of matrilysin in this location is currently unknown. Our immunohistochemical data demonstrate gelatinase A in the cytoplasm of normal basal cells and focally in malignant epithelium; however, the message is found exclusively in the surrounding stromal fibroblasts (Fig 6, C and D). The message for the 92-kD collagenase IV, gelatinase B, was found exclusively in mononuclear cells.

Recent research has revealed a dynamic interaction between malignant cells and their surrounding ECM. Nontumorigenic LNCaP cells become tumorigenic when injected into immunodeficient mice if they are coinjected with the basement membrane extract Matrigel.[73] Even NIH-3T3 cells will become tumorigenic, locally invasive, and highly vascularized when they are subcutaneously injected along with Matrigel.[74] Gleave et al. have shown that the nontumorigenic cell line LNCaP becomes tumorigenic in male athymic mice when inoculated with either normal prostate or bone fibroblasts but not with lung or mouse embryonic fibroblasts.[75] The reciprocal mesenchymal-epithelial interaction affecting prostate tumor growth and responsiveness has recently been reviewed by Chung et al.[76]

Several surface-associated molecules have been shown to modulate cell-matrix interactions, including the 67-kD laminin-binding protein and the integrin receptors.[25] The metalloproteinase genes appear to be regulated in part by contact of cells with ECM proteins and their fragments through integrin receptors.[77, 78] The role of integrins in these processes is supported by the observation that ligand binding by integrins mediates tyrosine phosphorylation of an intracellular 130-kD protein.[79]

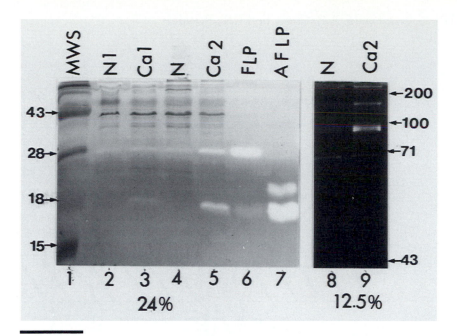

FIGURE 5.

Zymograms of proteins extracted from microdissected human prostate tissue. *Left panel,* 24% acrylamide-casein; *right panel,* 12.5% acrylamide-gelatin. Lane 1, molecular weight standard; lanes 2, 4 and 8, noncarcinomatous tissues; lanes 3, 5, and 9: invasive carcinoma; lane 6, control matrilysin generated in the baculovirus system; lane 7, baculovirus matrilysin activated with APMA. Note that Ca2 (lanes 5 and 9) contains both the 72- and 92-kD gelatinase proenzymes (lane 9), as well as both the inactive (31-kDA) and active (19 to 21-kDa) form of matrilysin (lane 5). (From Nagle RB, Knox JD, Wolf C, et al: *J Cell Biochem* 19(suppl):236, 1994. Used by permission.)

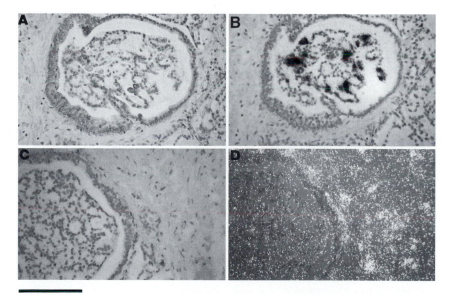

FIGURE 6.

Immunohistochemical and in situ localization of metalloproteinases. **A** and **B,** localization of matrilysin protein **(A)** and matrilysin message **(B).** Note the exact colocalization of the message in protein. **C** and **D,** lightfield and darkfield views of in situ hybridization of a similar field probing with antisense cDNA labeled with S35 specific for gelatinase A message. Note the localization of the message for gelatinase A over the interstitial fibroblasts (original magnification, ×350).

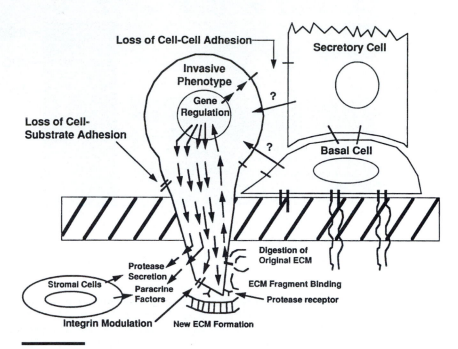

FIGURE 7.

Diagrammatic representation of the major events during prostate carcinoma invasion.

The fact that gelatinase A in synthesized by mesenchymal cells and is secondarily bound to epithelial cells where it becomes further activated underscores the complex nature of the interactions that occur between invading malignant cells and their surrounding stroma. These interactions are summarized in Figure 7. It is clear that the understanding and ultimate ability to intervene in the metastatic spread of prostate cancer will require a thorough knowledge of the genetic control mechanism of the molecules discussed in this review, not only in malignant cells but also in the supporting stroma.

ACKNOWLEDGMENTS

The authors wish to thank Kathleen McDaniel, Virginia Clark, Junshan Hao, and Joanne Finch for their excellent technical assistance, J. David Knox, Ph.D., for reviewing the manuscript, and Nancy E. Suttle for assistance with manuscript preparation. This work was supported by National Institutes of Health grant 5PO1 CA56666-O2.

REFERENCES

1. Silverberg E, Boring CC, Squires TS, et al: Cancer statistics, 1993, *Cancer J Clin* 43:;7–26, 1993.
2. Henson DE, Fielding LP, Grigon DJ, et al: Summary: CAP National Conference XXVI "Prognostic Markers in Solid Tumors." Snowbird, Utah, July 1994.
3. Ware JL: Prostate cancer progression: Implications of histopathology. *Am J Pathol* 145:983–993, 1994.

4. Kovi J: *Surgical Pathology of Prostate and Seminal Vesicles.* Boca Raton, Fla, CRC Press, 1989.

5. Horoszewicz JS, Leong SS, Kawinski E, et al: LNCaP model of human prostatic carcinoma. *Cancer Res* 43:1809–1818, 1983.

6. Stone KR, Mickey DD, Wunderli H, et al: Isolation of a human prostate carcinoma cell line (DU-145). *Int J Cancer* 21:274–281, 1978.

7. Kaighn ME, Narayan KS, Ohnuki Y, et al: Establishment and characterization of a human prostatic carcinoma cell line (PC-3). *Invest Urol* 17:16–23, 1979.

8. Cohen MB, Heidger PM, Lubaroff DM: Gross and microscopic pathology of induced prostatic complex tumors arising in Lobund-Wister rats. *Cancer Res* 54:626–628, 1994.

9. Aumüller G, Gröschel-Stewart U, Altmannsberger M, et al: Basal cells of H-Dunning tumor are myoepithelial cells. A comparative immunohisto-chemical and ultrastructural study with male accessory sex glands and mammary gland. *Histochemistry* 95:341–349, 1991.

10. Liotta LA, Steeg PS, Stetler-Stevenson WG: Cancer metastasis and angiogenesis: An imbalance of positive and negative regulation. *Cell* 64:327–336, 1991.

11. Villers A, McNeal JE, Redwine EA, et al: The role of perineural space in the local spread of prostatic adenocarcinoma. *J Urol* 142:763–768, 1989.

12. McNeal JE: Normal histology of the prostate. *Am J Surg Pathol* 12:619–633, 1988.

13. Fuchs ME, Brawer MK, Rennels MA, et al: The relationship of basement membrane to histologic grade of human prostatic carcinoma. *Mod Pathol* 2:105–111, 1989.

14. Bonkhoff H, Wernert N, Dhom G, et al: Distribution of basement membranes in primary and metastatic carcinomas of the prostate. *Hum Pathol* 23:934–939, 1992.

15. Knox JD, Cress AE, Clark V, et al: Differential expression of extracellular matrix molecules and the α-6 integrins in the normal and neoplastic prostate. *Am J Pathol* 145:167–174, 1994.

16. Nagle RB, Knox JD, Wolf C, et al: Adhesion molecules, extracellular matrix, and proteases in prostate carcinoma. *J Cellular Biochem* 19(suppl):232–237, 1994.

17. Burgeson RE, Chiquet M, Deutzmann R, et al: A new nomenclature for the laminins. *Matrix Biol* 14:209–211, 1994.

18. Rabinovitz I, Cress AE, Nagle RB: Biosynthesis and secretion of laminin and S-laminin by human prostate carcinoma cell lines. *Prostate* 25:97–107, 1994.

19. Birchmeier W, Weidner KM, Hulsken J, et al: Molecular mechanisms leading to cell junction (cadherin) deficiency in invasive carcinomas. *Semin Cancer Biol* 4:231–239, 1993.

20. Carter BS, Ewing CM, Ward WS, et al: Allelic loss of chromosomes 16q and 10q in human prostate carcinoma. *Proc Natl Acad Sci U S A* 87:8751–8755, 1990.

21. Bergenheim US, Kunimi K, Collins VP, et al: Deletion mapping of chromosomes 8, 10, and 16 in human prostatic carcinoma. *Genes Chromosome Cancer* 3:215–220, 1991.

22. Umbas R, Schalken JA, Aalders TW, et al: Expression of the cellular adhesion molecule, E-cadherin, is reduced or absent in high grade prostate cancer. *Cancer Res* 52:5104–5109, 1992.

23. Umbas R, Isaacs WB, Bringuier PP, et al: Decreased E-cadherin expression is associated with poor prognosis in patients with prostate cancer. *Cancer Res* 54:3929–3933, 1994.

24. Hynes RO: Integrins: A family of cell surface receptors. *Cell* 48:549–554, 1987.

25. Albeda SM: Biology of disease: Role of integrins and other cell adhesion molecules in tumor progression and metastasis. *Lab Invest* 68:4–17, 1993.

26. D'Errico A, Barbisa S, Liotta LA, et al: Augmentaiton of type IV collagenase, laminin receptor, and Ki67 proliferation antigen associated with human colon, gastric, and breast carcinoma progression. *Mod Pathol* 4:239–249, 1991.

27. Dedhar S, Saulnier R: Alteration in integrin expression on chemically transformed human cells: Specific enhancement of laminin and collagen receptor complexes. *J Cell Biol* 110:481–489, 1990.

28. Zutter MM, Mazoujian G, Santoro SA: Decreased expressino of integrin adhesive protein receptors in adenocarcinoma of the breast. *Am J Pathol* 137:863–870, 1990.

29. Ruiz P, Dunon D, Sonnenberg A, et al: Suppression of mouse melanoma metastasis by EA-1, a monoclonal antibody specific for $\alpha6$ integrins. *Cell Adhesion Commun* 1:67–81, 1993.

30. Witkowski CM, Rabinovitz I, Nagle RB, et al: Characterization of integrin subunits, cellular adhesion and tumorigenicity of four human prostate cell lines. *J Cancer Res Clin Oncol* 119:637–644, 1993.

31. Bonkhoff H, Stein U, Remberger K: Differential expression of $\alpha6$ and $\alpha2$ very late antigen integrins in the normal, hyperplastic, and neoplastic prostate: Simultaneous demonstration of cell surface receptors and their extracellular ligands. *Hum Pathol* 24:243–248, 1993.

32. Jones JC, Kurkapus MA, Cooper HM, et al: A function for the integrin $\alpha6\beta4$ in the hemidesmosome. *Cell Regul* 2:427–438, 1991.

33. Bostwick DG: Prostatic intraepithelial neoplasia (PIN). *Urology* 6(suppl):16–22, 1989.

34. Petein M, Michel P, Van Velthoven R, et al: Morphonuclear relationship between prostatic intraepithelial neoplasia and cancers as assessed by digital cell image analysis. *Am J Clin Pathol* 96:628–634, 1991.

35. Nagle RB, Brawer MK, Kittelson J, et al: Phenotypic relationships of prostatic intraepithelial neoplasia to invasive prostatic carcinoma. *Am J Pathol* 138:119–128, 1991.

36. Nagle RB, Bocker W, Davis JR, et al: Characterization of breast carcinomas by two monoclonal antibodies distinguishing myoepithelial from luminal epithelial cells. *J Histochem Cytochem* 34:;869–881, 1986.

37. Nagle RB, Cress AE, Knox JD, et al: Studies of hemidesmosome structures in normal and malignant prostate glands (abstract). *Mol Biol Cell* 4(suppl):409, 1993.

38. Klatte DH, Kurkapus MA, Grelling KA, et al: Immunochemical characterization of three components of the hemidesmosome and their expression in cultured epithelial cells. *J Cell Biol* 109:3377–3390, 1989.

39. Hieda Y, Nishizawa Y, Uematsu J, et al: Identificaiton of a new hemidesmosomal protein, HD1: A major, high molecular mass component of isolated hemidesmosomes. *J Cell Biol* 116:1497–1506, 1992.

40. Foisner R, Feldman B, Sander L, et al: Monoclonal antibody mapping of structural and functional plectin epitopes. *J Cell Biol* 112:397–405, 1991.

41. Kallunki P, Sainio K, Eddy R, et al: A truncated laminin chain homologous to the B2 chain: Structure, spatial expression, and chromosomal assignment. *J Cell Biol* 119:679–693, 1992.

42. Garrod DR: Desmosomes and hemidesmosomes. *Curr Opin Cell Biol* 5:30–40, 1993.

43. Jones JCR, Green KJ: Intermediate filament–plasma membrane interactions. *Curr Opin Cell Biol* 3:127–132, 1991.

44. Verhagen APM, Ramaekers FCS, Aalders TW, et al: Colocalization of basal and luminal cell–type cytokeratins in human prostate cancer. *Cancer Red* 52:6182–6187, 1992.

45. Bonkhoff H, Stein U, Remberger K: Multidirectional differentiation in the normal, hyperplastic, and neoplastic human prostate: Simultaneous demonstration of cell-specific epithelial markers. *Hum Pathol* 25:42–46, 1994.

46. Sinha A, Gleason DF, Deleon OF, et al: Localization of a biotinylated cathepsin B olignucleotide probe in human prostate including invasive cells and invasive edges by in situ hybridization. *Anat Red* 235:233–240, 1993.

47. Makar R, Mason A, Kittelson JM, et al: Immunohistochemical analysis of cathepsin D in prostate carcinoma. *Mod Pathol* 7:747–751, 1994.

48. Gaylis FD, Keer HN, Wilson MJ, et al: Plasminogen activators in human prostate cancer cell lines and tumors: Correlation with the aggressive phenotype. *J Urol* 142:193–198, 1989.

49. Camiolo SM, Markus G, Evers JL, et al: Plasminogen activator content of neoplastic and benign human prostate tissues: Fibrin activation of an activator activity. *Int J Cancer* 27:191–198, 1981.

50. Siadat-Pajouh M, Nagle RB, Breathnach R, et al: Expression of metalloproteinase genes in human prostate cancer. *J Cancer Res Clin Oncol* 117:144–150, 1991.

51. Stearns ME, Wang M: Type IV collagenase (M_r 72,000) expression in human prostate: Benign and malignant tissue. *Cancer Res* 53:878–883, 1993.

52. Woessner JF: Matrix metalloproteinases and their inhibitors in connective tissue remodeling. *FASEB J* 5:2145–2154, 1991.

53. Matrisian LM: The matrix-degrading metalloproteinases. *Bioessays* 14:455–462, 1992.

54. Birkedal-Hansen H, Moore WGI, Bodden MK, et al: Matrix metalloproteinases: A review. *Crit Rev Oral Biol Med* 4:197–250, 1993.

55. Basset P, Bellocq JP, Wolf C, et al: A novel metalloproteinase gene specifically expressed in stromal cells of breast carcinoma. *Nature* 348:699–704, 1990.

56. Basset P, Wolf C, Chambon P: Expression of the stromelysin-3 gene in fibroblastic cells of invasive carcinomas of the breast and other human tissues: A review. *Breast Cancer Res Treat* 24:185–193, 1993.

57. Sato H, Takino T, Okada Y, et al: A matrix metalloproteinase expressed on the surface of invasive tumour cells. *Nature* 370:61–65, 1994.

58. Stetler-Stevenson WG, Liotta LA, Kleiner DE: Extracellular matrix 6: Role of matrix metalloproteinases in tumor invasion and metastasis. *FASEB J* 7:1434–1441, 1993.

59. Monsky WL, Kelly T, Lin CY, et al: Binding and localization of M(r) 72,000 matrix metalloproteinase at cell surface invadapodia. *Cancer Res* 53:3159–3164, 1993.

60. Brown PD, Kleiner DE, Unsworth EJ, et al: Cellular activation of the 72 kDa type IV procollagenase/TIMP-2 complex. *Kidney Int* 43:163–170, 1993.

61. Sreenath T, Matrisian LM, Stetler-Stevenson W, et al: Expression of matrix metalloproteinase genes in transformed rat cell lines of high and low metastatic potential. *Cancer Res* 52:4942–4947, 1992.

62. Powell WC, Knox JD, Navre M, et al: Expression of the metalloproteinase matrilysin in DU-145 increases their invasive potential in severe combined immunodeficient mice. *Cancer Res* 53:417–422, 1993.

63. Bonfil RD, Reddel RR, Ura H, et al: Invasive and metastatic potential of a v-Ha-ras–transformed human bronchila epithelial cell line. *J Natl Cancer Inst* 81:587–594, 1989.

64. Clavel C, Polette M, Doco M, et al: Immunolocalization of matrix metallo-

proteinases and their tissue inhibitor in human mammary pathology. *Bull Cancer (Paris)* 79:261–270, 1992.

65. Basset P, Bellocq JP, Wolf C, et al: A novel metalloproteinase gene specifically expressed in stromal cells of breast carcinoma. *Nature* 348:699–704, 1990.

66. Monteagudo C, Merino MJ, San-Juan J, et al: Immunohistochemical distribution of type IV collagenase in normal, benign, and malignant breast tissue. *Am J Pathol* 136:585–592, 1990.

67. Höyhtyä M, Fridman R, Komarek D, et al: Immunohistochemical localization of matrix metalloproteinase 2 and its specific inhibitor TIMP-2 in neoplastic tissues with monoclonal antibodies. *Int J Cancer* 56:500–505, 1994.

68. Poulsom R, Pignatelli M, Stetler-Stevenson WG, et al: Stromal expression of 72 kDa type IV collagenase (MMP-2) and TIMP-2 mRNAs in colorectal neoplasia. *Am J Pathol* 141:389–396, 1992.

69. McDonnell S, Navre M, Coffey RJ, et al: Expression and localization of the matrix metalloproteinase PUMP-1 (MMP-7) in human gastric and colon carcinomas. *Mol Carcinog* 4:527–533, 1991.

70. Urbansky SJ, Edwards DR, Maitland A, et al: Expression of metalloproteinases and their inhibitors in primary pulmonary carcinomas. *Br J Cancer* 66:1188–1194, 1992.

71. Campo E, Merino MJ, Tavassoli FA, et al: Evaluation of basement membrane components and the 72 kDA type IV collagenase in serous tumors of the ovary. *Am J Surg Pathol* 16:500–507, 1992.

72. Campo E, Merino MJ, Liotta L, et al: Distribution of the 72-kd type IV collagenase in nonneoplastic and neoplastic thyroid tissue. *Hum Pathol* 23:1395–1401, 1992.

73. Pretlow TG, Delmoro CM, Dilley GG, et al: Transplantation of human prostatic carcinoma into nude mice in matrigel. *Cancer Res* 51:3814–3817, 1991.

74. Fridman R, Sweeney TM, Zain M, et al: Malignant transformation of NIH-3T3 cells after subcutaneous co-injection with a reconstituted basement membrane (Matrigel). *Int J Cancer* 51:740–744, 1992.

75. Gleave M, Hseih JT, Gao C, et al: Acceleration of human prostate cancer growth in vivo by factors produced by prostate and bone fibroblasts. *Cancer Res* 51:3753–3761, 1991.

76. Chung LWK, Gleave ME, Hsieh J-T, et al: Reciprocal mesenchymal-epithelial interaction affecting prostate tumour growth and hormonal responsiveness. *Cancer Surv* 11:91–121, 1991.

77. Werb Z, Tremble PM, Behrendtsen O, et al: Signal transduction through the fibronectin receptor induces collagenase and stromelysin gene expression. *J Cell Biol* 109:877–889, 1989.

78. Seftor REB, Seftor EA, Gehlsen KR, et al: Role of $\alpha v \beta 3$ integrin in human melanoma cell invasion. *Proc Natl Acad Sci U S A* 89:1557–1561, 1992.

79. Kornberg LJ, Earp HS, Turner CE, et al: Signal transduction by integrins: Increased protein tyrosine phosphorylation caused by clustering of beta 1 integrins. *Proc Natl Acad Sci U S A* 88:8392–8396, 1991.

Emerging Concepts in the Pathogenesis of IgA Nephropathy

Steven N. Emancipator, M.D.
Institute of Pathology, Case Western Reserve University, Cleveland, Ohio

Michael E. Lamm, M.D.
Institute of Pathology, Case Western Reserve University, Cleveland, Ohio

IgA nephropathy (IgAN), a glomerular disease in which IgA is the predominant immunoglobulin deposited according to immunohistochemical findings, is likely the most common form of glomerulonephritis worldwide.[1-7] However, the incidence of IgAN differs from country to country, probably due primarily to regional differences in defining which conditions/symptoms merit a renal biopsy (and a precise diagnosis of renal disease) and to genetic factors.[1-8] Wide variations in environmental conditions almost certainly also play a role.[9] The characteristics of IgAN, which have been reviewed recently with respect to clinical, morphologic, and immunologic features,[1-7] are summarized here. Subsequently, we present emerging concepts regarding the pathogenesis and pathophysiology of IgA nephropathy.

CHARACTERISTICS OF IGA NEPHROPATHY

CLINICAL FEATURES

Approximately 60% of patients have episodic macrohematuria (bloody urine) and low-grade proteinuria, below 1 g/day, whereas 30% of patients with IgAN (as determined by biopsy) show only microscopic hematuria (red blood cells seen in the urine sediment under a microscope), often with protein excretion in the 1- to 3-g/day range. Especially in individuals with microhematuria, a wide range of proteinuria, from undetectable to nephrotic, can be encountered, and transient acute renal failure is also seen in some patients. The process advances to end-stage renal disease in approximately 30% of patients over a 20-year period. Among a variety of clinical markers of progression, the rate of urinary protein excretion is the most accurate and sometimes the only predictor of how the disease will progress over the long term.

Advances in Pathology and Laboratory Medicine®, vol. 8
© 1995, Mosby–Year Book, Inc.

MORPHOLOGIC FEATURES

The elements of IgAN occur to varying degrees among individual renal biopsy specimens and within different sites in the same specimen as well. Most consistently there is expansion of the glomerular mesangium, a stalk of connective tissue supporting the glomerular capillaries that contains mesenchymal cells with contractile and phagocytic properties. IgA deposits can be found in the mesangium in almost all (95%) patients with IgAN by immunofluorescence, immunoenzymatic histology, electron microscopy, and/or immunoelectron microscopy. Codeposits of IgG and/or IgM are also evident in most (75%) of the cases, with the same pattern as IgA. Complement components are seen with a wide degree of variability. Biopsy specimens from nearly all (95%) of patients with IgAN prominently show common final pathway and alternative pathway complement components. A few patients (15%) also show relatively minor deposits of classical pathway complement components, but 80% of patients show no classical pathway complement components. Immune deposits are found outside the mesangium within the walls of filtering capillaries in 20% of all patients with IgAN and have a composition that mirrors the deposits in mesangium. Features such as cellular proliferation and thickening of the extracellular mesangial matrix and/or the glomerular basement membrane can generally be found where immunoglobulin is deposited, in similar patterns of distribution. However, in the 15% of patients in whom immunohistologic or ultrastructural techniques reveal conspicuous evidence of immunoglobulin deposits, tissue samples reveal only mild or equivocal changes in cell number and extracellular matrix in glomerular mesangial areas. Overall, the severity of injury in IgAN reflects that of glomerulonephritis in general, and variations in severity appear to be directly related to the amount of IgA deposits. None of the other histologic changes that are often (20% to 40%) seen in patients with IgAN, such as tubular degeneration or atrophy and/or interstitial mononuclear infiltrates, are specific to IgAN.

IMMUNOLOGIC FEATURES

Patients with IgAN show a significant overabundance of high-molecular-weight immunoglobulin and/or complement components associated with immunoglobulin in the serum. Serologic examination shows the presence of a variety of antigens derived from or associated with dietary or inhaled substances or infectious mucosal pathogens within circulating macromolecular aggregates and less frequently in glomerular immune deposits. However, although elevated titers of IgA and IgG antibodies specific for a variety of commensal, infectious, or environmental components have been detected in the circulation of patients with IgAN, most have also been observed in other forms of glomerulonephritis,[10] which suggests that these antibody titers are associated with glomerulonephritis in general rather than specifically with IgAN. Based on this evidence and the fact that the antigens implicated in an individual seldom correspond to antibodies specific for those antigens, one might suppose that IgAN does not reflect a specific change in immune complex activity. However, the wide variety of polyclonal antibodies and antigens implicated makes it difficult to evaluate this issue.

Elevated levels of serum IgA and/or increased numbers of IgA-bearing lymphocytes or plasma cells, in mucosal sites as well as in the circulation, are observed in most patients with IgAN vs. controls, although sometimes only transiently. Studies quantifying gastrointestinal lamina propria plasmacytes report conflicting results with respect to IgA-positive cells: two groups have found modest decreases,[11, 12] whereas another detected normal numbers of IgA-, IgG-, and IgM-positive cells.[13] Almost all of the increased content of circulating IgA is IgA1 subclass, which is further characterized by a relatively large proportion of oligomeric (mostly dimeric) IgA containing J chain. These features are very similar to the IgA seen in glomerular deposits. The total IgG concentration shows no such increase over the long-term course of IgAN except in exacerbation, when sharp increases occur in the amount of serum IgG and the number of IgG positive cells in peripheral blood. The tonsils of patients with IgAN have decreased IgG-bearing cells relative to controls.[14] One study suggests that in IgAN, the IgG1 and IgG3 subclasses appear at higher than normal levels, whereas IgG2 is seen at lower than normal levels,[15] but we and others have found no differences in IgG subclasses.[16, 17] Research on IgM yields more variation in data without clear abnormality.[6, 17]

Both the absolute and relative numbers of cells bearing CD4 and CD8 appear to be unaffected in patients as compared with normal individuals. Although the CD4/CD8 ratio has been shown by some to increase during exacerbation of IgAN in some patients, there are conflicting data on the origin of the increase of this ratio.[6] Specifically, is it due to a rise in CD4-positive cells, a decrease in CD8-positive cells, or a combination of the two? Taken together, the data on the numbers of CD4- and CD8-bearing cells in combination with the more equivocal data on the CD4/CD8 ratio suggest that IgAN is not significantly affected by CD4 and CD8 expression. There is no demonstrable causal relationship, nor is the disease notably ameliorated or exacerbated. Only one other type of T-cell marker has been closely studied, that is, increased expression of receptors for IgA.[6, 7] The high circulating IgA concentration common in IgAN probably causes this response in T-cell IgA receptor expression.

PATHOGENESIS

The two primary issues relating to the pathogenesis of IgAN remain very controversial, namely, (1) the site of its genesis (the mucosal or systemic immune system) and (2) the nature of the mesangial deposits (immune complexes or not). There have been some recent observations on regulation of the immune response and on mucosal immunity that could prove useful in understanding IgAN.

DYSREGULATED IMMUNE RESPONSE

Polymeric IgA and IgA1 seem to be overproduced to a greater degree than other immunoglobulins in vitro and in vivo in patients with IgAN. There are some reports of increased IgG production in vitro, but this phenomenon seems to appear in only a small minority of patients with extraordinarily high levels of immunoglobulin synthesis in general.[17−20] Limited evidence suggests that specific humoral responses to antigen are hyperkinetic in patients with IgAN.[21−26]

In patients with IgAN there is abnormal suppression of IgA synthesis relative to controls in response to concanavalin A (Con A),[6, 27] although interleukin-2 (IL-2) production and T-cell proliferation normally take place in response to mitogen. Patients' T cells are better at IgA suppression than those of controls at low doses, but as the dose of Con A increases, this suppression becomes progressively less effective relative to controls. This is demonstrated by the control T cells responding to an increasing degree at higher doses (progressively more effectively suppressing IgA synthesis), contrasted with the T cells of patients with IgAN, which respond to the same degree regardless of the dose. The T cells of most patients with IgAN seem to selectively aid IgA secretion in vitro, apparently according to differences in the relative number of T cells in the differing functional subsets rather than to the efficiency of individual T cells.[20, 28−30]

Mixing and depletion experiments comparing the coculture of B and T cells of patients with IgAN vs. normal subjects indicate that defective T-cell function consistently occurs in IgAN whereas there are inconsistent alterations in B-cell function. Normal B cells do consistently produce unusually high levels of IgA when cocultured with histocompatible T cells from patients with IgAN;[20, 28−31] however, only some of the patients' B cells have been observed to secrete heightened levels of IgA when coincubated with normal histocompatible T cells, with approximately 50% of the patients showing evidence of normal B-cell function.[20, 28−31] The secretion of IgA by patients' B cells is similarly affected when the population of autologous T cells is reduced in suspension before the culture phase of the experiment.[32] Faulty regulation of B-cell function may well be related to the aberrant production of lymphokines by T cells observed in at least a subpopulation of patients with IgAN.[27]

The imbalance in the IgA/IgG ratio observed when lymphocytes of patients with IgAN are maintained in vitro resembles the defect seen in experimental IgAN.[33] Conceivably, this altered IgA/IgG ratio could be due to a defect in mucosal tolerance, as it is in mice. The aberrant immunoglobulin ratio might play an important role in reducing complement-mediated solubilization and complement receptor (CR1)-mediated erythrocyte transport of immune complexes by diminishing their splenic and hepatic uptake and thereby enhancing immune complex deposition in glomeruli.[6, 34] IgA in the immune lattice increases the anionic charge and would therefore promote mesangial delivery[35]; mesangial delivery is also promoted by IgA's affinity for fibronectin[36] and perhaps other mesangial components that act as acceptors for immune complexes containing IgA. Normal mesangial function might be altered by the interaction of IgA immune complexes with mesangial fibronectin or mesangial glycoproteins. Moreover, codeposited IgG could promote mesangial complement deposition, which can lead to glomerular dysfunction.[33]

DEFECTIVE NEUTRALIZATION OF INTRACELLULAR PATHOGENS BY IGA

In order for mucosal IgA to reach the luminal secretions, dimeric IgA is first secreted by local plasma cells in the mucosal lamina propria (Fig 1). Next, because the IgA cannot go through the tight junctions between the lining epithelial cells, it must instead traverse the interior of the epithelial cells. The IgA binds to the polymeric immunoglobulin receptor expressed on the basolateral surface of mucosal epithelial cells. Subsequently, the IgA-receptor complex is internalized via constitutive endocytosis of the receptor. The internalized IgA migrates in vesicles through the epithelial cell to the apical surface, where it is released into the lumen by proteolytic cleavage of the exoplasmic domain of the polymeric immunoglobulin receptor, now called secretory component.[37] This passage of IgA through epithelial cells allows IgA antibodies specific for a viral antigen the opportunity to disrupt synthesis of that virus in an infected cell if the transcytotic pathway of the IgA intersects with pathways of viral replication (see Fig 1). Recent in vitro evidence supports this idea.[38, 39]

Impairment of this intracellular virus neutralization function could result in more severe or more prolonged mucosal viral infections. For instance, certain cytokines such as interferon-γ (IFN-γ), tumor necrosis factor α (TNF-α) and IL-4 upregulate the polymeric immunoglobulin receptor when IgA is particularly needed to promote the mucosal immune response.[40-43] Upregulation of the polymeric immunoglobulin receptor would permit more IgA to be internalized and transported at times when the rate-limiting factor would be the expression of the receptor on mucosal epithelial cells. It is possible that some individuals are unable to increase the expression of polymeric immunoglobulin receptors enough to combat mucosal infection and inflammation, which makes them more prone to more chronic and more severe mucosal infection. The development of IgAN might be more likely in such individuals by virtue of increased penetration of the mucosa by antigen, which would favor a more vigorous systemic immune response and the generation of increased amounts of immune complexes.[6] In point of fact, an analogous defect in transepithelial IgA transport, related to a lack of synthesis by mucosal plasma cells of the J chain required for binding of IgA to the polymeric immunoglobulin receptor, was recently recognized as prevalent among patients with IgAN.[44]

DEFECTIVE REMOVAL OF IGA IMMUNE COMPLEXES

Although one group reports that patients with IgAN have normal clearance of immune complexes,[45] others find that patients with IgAN have evidence of defective clearance of IgG-coated particles,[46] heat-aggregated IgA,[47] or IgA-IgG complexes[48] in the liver and spleen. The discrepancy among these studies could be attributed to variations in reagents, and nonspecific aberration in the removal of immune complexes can account for this problem in at least a few of the patients with IgAN.[34]

To date it is not clear why this defect in clearance occurs, although

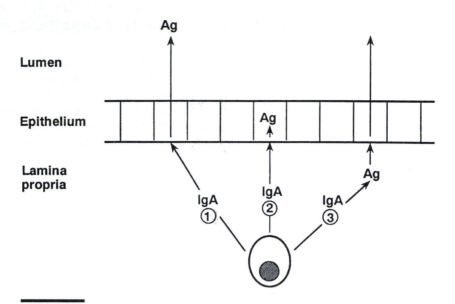

FIGURE 1.

The three proposed host defense functions of mucosal IgA. The drawing shows a plasma cell in the lamina propria secreting IgA antibody, which can potentially encounter its specific antigen in three places. In 1 *(left)*, the IgA is transported through a lining epithelial cell into the luminal secretions, where it can bind antigen and perform its immune exclusion function. In 2 *(center)*, during its transepithelial transport stage, anti–viral IgA can potentially neutralize virus that infects the same cell. In 3 *(right)*, IgA antibody complexes with antigen in the lamina propria; the entire complex is then excreted into the lumen. It is suggested that if for any reason route 3 cannot keep up with the demand, the excess IgA immune complexes could instead reach the circulation and be deposited in the kidney. (From Lamm ME, Mazanec MB, Nedrud JG, et al: *Vaccine Res* 1:169–173, 1992. Used by permission.)

there have been studies on one possible answer based on evidence that IgA binds complement poorly and inhibits IgG immune complex–induced complement activation.[6] These characteristics of IgA might enable it to promote glomerular immune deposition since complement helps to take immune complexes out of the circulation by solubilizing immune lattices and promotes transport to splenic, hepatic and circulating phagocytes via complement receptor (CR1) on the erythrocyte surface.[34] Sera from patients with IgAN have been shown to inhibit complement-mediated solubilization of IgG immune complexes, presumably because the incorporation of complement into the lattice is inhibited when small amounts of IgA are added to an IgG immune lattice.[6, 34]

Recent research suggests that mucosal IgA may act as an excretory antibody in host defense (see Fig 1).[49] Small but tangible amounts of inhaled or ingested substances can be absorbed intact across the mucosal epithelium in normal individuals.[50] In the presence of local infection, the quantity of antigens reaching the mucosal lamina propria should be even greater if injury to the mucosa increases penetration by antigen. Moreover, antigens from infectious mucosal pathogens could also reach the lamina propria. Therefore, when the mucosal immune response is mounted and locally secreted specific IgA antibodies are generated, the production of significant amounts of IgA-containing immune complexes could in turn be stimulated within the lamina propria by the binding of such antigens. In vitro experiments suggest that IgA immune complexes in the lamina propria can be readily transported through the mucosal epithelium by the same route and mechanism as free dimeric IgA, regardless of whether such complexes are present in the background amounts that would be produced under normal conditions or the increased amounts produced in response to mucosal infection.[49] Mucosal IgA bound to antigen and traveling in this transport mechanism would then operate as an "excretory" and not a "secretory" antibody.

An excretory immune system such as this could be a key to keeping local immune complexes out of the systemic circulation, thus reducing the risk of immune complex diseases developing. This is another case wherein individuals who are unable to adequately increase the expression of polymeric immunoglobulin receptor could consequently have impaired intraepithelial virus neutralization, be at greater risk for mucosal infections, and in turn have more viral antigens being shunted into the lamina propria and forming IgA immune complexes that are not efficiently excreted locally. Patients with IgAN who are deficient in J-chain production[44] might also generate greater quantities of IgA immune complexes in the lamina propria to such a degree that the immune complexes might overflow into the circulation.

The rodent hepatocyte provides an additional means for clearing IgA immune complexes from the circulation since dimeric IgA and IgA immune complexes can be transported through the liver from blood to bile. This occurs because rodent hepatocytes express the polymeric immunoglobulin receptor on their sinusoidal surface.[6, 49] However, this does not hold true for humans, so by comparison they are more likely to accumulate renal deposits of circulating IgA immune complexes, particularly at times when more complexes are being formed, as during mucosal infections.

ABNORMALLY STRUCTURED IGA

Although patients with IgAN have abnormally high levels of circulating IgA and/or IgA immune complexes, often higher still during exacerbations of disease,[51–53] there is not necessarily an accompanying increment in IgA deposition in glomeruli. Moreover, patients with acquired immunodeficiency syndrome, celiac disease, IgA multiple myeloma, dermatitis herpetiformis, or liver cirrhosis all have increased levels of IgA or IgA immune complexes in serum.[6, 54–57] Few such individuals have IgA deposits in glomeruli, and fewer still have signs of renal disease.[6, 57] None of the aforementioned immunologic aberrations encountered in IgAN are typically seen in such patients. These data suggest that there are still unknown factors affecting the interactions between circulating IgA immune complexes and mesangial cells and/or matrix in patients with IgAN.[5, 6] Moreover, there seem to be two interrelated immediate precursors to IgAN: (1) at least a portion of the IgA or IgA immune complex must have properties that favor entry to or persistence in the mesangium, and (2) the resulting deposit must have some direct or indirect effect on mesangial cell metabolism. When these conditions are both in evidence, one might see the development and progression of IgAN.

Regarding the first requirement, there are two sets of determinants promoting a tendency for IgA molecules to be deposited and remain in the mesangium. First are the particular properties of IgA, including the greater molecular weight of the polymeric form that is enriched in mesangial deposits,[58, 59] its tendency (enhanced during episodes of IgAN) to form complexes that are not easily removed from the bloodstream,[9, 34, 45] and the anionic properties of IgA relative to IgG and IgM, again with the mesangial IgA more anionic than that in serum.[35, 60, 61] However, we must consider that large amounts of polymeric IgA are often produced in the absence of any mesangial deposition of IgA. Also, mesangial deposition of IgM is rare even though it is significantly larger than dimeric IgA. Perhaps some of the IgA synthesized by patients with IgAN has a greater affinity for mesangium and/or is cleared from the mesangium less readily as a consequence of an altered structure.

The second set of determinants involves interactions of circulating macromolecular IgA with a nonimmunoglobulin component of the immune deposits. Experimental evidence shows that IgA can be linked by several molecules with lectinic properties to mesangial cells in culture.[62-64] Note that IgA1, the predominant subclass of IgA found in mesangial deposits in IgAN, has a greater capacity for carbohydrate interactions with lectins.[65] Viruses that target mammalian cells might bind preferentially to mesangial cells[63, 66] and then stimulate immune responses, including specific IgA antibody production. Therefore, mesangial localization of IgA immune complexes or in situ formation might be fostered by the mesangial affinity of an antigen and/or a nonantigen macromolecule that binds to IgA such as a lectin. These two potential affinities of immune or nonimmune IgA aggregates for the mesangium based on the nonimmunoglobulin component quite possibly play a synergistic role in the mesangial deposition of IgA. Differences in glycosylation and/or electrical charge of the IgA component that have been recognized in patients with IgAN vs. controls[35, 60, 67-70] may be additional factors in IgA immune complex affinity for mesangial matrix components or cells.

One hypothesis posits an altered glycosylation of IgA in patients with IgAN and perhaps a second defect in mesangial matrix or mesangial cells. Serum IgA as well as circulating macromolecular IgA (obtained by precipitation in 2.5% polyethylene glycol) in patients with IgAN has an increased affinity for mesangial matrix components, especially the glycoprotein components fibronectin and laminin.[67] Rather than occurring on an immune basis, this affinity seems to result from changes in the way the highly glycosylated IgA molecules and the mesangial matrix glycoproteins interact. Altered glycosylation of IgA, especially in the O-linked hinge oligosaccharides that are abundant on human IgA1 but rare on other circulating proteins, has been recently recognized on IgA1 derived from the serum of patients with IgAN.[68-70] The finding that IgAN disappears from some donor kidneys post-transplant and/or recurs in allografts[6, 71] suggests that an intrinsically altered IgA structure exists in patients with IgAN without a generalized defect in renal tissue. In fact, the alterations in IgA glycosylation confirmed in patients with IgAN studied in our laboratory can be selectively elicited by lymphokines (IL-4 and IL-5) derived from Th2-class helper cells.[72] These same lymphokines tend to be overproduced by T cells derived from patients with IgAN and maintained in short-term culture.[27] In a passive murine model, the kinetics of clearance from the blood of model IgA immune complexes and their uptake into the kidney are heavily influenced by glycosylation of the IgA antibody; glomerular deposition of the aberrantly glycosylated IgA is favored.[72] On the other hand, the increased risk for recurrence of IgAN in living related donor kidneys[71] and the recurrence of IgA deposits in the absence of renal injury in patients with IgAN after allografting suggest that some feature of the mesangium favors a pathophysiologic response to the deposited IgA.

PATHOPHYSIOLOGY

HEMODYNAMIC ALTERATIONS IN IGA NEPHROPATHY

Oral immunization of rats results in both high titers of specific IgA antibody in the circulation and mesangial immune deposits containing primarily IgA. Immunized rats challenged parenterally with antigen to promote increased generation of immune complexes and emulate antigen penetration of the mucosal barrier show signs of hematuria and low-grade proteinuria associated with equivocal or mild histologic changes.[73] The glomerular filtration rate (GFR) and effective renal plasma flow (RPF) decrease by 20% in these rats. The pattern of glomerular eicosanoid synthesis inverts: thromboxane A_2 (TxA_2) production increases, whereas prostaglandin E_2 (PGE_2) synthesis remains normal or is minimally reduced. Experimental therapy that reduces thromboxane or its effects prevents hematuria and normalizes RPF but does not improve GFR.[73]

In this model of IgAN and possibly also in patients with IgAN, it may be that contraction of both efferent arterioles and glomeruli (via mesangial cells) occurs. However, efferent arteriolar constriction seems to be thromboxane-sensitive since these arterioles most resist glomerular flow. It is conceivable that mesangial contraction, possibly controlled to some degree by angiotensin II, is thromboxane independent. In the absence of pharmacologic agents, mesangial contraction and attendant diminution of the filtering surface area would be counteracted by efferent arteriolar constriction. Blockade of efferent arteriolar constriction by antithromboxane agents decreases the glomerular filtration fraction since RPF remains normal while the filtering surface area and glomerular capillary pressure are lowered. In this hypothetical scheme, the GFR reflects mesangial contraction whereas microhematuria reflects efferent arteriolar constriction. This hypothesis generates the possible therapeutic goal of reversing mesangial contraction independently from glomerular thromboxane synthesis.

One of the most important hemodynamic mechanisms contributing to the progression of IgAN may be local activation of the renin-angiotensin system. This mechanism must work synergistically with immunologic factors in order to have this pathogenetic effect.[74] Among 27 patients with IgAN who were given an intense course of angiotensin converting enzyme inhibitor, the 18 with normal initial renal function exhibited a slight increase in GFR but a more profound increase in RPF and consequently a decreased filtration fraction. Nine patients with initial renal failure again showed similar but more profound changes, and the more heavily proteinuric patients with IgAN and normal renal function also had similar but numerically larger changes.[74]

These effects of angiotensin converting enzyme inhibitors are similar to what is seen in rat studies[73] and implicate glomerular hyperactivity of the renin-angiotensin system. Since this finding applies to patients with early renal failure and those with patent proteinuria, angiotensin II could possibly contribute to the progression of IgAN.[74]

INTERACTIONS BETWEEN VIRUSES AND MESANGIAL CELLS IN VITRO

Certain DNA and RNA viruses can alter cellular metabolism when added to mesangial cell cultures. The synthesis and secretion of TNF and IL-1β are stimulated and supported by adenovirus, herpesvirus, and Sendai virus, which also elicit doubling or tripling of TxA_2 to the detriment of PGE_2. The number of virions added affects the cellular responses over a range of 4 to 6 log plaque-forming units.[63, 64] These changes are not a result of viral infection of the cells, at least with Sendai virus, as judged by immunofluorescence with anti–Sendai virus antibodies and by Northern analysis for viral genome in proportion to the amount of virus added (unpublished observations). Clearly, neither viral replication nor viral infection takes place in mesangial cells.

Furthermore, virus deactivated by ultraviolet irradiation retains as much potency as infectious virions with respect to both changes in eicosanoid synthesis and binding to mesangial cells. Isolated viral protein, on the other hand, when introduced in quantities similar to the protein present in intact virions, had no discernible effect on mesangial cell eicosanoid metabolism and substantially retarded the increase in TxA_2 when coincubated with intact virions despite comparable degrees of binding to the cells.[64] It seems that the cytoplasmic membrane must be the site of some macromolecular aggregation, perhaps via cross-linking since soluble viral proteins are known to decrease cellular responses to virus rather than imitate them. Viruses targeted to the mesangium by virtue of their presence in IgA immune complexes may promote parallel changes in cell function in vivo. Such potential effects of Sendai virus on mesangial cells may explain the dichotomy between immunized mice in which hematuria develops after challenge with intact virus as opposed to immunized mice in which hematuria does not develop after experimental challenge with solubilized viral protein despite comparable glomerular deposits of complexes of Sendai virus and specific antibody in both groups.[66, 75]

INTERACTIONS BETWEEN EXOGENOUS LECTINS, IGA, AND MESANGIAL CELLS

IgA can be converted into macromolecular aggregates through an antigen-antibody reaction or via an interaction between the carbohydrate moiety of IgA and lectinic molecules. Lectins are animal, plant, bacterial, or viral proteins that bind to specific carbohydrate domains; most lectins interact with the terminal end of nonreducing sugars of glycoprotein or glycolipid portions of the cell membranes.[62–64] Several lectins, particularly jacalin, can bind IgA, primarily IgA1,[65] the hinge region of which bears an O-linked N-acetyl-galactosamine-galactoside that is unusual among proteins circulating in mammalian plasma. Several lectins can bind polymeric IgA, which has many terminal galactosyl residues. These interactions guide the development of macromolecular aggregates of IgA with lectins. Gliadin is conspicuous among IgA-binding lectins as the cause of celiac disease in susceptible individuals,[76] and furthermore IgAN sometimes develops in patients with celiac disease as well.[77]

The in vitro binding of human polymeric IgA to gliadin is inhibitable by certain sugars (GalNac > Gal > GlcNac > Glc).[62, 78] Since complement fixation by an immune complex is inhibited by the presence of IgA in the immune lattice via saccharides on the IgA,[79] interaction of gliadin with the carbohydrate side chains of IgA might allow more C3 to enter IgA-IgG immune deposits, hence promoting C3's adverse effects, specifically hematuria and kidney tissue damage. Furthermore, gliadin and other lectins bind to cultured mesangial cells in a monotonic fashion that is selectively repressed by GlcNac.[62, 63] Because IgA and mesangial cells have binding sites such that the distinct lectin domains on gliadin can bridge the two together, the incorporation of gliadin or perhaps other lectin molecules into an immune lattice could increase immune complex deposition within glomeruli.[62, 63, 80]

Renal tissue has been shown to have lectin binding sites, particularly in mesangial matrix and podocyte glycocalyx.[81] We surmised that the functional characteristics of mesangial cells might be altered via interaction with lectins. In fact, lectins such as wheat germ agglutinin, soybean lectin, *Limulus polyphemus* lectin, Con A, and particularly gliadin augmented mRNA expression of the protooncogenes c-*myc* and c-*fos* in mesangial cells.[64] C-*myc* and c-*fos* are markers of cell growth, differentiation, and mitosis and play a role in transcriptional enhancement. A 46-fold increase in mRNA encoding for c-*myc* and a 3.5 fold increase in c-*fos* mRNA were generated upon incubation of mesangial cells for 4 hours with gliadin. Expression of c-*myc* and c-*fos* diminished upon coincubation with GlcNAc, a sugar that competitively inhibits IgA binding to gliadin.[64] Four hours after the addition of gliadin, TNF-α and IL-6 mRNA expression was augmented in mesangial cells (10- and 3-fold, respectively), and both increases were nearly totally counteracted by the addition of GlcNAc.[64] Similarly, bioactive TNF protein release was augmented by incubation with gliadin but was specifically inhibited when the appropriate competitive sugars were coincubated. Other lectins evoked a similar response and affected the expression of TNF mRNA and/or release of protein. For example, both mRNA and protein expression were increased severalfold in the presence of *Limulus polyphemus* or *Ulex I* lectins. Wheat germ agglutinin and Con A also had statistically significant effects, although to a lesser degree. Soybean lectin did not affect TNF production.[64] Interleukin-1β mRNA was undetectable in initial readings, and lectin conditioning had no discernible effect, but *Ulex I* heightened the concentration of IL-1β protein in culture supernatant. Con A and *Limulus polyphemus* lectin had little effect on IL-1 protein content, but it was reduced by soybean lectin, gliadin, and wheat germ agglutinin. Gliadin's effect on the release of IL-1β by mesangial cells was not affected by co-incubation of the competitive sugar for lectinic binding to the cells.[64]

Although gliadin did not increase platelet activating factor synthesis or activity above the detection limit in conditioned mesangial cell supernatants over a range of times, the lectin greatly hindered PGE_2 production in mesangial cell cultures while increasing TxA_2 production.[62-64] The introduction of a competitive sugar again totally reversed these effects and validated the lectin specificity to account for our previous findings. A similar depression in PGE_2 production was evoked by soybean and *Limulus polyphemus* lectins, with Con A causing a modest rise in TxA_2. Neither *Ulex I* nor wheat germ agglutinin had an effect on either eicosanoid.[62, 64]

Apparently, lectins are capable of modifying mesangial cell functions such as the production of potent cytokines and eicosanoids by virtue of binding to saccharides on the cells, in turn potentially leading to vasoconstriction, mesangial cell contraction, and mesangial matrix expansion and proliferation. These effects by which lectins might instigate and/or further the progression of IgAN are in addition to the enhanced formation of mesangial deposits of IgA immune complexes containing such lectins and/or nonimmune IgA-lectin aggregates mediated through lectin binding to mesangial cells. Therefore, IgA-lectin aggregates have properties that may synergize to evoke IgAN.

SUMMARY AND PERSPECTIVE

From the foregoing, several issues should be apparent. IgA nephropathy is variable in its mode of presentation, its histologic appearance, and its clinical course. Although it clearly represents an accumulation of noncovalently bound aggregates of immunoglobulin with other macromolecules, the identity and nature of the nonimmunoglobulin component(s) are controversial and probably heterogeneous, even within a given afflicted individual. Conceivably, some or all of the aggregates form on the basis of affinity other than antibody for antigen. Notwithstanding the fact that production of macromolecular aggregates containing IgA is required for the genesis of this disease, increased steady-state levels of circulating IgA-containing aggregates is neither necessary nor sufficient for the development of IgAN. Rather, the pathogenic contributions of an increased rate of formation and/or diminished rate of clearance of IgA complexes prevalent among patients with IgAN seem to be less important than the specific mechanism(s) that alter(s) these rates.

Apparently, in order for IgAN to ensue, the aggregates must have features that both favor glomerular deposition and promote a mesangial cellular response. We have discussed the potential for IgA that is more anionic and/or aberrantly glycosylated to bind better to the mesangium. At present there is no evidence to suggest that alternate IgA structures influence the mesangial cellular response to IgA aggregates, but this is an area that merits further scrutiny. In contrast, several viruses and lectins that are potentially antigenic components of an IgA immune complex can bind to mesangium and/or mesangial cells in culture and consequently modulate cellular metabolism. To the extent that these binding activities are preserved in an immune complex, such infectious and environmental agents can also promote the binding of IgA to the mesangium. With lectins, at least, the IgA aggregates need not be immune complexes in that lectins can bind to mesangium and to IgA via distinct domains.

Therefore we predict two general routes to IgAN, not mutually exclusive and indeed likely synergistic. First, an altered IgA structure can derive from the influence of lymphokines produced by T cells upon developing IgA B cells. Similar effects on B cells can be elicited by cytokines derived from other cells, such as the IL-10 homologue produced by virally infected epithelium. Although increased IgA production would result, the IgA produced would also be distinct in that it bears oligosaccharides that for some reason promote glomerular deposition and injury.[72] This mechanism could, in some patients, be genetic in origin. Among those with an acquired defect, direct modification of normally structured IgA by enzymes produced or evoked by infectious agents is also possible. Second, the nonimmunoglobulin component of the deposited IgA complex confers both the mesangial deposition and the requisite cellular response.

Viral infection and entry of environmental agents such as lectins therefore remain the major risk factors for the development of IgAN, as has been postulated since the recognition of the disease by Jean Berger 25 years ago. The evolution of our understanding has led, however, to an appreciation of such infection and/or penetration of environmental agents beyond the simple roles of antigen. Rather, these elements seem to encompass effects on IgA structure, affinity for mesangium, and potency on mesangial cellular metabolism. Presumably, the degree to which these elements act and interact underlies the variation in the population of patients with IgAN. As recognition and prognostication in IgAN move away from traditional morphologic and immunohistochemical criteria toward chemical and immunochemical criteria, measures of anionicity or glycosylation of IgA, the binding affinity of IgA aggregates for extracellular matrix proteins and/or oligosaccharides, and the capacity for specific oligosaccharides to dissociate IgA-containing macromolecular aggregates will likely become important. If, indeed, patients with IgAN can be grouped into more cohesive subpopulations based on chemical or immunochemical classification, such tests will become valuable not only for their capacity for diagnosis and prognosis but also as guides to the selection of specific therapy. The critical goals will then center around defining criteria with strong predictive value that also offer insight to pathogenesis and the likely response to therapeutic algorithms. Clearly, research into the mechanism(s) of IgAN will provide opportunities to the diagnostic laboratory that affect the practical management of patients.

REFERENCES

1. D'Amico G: The commonest glomerulonephritis in the world: IgA nephropathy. *Q J Med* 64:709–727, 1987.
2. Clarkson AR: *IgA Nephropathy.* Boston, Martinus Nijhoff, 1987.
3. Julian BA: IgA nephropathy: [Proceedings of] A national symposium. *Am J Kidney Dis* 12:1–457, 1988.
4. Schena FP: A retrospective analysis of the natural history of primary IgA nephropathy worldwide. *Am J Med* 89:209–215, 1990.

5. Emancipator SN: Primary and secondary forms of IgA nephritis, Schönlein-Henoch syndrome, in Heptinstall RH (ed): *Pathology of the Kidney*, vol 1. Boston, Little Brown, 1992, pp 389–476.

6. Emancipator SN, Lamm ME: IgA nephropathy and related diseases, in Ogra PL, Mestecky J, Lamm ME, et al (eds): *Handbook of Mucosal Immunology*. San Diego, Academic Press, 1994, pp 663–676.

7. Sakai H, Sakai O, Nomoto Y: *Pathogenesis of IgA Nephropathy*. Tokyo, Harcourt Brace Jovanovich, 1990.

8. Julian BA, Woodford SY, Baehler RW, et al: Familial clustering and immunogenetic aspects of IgA nephropathy. *Am J Kidney Dis* 12:366–370, 1988.

9. Emancipator SN, Lamm ME: Biology of disease: IgA nephropathy: Pathogenesis of the most common form of glomerulonephritis. *Lab Invest* 60:168–183, 1989.

10. Rostoker G, Petit-Phar M, Delprato S, et al: Mucosal immunity in primary glomerulonephritis: II. Study of the serum IgA subclass repertoire to food and airborne antigens. *Nephron* 59:561–566, 1991.

11. Harper SJ, Pringle JH, Wicks ACB, et al: Expression of J chain mRNA in duodenal IgA plasma cells in IgA nephropathy. *Kidney Int* 45:836–844, 1994.

12. Hené RJ, Schuurman JH, Kater L: Immunoglobulin A subclass–containing plasma cells in the jejunum in primary IgA nephropathy and in Henoch-Schölein purpura. *Nephron* 48:4–7, 1988.

13. Westberg NG, Baklien K, Schmekel B, et al: Quantitation of immunoglobulin-producing cells in small intestinal mucosa of patients with IgAN nephropathy. *Clin Immunol Immunopathol* 26:442–445, 1983.

14. Béné MC, Hurault de Ligny B, Kessler M, et al: Confirmation of tonsillar anomalies in IgA nephropathy: A multicenter study. *Nephron* 58:425–428, 1991.

15. Rostoker G, Pech MA, del Prato S, et al: Serum IgG subclasses and IgM imbalances in adult IgA mesangial glomerulonephritis and idiopathic Henoch-Schoenlein purpura. *Clin Exp Immunol* 75:30–34, 1989.

16. Aucouturier P, Monteiro RC, Noel LH, et al: Glomerular and serum immunoglobulin G subclasses in IgA nephropathy. *Clin Immunol Immunopathol* 51:338–347, 1989.

17. Scivittaro V, Ranieri E, DiCillo M, et al: In vitro immunoglobulin production in relatives of patients with IgA nephropathy. *Clin Nephrol* 42:1–8, 1994.

18. Bannister KM, Drew PA, Clarkson AR, et al: Immunoregulation in glomerulonephritis, Henoch-Schoenlein purpura and lupus nephritis. *Clin Exp Immunol* 53:384–390, 1983.

19. Cosio FG, Lam S, Folami AO, et al: Immune regulation of immunoglobulin production in IgA nephropathy. *Clin Immunol Immunopathol* 23:430–436, 1982.

20. Hale GM, McIntosh SL, Hiki Y, et al: Evidence for IgA-specific B cell hyperactivity in patients with IgA nephropathy. *Kidney Int* 29:718–724, 1986.

21. Endoh M, Suga T, Miura M, et al: In vivo alteration of antibody production in patients with IgA nephropathy. *Clin Exp Immunol* 57:564–570, 1984.

22. Pasternack A, Mustonen J, Leinikki P: Humoral immune response in patients with IgA and IgM glomerulonephritis. *Clin Exp Immunol* 63:228–233, 1986.

23. Leinikki PO, Mustonen J, Pasternack A: Immune response to oral polio vaccine in patients with IgA glomerulonephritis. *Clin Exp Immunol* 68:33–38, 1987.

24. van den Wall Bake AWL, Beyer WEP, Evers-Schouten JH, et al: Humoral immune response to influenza vaccination in patients with primary immunoglobulin A nephropathy. *J Clin Invest* 84:1070–1075, 1989.

25. Waldo FB: Systemic immune response after mucosal immunization in patients with IgA nephropathy. *J Clin Immunol* 12:21–26, 1992.

26. Waldo FB, Cochran AM: Systemic immune response to oral polio immunization in patients with IgA nephropathy. *J Clin Lab Immunol* 28:109–114, 1987.
27. Scivittaro V, Gesualdo L, Ranieri E, et al: Profiles of immunoregulatory cytokine production in vitro in patients with IgA nephropathy and their kindred. *Clin Exp Immunol* 96:311–316, 1994.
28. Cagnoli L, Beltrandi E, Pasquali S, et al: B and T cell abnormalities in patients with primary IgA nephropathy. *Kidney Int* 28:646–651, 1985.
29. Egido J, Blasco R, Sancho J, et al: T-cell dysfunctions in IgA nephropathy: Specific abnormalities in the regulation of IgA synthesis. *Clin Immunol Immunopathol* 26:201–212, 1983.
30. Sakai H, Endoh M, Tomino Y, et al: Increase of IgA specific helper T cells in patients with IgA nephropathy. *Clin Exp Immunol* 50:77–82, 1982.
31. Sakai H, Nomoto Y, Arimori S: Decrease of IgA specific suppressor T cell activity in patients with IgA nephropathy. *Clin Exp Immunol* 38:243–248, 1979.
32. Rothschild E, Chatenoud L: T cell subset modulation of immunoglobulin production in IgA nephropathy and membranous glomerulonephritis. *Kidney Int* 25:557–564, 1984.
33. Gesualdo L, Lamm ME, Emancipator SN: Defective oral tolerance promotes nephritogenesis in experimental IgA nephropathy induced by oral immunization. *J Immunol* 145:3684–3691, 1990.
34. Emancipator SN, Lamm ME: IgA nephropathy: Overproduction or decreased clearance of immune complexes? *Lab Invest* 61:365–367, 1989.
35. Montiero RC, Halbwachs-Mecarelli L, Roque-Barreira MC, et al: Charge and size and mesangial IgA in IgA nephropathy. *Kidney Int* 28:666–671, 1985.
36. Baldree LA, Wyatt RJ, Julian BA, et al: Immunoglobulin A–fibronectin aggregate levels in children and adults with immunoglobulin A nephropathy. *Am J Kidney Dis* 22:1–4, 1993.
37. Solari R, Kraehenbuhl J-P: The biosynthesis of secretory component and its role in the transepithelial transport of IgA dimer. *Immunol Today* 6:17–20, 1985.
38. Mazanec MB, Nedrud JG, Kaetzel CS, et al: A three-tiered view of the role of IgA in mucosal defense. *Immunol Today* 14:430–435, 1993.
39. Mazanec MB, Kaetzel CS, Lamm ME, et al: Intracellular neutralization of virus by immunoglobulin A antibodies. *Proc Natl Acad Sci U S A* 89:6901–6905, 1992.
40. Sollid LM, Kvale D, Brandtzaeg P, et al: Interferon-γ enhances expression of secretory component, the epithelial receptor for polymeric immunoglobulins. *J Immunol* 138:4304–4306, 1987.
41. Kvale D, Løvhaug D, Sollid LM, et al: Tumor necrosis factor-α up-regulates expression of secretory component, the epithelial receptor for polymeric Ig. *J Immunol* 140:3086–3089, 1988.
42. Phillips JO, Everson MP, Moldoveanu Z, et al: Synergistic effect of IL-4 and IFN-γ on the expressin of polymeric Ig receptor (secretory component) and IgA binding by human epithelial cells. *J Immunol* 145:1740–1744, 1990.
43. Youngman KR, Fiocchi C, Kaetzel CS: Inhibition of interferon-γ activity in supernatants from stimulated human intestinal mononuclear cells prevents up-regulation of the polymeric immunoglobulin receptor in an intestinal epithelial cell line. *J Immunol* 153:675–681, 1994.
44. Harper SJ, Pringle JH, Wicks ACB, et al: Expression of J chain mRNA in duodenal IgA plasma cells in IgA nephropathy. *Kidney Int* 45:836–844, 1994.
45. Rifai A, Schena FP, Montinaro V, et al: Clearance kinetics and fate of macromolecular IgA in patients with IgA nephropathy. *Lab Invest* 61:381–388, 1989.

46. Roccatello D, Coppo R, Piccoli G, et al: Circulating Fc-receptor blocking factors in IgA nephropathies. *Clin Nephrol* 23:159–168, 1985.

47. Roccatello D, Picciotto G, Coppo R, et al: Clearance of polymeric IgA aggregates in humans. *Am J Kidney Dis* 14:354–360, 1989.

48. Roccatello D, Picciotto G, Ropolo R, et al: Kinetics and fate of IgA-IgG aggregates as a model of naturally occurring immune complexes in IgA nephropathy. *Lab Invest* 66:86–95, 1992.

49. Kaetzel CS, Robinson JK, Chintalacharuvu KR, et al: The polymeric immunoglobulin receptor (secretory component) mediates transport of immune complexes across epithelial cells: A local defense function for IgA. *Proc Natl Acad Sci U S A* 88:8796–8800, 1991.

50. Husby S, Jensenius JC, Svehag SE: Passage of undegraded dietary antigen into the blood of healthy adults. Quantitation, estimation of size distribution, and relation of uptake to levels of specific antibodies. *Scand J Immunol* 22:83–92, 1985.

51. Coppo R, Basolo B, Martina G, et al: Circulating immune complexes containing IgA, IgG, and IgM in patients with primary IgA nephropathy and with Henoch-Schoenlein nephritis. Correlation with clinical and histologic signs of activity. *Clin Nephrol* 18:230-239, 1982.

52. Jones CL, Powell HR, Kincaid-Smith P, et al: Polymeric IgA and immune complex concentration in IgA-related renal disease. *Kidney Int* 38:323–331, 1990.

53. Coppo R, Basolo B, Roccatello D, et al: Immunological monitoring of plasma exchange in primary IgA nephropathy. *Artif Organs* 9:351–358, 1985.

54. Coppo R, Arico S, Basolo B, et al: Presence and origin of IgA1 and IgA2 containing immune complexes in chronic alcoholic liver disease with and without glomerulonephritis. *Clin Immunol Immunopathol* 35:1–8, 1985.

55. Van den Wall Bake AWL, Kirk KA, Gay RE, et al: Binding of serum immunoglobulins to collagen in IgA nephropathy and HIV infection. *Kidney Int* 42:374–382, 1992.

56. Moorthy AV, Zimmerman SW, Maxim PE: Dermatitis herpetiformis and coeliac disease: Association with glomerulonephritis, hypocomplementemia and circulating immune complexes. *JAMA* 239:2019–2020, 1978.

57. Sinniah R: Occurrence of mesangial IgA and IgM deposits in a control necropsy population. *J Clin Pathol* 36:276–279, 1983.

58. Lomax-Smith JD, Zabrowarny LA, Howarth GS, et al: The immunochemical characterization of mesangial IgA deposits. *Am J Pathol* 113:359–364, 1983.

59. Rifai A, Millard K: Glomerular deposition of immune complexes prepared with monomeric or polymeric IgA. *Clin Exp Immunol* 60:363–368, 1985.

60. Monteiro RC, Chavailler A, Noel L, et al: Serum IgA preferentially binds to cationic polypepties in IgA nephropathy. *Clin Exp Immunol* 73:300–306, 1988.

61. Gallo GR, Caulin-Glaser T, Emancipator SN, et al: Nephritogenicity and differential distribution of glomerular immune complexes related to immunogen charge. *Lab Invest* 48:353–362, 1983.

62. Amore A, Emancipator SN, Roccatello D, et al: Functional consequences of the binding of gliadin to cultured rat mesangial cells: Bridging immunoglobulin A cells and modulation of eicosanoid synthesis and altered cytokine production. *Am J Kidney Dis* 23:290–301, 1994.

63. Emancipator SN, Rao CS, Amore A, et al: Macromolecular properties that promote mesangial binding and mesangiopathic nephritis. *J Am Soc Nephrol* 2(suppl):149–158, 1992.

64. Amore A, Cavallo F, Bocchietto E, et al: Cytokine mRNA expression by cultured rat mesangial cells after contact with environmental lectins. *Kidney Int* 43(suppl):41–46, 1993.

65. Kondoh H, Kobayashi K, Hagiwara K, et al: Jacalin, a jack-fruit lectin, precipitates IgA1 but not IgA2 subclass on gel diffusion reaction. *J Immunol Methods* 80:171–173, 1986.
66. Amore A, Coppo R, Nedrud J, et al: Mucosal tolerance failure in an experimental model of IgA nephropathy in mice induced by Sendai virus. *Kidney Int*, in press.
67. Coppo R, Amore A, Gianoglio B, et al: Serum IgA and macromolecular IgA reactive with mesangial matrix components. *Contrib Nephrol* 104:162–172, 1993.
68. Coppo R, Amore A, Cirina P, et al: Characteristics of IgA and macromolecular IgA in sera from IgA nephropathy transplanted patients with and without IgA nephropathy recurrence. *Contrib Nephrol* III:85–92, 1995.
69. Allen AC, Harper SJ, Feehally J: Reduced IgA 1 galactosylation and increased β1, 3 galactosyl transferase activity in IgA nephropathy (abstract). *J Am Soc Nephrol* 5:739, 1994.
70. Mestecky J, Oh H, Tomana M: Alterations in the IgA carbohydrate chains influence the cellular distribution of IgA. *Contrib Nephrol* 111:66–72, 1995.
71. Brensilver JN, Mallat S, Scholes J, et al: Recurrent IgA nephropathy in living-related donors transplanation: Recurrence or transmission of familial disease? *Am J Kidney Dis* 2:147–151, 1988.
72. Rao CS, Emancipator SN: Interleukins 4 and 5 alter oligosaccharides on IgA in mice and humans: Ramifications for kinetics of deposition and complement fixation (abstract). *J Am Soc Nephrol* 5:771, 1994.
73. Gesualdo L, Emancipator SN, Kesselheim C, et al: Glomerular hemodynamics and eicosanoid synthesis in a rat model of IgA nephropathy. *Kidney Int* 42:106–114, 1992.
74. Coppo R, Amore A, Gianoglio B, et al: Angiotensin II local hyperreactivity in the progression of IgA nephropathy. *Am J Kidney Dis* 21:593–602, 1993.
75. Jessen RH, Emancipator SN, Jacobs GH, et al: Experimental IgA-IgG nephropathy induced by a viral respiratory pathogen: Dependence on antigen form and immune status. *Lab Invest* 67:379–386, 1992.
76. Douglas AP: The binding of a glycopeptide component of wheat gluten to intestinal mucosa of normal and coeliac human subjects. *Clin Chim Acta* 73:357–361, 1976.
77. Fornasieri A, Sinico AR, Maldifassi P, et al: IgA-antigliadin antibodies in IgA mesangial nephropathy (Berger's disease). *BMJ* 295:78–79, 1987.
78. Coppo R, Amore A, Roccatello D: Dietary antigens and primary immunoglobulin A nephropathy. *J Am Soc Nephrol* 2(suppl):173–180, 1992.
79. Russell MW, Reinholdt J, Killian L: Anti-inflammatory activity of human IgA antibodies and the Fab alpha fragments: Inhibition of IgG-mediated complement activation. *Eur J Immunol* 19:2243–2248, 1989.
80. Davin JC, Dechenne C, Lombet J, et al: Acute experimental glomerulonephritis induced by the glomerular deposition of circulating polymeric IgA concanavalin A complexes. *Virchows Arch A Pathol Anat Histopathol* 415:7–20, 1989.
81. Holthofer H: Lectin binding sites in kidney. A comparative study of 14 animal species. *J Histochem Cytochem* 31:531–537, 1983.

Rheumatoid Arthritis: Update on Molecular Studies

Ralph C. Williams, Jr., M.D.
Eminent Scholar, Marcia Whitney Schott Chair in Rheumatoid Arthritis
Research and Professor and Chief, Division of Rheumatology, Department of
Medicine, University of Florida College of Medicine, Gainesville, Florida

Rheumatoid arthritis (RA) continues to be an important chronic disabling disease that affects between 4 and 5 million people in the United States—approximately 2% of our population. Unlike acquired immunodeficiency syndrome (AIDS) or new ailments like Hantavirus respiratory distress syndrome,[1, 2] which have sometimes emerged in major or minor epidemic proportions throughout the world, RA still stands as a major chronic disorder afflicting a substantial proportion of our population. Although a number of new approaches to treatment have emerged during the past several years, unfortunately there has been no recent important major breakthrough in our understanding of disease pathogenesis or any dramatic new therapeutic approaches that have provided major advances in understanding the primary etiology of the disease itself.

EPIDEMIOLOGY AND DISEASE COURSE

Recent extensive epidemiologic studies have confirmed the fact that RA appears to affect a broad range of population groups throughout the world.[3-6] Of considerable interest in this regard is the fact that newer treatment programs such as weekly methotrexate have been very effective in many patients since their reintroduction to the modern therapeutic armamentarium. However, studies of the overall effect of the disease itself on actual morbidity and mortality have now indicated that merely having the disease definitely shortens patients' life spans.[7, 8] Thus in view of a number of different immediate causes of death such as coronary artery disease, arteriosclerosis, pneumonia, or malignancy, patients with RA die sooner of these conditions than do other age- and sex-matched control groups.[7, 8] There seems to be some sort of accelerating or ominous negative influence associated with RA that shortens a patient's life and that often cannot be obviously linked to specific pathogenic mechanisms directly associated with the disease such as vasculitis, release of waves of proinflammatory cytokines, or the intense synovitis present in multiple joints.

Advances in Pathology and Laboratory Medicine®, vol. 8
© 1995, Mosby–Year Book, Inc.

STUDIES OF RHEUMATOID FACTOR

Rheumatoid factors (RFs), which are among the very first autoantibodies ever recognized and were named after the very disease, were initially described by Waaler more than five decades ago.[9] Since their initial description (and several years later, their rediscovery) by Rose et al.,[10] literally thousands of papers have appeared that have defined RF specificities, mechanisms that could amplify a destructive series of inflammatory reactions within the affected synovium, as well as genetic reactivities and altered immune reactions, which appeared to play a central role in the actual RA inflammatory process. The initial studies of human RF appeared to confirm that this group of autoantibodies behaved like IgM, IgA, or IgG antiglobulins that reacted with antigens on the Fc portion of IgG, including epitopes on the CH2 and CH3 domains.[11-15] Studies of RF specificity frequently demonstrated a peculiar heteroclitic pattern of reaction for genetically determined antigenic sites on the CH2 or the CH3

TABLE 1.

Gm Phenotypes and Anti-Gm Specificities of IgM Rheumatoid Factor Isolated From Patients with Rheumatoid Arthritis*

Gm IgG Phenotype and Patient Number	Anti-Gm(a) Activity	Anti-Gm(b) Activity	Anti-Gm(g) Activity	Anti-Gm(f) Activity
Gm(a−), (b+), (g−), (f+)				
1	40,960†	1,280	40,960	20,480
2	5,120	80	5,120	10,240
3	5,120	160	10,240	20,480
4	5,120	320	10,240	10,240
5	2,560	160	5,120	10,240
6	2,560	5,120	1,280	2,560
7	2,560	5,120	1,280	10,240
8	2,560	2,560	1,280	10,240
9	160	20	160	2,560
Gm(a+), (x+), (b+), (g+), (f+)				
10	40,960	2,560	40,960	320,000
11	20,480	160	20,480	20,480
12	5,120	80	5,120	10,240
13	320	0	40	320
14	160	0	0	20
Gm(a+), (x−), (b+), (g+), (f+)				
15	80	0	80	160
16	80	0	40	0
Gm(a+), (x+), (b−), (g+), (f−)				
17	40	0	0	0

*From Williams RC Jr, Malone CC, Casali P: J Immunol 149:1817–1824, 1992. Used by permission.
†Numbers represent reciprocal values of the highest dilution at which hemagglutination was still observed. All isolated IgM rheumatoid factors tested were adjusted to the same concentration (5μg/mL) before the titrations were carried out with Gm-specific IgG-coated erythrocytes.

IgG domains *not* present on the affected host's autologous IgG molecules.[14-18] Thus RFs from patients with RA who were Gm(a-) or Gm(g-) often showed specificity for IgG allotypes not present on the patient's own autologous IgG (Table 1). If indeed RFs were true autoantibodies, then how could such strange heteroclitic reactions occur? A number of imaginative explanations or hypotheses were suggested, including viral transduction of new Gm-determinant genes within the patient's germ line, possibly suggesting an ongoing subclinical viral infection associated with the disease[19] or a slight physical alteration of IgG during the process of endogenous immune complex formation[20] that exposed antigenic determinants on autologous IgG very similar to or conformationally mimicking the heteroclitic Gm(a) or Gm(g) determinants. In fact, the latter explanation for heteroclitic RF specificity was indeed shown to be the case since monoclonal RF generated by Epstein-Barr virus (EBV) transformation from a Gm(a-), GM(g-) patient with RA could be shown to react with origi-

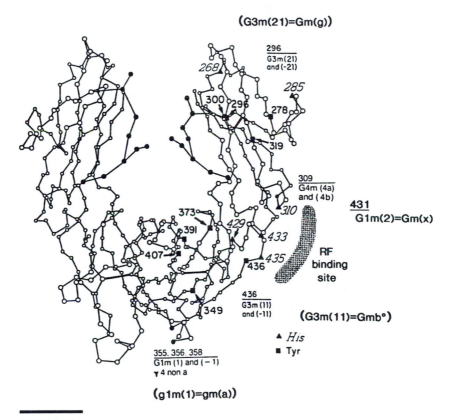

FIGURE 1.

X-ray crystallographic model of the $C_\gamma 2 - C_\gamma 3$ domains of human IgG. The rheumatoid factor binding site at the C_γ-2 – C_γ3 interface is shown by the *shaded area*. The relative distribution of several single or double amino acid substitutions determining the Gm(a), Gm(x), Gm(b), or Gm(g) allotype is also shown. Histadyl and tyrosyl residues are indicted by the *filled triangles* and *filled squares*, respectively. The Gm(f) allotype–specific residues Arg 214 and Ser 219 are not shown in this view of IgG since they are located beyond the hinge region within the $C_\gamma 1$ domain. (Adapted from Deisenhofer J, Jones TA, Huber R, et al: *Hoppe-Seyler Z Physiol Chem* 359:975–985, 1978. Used by permission.)

CH₂ Region of IgG-1

CH₃ Region of IgG-1

CH₂ Region of IgG-1

```
          PRO  SER
240 VAL
241–250   PHE  LEU  PHE  PRO  PRO  LYS  PRO  LYS  ASP  THR
251–260   LEU  MET  ILE  SER  ARG  THR  PRO  GLU  VAL  THR
261–270   CYS  VAL  VAL  VAL  ASP  VAL  SER  HIS  GLU  ASP
271–280   PRO  GLU  VAL  LYS  PHE  ASN  TRP  TYR  VAL  ASP
281–290   GLY  VAL  GLU  VAL  HIS  ASN  ALA  LYS  THR  LYS
291–300   PRO(LEU)  ARG  GLU  GLN  GLN  TYR(TYR)  ASX  SER  THR  TYR   (G)
301–310   ARG  VAL  VAL  SER  VAL  LEU  THR  VAL  LEU  HIS
311–320   GLN  ASP  TRP  LEU  ASN  GLY  LYS  GLU  TYR  LYS
321–330   CYS  LYS  VAL  SER  ASN  LYS  ALA  LEU  PRO  ALA
331–340   PRO  ILE  GLU  LYS  THR  ILE  SER  LYS  ALA  LYS
341       GLY
```

Boxed residues: 291 PRO(LEU), 296 TYR(TYR)

CH₃ Region of IgG-1

```
341–350   GLY  GLN  PRO  ARG  GLU  PRO  GLN  VAL  TYR  THR          (A)
351–360   LEU  PRO  PRO  SER  ARG  GLU(ASP)  GLU  MET(LEU)  THR  LYS
361–370   ASN  GLN  VAL  SER  LEU  THR  CYS  LEU  VAL  LYS
371–380   GLY  PHE  TYR  PRO  SER  ASP  ILE  ALA  VAL  GLU
381–390   TRP  GLU  SER  ASN  GLY  GLN  PRO  GLU  ASN  ASN
391–400   TYR  LYS  THR  THR  PRO  PRO  VAL  LEU  ASP  SER
401–410   ASP  GLY  SER  PHE  PHE  LEU  TYR  SER  LYS  LEU
411–420   THR  VAL  ASP  LYS  SER  ARG  TRP  GLN  GLN(GLN)  GLY     (B⁵)
421–430   ASN  VAL(ILE)  PHE  SER  CYS  SER  VAL  MET  HIS  GLU     (B⁵)
431–440   ALA(GLY)  LEU  HIS  ASN  HIS  TYR  THR  GLN  LYS  SER     (X)
441–446   LEU  SER  LEU  SER  PRO  GLY(446)
```

Dashed boxes: 356 GLU(ASP), 358 MET(LEU)
Dotted boxes: 419 GLN(GLN), 422 VAL(ILE)
Solid box: 431 ALA(GLY)

FIGURE 2.

Sequences of CH2 and CH3 region of IgG1 showing single or double amino acid substitutions at key residues that have been linked to the Gm allotypic markers Gm(a), Gm(x), Gm(b⁵), Gm(f) and Gm(g). Gm(f) and Gm(z) are not shown since these allotypes depend on the presence of an arginine at position 214 in CH1 (Gm(f)); the allele of Gm(f), which is Gm(z), has a lysine at position 214. The CH2 sequence (left) shows the Gm(g)-specific residues leucine at position 291 and tyrosine at position 296 in boxes. When a proline is present at position 291, the Gm(g) allotype is not detected. On the right is shown the CH3 region of IgG1. The allotype-specific amino acids aspartic acid at position 356 and leucine at 358 (dashed boxes) confer Gm(a) specificity. With glutamic acid and methionine at positions 356 and 358, Gm(a) is not expressed. Glutamine at position 419 and isoleucine at 422 constitute the allotype residues associated with Gm(b⁵) (dotted boxes). Finally, the allotype-specific residue for Gm(x) is a glycine at position 431 (solid box). If alanine occurs at this residue, the Gm(x) allotype is not detected. The interface between CH2 and CH3 contains rheumatoid factor–reactive epitopes.

nally Gm(a-) IgG after it had formed tetanus-antitetanus IgG immune complexes in vitro.[21] During the course of this work a more precise understanding of the actual structural basis for IgG Gm allotypic antigenic determinants emerged that was based on chemical modification studies of isolated IgG myeloma proteins and various truncated IgG fragments recovered from the serum and urine of patients with several forms of hematopoietic malignancy.[22] Thus it had been known for some time that the Gm(a) allotypic marker consisted of single amino acid differences at positions 356 and 358 within the IgG1 CH3 domain.[16, 23] It was also known that RF reacting with IgG and showing clear-cut anti-Gm(a) specificity actually reacted with the IgG molecule at sites along the CH3-CH2 domain interface[24, 25, 26] some distance away from the actual site of the two Gm(a)-specific amino acid substitutions at positions 356 and 358 (Fig 1). Thus "Gm(a)-ness" seemed to depend on conformational determinants somehow allosterically induced by the two simple amino acid substitutions at positions 356 and 358 (Fig 2). Moreover, conformational determinants within the CH3 domains essential for Gm(a) antigenic expression also appeared to depend on the structural influence of other contiguous IgG domains since mutant IgG fragments bearing the two Gm(a)-specific residues at positions 356 and 358 also did not express the Gm(a) antigen if they showed a complete deletion of the contiguous CH1 domain.[22] These observations were of considerable interest since they also demonstrated that IgG genetic allotypic markers were highly dependent on the shape or conformational aspects of the tertiary structure of the immunoglobulin CH3 or CH2 domains and that isolated single allotypic amino acid differences within the structure of a very large molecule like IgG1 could in turn produce major allosteric differences in conformation and expression of "Gm(a)-ness" or "Gm(g)-ness."

DEFINITION OF SITES ON IGG REACTING WITH RHEUMATOID FACTOR

For some time it had been known that RF appeared to show major reactive epitopes on regions of IgG at the CH3-CH2 interface.[24, 25, 26] Recently our group has focused on attempts to define exact regions on both CH3 and CH2 that actually participate in such RF reactivity by using the epitope-mapping strategy originally introduced by Geysen and coworkers.[27, 28]

This approach uses synthesis of the primary amino acid sequence of a protein domain of interest as overlapping heptamers on small polypropylene rods arranged in rows on a microtiter-sized plastic plate. After the synthesis of the heptamers derived from the primary sequence has been completed, the set of pins containing overlapping peptides derived from the original sequence can be used as a test substrate over and over again in enzyme-linked immunosorbent assays (ELISA) with test monoclonal or polyclonal antibodies.[29] This technology is illustrated in Figure 3. Identification of reactive regions within the primary linear sequence can be focused even more precisely by resynthesizing antibody-reactive regions over again followed by heptamers in which a neutral glycine or alanine is substituted for each amino acid residue.[29] A fall in reactivity of more than 50% after glycine or alanine substitution indicates that the sub-

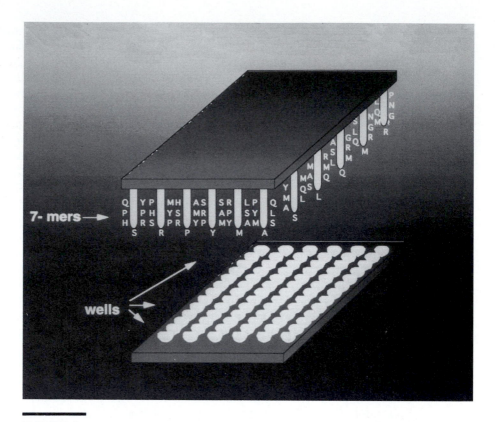

FIGURE 3.

Overlapping heptamers of the primary amino acid sequence are synthesized on small polypropylene rods or pins arranged on a standard microtiter plate support (*above*). When synthesis of the peptides on each pin has been completed, the pins bearing the peptides can be used to test each heptamer of the primary sequence by using an enzyme-linked immunosorbent assay with either polyclonal or monoclonal antibody. During the course of the heptamer synthesis, two standard pins containing the sequences PLAC and GLAC are also synthesized and used with a standard monoclonal mouse antibody recognizing only the peptide PLAC. Reactivity with the standard peptide is used with each assay to establish an internal control for reproducibility.

stituted residue represents a relatively important antigenic site in the area in question. Lesser degrees of decreased ELISA reactivity on glycine/alanine substitution such as a 25% to 49% reduction are interpreted as indicating antigenic contributions of lesser importance by the substituted residue. Regions of protein structure analyzed in this way by using overlapping heptamers of primary sequence must be known to be solvent accessible and therefore not completely buried within the tertiary structure of the molecules under study. With this important caveat in mind, most of the protein domains we have recently examined with this strategy have been proteins in which the three-dimensional structure has already been completely elucidated by previous high-resolution studies of crystal structure.[30, 31]

When we applied this approach to the CH3 and CH2 domains of IgG1 to define the major RF-reactive regions of the molecule, a surprising multiplicity of regions both on the CH3 and CH2 domains were identi-

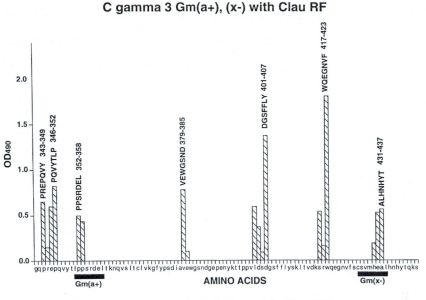

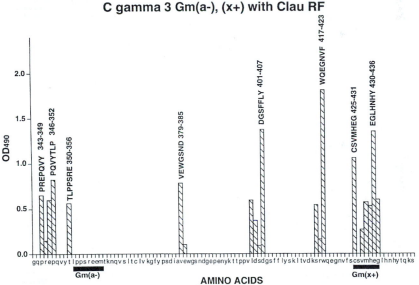

FIGURE 4.

Overlapping heptamers of IgG CH3 sequence were synthesized on polypropylene pins and tested for reactivity with polyclonal IgM rheumatoid factor *(RF)* Clau from a patient with rheumatoid arthritis. Reactions with individual regions of primary sequence are showed as *vertical bars.* The CH3 sequence was synthesized *(above)* to include the Gm(a+) allotypic substitutions but not those for Gm(x). The sequence *below* includes the Gm(a−) amino acid sequence and contains the allotypic amino acids governing Gm(x). (From Peterson C, Malone CC, Williams RC Jr: Rheumatoid-factor−reactive sites on CH3 established by overlapping 7-mer peptide epitope analyses. *Mol Immunol,* 32:57, 1995. Used by permission.)

fied.[32, 33] Each affinity-isolated polyclonal human IgM RF seemed to display a slightly different set of major CH3 and CH2 domain reactivities. Moreover, these slight differences in IgG Fc domain–reactive patterns showed no clear correlation with anti-Gm or anti-IgG H-chain subgroup RF specificities. Examples of reactive patterns for polyclonal and mono-

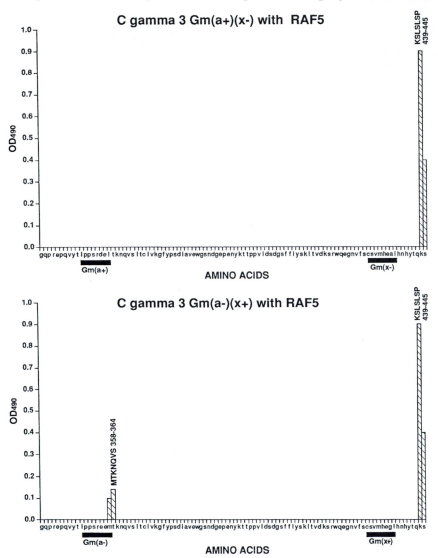

FIGURE 5.

The reactions illustrated here show a monoclonal IgM rheumatoid factor (RF) from a patient with rheumatoid arthritis who is Gm(a−) and Gm(g−). The RF tested in this pin enzyme-linked immunosorbent assay reaction shows primary anti-Gm(a) and anti-Gm(g) specificity; however, on the reactivity with the actual CH3 IgG sequence, only one small peak of minimal reactivity is seen near the Gm(a−) region to the left and a high peak of reactivity at KSLSLSP at positions 439 to 445 far from the actual Gm(a) or Gm(g) allotype substitutions. (From Peterson C, Malone CC, Williams RC Jr: Rheumatoid-factor–reactive sites on CH3 established by overlapping 7-mer peptide epitope analyses. *Mol Immunol,* 32:57, 1995. Used by permission.)

clonal IgM RF from patients with active seropositive RA are shown in Figures 4 and 5. A composite view of all of the solvent-accessible RF-reactive regions within the IgG CH2 and CH3 domains is shown in Figure 6.

Of great interest during the course of these studies, which were greatly extended by using a large panel of both polyclonal and monoclonal human IgM RF, was our finding that the actual RF-reactive epitopes identified within the CH3 or CH2 domains showed no obvious exact sequence

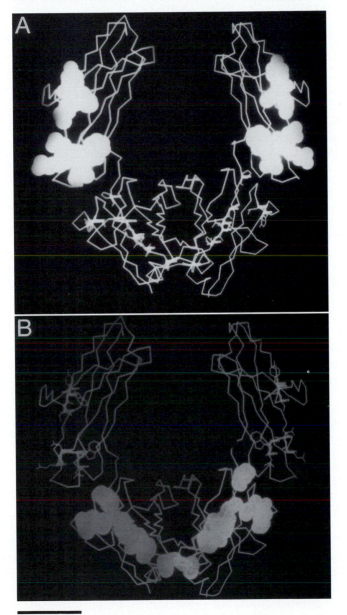

FIGURE 6.

Composite view of all rheumatoid factor–reactive sties on the CH2 **(A)** and CH3 **(B)** domains of IgG as identified by the overlapping heptamer strategy described in the text and elsewhere.[29, 32, 33]

TABLE 2.

Rheumatoid Factor–Reactive Antigenic Epitopes on the CH3 and CH2 Domains of Human IgG

Domain	Primary Squence	Residue
CH3	P R E P Q V Y*	343–349
	P Q V Y T L P	346–352
	T L P P S R E	350–356
	D G S F F L Y	401–407
	W Q Q G N V F	417–423
	C S V M H E G	425–431
	E G L H N H Y	430–436
CH2	S V F L F P P	239–245
	K F N W Y V D	274–280
	N S T Y R V V S V	297–305
	V L T V L H Q N W L	305–314

*Residues underlined represent immunodominant amino acids making a major contribution to the antigenicity of IgG at this site as established by the glycine/alanine substitution strategy.

homologies. This can be quickly appreciated when one compares the spectrum of CH3 and CH2 RF-reactive heptamers shown in Table 2. Presently we believe that this is the case because although the primary sequences of RF-reactive linear regions of CH3 or CH2 are indeed quite different, their actual shapes or conformations may actually be very similar. This is strongly supported by our recent studies using rabbit antisera made against a number of these CH3 or CH2 RF-reactive peptides. In these latter experiments, many strong cross-reactions have been recorded that confirm the impression that similar small RF-reactive regions on IgG without any clear sequence identity may actually share remarkable similarities in conformation.

RHEUMATOID FACTORS ALSO REACT WITH HUMAN β_2-MICROGLOBULIN AND CLASS I AND CLASS II HLA MOLECULES

As an extension of our epitope-mapping studies on the CH2 and CH3 domains of IgG we next examined RF reactivity with other members of the immunoglobulin gene superfamily, including β_2-microglobulin $(\beta_2 M)$[31, 34] and class I as well as class II HLA molecules.[35] To our great surprise, both affinity-isolated polyclonal IgM RFs from RA patients' serum as well as monoclonal RF generated by direct hybridoma cell line fusion with rheumatoid synovial B cells[36] also often showed strong ELISA reactivities with $\beta_2 M$ and class I HLA molecules.[34–36] In the case of $\beta_2 M$, the invariant light chain of class I HLA molecules, the RF-reactive regions encompassed two small linear $\beta_2 M$ segments at solvent-exposed positions

57 to 63 and 87 to 97. An example of this strong RF reactivity for β_2M is shown in Figure 7. Again, use of the glycine/alanine substitution strategy identified a limited number of immunodominant RF-reactive residues, including lysine residues at positions 58 and 94 and aspartic acid at 59 and 96, as well as arginine at position 95. Moreover, again when the actual linear RF-reactive peptides themselves were examined, a remarkable antigenic cross-reactivity became apparent since rabbit antisera produced by immunization with the β_2M peptide SKDWSFY showed strong ELISA reactivity with the other RF-reactive β_2M epitope LSQPKIVKWDR and vice versa. These findings again led us to the conclusion that these two RF-reactive regions on β_2M probably shared considerable shape homology despite their apparent nonidentity when their primary sequences were compared directly.

Studies of RF reactivity with class I HLA molecules are still ongoing and thus far have shown the same striking patterns of reactivity within extremely localized solvent-accessible regions of class I molecules. Work demonstrating RF reactivity with HLA class I antigens is currently in progress in our laboratory.

When immunodominant RF-reactive residues identified by glycine/

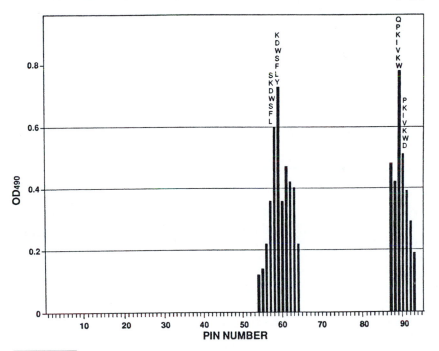

FIGURE 7.

Results of pin enzyme-linked immunosorbent assays (ELISA) of rheumatoid factor (RF) Har binding to pins containing overlapping heptamers of the entire β_2-microglobulin (β_2m) amino acid sequence. The two major peaks of positive RF reactivity with β_2m noted at pins 58 and 59 and pins 87 to 90 represent overlapping heptamers that encompass the sequences SKDWSFY (residues 57 to 63) and LSQPKIVKWDR (residues 87 to 97). The positive reactions shown here were also maintained when pin ELISA was run under 300mM or 400mM NaCl (high salt) conditions. OD_{490} = optical density at 490nm. (From Williams RC Jr, Malone CC, Harley JB: *Arthritis Rheum* 36:916−926, 1993. Used by permission.)

alanine substitution were compared in CH3, CH2, and β_2M structures, a remarkable relative restriction of amino acids important for RF reactivity was identified. Thus valines, leucines, lysines, tryptophanes, arginines, glutamines, and to a lesser extent, histidines, threonines, and prolines appeared to be extremely important for the antigenicity of RF-reactive epitopes. These findings are summarized in Table 3.

Work presented in detail here concerning our attempts to identify exact reactive sites for RF on the CH2 and CH3 domains of IgG as well as on β_2M and class I molecules has been directed at precise insight into what a certain group of so-called autoantibodies (RF) actually react with. For years, because RFs were originally demonstrated to react with the Fc portion of IgG, it was assumed that they functioned only as antibodies reacting with autologous or self-IgG. Our demonstration that RFs from patients with RA also react with solvent-accessible structures on β_2M as well as class I molecules indicates that RF can be considered a class of autoantibodies with multiple overlapping specificities, and *not* merely an autoantibody to the Fc portions of IgG. How the cross-reactivity of RF with other immunoglobulin gene superfamily products affects a number of basic biological functions that may be thus influenced through such reactivity remains to be determined. Another alternative important question raised by our findings that RFs react with several other salient molecules such as β_2M and HLA class I structures is the distinct possibility that the original antigenic stimulus initiating RF production may indicate that

---

TABLE 3.

Relatively Restricted Spectrum of Rheumatoid Factor–Reactive Immunodominant Amino Acid Residues on CH3, CH2, and β_2-Microglobulin as Determined by Glycine/Alanine Substitution*

CH3 Domain	CH2 Domain	β_2-Microglobulin
Tyrosine 349,† 407, 436	Tyrosine 278	
Proline 343, 346, 352	Tryptophane 277, 313	Tryptophane 60, 95; proline 90
Glutamine 347	Glutamine 311	
Valine 348	Valine 279, 305	Valine 93
Threonine 350		
Leucine 351, 432	Leucine 314	
Arginine 354		Arginine 97
Aspartic acid 401	Aspartic acid 315	Aspartic acid 59, 96
Serine 426		Serine 57
Histidine 429		
Lysine 439		Lysine 58, 91

*Epitopes synthesized as overlapping heptamers on polypropylene pins and tested by enzyme-linked immunosorbent assay in parallel with the same sequence in which a neutral glycine or alanine was substituted for the native residue. More than a 50% decrease in reactivity after such single-residue substitution was interpreted to indicate an immunodominant contribution of that amino acid to antigenicity for rheumatoid factor.

†Residues underlined were clearly immunodominant for rheumatoid factor reactivity of the domain or protein tested.

some other external antigen actually represents the initiating factor for RF production during the development of RA as a systemic disease. With this alternative possibility in mind and with the immunodominant RF-reactive amino acid residues shown in Table 3, eventually it might be possible to construct a theoretical model of composite antigenic structures capable of initiating RF production. Such a model could then serve as a hypothetical paradigm for antigens actually causally associated with the underlying disease process. It is for these reasons that we consider the definition of antigenic epitopes capable of reacting with general classes of autoantibodies such as RF or antinuclear antibodies of great theoretical and practical importance.

ASSOCIATION OF SEROPOSITIVE RHEUMATOID ARTHRITIS WITH HLA-DR4

Perhaps the most important step forward toward eventual clear understanding of the basic pathogenesis of RA was the discovery by Stastny of a strong association between seropositive RA and HLA-DR4.[37, 38] This observation was subsequently expanded by a large number of groups throughout the world to help define distinct DR4 subgroups—particularly DR4, Dw4, Dw14, and Dw10 as well as DR1—as being highly associated with RF-positive RA. The HLA-DR4 allelic variants have recently been designated HLA-DR B1, and the former Dw designations have now been replaced by the DR B1 allelic nomenclature, which is illustrated in Table 4. It has been clearly established that those variants that are closely associated with RA all share modification of a common sequence motif (QK/RAA) in the third hypervariable region of the β chain. This shared-sequence motif has been referred to as the shared epitope and originally generated what has been called the shared-epitope hypothesis.[39] An extension of these original findings has been presented by Weyand and Goronzy,[40] who analyzed 102 patients with RA who showed RF along with

TABLE 4.
Disease-Linked Sequence Motifs of HLA-DR B1 Alleles in Rheumatoid Arthritis

Allele	HVR1*	HVR2	HVR3
AA pos	4 9 10 11 12 13 14	26 28 30 31 32 33 37	57 58 60 67 70 71 73 74 78 86
Disease-associated DR B1 alleles			
0401	R E Q V L H E	F D Y F Y H Y	D A Y L Q K A A Y G
0404/8	R E Q V K H E	F D Y F Y H Y	D A Y L Q R A A Y V
0101	R W A L K F E	L E C I Y N S	D A Y L Q R A A Y G
1402	R E Y S T S E	F D Y F H N N	D A Y L Q R A A Y V
Disease-nonassociated DR B1 alleles			
0402	R E Q V K H E	F D Y F Y H Y	D A Y I D E A A Y V
1301	R E Y S T S E	F D Y F H N N	D A Y I D E A A Y V

*HVR1 = hypervariable region of the β chain; AA pos = position of amino acids.

erosive joint disease. Within this group 98% showed at least one of the RA-associated HLA-DR B1 alleles. Moreover, over 50% of these patients showed disease-associated alleles on both parental haplotypes. Patients with mild disease had only one disease-associated allelic marker, and patients with the most severe aggressive crippling disease were predominantly homozygous for HLA-DR B1 *0404 or 0401 alleles. Thus there appeared to be a gene-dosage effect in RA. Moreover, the presence of the shared epitope might directly determine disease severity rather than merely disease susceptibility. Such a hypothesis seems reasonable at present, particularly since roughly 24% of the average general population in this country is HLA-DR4–positive.

As an extension of the shared-epitope hypothesis, Albani and coworkers[41] have reported that the QK/RAA shared epitope is also present in heat shock proteins from relatively common Gram-negative bacteria, including dnaJ of *Escherichia coli* as well as gp110 of EBV. Serum antibodies to dnaJ were present in normal individuals, as well as patients with chronic juvenile rheumatoid arthritis (JRA) and patients with untreated RA. However, when Albani and coworkers examined nine pairs of monozygotic twins discordant for RA, the affected twin had a higher level of anti-dnaJ in every case. Additional studies indicated that synovial fluid and peripheral blood T-cell responsiveness was present to a test peptide encompassed in the QK/RAA peptide in 21 RA patients with untreated early disease who possessed one of the HLA-DR B1 haplotypes, whereas *no* significant response was recorded to a peptide from the same region of HLA-DR B1 *0402, an allele *not* associated with RA. It was therefore postulated that the HLA-DR B1 molecule itself might somehow act as an antigen and that low-affinity interactions between T cells and such distinct structures on HLA molecules could function in some way to provide an ongoing, chronic immunostimulatory mechanism to perpetuate the disease.[42]

A number of other groups of workers have studied various isolated, genetically distinct subsets of patients as far as HLA-DR4 or HLA-DR B1 allelic influence on disease occurrence or severity are concerned and have recorded a number of interesting variations on the basic shared-epitope theme. In one study a group of Japanese researchers reported that Japanese patients with RA showed much higher levels of serum IgG antibody to an HLA-DR4 peptide from the hypervariable region of the β chain than did normal Japanese controls.[43] By contrast, a recent study by Salvat et al. seemed to support an opposite type of phenomenon in which relative anergy or unresponsiveness to β-chain hypervariable region QK/RAA-containing peptides studied as T-cell stimulators was recorded in a group of seropositive patients.[44] How the definite HLA-DR B1 allelic association between seropositive RA as well as disease severity will finally be resolved must await further investigation.

T-CELL RECEPTOR REPERTOIRES

Since T cells represent a major cellular constituent of the basic inflammatory response within RA synovium, it has been a rather natural avenue for many groups of investigators to explore in terms of searching for clues to the etiology of the disease itself. Indeed, one of the most characteristic histologic features of rheumatoid inflammation within the joint is large collections of small T lymphocytes—most of them helper-inducer or OKT4-positive cells—arranged in sometimes massive collections within the synovium and representing perhaps as much as 50% of the inflammatory component in the affected synovial tissues (Fig 8). It was therefore not at all surprising that when it became apparent (largely through molecular characterizations of various families of T-cell receptors) that certain T-cell receptor triggering mechanisms could indeed activate large proportions of cells through superantigen-driven mechanisms, the search was on for evidence that might support such a scenario in terms of driving the disease in RA. The first reports suggesting a marked restriction in synovial T-cell repertoire appeared in 1991.[45, 46] These workers recorded a distinct apparent restriction of T-cell receptor profiles by using fluorescence-activated cell sorter analysis of T-cell subsets from the peripheral blood as well as synovial tissue of patients with RA. Subsequent similar attempts to document consistent reproducible T-cell receptor family RA-associated profiles have produced a large number of reports but very little in the way of consistent or uniform data. It was, of course, hoped from the beginning that an apparent uniform restriction in T-cell receptor usage might provide some sort of clue as to the characteristics of the underlying antigenic stimulus that must be the basic driving mechanism for the disease itself. Thus far no uniform confirmation of any characteristic rheumatoid T-cell receptor profile or subfamily has yet emerged, although some interesting recent evidence does suggest selective expansion of particular T-cell clones.[47]

Many elements of RA as a systemic disease affecting millions of patients within the very prime of their lives—ages 16 to 50—suggest that

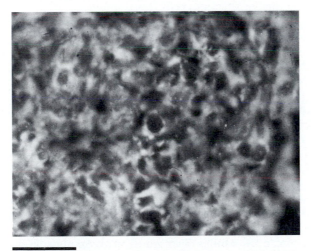

FIGURE 8.
Immunofluorescence photomicrograph of synovial tissue from a patient with rheumatoid arthritis that was stained with anti–T-cell antibody shows the massive numbers of T cells making up the cellular infiltrates in these tissues. All cells showing bright surface membrane immunofluorescence represent T cells. Subset studies of such T cells indicate that most are OKT4-positive or helper-inducer cells.

the disease represents an immune reaction of some kind. First of all, the synovial tissue lesions—filled as they are with millions of activated helper-inducer T-cells interspersed with nests of B-cells producing RF— suggest an immunologic process. Second, the now clear association of the disease with the HLA-DR B1 allelic complex containing the shared QK/ RAA epitope also suggests a major histocompatibility complex–restricted immune reaction. Finally, the fact that RF—the autoantibody character-istically associated with active erosive disease and many of the cata-strophic extra-articular disease complications—has now been demon-strated to function as a superantibody that reacts not only with the CH2 and CH3 IgG domains but also with $\beta_2 M$ and HLA class I molecules also supports the role of a fundamental immunologic process at the root of the disease. Much has been learned, but there still remains a great deal to be understood regarding this fascinating disorder.

REFERENCES

1. Nichol ST, Spiropoulou CF, Morzunov S, et al: Identifcation of a Hantavirus associated with an outbreak of acute respiratory illness. *Science* 262:914–917, 1993.
2. Hughes JM, Peters CJ, Cohen ML, et al: Hantavirus pulmonary syndrome: An emerging infectious disease. *Science* 262:850–851, 1992.
3. Kellgren JH, Jeffrey MR, Ball JF: *The Epidemiology of Chronic Rheumatism*, vol 1. Philadelphia, FA Davis, 1963.
4. Del Puente A, Knowler WC, Pettit DJ, et al: High incidence and prevalence of rheumatoid arthritis in Pima Indians. *Am J Epidemiol* 129:1170–1178, 1989.
5. Jacobsson LTH, Hanson RL, Knowler WC, et al: Decreasing incidence and prevalence of rheumatoid arthritis in Pima Indians over a twenty-five year period. *Arthritis Rheum* 37:1158–1165, 1994.
6. Hochberg MC: Changes in the incidence and prevalence of rheumatoid ar-thritis in England and Wales, 1970–1982. *Semin Arthritis Rheum* 19:294–302, 1990.
7. Pincus T, Callahan LF: The "side effects" of rheumatoid arthritis: Joint de-struction, disability and early mortality. *Br J Rheumatol* 32(suppl 1):28–38, 1993.
8. Pincus T, Callahan L, Sale WG, et al: Severe functional declines, work dis-ability, and increased mortality in seventy-five rheumatoid arthritis patients studied over nine years. *Arthritis Rheum* 27:864–872, 1984.
9. Waaler E: On occurrence of a factor in human serum activating the specific agglutination of sheep blood corpuscles. *Acta Pathol Microbiol Scand* 17:172–188, 1940.
10. Rose HM, Ragan C, Pearce E, et al: Differential agglutination of normal and sensitized sheep erythrocytes by sera of patients with rheumatoid arthritis. *Proc Soc Exp Biol Med* 68:1–6, 1948.
11. Franklin EC, Holman HR, Müller-Eberhard HJ, et al: An unusual protein com-ponent of high molecular weight in the serum of patients with rheumatoid arthritis. *J Exp Med* 105:425–438, 1957.
12. Munthe E, Natvig JB: Immunoglobulin classes, subclasses, and complexes of IgG rheumatoid factor in rheumatoid plasma cells. *Clin Exp Immunol* 12:55–70, 1972.
13. Kunkel HG, Franklin EC, Müller-Eberhard HJ: Studies on the isolation and characterization of the "rheumatoid factor." *J Clin Invest* 38:424–434, 1959.

14. Harboe M: Relation between Gm types and hamgglutinating substance in rheumatoid sera. *Acta Pathol Microbiol Scand* 50:89–105, 1960.
15. Fudenberg HH, Kunkel HG: Specificity of the reaction between rheumatoid factors and gammaglobulin. *J Exp Med* 114:257–278, 1961.
16. Grubb R, Laurell AB: Hereditary serological human serum groups. *Acta Pathol Microbiol Immunol Scand* 39:390–398, 1956.
17. Grubb R, Kronvall G, Martensson L: Some aspects of the relations between rheumatoid arthritis, anti-gammaglobulin factors and the polymorphism of human gammaglobulin. *Ann N Y Acad Sci* 124:865–872, 1965.
18. Grubb R, Matsumoto H, Sattar M: Incidence of anti-human Ig with restricted specificity in Japanese, Kuwaiti, and Swedish patients with rheumatoid arthritis. *Arthritis Rheum* 31:60–62, 1988.
19. Grubb R, Kjellen L: On the origin of antibodies to immunoglobulin genetic markers in rheumatoid arthritis. An outline of a novel concept of the nature of rheumatoid arthritis–transduction in man. *Exp Clin Immunogenet* 6:88–98, 1989.
20. Aho K, Simons K: Studies of the antibody nature of the rheumatoid factor reaction of the rheumatoid factor with human specific precipitates and with native human gammaglobulin. *Arthritis Rheum* 6:676–688, 1963.
21. Williams RC Jr, Malone CC, Casali P: Antigen-induced aggregation of Gm(a)(-), Gm(g)(-) IgG results in exposure of determinants recognized by heteroclitic polyclonal and monoclonal anti-Gm(a) and Gm(g) human rheumatoid factors. Relevance to the in vivo induction of high affinity anti-IgG autoantibodies. *J Immunol* 149:1817–1824, 1992.
22. Williams RC Jr, Malone CC, Solomon A: Conformational dependency of human IgG heavy-chain associated Gm allotypes. *Mol Immunol* 30:341-351, 1993.
23. Grubb R: Interpretation of immunological concepts and of notational terms in structural concepts, in *The Genetic Markers of Human Immunoglobulins*. New York, Springer-Verlag, 1970, pp 13–24.
24. Nardella RA, Teller DC, Barber CV: IgG rheumatoid factors and staphylococcal protein A bind to a common molecular site on IgG. *J Exp Med* 162:1811–1824, 1985.
25. Nelson JL, Nardella RA, Oppliger IR, et al: Rheumatoid factors from patients with rheumatoid arthritis possess private repertoires of idiotypes. *J Immunol* 138:1391–1396, 1987.
26. Sasso EH, Barber CV, Nardella FA, et al: Antigenic specificities of human monoclonal and polyclonal IgM rheumatoid factors. The $C_\gamma 2$–$C_\gamma 3$ interface contains the major determinants. *J Immunol* 140:3098–3107, 1988.
27. Geysen HM, Rodda SJ, Mason TJ, et al: Strategies for epitope analysis using peptide synthesis. *J Immunol Methods* 102:259–274, 1987.
28. Getzoff ED, Geysen HM, Rodda SJ, et al: Mechanisms of antibody binding to a protein. *Science* 235:1191–1196, 1987.
29. Williams RC Jr, Kievit E, Tsuchiya N, et al: Differential mapping of Fcγ-binding and monoclonal antibody–reactive epitopes on gE, the Fcγ-binding glycoprotein of herpes simplex virus type 1. *J Immunol* 149:2415–2427, 1992.
30. Deisenhofer J, Jones TA, Huber R, et al: Crystallization, crystal structure analysis, and atomic model of the complex formed by a human Fc fragment and fragment B of protein A from *Staphylococcus aureus*. *Hoppe-Seyler Z Physiol Chem* 359:975–985, 1978.
31. Williams RC Jr, Malone CC, Tsuchiya N: Rheumatoid factors from patients with rheumatoid arthritis react with β_2-microglobulin. *J Immunol* 149:1104–1113, 1992.
32. Williams RC, Malone CC: Rheumatoid-factor–reactive sites on CH2 estab-

lished by analysis of overlapping peptides of primary sequence. *Scand J Immunol* 40:443–456, 1994.

33. Peterson C, Malone CC, Williams RC Jr; Rheumatoid-factor–reactive sites on CH3 established by overlapping 7-mer peptide epitope analyses. *Mol Immunol*, 32:57–75, 1995.

34. Williams RC Jr, Malone CC, Harley JB: Rheumatoid factors from patients with rheumatoid arthritis react with tryptophane 60 and 95, lysine 58 and arginine 97 on human β_2-microglobulin. *Arthritis Rheum* 36:916–926, 1993.

35. Williams RC Jr, Malone CC: Human IgM rheumatoid factors react with class I HLA molecules. *Arthritis Rheum* 36(suppl):S265, D203, 1993.

36. Williams RC Jr, Malone CC, Kenny T, et al: Monoclonal IgM rheumatoid factors generated from synovial B cells of rheumatoid arthritis patients react with β_2-microglobulin. *Autoimmunity* 16:103–114, 1993.

37. Stastny P: Mixed lymphocyte culture typing cells from patients with rheumatoid arthritis. *Tissue Antigens* 4:572–579, 1974.

38. Stastny P: Association of the B-cell alloantigen DRw4 with rheumatoid arthritis. *N Engl J Med* 298:869–871, 1978.

39. Gregersen PK, Silver J, Winchester RJ: The shared epitope hypothesis: An approach to understanding the molecular genetics of susceptibility to rheumatoid arthritis. *Arthritis Rheum* 30:1205–1213, 1987.

40. Weyand CM, Goronzy JJ: Functional domains on HLA-DR molecules: Implications for the linkage of HLA-DR genes to different autoimmune diseases. *Clin Immunol Immunopathol* 70:91–98, 1994.

41. Albani S, Tuckwell JE, Esparza L, et al: The susceptibility sequence to rheumatoid arthritis is a cross-reactive B cell epitope shared by the *Escherichia coli* heat shock protein dnaJ and the histocompatibility leukocyte antigen DR B10401 molecule. *J Clin Invest* 89:327–331, 1992.

42. Wicks I, McColl G, Harrison L: New perspectives on rheumatoid arthritis. *Immunol Today* 15:553–556, 1994.

43. Takeuchi F, Kosuge E, Matsuta K, et al: Antibody to a specific HLA DR β1 sequence in Japanese patients with rheumatoid arthritis. *Arthritis Rheum* 33:1867–1868, 1990.

44. Salvat S, Auger I, Rochelle L, et al: Tolerance to a self-peptide from the third hypervariable region of HLA DR B0401 in rheumatoid arthritis patients and normal subjects. *J Immunol* 153:5321–5329, 1994.

45. Paliard X, West SG, Lafferty JA, et al: Evidence for the effects of a superantigen in rheumatoid arthritis. *Science* 253:325–329, 1991.

46. Howell MD, Diveley JP, Lundeen KA, et al: Limited T-cell receptor β-chain heterogeneity among interleukin 2 receptor–positive synovial T cells suggests a role for superantigen in rheumatoid arthritis. *Proc Natl Acad Sci U S A* 88:10921–10925, 1991.

47. Li Y, Sun GR, Tumang JR, et al: CDR3 sequence motifs shared by oligoclonal rheumatoid arthritis synovial T cells. Evidence for an antigen-driven response. *J Clin Invest* 94:2525–2531, 1994.

Impact of Molecular Biology on the Practice of Transfusion Medicine

Anne L. Frattali, M.D., Ph.D.

Assistant Instructor, The University of Pennsylvania Medical Center, Hospital of the University of Pennsylvania, Department of Pathology and Laboratory Medicine, Philadelphia, Pennsylvania

Robert B. Wilson, M.D., Ph.D.

Assistant Professor, Division of Molecular Diagnosis, The University of Pennsylvania Medical Center, Hospital of the University of Pennsylvania, Department of Pathology and Laboratory Medicine, Philadelphia, Pennsylvania

Steven L. Spitalnik, M.D.

Co–Vice Chair, Division of Laboratory Medicine, Associate Professor, The University of Pennsylvania Medical Center, Hospital of the University of Pennsylvania, Department of Pathology and Laboratory Medicine, Philadelphia, Pennsylvania

The molecular biology revolution has influenced all areas of medicine. Investigating the molecular basis of disease has inspired novel treatment of inherited diseases caused by mutations in a single gene such as cystic fibrosis, as well as multifactorial disease processes such as atherosclerosis and oncogenesis.[1-3] The practice of transfusion medicine will also benefit from new diagnostic tests and therapeutic procedures resulting from insight gained from the application of molecular biology. These innovations include the production of recombinant red blood cell (RBC) antigens and antibodies for use in serologic blood typing reactions, molecular typing of genes encoding RBC and platelet antigens, screening of blood products for infectious diseases, production of recombinant clotting factors and hematopoietic growth factors, and manipulation of bone marrow and hematopoietic stem cell products for transplantation.

RECOMBINANT REAGENTS IN BLOOD GROUP SEROLOGY

Karl Landsteiner discovered the ABO blood group system in humans at the turn of the century. Subsequently, the Rhesus, MNSs, Lewis, Kell, Duffy, and Kidd blood group systems and numerous other RBC antigens have been investigated at the serologic and biochemical level. Not until recently, however, has information about the molecular basis of many of these antigens been obtained.[4] These seminal discoveries include the cloning of many of the genes encoding RBC antigens and antibodies and

Advances in Pathology and Laboratory Medicine®, vol. 8

© 1995, Mosby–Year Book, Inc.

have led to the potential for producing recombinant reagents for use in serologic blood typing. Classic serology is based on observing hemagglutination reactions that occur when serum from one source is mixed with RBCs from another source. A screen is performed first to detect the presence of reactive, potentially clinically significant antibodies directed against any of an extraordinary number of carbohydrate and protein antigens on the surface of the reagent red cells. The specificity of detected antibodies is deduced from the pattern of serum reactivity against a panel of reagent red cells representing all known clinically significant antigens. Conversely, patients' RBC phenotypes are defined when their RBCs are mixed with antibodies of defined specificity. Recombinant antigen and antibody reagents have recently been produced and can be used in conjunction with the screening techniques to improve the specificity of these methods.[5-9] For example, recombinant glycophorin A, which contains the M or N antigen, was expressed in a cultured cell line.[5, 6] Acetone powders containing the recombinant protein were produced that specifically adsorbed serum antibodies directed against glycophorin A antigens. When such an adsorption removes serum reactivity against appropriate reagent RBCs, the specificity of a patient's antibody can be inferred to be against an antigen on glycophorin A. Acetone powders have several advantages, including high specificity, long-term stability at room temperature, potential for mass production and low cost, and availability of rare antigens. Similar approaches using insoluble immunoadsorbents of silica particles coupled to synthetic oligosaccharides have been used previously for analyzing human antibodies to carbohydrate antigens in the Lewis and P blood group systems.[8, 9] In theory, these methods can be applied to any blood group protein or glycoprotein antigen that has been cloned, sequenced, and expressed in vitro.[4] This approach may be problematic, however, for antigens such as Rh antigens, which may require association with phospholipids to maintain appropriate antigenicity and may require the presence of other membrane proteins for efficient cell surface expression.

In addition to RBC antigens, RBC-specific human and murine monoclonal antibodies can be isolated by the molecular technique known as repertoire cloning.[10-12] This method takes advantage of the properties of phagemid expression vectors, which exist as either plasmids or bacteriophage depending on the experimental conditions. Briefly, immunoglobulin gene sequences from donor B cells are isolated and cloned into a phagemid expression vector. Upon coinfection with M13 helper phage, phagemid particles with immunoglobulin DNA sequences and copies of the encoded Fab fragment incorporated into their coat protein are released. The Fab fragment containing the desired specificity, as well as the cDNA encoding this polypeptide, can be simultaneously identified since the phage provides a physical association between each recombinant protein and its nucleotide coding sequence (Fig 1). This technique has been used to express and characterize antibody fragments directed against blood group antigens in the ABO, Ii, Rhesus, MN, and Kell blood group systems as well as against numerous other polypeptides.[13-15] Repertoire cloning provides an attractive alternative to conventional hybridoma technology for producing antibodies to cell surface antigens. This

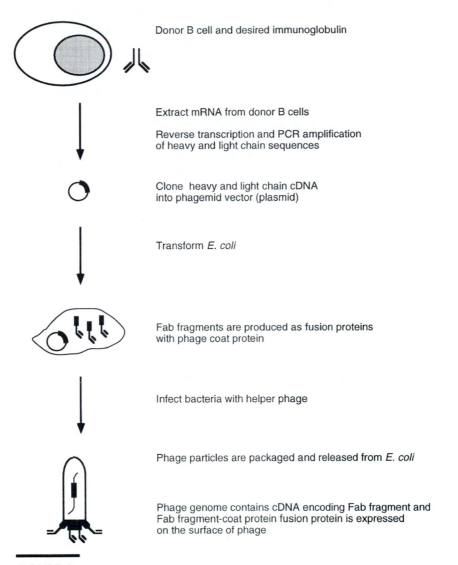

Donor B cell and desired immunoglobulin

Extract mRNA from donor B cells

Reverse transcription and PCR amplification
of heavy and light chain sequences

Clone heavy and light chain cDNA
into phagemid vector (plasmid)

Transform *E. coli*

Fab fragments are produced as fusion proteins
with phage coat protein

Infect bacteria with helper phage

Phage particles are packaged and released from *E. coli*

Phage genome contains cDNA encoding Fab fragment and
Fab fragment-coat protein fusion protein is expressed
on the surface of phage

FIGURE 1.
Repertoire cloning to isolate red blood cell–specific human monoclonal antibodies. PCR = polymerase chain reaction.

is particularly true for producing human monoclonal antibodies since hybridoma, heterohybridoma, and Epstein-Barr virus transformation methods have proved to be difficult and less than satisfactory. Repertoire cloning will facilitate the investigation of human autoimmune and alloimmune responses to Rh and other RBC antigens and could potentially provide an endless supply of useful serologic reagents.

In addition to stimulating the development of recombinant typing reagents, knowledge of the molecular basis of RBC antigen expression provides an alternate method to deduce the RBC phenotype by determining the RBC genotype. Serologic methods used to identify blood group antigens on the surface of RBCs are based on direct visualization of RBC agglutination. In certain clinical situations, determining the RBC phenotype by serologic methods is problematic. After massive transfusion, for example, blood obtained from the patient for serologic typing is a heterogeneous mixture of transfused and native RBCs. Attempts to purify sufficient quantities of the patient's reticulocytes for typing can be difficult or impossible. Another serologic challenge involves patients with warm autoimmune hemolytic anemia, in whom IgG autoantibodies coat their own erythrocytes, thus blocking the ability of many typing sera to detect RBC antigens. Finally, determining fetal RBC antigen composition could identify those at risk for hemolytic disease of the newborn. Currently, routine agglutination methods are of limited use for this purpose because periumbilical blood sampling must be performed to obtain fetal cells. Similarly, new approaches would be helpful in determining the platelet antigen type in the setting of post-transfusion purpura or suspected neonatal isoimmune thrombocytopenia.

Since anti-Rh(D) antibodies are most commonly implicated in hemolytic disease of the newborn, molecular typing of the Rhesus genetic locus would be advantageous. The Rh genetic locus resides on chromosome 1p34-p36 and contains two adjacent, homologous structural genes designated *Rh(CcEe)* and *Rh(D)*.[16] Rh(D)-positive individuals have both genes, whereas Rh(D)-negative individuals lack the *Rh(D)* gene. In addition, the sequence polymorphisms in the *Rh(CcEe)* genes that most likely determine C, c, E, and e antigenicity have recently been defined.[16] Knowledge of the genomic organization and sequences of the *Rh(CcEe)* and *Rh(D)* genes in Rh(D)-positive and Rh(D)-negative individuals allows the detection of *Rh(D)* genomic sequences with the polymerase chain reaction (PCR).[17] Two pairs of oligonucleotide primers are used. One pair hybridizes to both the *Rh(D)* gene and the *Rh(CcEe)* gene to yield a 136-bp product. With the second pair, the 5' primer hybridizes to both genes, whereas the 3' primer hybridizes only to the *Rh(D)* gene. A 186-bp product is formed only if the *Rh(D)* gene is present. Consequently, in Rh(D)-positive samples, two amplified products are detected on agarose gels, whereas in Rh(D)-negative samples, only one amplified product from the *Rh(CcEe)* gene is detected (Fig 2).

Allelic polymorphism in genes encoding other RBC antigens is usually more subtle than complete deletions; many alleles differ by single point mutations. Allele-specific PCR (AS-PCR) has been used to detect these allelic differences in the ABO and MNSs blood group systems.[18−21] In AS-PCR, one oligonucleotide primer, the allele-specific primer, is designed to hybridize perfectly to the sequence of only one of two alleles, whereas the second oligonucleotide primer is designed to hybridize to both alleles at a nearby site. The allele-specific primer forms an incomplete match with the alternative allele, usually involving a terminal 3' base pair mismatch that interferes with effective amplification. Consequently, only the allele to which the allele-specific primer hybridizes perfectly is efficiently amplified and detected by this method.

Neonatal isoimmune thrombocytopenia is similar to hemolytic disease of the newborn in that a maternal IgG antibody is directed against a fetal antigen inherited from the father. The genes encoding platelet antigens that are frequently involved in neonatal isoimmune thrombocytopenia, such as Pl^{A1} and Br^a, have been cloned and sequenced. With this

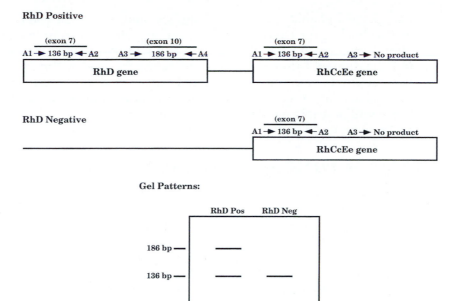

FIGURE 2.

Polymerase chain reaction (PCR) to distinguish Rh(D)-positive from Rh(D)-negative individuals. A1, A2, A3, and A4 are the primers used for PCR. The A4 primer hybridizes only to the *Rh(D)* gene. Hence, only the 136-bp product is amplified from Rh(D)-negative individuals, whereas both the 136-bp and 186-bp products are amplified from Rh(D)-positive individuals. (Adapted from Bennett PR, Le Van Kim C, Colin Y, et al: *N Engl J Med* 329:607–660, 1993. Used by permission.)

information, AS-PCR has been applied to prenatal screening for this condition.[22, 23]

The major advantage of PCR is its exquisite sensitivity. Minute quantities of nucleated fetal erythrocytes in the maternal circulation have been detected as early as 9 weeks of gestation, and populations enriched in fetal cells have been obtained by using multiparameter flow cytometry.[24] This technology, combined with AS-PCR, may obviate the need for either periumbilical blood sampling, currently required to obtain fetal RBCs for antigen typing, or chorionic villus sampling or amniocentesis, which are required to obtain nucleated cells for genotyping.

The major limitation of molecular blood typing is that the most probable genotype rather than the actual phenotype of the RBCs or platelets is determined.[19] Possible discrepancies between the deduced phenotype and actual phenotype could arise for several reasons. For example, an allele may be detected but its protein product may not be produced because of mutations present in the promoter or in other regions distant from the allele-specific oligonucleotide primer. Conversely, an allele may not be detected but the protein may be present because of a silent polymorphism that interferes with hybridization of the allele-specific oligonucleotide primer but does not alter the encoded amino acid sequence of the protein. Finally, genetic heterogeneity of some loci may preclude the use of AS-PCR for typing. For example, more than one mutation in a given gene may cause a phenotype or altered antigen, and more than one gene may be involved in the expression of a given antigen. Therefore, many more clinical samples need to be analyzed and large population studies need to be performed before these approaches can be used routinely in clinical practice. In addition, although molecular blood typing may be useful in specific clinical settings such as massive transfusion or prenatal screening, it will probably not replace routine serologic methods, which are currently more rapid and less expensive.

PREVENTION OF TRANSFUSION-TRANSMITTED DISEASE

In contrast to the aforementioned serologic results, molecular techniques have already become established in routine confirmatory testing for infectious agents in blood products. Before 1985, the only infectious diseases for which screening tests existed were syphilis and hepatitis B. Although transfusion-transmitted syphilis is primarily a theoretical concern, transfusion-transmitted hepatitis is historically and arguably still the most serious threat to the safety of the nation's blood supply. Interestingly, institution of an assay to detect the hepatitis B surface antigen did not eradicate transfusion-transmitted hepatitis. In fact, studies conducted during the late 1970s revealed that hepatitis B accounted for only approximately 10% of post-transfusion hepatitis cases.[25-27] Indirect or surrogate testing for non-A, non-B hepatitis, including alanine aminotransferase (ALT) and hepatitis B core antibody, reduced the incidence of non-A, non-B hepatitis significantly.[28-31] The failure to eradicate transfusion-associated hepatitis, however, inspired researchers to search for additional etiologic agents causing this disorder.

A major coup of the molecular approach was the cloning in 1989 of the nucleotide sequence of a viral antigen associated with non-A, non-B hepatitis before the etiologic agent was isolated and characterized.[32] Briefly, nucleic acids were extracted from plasma prepared from infected chimpanzees. Since the nature of the infectious particle was not known, the purified nucleic acid was fully denatured and reverse transcription with random primers was performed to allow amplification of RNA as well as DNA by PCR. A bacterial expression library was constructed with the resulting cDNA and screened for rare clones expressing viral antigen with sera from patients with chronic non-A, non-B hepatitis. One clone was identified whose full-length counterpart encoded a 363−amino acid polypeptide, c100-3. This discovery resulted in the immediate development of a screening test for circulating antibodies to hepatitis C virus.[33] Recombinant polypeptide containing the c100-3 antigen was used in the first-generation enzyme immunoassay (EIA) for hepatitis C virus licensed in the United States in May 1990. By using this approach, circulating antibodies to hepatitis C virus in blood samples could be captured and detected in the wells of microtiter plates coated with c100-3.

The first-generation EIA reduced the incidence of post-transfusion non-A, non-B hepatitis by approximately 60% to 80%.[34-37] With this screening test the overall risk of contracting hepatitis C from transfusion was estimated as 3 per 10,000 units transfused.[36, 37] Although development of a screening test for hepatitis C virus was an enormous advance, the first-generation EIA suffered from several disadvantages, including poor diagnostic accuracy. The false-positive rate in the low-prevalence donor population was high, and the positive predictive value for the viral carrier state was low.[38–40] The false-positive rate in other populations, such as patients with autoimmune diseases, was also high. The c100-3 polypeptide was later defined to be the product of a nonstructural gene and represented epitopes encoded by only 12% of the hepatitis C viral genome. Improved serodiagnosis of hepatitis C infection was reported with synthetic or recombinant capsid antigen.[39, 41, 42] A second-generation hepatitis C EIA was licensed in March 1992 and used additional epitopes from nucleocapsid protein and another nonstructural antigen; this represented epitopes from 26% of the genome. This test detected approximately 10% to 20% more patients with acute post-transfusion hepatitis and became positive 30 to 120 days earlier than the first-generation test[43–46] (Fig 3). With this screening test, one additional hepatitis C virus–infected unit per 1,000 donations may be detected.[44] An estimated 91% of cases of non-A, non-B transfusion-associated hepatitis are caused by hepatitis C virus.[47] The remainder may represent false negatives in the first- and second-generation EIAs that are due to different, undetectable antibody variants or another etiologic agent of hepatitis. Third-generation EIAs, which use epitopes encoded by 60% of the hepatitis C viral genome, are currently available and may additionally lower the overall risk.[48] Improved EIAs are also currently available for detecting human immunodeficiency virus (HIV) antibody and hepatitis B core antibody. The current estimate of the risk of transfusion-transmitted HIV infection is 1 per 225,000 units transfused; the risk of hepatitis B infection is 1 per 200,000 units transfused.[36]

Despite this progress, EIAs for detecting antibodies generally have low predictive values in a low-prevalence blood donor population. False-positive results obtained in screening tests and confirmatory tests for antiviral antibodies result in unnecessarily discarded donor units and in un-

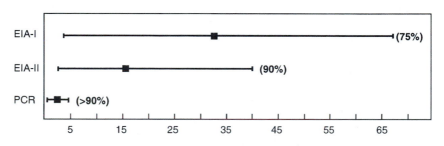

TIME AFTER EXPOSURE (WEEKS)

FIGURE 3.

Temporal detection of hepatitis C–specific antibodies or viral RNA in infected individuals: comparison of first-generation enzyme immunoassay *(EIA-I)*, *second-generation enzyme immunoassay (EIA-II)*, and polymerase chain reaction *(PCR)*. The mean time to development of a positive test *(closed squares)* and approximate percentages of exposed individuals in whom a positive test result develops over the indicated interval are given. (Data from Alter J: *Hepatology* 15:350–353, 1992; Peters T, Mohr L, Scheiffele F, et al: *J Med Virol* 42:420–427, 1994.)

necessary medical evaluation and concern among those erroneously testing positive.[38] Confirmatory testing is required to demonstrate the specificity of the reaction and usually involves visualizing the number of reactive viral antigens against which antibodies have been produced by using a Western blot or recombinant immunoblot assay. Screening tests and confirmatory tests based on detection of antiviral antibodies suffer from the major disadvantage that time is required after infection to generate a detectable immune response. Enzyme immunoassays for viral antigens, such as those for HIV p24 and hepatitis B surface antigen, become positive before the EIAs for antiviral antibodies. There is currently a debate over whether to incorporate the HIV p24 assay into the routine screening process for blood product donation. Polymerase chain reaction can also be used to detect both RNA viruses such as hepatitis C virus and HIV as well as DNA viruses such as hepatitis B virus and cytomegalovirus early in the course of infection. In fact, PCR detects hepatitis C RNA in sera within 1 to 2 weeks after infection[49, 50] (Fig 3). The exquisite sensitivity of PCR detection of viral RNA allows for the screening of pools of sera from numerous units rather than individual units.[51, 52] As a cautionary note, standardization of PCR assays is still necessary to improve their reliability.[53]

RED BLOOD CELL ANTIGENS AND PATHOGENESIS OF VIRAL AND PARASITIC DISEASE

Molecular technology has also enabled the cloning of RBC antigens and the delineation of their involvement in the pathogenesis of certain viral and parasitic diseases. The Duffy polypeptide, for example, is involved in attachment and invasion of the malarial parasite *Plasmodium knowlesi*, and glycophorin A, which contains the M/N antigens, serves as the membrane receptor for *Plasmodium falciparum*.[54, 55] The P antigen is the membrane receptor for parvovirus.[56] Defining the receptor and ligand domains involved in viral or parasitic infection may suggest targets for vaccines and lead to rational design of products that can block attachment to the erythrocyte.

RECOMBINANT COAGULATION FACTORS

The purified coagulation factor concentrates available in the 1970s were an important advance in the treatment of hemophilia. These products enabled patients with hemophilia A, caused by a deficiency of factor VIII, and hemophilia B, caused by a deficiency of factor IX, to live relatively normal lives. Since the 1980s, however, the hemophiliac community has been devastated by the advent of the acquired immunodeficiency syndrome (AIDS). Approximately half of all patients with hemophilia are HIV-positive.[57] Screening tests for blood-borne viruses and viral inactivation strategies have greatly improved the safety of factor concentrates but have not eliminated the risk of infection. Cloning of the cDNAs for factor VIII and factor IX raised the possibility that safe, inexpensive, highly purified recombinant factors could be produced in vitro and that gene therapy trials could be initiated for treating hemophilia. Factor VIII was the first recombinant clotting factor produced in sufficient quantities for clinical trials.[57] Interestingly, coexpression of von Willebrand factor or deletions within a nonessential domain of factor VIII significantly increase the yield of factor VIII. Recombinant factor VIII is biochemically indistinguishable from purified, plasma-derived factor VIII. The overwhelming consensus reached from clinical trials is that recombinant factor VIII is safe and efficacious. An unresolved controversy, however, is whether recombinant factor VIII is more likely to induce production of inhibitors than plasma-derived factor VIII. Although truncated factor VIII retains normal biochemical activity and can be produced more efficiently by transfected cells than full-length factor VIII, the antigenicity of the truncated protein has not been determined.

Production of recombinant factor IX to treat the second most common inherited bleeding disorder, hemophilia B, proved technically more difficult.[57, 58] Factor IX undergoes extensive post-translational modification, including proteolytic cleavage of the signal peptide and propeptide, O- and N-linked glycosylation, hydroxylation of an aspartic acid residue, and vitamin K–dependent γ-carboxylation of amino-terminal glutamic acid residues. Expression in various eukaryotic cultured cell lines was successful; however, the majority of factor IX recovered was functionally inert because of the limited capacity of the host cells to enzymatically process the polypeptide. Consequently, active factor IX must be separated from inactive factor IX after purification from the host cells. Since production of biologically active factor IX is currently limited by the ability of the host cells to perform the requisite post-translational processing, modification of the host cell by introducing the necessary enzymes for carboxylation and proteolytic cleavage may result in adequate expression of clinically useful recombinant factor IX. The enzyme that mediates vitamin K–dependent γ-carboxylation has recently been cloned.[59] Alternatively, transgenic animals designed to secrete recombinant factor IX in their milk are being developed.[57]

Given the obstacles encountered in producing large amounts of recombinant factor IX for replacement therapy, somatic gene therapy for hemophilia B has been pursued with vigor and impressive success in animal models. Factor IX cDNA has been introduced into a number of cell types, including fibroblasts, myoblasts, endothelial cells, keratinocytes, and hepatocytes.[60] Gene transfer into hepatocytes and myoblasts may eventually allow at least transient expression of therapeutic levels of recombinant factor IX. Recently, a recombinant adenoviral vector containing canine factor IX cDNA was used to treat dogs with hemophilia B by direct vector infusion into the portal vasculature of deficient animals.[61] Therapeutic levels of factor IX persisted for 1 to 2 months in these treated animals.

HEMATOPOIETIC GROWTH FACTORS

Molecular approaches to therapies for other hematologic disorders are under investigation. Discovery of the growth factors involved in hematopoietic cell proliferation and differentiation has led to their cloning and subsequent production as recombinant pharmaceuticals. Erythropoietin was the first such growth factor developed as a therapy for anemia in certain clinical situations.[62] Patients with chronic renal disease and nonfunctioning kidneys fail to produce erythropoietin in sufficient quantity to support RBC production. Administration of recombinant erythropoietin corrects the anemia associated with chronic renal disease and virtually eliminates the need for erythrocyte transfusion[63-68] (Fig 4). Additional therapeutic applications for erythropoietin include the treatment of anemia in HIV-infected patients receiving the myelosuppressive antiviral drug azidothymidine and in cancer patients receiving myeloablative chemotherapy.[69, 70] Recombinant erythropoietin can also be used in selected patient populations to augment the hematocrit before repetitive autologous blood donation for elective surgical procedures and in the postoperative recovery period.[71, 72] In addition, increasing the red cell volume with erythropoietin may be an effective treatment for orthostatic hypotension caused by autonomic neuropathy as well as for the anemia of prematurity.[73-76] Large-scale clinical trials to establish appropriate dose regimens for these different therapeutic applications have not yet been reported.

Unfortunately, erythropoietin is not effective for every anemic patient. For example, although a subset of patients with rheumatoid arthri-

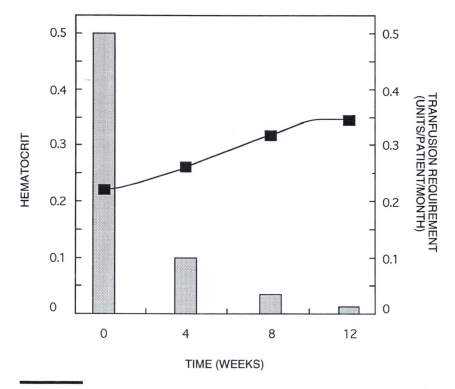

FIGURE 4.

Relationship between hematocrit and transfusion requirements in patients following initiation of recombinant human erythropoietin therapy. Hematocrit, *closed squares*; transfusion requirement (mean units per patient per month), *shaded bars*. (Adapted from Eschbach JW, Abdulhadi MH, Browne JK, et al: *Ann Intern Med* 111:992–1000, 1989.)

tis demonstrate an increased hematocrit after erythropoietin therapy, few report subjective improvement.[77-79] Recombinant erythropoietin therapy in this population may be limited to the minority of those patients significantly anemic to require transfusion or to augment the hematocrit before autologous transfusion for elective surgery.[79] The refractory anemia associated with myelodysplastic syndromes is also rarely ameliorated by erythropoietin but may respond to combination therapy consisting of erythropoietin and other cytokines.[80] Similarly, erythropoietin alone is not an effective therapy for sickle cell anemia; however, it may be useful when administered in conjunction with hydroxyurea.[81-83] Side effects of erythropoietin therapy include thromboembolic events, hypertension, and seizures in patients with chronic renal failure. These complications are generally not observed in predialysis patients, in postoperative patients, or in patients with myelodysplastic syndrome or other types of anemia.[72]

Following the discovery of erythropoietin, additional glycoprotein cytokines were identified that stimulate the proliferation and differentiation of hematopoietic progenitors in vivo and in vitro.[84-91] Factors such as granulocyte (G-CSF), macrophage (M-CSF), granulocyte-macrophage (GM-CSF) colony-stimulating factors, and thrombopoietin stimulate lineage-restricted progenitors, whereas factors such as interleukin-1 (IL-1), IL-3, IL-6, and c-kit ligand (stem cell factor, steel factor) stimulate pluripotent cells. These cytokines can be produced in vitro and have numerous potential clinical applications.

Recombinant G-CSF and GM-CSF are administered to patients undergoing autologous bone marrow transplantation. When given during recovery from high-dose chemotherapy, these factors accelerate granulocyte production, effectively shortening the period of severe neutropenia.[92-95] Although some studies have revealed that patients treated with hematopoietic growth factors had fewer days of bacteremia and fewer hospital days, other studies have revealed no significant differences in chemotherapeutic toxicity and generally no increase in overall patient survival.[95-97] The lack of effect in the early post-transplant period is presumably due to limiting numbers of committed progenitors present in the transplanted bone marrow. In contrast, undisputed benefit has been demonstrated in certain circumstances when G-CSF and GM-CSF are given pretransplant. These factors increase the number of circulating progenitors, thereby enhancing the yield of peripheral blood stem cells harvested by leukapheresis.[98-101] Infusing both peripheral committed progenitors and bone marrow stem cells affords more rapid hematologic recovery after myeloablative chemotherapy and may allow for administration of intensified doses of chemotherapeutic agents to be administered.[96, 97] Additional clinical applications include the treatment of congenital defects of granulocyte production and acquired disorders such as idiopathic neutropenia, aplastic anemia, and possibly myelodysplastic syndromes and AIDS-related toxicity.[80, 86, 102]

Numerous studies suggest that platelet production is regulated by humoral factors, but for 30 years a megakaryocyte-specific growth factor eluded researchers.[103] After myeloablative therapy, the hematopoietic lineages typically recover in the following sequence: erythrocytes, granulocytes and lymphocytes, and finally, platelets. Megakaryocyte recovery may take as long as 4 to 6 weeks, thus necessitating numerous platelet transfusions. Since platelet transfusion therapy is often complicated by the development of refractoriness caused by antibodies directed against HLA antigens or platelet antigens, strategies to accelerate platelet recovery would be highly beneficial. Recombinant GM-CSF and IL-3 both possess megakaryocyte-stimulating activity, which suggested to many that megakaryocytopoiesis and thrombopoiesis require a combination of cytokines. The existence of a cytokine specific for the megakaryocytic lineage was first suggested by the identification of a receptor, c-*mpl*, that possesses striking homology to the highly conserved hematopoietin receptor superfamily and is restricted to stem cells, megakaryocytes, and platelets.[104] Biochemical purification, cloning, and characterization of the c-*mpl* ligand thrombopoietin revealed that it stimulated megakaryocytopoiesis and thrombopoiesis as predicted.[88–91] Conversely, antisense oligodeoxynucleotides that interfere with c-*mpl* expression inhibit megakaryocytopoiesis in vitro.[105] Exciting prospects for clinical applications of thrombopoietin include the acceleration of platelet recovery following myeloablative therapy.

In addition to stimulating hematopoiesis in vivo, these growth factors also stimulate the growth of long-term bone marrow cultures in vitro. Several systems have been developed that support the growth of hematopoietic progenitor cells.[106–113] Common to all these systems are surfaces coated with extracellular matrix, cocultivation with stromal cells, and mixtures of hematopoietic growth factors. A future goal of transfusion therapy is to maintain continuous hematopoietic progenitor and stem cell cultures in vitro. With this approach, long-term bone marrow culture systems may eventually permit the unlimited production of functional RBCs, platelets, granulocytes, lymphocytes, and monocytes in vitro. Functional natural killer (NK) cell populations have also been produced in vitro by culturing CD34+/HLA-DR− progenitor cells in a stroma-dependent system supplemented with IL-2 and serum.[114] These NK cells are cytotoxic against K562 and Raji target cell lines. Moreover, tumor-infiltrating leukocytes have been prepared from solid tumors, and cytotoxic lymphocytes have been expanded in vitro with IL-2.[115, 116] Cellular gene therapy with tumor-infiltrating leukocytes and IL-2 has been effectively administered to patients with melanoma and other malignancies.[115, 116] Production of cell populations with antitumor activity and engineering antigenically null, functional blood components for transfusion are exciting potential extensions of in vitro culturing techniques. Moreover, an abundant supply of autologous hematopoietic progenitors maintained in long-term culture will facilitate human somatic gene therapy by providing a vehicle to deliver transduced genes to deficient individuals. Treatment of the inherited deficiency in adenosine deaminase, which results in severe combined immunodeficiency, is one model for this approach.[117]

Hematopoiesis is stimulated not only by the addition of positive regulators but also by the removal of inhibitors. The most widely studied inhibitory factors belong to the transforming growth factor β (TGF-β) family.[85] Proliferation of primitive hematopoietic cells is selectively inhibited by TGF-β_1. Consequently, the proliferative capacity of stem cells is enhanced by interfering with TGF-β_1 expression or TGF-β_1 activity.[118] Human umbilical cord blood is enriched in stem cells, specifically the subset thought to contain the primitive hematopoietic stem cells required for long-term engraftment. A high proportion of these cells, however, are quiescent. Incubation with TGF-β_1 antisense oligonucleotides or anti–TGF-β_1 antibodies stimulated early progenitors in long-term cultures of bone marrow and umbilical cord blood cells.[118] Since umbilical cord blood has been used successfully in pediatric transplantation, enhancing the proliferative capacity of hematopoietic stem cells may facilitate transplantation in adults and may further improve long-term engraftment.[119-124]

BONE MARROW AND PERIPHERAL STEM CELL TRANSPLANTATION

As described earlier, growth factors can aid in the production of hematopoietic progenitors in vitro and in vivo. In contrast to nurturing cellular growth, eliminating certain cell populations is often desirable in bone marrow and peripheral blood stem cell transportation.[125, 126] For example, strategies have been developed to eliminate malignant cells selectively from autografts in vitro. Progress in autologous bone marrow transplantation for treating chronic myelogenous leukemia has the potential to eliminate the need for histocompatible donors and complications associated with rejection or graft-vs.-host disease. A major obstacle, however, is contamination of the graft with leukemic cells. Chronic myelogenous leukemia arises from malignant transformation of a pluripotent hematopoietic stem cell.[127] The disease is characterized by expansion of the myeloid compartment with retention of full differentiation in the chronic phase followed by the inevitable progression to acute leukemia and blast crisis. More than 95% of patients with chronic myelogenous leukemia demonstrate the Philadelphia chromosome by cytogenetic analysis. The Philadelphia chromosome is a 9:22 reciprocal translocation that juxtaposes the c-*abl* gene on chromosome 9 with the break point cluster region (*bcr*) on chromosome 22. Expression of the hybrid gene resulting from this translocation, *bcr-abl*, not only serves as a marker for the disease but also likely plays a significant role in its pathogenesis.[128, 129] Expression of *bcr-abl* has been disrupted by using antisense oligonucleotides and retroviral-transduced antisense RNA. This inhibition of *bcr-abl* expression suppresses the growth of leukemic cells.[130, 131]

Another target for antisense therapy is the proto-oncogene c-*myb*, which is preferentially expressed in primitive hematopoietic cell lines and regulates hematopoietic cell proliferation and differentiation.[132] Blocking c-*myb* expression with antisense oligonucleotides inhibits the proliferation of normal and malignant human hematopoietic cells.[132, 133] Leukemic cells, however, are more sensitive to antisense c-*myb* oligonucleotides in vitro than are normal cells.[134] Antisense oligonucleotide treatment of peripheral blood mononuclear cells from patients with chronic myelogenous leukemia may effectively eliminate malignant cells. The advantages of antisense oligonucleotide treatment of bone marrow in vitro include minimal risk and toxicity because antisense oligonucleotides are not directly administered to the patient. Ideally, the malignant population is purged entirely in vitro and only normal cells are reinfused into the patient. Clinical trials to evaluate the effectiveness of the c-myb antisense oligonucleotide in a purging protocol in vitro are currently under way.

In these antisense trials, reverse transcription and amplification by PCR (RT-PCR) is used to detect the hybrid bcr-abl mRNA and determine the efficiency of the antisense therapy in removing malignant cells from the autograft. In addition, RT-PCR is used clinically to detect leukemic recurrence in patients after bone marrow transplantation. Of course, this strategy is limited to detecting residual disease for those malignancies associated with known chromosomal markers or translocations such as chronic myelogenous leukemia and acute myelogenous leukemia (9;22), acute promyelocytic leukemia (15;17), follicular lymphoma (14;18), multiple myeloma (immunoglobulin gene rearrangement), and others.[135,136]

CONCLUSIONS AND FUTURE PROSPECTS

In conclusion, molecular biology has already had a significant impact on the practice of transfusion medicine and will continue to influence the development of additional applications in the future. Advances in diagnostic procedures include molecular blood typing and improved methods for infectious disease screening. Innovations in therapeutic blood products derive from manipulating hematopoiesis in vivo and in vitro. Exciting future prospects include gene therapy for hemophilia and other inherited diseases, genetically engineered null-antigen RBCs and platelets, and improved autologous bone marrow and peripheral blood stem cell products for transplantation.

REFERENCES

1. Collins FS: Cystic fibrosis: Molecular biology and therapeutic implications. *Science* 256:774–779, 1992.
2. Ohno T, Gordon D, San H, et al: Gene therapy for vascular smooth muscle cell proliferation after arterial injury. *Science* 265:781–784, 1994.
3. Culver KW, Ram Z, Wallbridge S, et al: In vivo gene transfer with retroviral vector-producer cells for treatment of experimental brain tumors. *Science* 256:1550–1552, 1992.
4. Lutz P, Dzik WH: Molecular biology of red cell blood group genes. *Transfusion* 32:467–483, 1992.
5. Blackall DP, Ugorski M, Smith ME, et al: The binding of human alloantibodies to recombinant glycophorin A. *Transfusion* 32:629–632, 1992.
6. Blackall DP, Ugorski M, Pahlsson P, et al: A molecular biologic approach to study the fine specificity of antibodies directed to the MN human blood group antigens. *J Immunol* 152:2241–2247, 1994.
7. Lublin DM, Thompson ES, Green AM, et al: Dr(a−) polymorphism of decay accelerating factor. Biochemical, functional, and molecular characterization and production of allele-specific transfectants. *J Clin Invest* 87:1945–1952, 1991.
8. Spitalnik S, Cowles J, Cox MT, et al: Neutralization of Lewis blood group

antibodies by synthetic immunoadsorbents. *Am J Clin Pathol* 80:63–65, 1983.

9. Cowles JW, Blumberg N: Neutralization of P blood group antibodies by synthetic solid-phase antigens. *Transfusion* 27:272–275, 1987.
10. Winter G, Milstein C: Man made antibodies. *Nature* 349:293–299, 1991.
11. Lerner RA, Barbas CF, Kang AS, et al: On the use of combinatorial antibody libraries to clone the "fossil record" of an individual's immune response. *Proc Natl Acad Sci U S A* 88:9705–9706, 1991.
12. Hoogenboom HR, Marks JD, Griffiths AD, et al: Building antibodies from their genes. *Immunol Rev* 130:41–68, 1992.
13. Czerwinski M, Siegel DL, Moore JS, et al: Construction of bacteriophage expressing mouse monoclonal Fab fragments directed against the human MN glycophorin blood group antigens. *Transfusion,* 35:137–144, 1995.
14. Siegel DL, Silberstein LE: Expression and characterization of recombinant anti-Rh(D) antibodies on filamentous phage: A model system for isolating human red blood cell antibodies by repertoire cloning. *Blood* 83:2334–2344, 1994.
15. Marks JD, Ouwehand WH, Bye JM, et al: Human antibody fragments specific for human blood group antigens from a phage display library. *Biotechnology* 11:1145–1149, 1993.
16. Mollison PL: The genetic basis of the Rh blood group system. *Transfusion* 34:539–541, 1994.
17. Bennett PR, Le Van Kim C, Colin Y, et al: Prenatal determination of fetal RhD type by DNA amplification. *N Engl J Med* 329:607–660, 1993.
18. Ugozzoli L, Wallace RB: Application of an allele-specific polymerase chain reaction to the direct determination of ABO blood group genotypes. *Genomics* 12:670–674, 1992.
19. Eshleman JR, Shakin-Eshleman SH, Church A, et al: DNA typing of the human MN and Ss blood group antigens in amniotic fluid and following massive transfusion. *Am J Clin Pathol* 103:353–357, 1995.
20. Corfield VA, Moolman JC, Martell R, et al: Polymerase chain reaction–based detection of MN blood group–specific sequences in the human genome. *Transfusion* 33:119–124, 1992.
21. Huang CH, Guizzo ML, McCreary J, et al: Typing of MNSs blood group specific sequences in the human genome and characterization of a restriction fragment tightly linked to S–s– alleles. *Blood* 77:381–386, 1991.
22. McFarland JG, Aster RH, Bussel JB, et al: Prenatal diagnosis of neonatal alloimmune thrombocytopenia using allele-specific oligonucleotide probes. *Blood* 78:2276–2282, 1991.
23. Santoso S, Kalb R, Walka M, et al: The human platelet alloantigens Br_a and Br_b are associated with a single amino acid polymorphism on glycoprotein Ia (integrin subunit $\alpha2$). *J Clin Invest* 92:2427–2432, 1993.
24. Wachtel S, Elias S, Price J, et al: Fetal cells in the maternal circulation: Isolation by multiparameter flow cytometry and confirmation by polymerase chain reaction. *Hum Reprod* 6:1466–1469, 1991.
25. Aach RD, Lander JJ, Sherman LA, et al: Transfusion-transmitted viruses: Interim analysis of hepatitis among transfused and non-transfused patients, in Vyas GM, Cohen SN, Schmid R (eds): *Viral Hepatitis.* Philadelphia, Franklin Institute Press, 1978, pp 383–396.
26. Alter HJ, Purcell RH, Feinstone SM, et al: Non-A/non-B hepatitis: A review and interim report of an ongoing prospective study, in Vyas GM, Cohen SN, Schmid R (eds): *Viral Hepatitis.* Philadelphia, Franklin Institute Press, 1978, pp 359–369.

27. Seeff LB, Wright EC, Zimmerman HJ, et al: Posttransfusion hepatitis among transfused and non-transfused patients, 1973–1975: A Veterans Administration cooperative study, in Vyas GM, Cohen SN, Schmid R (eds): *Viral Hepatitis*. Philadelphia, Franklin Institute Press, 1978, pp 371–381.
28. Aach RD, Szmuness W, Mosley JW, et al: Serum alanine aminotransferase of donors in relation to the risk of non-A, non-B hepatitis in recipients: The Transfusion-Transmitted Viruses Study. *N Engl J Med* 304:989–994, 1981.
29. Stevens CE, Aach RD, Hollinger FB, et al: Hepatitis B virus antibody in blood donors and the occurrence of non-A, non-B hepatitis in transfusion recipients: An analysis of the Transfusion-Transmitted Viruses Study. *Ann Intern Med* 101:733–738, 1984.
30. Koziol DE, Holland PV, Alling DW, et al: Antibody to hepatitis B core antigen as a paradoxical marker for non-A, non-B hepatitis agents in donated blood. *Ann Intern Med* 104:488–495, 1986.
31. Morris JA, Wilcox TR, Reed GW, et al: Safety of the blood supply: Surrogate testing and transmission of hepatitis C in patients after massive transfusion. *Ann Surg* 219:517–526, 1994.
32. Choo QL, Kuo G, Weiner AJ, et al: Isolation of a cDNA clone derived from a blood-borne non-A, non-B viral hepatitis genome. *Science* 244:359–361, 1989.
33. Kuo G, Choo Q-L, Alter HJ, et al: An assay for circulating antibodies to a major etiologic virus of human non-A, non-B hepatitis. *Science* 244:362–364, 1989.
34. Japanese Red Cross, Non-A, Non-B Hepatitis Research Group: Effect of screening for hepatitis C virus antibody and hepatitis B virus core antibody on incidence of post-transfusion hepatitis. *Lancet* 338:1040–1041, 1991.
35. Esteban JI, Gonzales A, Hernandez JM, et al: Evaluation of antibodies to hepatitis C virus in a contemporary study of transfusion associated hepatitis. *N Engl J Med* 323:1107–1112, 1991.
36. Dodd RY: The risk of transfusion-transmitted infection. *N Engl J Med* 327:419–421, 1992.
37. Donahue JG, Munoz A, Ness PM, et al: The declining risk of post-transfusion hepatitis C virus infection. *N Engl J Med* 327:370–373, 1992.
38. MacDonald KL, Mills WA, Wood RC, et al: Evaluation of clinical and laboratory aspects of antibody tests for detection of hepatitis C virus infection in blood donors and recipients from a low-risk population. *Transfusion* 34:202–208, 1994.
39. De Beenhouwer H, Verhaert H, Claeys H, et al: Confirmation of HCV positive blood donors by immunoblotting and PCR. *Vox Sang* 63:198–203, 1992.
40. Caspari G, Gerlich WH, Beyer J, et al: Variable results of first generation anti-HCV enzyme immunoassay during follow-up of blood donors. *Vox Sang* 64:61–62, 1993.
41. Nasoff MS, Zebedee SL, Inchauspe G, et al: Identification of an immunodominant epitope within the capsid protein of hepatitis C virus. *Proc Natl Acad Sci U S A* 88:5462–5466, 1991.
42. Hosein B, Fang CT, Popovsky MA, et al: Improved serodiagnosis of hepatitis C virus infection with synthetic antigen from capsid protein. *Proc Natl Acad Sci U S A* 88:3647–3651, 1991.
43. Alter J: New kit on the block: Evaluation of second-generation assays for detection of antibody to the hepatitis C virus. *Hepatology* 15:350–353, 1992.
44. Kleinman S, Alter H, Busch M, et al: Increased detection of hepatitis C virus (HCV)-infected blood donors by a multiple antigen HCV enzyme immunoassay. *Transfusion* 32:805–813, 1992.
45. Peters T, Mohr L, Scheiffele F, et al: Antibodies and viremia in acute post-transfusion hepatitis C: A prospective study. *J Med Virol* 42:420–427, 1994.

46. Alter HJ: Descartes before the horse: I clone, therefore I am: The hepatitis C virus in current perspective. *Ann Intern Med* 115:;644–649, 1991.
47. Aach RD, Stevens CE, Hollinger FB, et al: Hepatitis C virus infection in post-transfusion hepatitis. An analysis with first-and second-generation assays. *N Engl J Med* 325:1325–1329, 1991.
48. Uyttendaele S, Claeys H, Mertens W, et al: Evaluation of third-generation screening and confirmatory assays for HCV antibodies. *Vox Sang* 66:122–129, 1994.
49. Farci P, London WT, Wong DC: The natural history of infection with hepatitis C virus (HCV) in chimpanzees: Comparison of serologic responses measured with first and second generation assays and relationship to HCV viremia. *J Infect Dis* 165:1006–1011, 1992.
50. Farci P, Alter HF, Wong D, et al: A long-term study of hepatitis C virus replication in non-A, non-B hepatitis. *N Engl J Med* 325:98–104, 1991.
51. Ulrich PP, Romeo JM, Lane PK, et al: Detection, semiquantitation and genetic variation in hepatitis C virus sequences amplified from the plasma of blood donors with elevated alanine aminotransferase. *J Clin Invest* 86:1609–1614, 1990.
52. Sankary TM, Yang G, Romeo JM, et al: Rare detection of hepatitis B and hepatitis C virus genomes by polymerase chain reaction in seronegative donors with elevated alanine aminotransferase. *Transfusion* 34:656–660, 1993.
53. Zaaijer HL, Cuypers HTM, Reesink HW, et al: Reliability of polymerase chain reaction for detection of hepatitis C virus. *Lancet* 341:722–724, 1993.
54. Gratzer WB, Dluzewski AR: The red blood cell and malaria parasite invasion. *Semin Hematol* 30:232–247, 1993.
55. Sim KL, Chitnis CE, Wasniowska K, et al: Receptor and ligand domains for invasion of erythrocytes by Plasmodium falciparum. *Science* 264:1941–1944, 1994.
56. Brown KE, Hibbs JR, Gallinella G, et al: Resistance to parvovirus B19 infection due to lack of virus receptor (erythrocyte P antigen). *N Engl J Med* 330:1192–1196, 1994.
57. Mannucci PM: Modern treatment of hemophilia: From the shadows towards the light. *Thromb Haemost* 70:17–23, 1993.
58. Limentani SA, Roth DA, Furie BC, et al: Recombinant blood clotting proteins for hemophilia therapy. *Semin Thromb Hemost* 19:62–72, 1993.
59. Wu S-M, Cheung W-F, Frazier D, et al: Coning and expression of the cDNA for human γ-glutamyl carboxylase. *Science* 254:1634–1636, 1991.
60. Kurachi K, Yao SN: Gene therapy of hemophilia B. *Thromb Haemost* 70:193–197, 1993.
61. Kay MA, Landen CN, Rothenberg SR, et al: In vivo hepatic gene therapy: Complete albeit transient correction of factor IX deficiency in hemophilia B dogs. *Proc Natl Acad Sci U S A* 91:2353–2357, 1994.
62. Zanjani ED, Ascensae JL: Erythropoietin. *Transfusion* 29:46–57, 1989.
63. Eschbach JW, Egrie JC, Downing MR, et al: Correction of the anemia of end stage renal disease with recombinant human erythropoietin. *N Engl J Med* 316:73–78, 1987.
64. Eschbach JW, Abdulhadi MH, Browne JK, et al: Recombinant human erythropoietin in anemic patients with end-stage renal disease. Results of a Phase III Multicenter Clinical Trial. *Ann Intern Med* 111:992–1000, 1989.
65. Eschbach JW, Kelly MR, Haley N, et al: Treatment of the anemia of progressive renal failure with recombinant human erythropoietin. *N Engl J Med* 321:158–163, 1989.
66. Lim VS, DeGowin RL, Zavala D, et al: Recombinant human erythropoietin

treatment in pre-dialysis patients. A double-blind placebo-controlled trial. *Ann Intern Med* 110:108–114, 1989.

67. Stone WB, Graber SE, Drantz SB, et al: Treatment of the anemia of predialysis patients with recombinant human erythropoietin: A randomized placebo controlled trial. *Am J Med Sci* 31:171–179, 1989.

68. US Recombinant Human Erythropoietin Predialysis Study Group: Double-blind placebo-controlled study of the therapeutic use of recombinant human erythropoietin for anemia associated with chronic renal failure in predialysis patients. *Am J Kidney Dis* 18:50–59, 1991.

69. Fischl M, Richman D, Grieco MH, et al: Recombinant human erythropoietin therapy for AIDs patients treated with AZT: A double-blind, placebo controlled clinical study. *N Engl J Med* 322:1488–1493, 1990.

70. Herrmann F, Brugger W, Lothar K, et al: In vivo biology and therapeutic potential of hematopoietic growth factor and circulating progenitor cells. *Semin Oncol* 19:422–431, 1992.

71. Goodnough LT, Rudnick S, Price T, et al: Increased autologous blood donation with recombinant human erythropoietin therapy. *N Engl J Med* 321:1163–1167, 1989.

72. Goodnough LT: Clinical application of recombinant erythropietin in the perioperative period. *Hematol Oncol Clin North Am* 8:1011–1019, 1994.

73. Hoeldtke RD, Streeten DHP: Treatment of orthostatic hypotension with erythropoietin. *N Engl J Med* 329:611–615, 1993.

74. Gallagher PG, Ehrenkranz RA: Erythropoietin therapy for anemia of prematurity. *Clin Perinatol* 20:169–191, 1993.

75. Shannon K: Recombinant erythropoietin in anemia of prematurity: Five years later. Pediatrics 92:614, 1993.

76. Maier RF, Obladen M, Scigalla P, et al: The effect of epoetin beta (recombinant human erythropoietin) on the need for transfusion in very-low-birth-weight infants. *N Engl J Med* 330:1173–1178, 1994.

77. Remacha AF, Rodriguez–De La Serna A, Garcia-Die F, et al: Erythroid abnormalities in rheumatoid arthritis: The role of erythropoietin. *J Rhematol* 19:1687–1691, 1992.

78. Baer AN, Dessypris EN, Krantz SB: The pathogenesis of anemia in rheumatoid arthritis: A clinical and laboratory analysis. *Semin Arthritis Rheum* 19:209–223, 1990.

79. Means RT: Clinical application of recombinant erythropoietin in the anemia of chronic disease. *Hematol Oncol Clin North Am* 8:933–945, 1994.

80. Mittelman M, Lessin LS: Clinical application of recombinant erythropoietin in myelodysplasia. *Hematol Oncol Clin North Am* 8:993–1009, 1994.

81. Alkhatti A, Veith RW, Papayannopoulou T, et al: Stimulation of fetal hemoglobin synthesis by erythropoietin in baboons. *N Engl J Med* 317:415–420, 1987.

82. Sherwood JB, Goldwasser E, Chilcote R, et al: Sickle cell anemia patients have low erythropoietin levels for their degree of anemia. *Blood* 67:46–49, 1986.

83. Rodgers GP, Dover GJ, Uyesaka M, et al: Augmentation by erythropoietin of the fetal-hemoglobin response to hydroxyurea in sickle cell disease. *N Engl J Med* 328:73–80, 1993.

84. Spangrude GJ: Biological and clinical aspects of hematopoietic stem cells. *Annu Rev Med* 45:93–104, 1994.

85. Moore MAS: Clinical implications of positive and negative hematopoietic stem cell regulators. *Blood* 78:1–19, 1991.

86. Moore MAS: The clinical use of colony stimulating factors. *Annu Rev Immunol* 9:159–191, 1991.

87. Peters WP, Ross M, Vredenburgh J, et al: Role of cytokines in autologous bone marrow transplantation. *Hematol Oncol Clin North Am* 7:737–747, 1993.

88. Kaushansky K, Lok S, Holly RD, et al: Promotion of megakaryocyte progenitor expansion and differentiation by the c-mpl ligand thrombopoietin. *Nature* 369:568–571, 1994.

89. Bartley TD, Bogenberger J, Hunt P, et al: Identification and cloning of a megakaryocyte growth and development factor that is a ligand for the cytokine receptor Mpl. *Cell* 77:1117–1124, 1994.

90. De Sauvage FJ, Hess PE, Spencer SD, et al: Stimulation of megakaryocytopoiesis and thrombopoesis by the c-Mpl ligand. *Nature* 369:533–538, 1994.

91. Erickson-Miller CL: Megakaryocyte colony stimulating factor (Meg-CSF) is a unique cytokine specific for the megakaryocyte lineage. *Br J Haematol* 84:197–203, 1993.

92. Brandt SJ, Peters WP, Atwater SK, et al: Effect of recombinant human granulocyte-macrophage colony-stimulating factor on hematopoietic reconstitution after high-dose chemotherapy and autologous bone marrow transplantation. *N Engl J Med* 318:869–876, 1988.

93. Neumanaitis J, Singer JW, Buckner CK, et al: Use of recombinant human granulocyte-macrophage colony-stimulating factor in autologous marrow transplantation for lymphoid malignancies. *Blood* 72:834–836, 1988.

94. Peters WP, Atwater S, Kurtzberg J, et al: The use of recombinant human granulocyte-macrophage colony stimulating factor in autologous bone marrow transplantation. *UCLA Symp Mol Cell Biol* 91:595–606, 1989.

95. Nemunaitis J, Rabinowe SN, Singer JW, et al: Recombinant granulocyte macrophage colony stimulating factor after autologous bone marrow transplantation for lymphoid cancer. *N Engl J Med* 324:1773–1778, 1991.

96. Nemunaitis J, Singer JW, Sanders JE: The use of recombinant human granulocyte macrophage colony-stimulating factor in autologous bone marrow transplantation. *Bone Marrow Transplant* 3(suppl 7):24–27, 1991.

97. Neidhart JA: Hematopoietic colony stimulating factors: Uses in combination with standard chemotherapeutic regimens and in support of dose intensification. *Cancer* 70:913–920, 1992.

98. Solinski MA, Cannistra SA, Elias A, et al: Granulocyte macrophage colony stimulating factor expands the circulating hematopoietic progenitor cell compartment in man. *Lancet* 1:1194–1198, 1988.

99. Gianni AM, Siena A, Bregni M, et al: Granulocyte-macrophage colony-stimulating factor to harvest circulating haemopoietic stem cells for autotransplantation. *Lancet* 2:580–585, 1989.

100. Siena S, Bregni M, Brando B, et al: Circulation of CD34+ hematopoietic stem cells in the peripheral blood of high-dose cyclophosphamide treated patients: Enhancement by intravenous recombinant human granulocyte-macrophage colony stimulation factor. *Blood* 74:1905–1914, 1989.

101. Chao NJ, Schriber JR, Grimes K, et al: Granulocyte colony-stimulating factor "mobilized" peripheral blood progenitor cells accelerate granulocyte and platelet recovery after high-dose chemotherapy. *Blood* 81:2031–2035, 1993.

102. Groopman JE, Feder D: Hematopoietic growth factors in AIDS. *Semin Oncol* 19:408–414, 1992.

103. Hoffman R: Regulation of megakaryocytopoiesis. *Blood* 74:1196–1212, 1989.

104. Vignon I, Mornon JP, Cocault L, et al: Molecular cloning and characterization of MPL, the human homolog of the v-*mpl* oncogene: Identification of a member of the hematopoietic growth factor receptor superfamily. *Proc Natl Acad Sci U S A* 89:5640–5644, 1992.

105. Methia N, Louache F, Vainchenker W, et al: Oligodeoxynucleotide antisense to the proto-oncogene c-*mpl* specifically inhibit in vitro megakaryocytopoiesis. *Blood* 82:1395–1401, 1993.

106. Dexter TM, Moore MAS, Sheridan APC: Maintenance of hemopoietic stem cells and production of differentiated progeny in allogeneic and semi-allogeneic bone marrow chimeras in vitro. *J Exp Med* 145:1612–1616, 1977.

107. Gartner S, Kaplan HS: Long term culture of bone marrow cells. *Proc Natl Acad Sci U S A* 77:4657–4659, 1980.

108. Andrews RG, Singer JW, Bernstein ID: Human hematopoietic precursors in long term culture: Single CD34+ cells that lack detectable T, B, and myeloid antigens produce multiple colony forming units when cultured with marrow stromal cells. *J Exp Med* 172:355–358, 1990.

109. Coutinho L, Wil A, Radford J, et al: Effects of recombinant human GCSF, GMCSF and gibbon IL3 on hematopoiesis in human long term bone marrow culture. *Blood* 75:2118–2129, 1990.

110. Palsson BO, Paek SW, Palsson M, et al: Expansion of human bone marrow progenitor cells in a continuous perfusion hematopoietic bioreactor. *Biotechnology* 11:268–313, 1993.

111. Koller MR, Emerson SG, Palsson BO: Large scale expansion of human hematopoietic stem and progenitor cells from bone marrow mononuclear cells in continuous perfusion culture. *Blood* 82:378–384, 1993.

112. Emerson SG, Palsson BO, Clarke MF: The construction of high efficiency human bone marrow tissue ex vivo. *J Cell Biochem* 3:268–272, 1991.

113. Wang TY, Wu JHD: A continuous perfusion bioreactor for long term bone marrow culture. *Ann N Y Acad Sci* 665:274–284, 1992.

114. Miller JS, Verfaillie C, McGlave P: The generation of human natural killer cells from CD34+/DR− primitive progenitors in long term bone marrow culture. *Blood* 80:2182–2187, 1992.

115. Rosenberg SA, Yannelli JR, Lopalian SL, et al: Treatment of patients with metastatic melanoma with autologous tumor-infiltrating lymphocytes and interleukin 2. *J Natl Cancer Inst* 86:1159–1166, 1994.

116. Schwarzentruber DJ, Hom SS, Dadmarz R, et al: In vitro predictors of therapeutic response in melanoma patients receiving tumor-infiltrating lymphocytes and interleukin-2. *J Clin Oncol* 12:1475–1483, 1994.

117. Cournoyer D, Scarpa M, Mitani K, et al: Gene transfer of adenosine deaminase into primitive human hematopoietic progenitor cells. *Hum Gene Ther* 2:203–213, 1991.

118. Cardoso AA, Li ML, Batard P, et al: Release from quiescence of CD34+CD38− human umbilical cord blood cells reveals their potentiality to engraft adults. *Proc Natl Acad Sci U S A* 90:8707–8711, 1993.

119. Gluckman E, Broxmeyer HE, Auerbach AD, et al: Hematopoietic reconstitution in a patient with Fanconi's anemia by means of umbilical cord blood from an HLA-identical sibling. *N Engl J Med* 321:1174, 1989.

120. Wagner JE: Umbilical cord blood stem cell transplantation: Current and future prospects. *J Hematother* 2:225–228, 1992.

121. Stone R: Banking on umbilical cords. *Science* 257:615, 1992.

122. Broxmeyer HE, Kurtzberg J, Gluckman E: Umbilical cord blood hematopoietic stem and repopulating cells in human clinical transplantation. *Blood Cells* 17:313–329, 1991.

123. Wagner JE: Umbilical cord blood stem cell transplantation. *Am J Pediatr Hematol Oncol* 15:169–174, 1993.

124. Broxmeyer HE, Hangoc G, Cooper S, et al: Growth characteristics and expansion of human umbilical cord blood and estimation of its potential for transplantation of adults. *Proc Natl Acad Sci U S A* 89:4109–4113, 1992.

125. Dunbar CE, Stewart FM: Separating the wheat from the chaff: Selection of benign hematopoietic cells in chronic myeloid leukemia. *Blood* 79:1107–1110, 1992.

126. Freedman AS, Nadler LM: Developments in purging in autotransplantation. *Hematol Oncol Clin North Am* 7:687–715, 1993.

127. Kurzrock R, Gutterman JU, Talpaz M: The molecular genetics of Philadelphia chromosome–positive leukemias. *N Engl J Med* 319:990–998, 1988.

128. Gewirtz AM, Calabretta B: Role of the c-*myb* and c-*abl* protooncogenes in human hematopoiesis. *Ann N Y Acad Sci* 628:63–73, 1991.

129. Sawyers CL: The *bcr-abl* gene in chronic myelogenous leukaemia, in Witte ON (ed): *Cancer Surveys 15: Oncogenes in the Development of Leukaemia.* Cold Spring Harbor, NY, Cold Spring Harbor Laboratory, 1992.

130. Szczylik C, Skorski T, Nicolaides NC, et al: Selective inhibition of leukemia cell proliferation by bcr-abl antisense oligodeoxynucleotides. *Science* 253:562–565, 1991.

131. Martiat P, Lewalle P, Taj AS, et al: Retrovirally transduced antisense sequences stably suppress p210 bcr-abl expression and inhibit the proliferation of BCR/ABL-containing cell lines. *Blood* 81:502–509, 1993.

132. Gewirtz AM, Anfossi G, Venturelli D, et al: G1/S transition in normal human T-lymphocytes requires the nuclear protein encoded by c-*myb*. *Science* 245:180–183, 1989.

133. Ratajczak MZ, Hijiya N, Catani L, et al: Acute and chronic phase chronic myelogenous leukemia colony-forming units are highly sensitive to the growth inhibitory effects of c-*myb* antisense oligodeoxynucleotides. *Blood* 79:1956–1961, 1992.

134. Calabretta B, Sims RB, Vatieri M, et al: Normal and leukemic hematopoietic cells manifest differential sensitivity to inhibitory effects of c-*myb* antisense oligodeoxynucleotides: An in vitro study relevant to bone marrow purging. *Proc Natl Acad Sci U S A* 88:2351–2355, 1991.

135. Miyanura K, Tanimoto M, Morishima Y, et al: Detection of Philadelphia chromosome–positive acute lymphoblastic leukemia by polymerase chain reaction: Possible eradication of minimal residual disease by marrow transplantation. *Blood* 79:1366–1370, 1992.

136. Gribben JG, Neuberg D, Barber M, et al: Detection of residual lymphoma cells by polymerase chain reaction in peripheral blood is significantly less predictive for relapse than detection in bone marrow. Blood 83:3800–3807, 1994.

Index

A

A band, 169

Absolute ethanol fixation, 101

ACE inhibitors, in IgA nephropathy, 531–532

Acetylcholinesterase, in Hirschsprung disease, 207

Acid maltase deficiency, 189

ACLAT syndrome, 389–390, 393–399

Acquired immunodeficiency syndrome (AIDS) (see also Gastrointestinal diseases, diagnosis in AIDS; HIV infection)
  hepatic granulomas in, 251–252

Actinomycosis, hepatic granulomas from, 260, 261–262

Activated partial thromboplastin time (aPTT), in detection of lupus anticoagulants, 412, 413

Adenoma-carcinoma sequence, in colon cancer, 482–483
  early changes, 485–492
  later changes, 492–497

Adenovirus, in gastrointestinal disease in AIDS, 465, 466

Adhesion molecules, in prostate cancer, 511–515

Adrenal hyperplasia, congenital, 435

Adrenogenital syndrome, 435

Aganglionosis coli (see Hirschsprung disease)

AIDS (see also Gastrointestinal diseases, diagnosis in AIDS; HIV infection)
  hepatic granulomas in, 251–252

Alkaline phosphatase detection cascade, 82, 83, 84

Allergic granulomatosis, hepatic granulomas in, 309

Alpha-fetoprotein testing, decision making on, 28, 29

Aluminum, hepatic granulomas from, 313–314

Alveolar rhabdoymosarcomas of childhood, 232–233

American College of Rheumatology, vasculitides classification and, 369

American Society of Clinical Pathologists, practice parameters and, 16, 17

Amino acids, rheumatoid factors and, 552

AmpliType PCR kit, 380–381

AmpliType Polymarker, 381

ANCAs (see Antineutrophil cytoplasmic autoantibodies)

Androgen excess, 435

Angiitis, leukocytoclastic, 365, 366, 371

Angiotensin converting enzyme inhibitors, in IgA nephropathy, 531–532

Anthracosilicosis, hepatic granulomas from, 322, 324–325

Antibodies
  antineutrophil cytoplasmic autoantibodies, 361–376
  antiphospholipid (see Anticardiolipin antibodies; Antiphospholipid thrombosis syndromes)
  heat-induced epitope retrieval and, 104, 106–108, 109
  monoclonal, red blood cellDspecific, 560–561
  protease-induced epitope retrieval and, 103

Anticardiolipin antibodies (see also Antiphospholipid thrombosis syndromes)
  cardiac disease and, 395–396
  collagen vascular disease and, 397
  cutaneous manifestations, 396–397
  detection, 410, 412
  lupus anticoagulants and, 392, 394
  miscellaneous disorders and, 399
  neurologic syndromes and, 397
  obstetric syndromes and, 398–399
  thrombosis and, 393–395

Anticardiolipin antibody thrombosis syndrome, 389–390, 393–399
  patient characteristics, 404–410, 411

Antigen retrieval (see Epitope retrieval in immunohistochemistry)

Antimicrobials for *Legionella* infection, 159

Antineutrophil cytoplasmic autoantibodies, 361–376
  antigen specificity, 362–363

581